Succinct Pediatrics

D1285535

Evaluation and Management for Infectious Diseases and Dermatologic Disorders

Editors

Leonard G. Feld, MD, PhD, MMM, FAAP
John D. Mahan, MD, FAAP

Associate Editor

Mary Anne Jackson, MD, FPIDS, FISSA, FAAP

American Academy
of Pediatrics

DEDICATED TO THE HEALTH OF ALL CHILDREN®

American Academy of Pediatrics Publishing Staff

Mark Grimes, *Director, Department of Publishing*
Chris Wiberg, *Senior Editor, Professional/Clinical Publishing*
Alain Park, *Senior Product Development Editor*
Carrie Peters, *Editor, Professional/Clinical Publishing*
Theresa Wiener, *Production Manager, Clinical and Professional Publications*
Linda Diamond, *Manager, Art Direction and Production*
Amanda Helmholz, *Editorial Specialist*
Mary Lou White, *Senior Vice President, Membership Engagement and Marketing & Sales*
Linda Smessaert, *Brand Manager, Clinical and Professional Publications*

141 Northwest Point Blvd
Elk Grove Village, IL 60007-1019
Telephone: 847/434-4000
Facsimile: 847/434-8000
www.aap.org

The recommendations in this publication do not indicate an exclusive course of treatment or serve as a standard of care. Variations, taking into account individual circumstances, may be appropriate.

Brand names are furnished for identification purposes only. No endorsement of the manufacturers or products mentioned is implied.

Every effort has been made to ensure that the drug selection and dosages set forth in this text are in accordance with the current recommendations and practice at the time of publication. It is the responsibility of the health care professional to check the package insert of each drug for any change in indications and dosages and for added warnings and precautions.

This publication has been developed by the American Academy of Pediatrics. The authors, editors, and contributors are expert authorities in the field of pediatrics. No commercial involvement of any kind has been solicited or accepted in the development of the content of this publication.

The publishers have made every effort to trace the copyright holders for borrowed material. If they have inadvertently overlooked any, they will be pleased to make the necessary arrangements at the first opportunity.

Every effort is made to keep *Succinct Pediatrics: Evaluation and Management for Infectious Diseases and Dermatologic Disorders* consistent with the most recent advice and information available from the American Academy of Pediatrics.

Special discounts are available for bulk purchases of this publication. E-mail our Special Sales Department at aapsales@aap.org for more information.

Printed in the United States of America

9-371/1216

1 2 3 4 5 6 7 8 9 10

MA0815

ISBN: 978-1-61002-076-3

eBook: 978-1-61002-077-0

Library of Congress Control Number: 2016936023

Disclosures: Dr Chatterjee indicated a consulting, clinical trials, and speakers' bureau relationship with Merck; a clinical trials relationship with GlaxoSmithKline; a speakers' bureau, advisory board relationship with Pfizer; an advisory board and clinical trials relationship with Astra Zeneca; and a speakers' bureau relationship with Sanofi Pasteur. Dr Kaplan indicated a consulting relationship with Pfizer. Dr Newland indicated an educational grant relationship with Pfizer. All other contributors disclosed no relevant financial relationships.

Contributors

Amina Ahmed, MD, FAAP
Department of Pediatrics
Division of Pediatric Infectious Disease
Levine Children's Hospital at Carolinas Medical Center
Charlotte, North Carolina

Krow Ampofo, MB, ChB, FPIDS, FIDSA, FAAP
Department of Pediatrics
Division of Pediatric Infectious Diseases
University of Utah School of Medicine
Salt Lake City, UT

Charalampos Antachopoulos, MD
3rd Department of Pediatrics
Aristotle University, Hippokration Hospital
Thessaloniki, Greece

Paul M. Arguin, MD
Domestic Malaria Unit Chief
Center for Global Health
Centers for Disease Control and Prevention
Atlanta, GA

Jeffrey R. Avner, MD, FAAP
Chief, Division of Pediatric Emergency Medicine
Professor of Clinical Pediatrics
Children's Hospital at Montefiore
Albert Einstein College of Medicine
Bronx, NY

Henry Bernstein, DO, MHCM, FAAP
Hofstra Northwell School of Medicine
Steven and Alexandra Cohen Children's Medical Center of New York
Department of Pediatrics, Division of General Pediatrics
New Hyde Park, NY

Joseph A. Bocchini Jr, MD, FAAP
Department of Pediatrics
Louisiana State University Health Sciences Center
Shreveport, LA

Kristina Bryant, MD, FAAP
Department of Pediatrics
Division of Pediatric Infectious Diseases
University of Louisville
Louisville, KY

Craig N. Burkhart, MD
Associate Professor
Department of Dermatology
University of North Carolina at Chapel Hill
Chapel Hill, NC

Jeana Bush, MD, FAAP
Levine Children's Hospital
Carolinas Medical Center
Charlotte, NC

Kristi Canty, MD, FAAP, FAAD
Department of Pediatrics
Division of Dermatology
Children's Mercy Kansas City
University of Missouri-Kansas City School of Medicine
Kansas City, MO

Cynthia Marie Carver DeKlotz, MD
Assistant Professor, Dermatology
Georgetown University School of Medicine
MedStar Washington Hospital Center/Georgetown University Hospital
Washington, DC

Shelley Cathcart, MD
Pediatric Dermatologist
Blue Ridge Dermatology Associates
Raleigh, North Carolina

Archana Chatterjee, MD, PhD, FAAP
Professor and Chair, Department of Pediatrics
Senior Associate Dean for Faculty Development
University of South Dakota Sanford School of Medicine
Sioux Falls, SD

Andrea T. Cruz, MD, MPH, FAAP
Department of Pediatrics
Sections of Infectious Diseases and Emergency Medicine
Baylor College of Medicine
Houston, TX

Rachel Dawkins, MD, FAAP
Assistant Professor of Pediatrics, Johns Hopkins School of Medicine
Medical Director, Pediatric and Adolescent Medicine Clinic
Johns Hopkins All Children's Hospital
St Petersburg, FL

James Christopher Day, MD, FAAP
Department of Pediatrics
Division of Infectious Diseases
Children's Mercy Hospitals and Clinics
Kansas City, MO

Penelope H. Dennehy, MD, FAAP
Director, Division of Pediatric Infectious Diseases
Hasbro Children's Hospital
Professor and Vice Chair for Academic Affairs
Department of Pediatrics
The Alpert Medical School of Brown University
Providence, RI

B. Keith English, MD, FAAP
Professor and Chair
Department of Pediatrics and Human Development
College of Human Medicine
Michigan State University

Janet A. Englund, MD
Professor, Department of Pediatrics
Seattle Children's Hospital
University of Washington
Seattle, WA

Claudia Espinosa, MD, MSc, FAAP
Department of Pediatrics
Division of Pediatric Infectious Diseases
University of Louisville
Louisville, KY

Lori Falcone, DO, FAAP
Priority Care Pediatrics
Kansas City, MO

Sheila Fallon Friedlander, MD, FAAP
Professor of Clinical Dermatology and Pediatrics
UC San Diego Medical Center
Director, Pediatric Dermatology Fellowship Training Program
Rady Children's Hospital
San Diego, CA

Marc Foca, MD
Associate Professor of Pediatrics
Division of Infectious Diseases
Department of Pediatrics
Children's Hospital of New York Presbyterian
New York, NY

Anne A. Gershon, MD, FAAP
Professor of Pediatrics
Division of Infectious Disease
Columbia University College of Physicians and Surgeons
New York, NY

Joan E. Giovanni, MD, FAAP
Department of Pediatrics
Division of Emergency and Urgent Care Services
Children's Mercy Hospitals and Clinics
Kansas City, MO

Andreas H. Groll, MD
Infectious Disease Research Program
Centre for Bone Marrow Transplantation
Department of Pediatric Hematology/Oncology
University Children's Hospital Münster
Münster, Germany

Benjamin R. Hanisch, MD
Department of Pediatric Infectious Diseases
University of Minnesota
Minneapolis, MN

Jason B. Harris, MD, MPH, FIDSA
Division of Infectious Diseases
Massachusetts General Hospital
Department of Pediatrics
Harvard Medical School

Jo-Ann S. Harris, MD, FAAP
Consultant, Pediatric Infectious Diseases
Hospital Epidemiologist
Stormont-Vail HealthCare
Adjunct Professor of Pediatrics
University of Kansas
Topeka, KS

Christopher Harrison, MD, FAAP, FPIDS, FIDSA
Department of Pediatrics
Director of Pediatric Infectious Diseases Laboratory
Division of Infectious Diseases
Children's Mercy Hospital of Kansas City
Professor of Pediatrics
University of Missouri at Kansas City School of Medicine

Kimberly A. Horii, MD, FAAP, FAAD
Department of Pediatrics
Division of Dermatology
Children's Mercy Hospitals and Clinics
Associate Professor of Pediatrics
University of Missouri-Kansas City School of Medicine
Kansas City, MO

Sadaf Hussain, MD
Fellow, Pediatric Dermatology
The Children's Hospital of Philadelphia
Philadelphia, PA

Christelle M. Ilboudo, MD, FAAP
Assistant Professor of Pediatrics
Division of Infectious Diseases
Department of Child Health
University of Missouri Health System

Jodi Jackson, MD, FAAP
Division of Neonatology
The Children's Mercy Hospitals and Clinics, Kansas City
Associate Professor of Pediatrics
University of Missouri-Kansas City School of Medicine
Kansas City, MO

Mary Anne Jackson, MD, FPIDS, FISSA, FAAP
Director, Division of Infectious Diseases
Associate Chair of Community and Regional Pediatric Collaboration
Children's Mercy, Kansas City
Professor of Pediatrics
University of Missouri-Kansas City School of Medicine
Kansas City, MO

Chandy C. John, MD, MS, FAAP
Department of Pediatrics
Director, Ryan White Center for Pediatric Infectious Disease and Global Health
Indiana University School of Medicine
Indianapolis, MN

Sheldon L. Kaplan, MD, FAAP
Department of Pediatrics
Section of Infectious Disease
Baylor College of Medicine
Texas Children's Hospital
Houston, TX

J. Michael Klatte, MD, FAAP
Assistant Professor of Pediatrics
Baystate Medical Center
Tufts University School of Medicine
Springfield, MA

Martin B. Kleiman, MD
Professor of Pediatrics Emeritus
University of Indiana
Riley Hospital for Children
Indianapolis, IN

Keren Z. Landman, MD
Atlanta, GA

Sarah S. Long, MD, FAAP
Professor of Pediatrics
Drexel University College of Medicine
Department of Pediatrics, Section of Infectious Diseases (Chief)
St. Christopher's Hospital for Children
Philadelphia, PA

Morgan Maier, PA-C
Division of Dermatology
Seattle Children's Hospital
Seattle, WA

Keith J. Mann, MD, MEd, FAAP
Department of Pediatrics
Division of General Pediatrics
Chief Medical Quality and Safety Officer
Associate Chair of Quality Improvement
Children's Mercy Hospitals and Clinics
Professor of Pediatrics
University of Missouri-Kansas City School of Medicine
Kansas City, MO

Gary S. Marshall, MD, FAAP
Division of Pediatric Infectious Diseases
University of Louisville School of Medicine
Louisville, KY

Kimberly C. Martin, DO, MPH, FAAP
Assistant Professor of Pediatrics
Division of Pediatric Infectious Diseases
University of Oklahoma School of Community Medicine
Tulsa, OK

J. Chase McNeil, MD, FAAP
Department of Pediatrics
Section of Infectious Disease
Baylor College of Medicine
Houston, TX

Shirley Molitor-Kirsch, RN, MSN, CPNP-AC
Infectious Diseases/International Travel Medicine
Children's Mercy Hospital & Clinics
Kansas City, MO

Dean S. Morrell, MD
Professor of Dermatology
Director of Pediatric and Adolescent Dermatology
University of North Carolina at Chapel Hill Department of Dermatology
Chapel Hill, NC

Angela L. Myers MD, MPH, FAAP
Associate Professor of Pediatrics
Division of Infectious Diseases
Director, Pediatric Infectious Diseases Fellowship Program
Children's Mercy Hospital, Kansas City
University of Missouri-Kansas City School of Medicine
Kansas City, MO

Kari Neemann, MD, FAAP
Assistant Professor, Adult and Pediatric Infectious Diseases
University of Nebraska Medical Center
Omaha, NE

Brandon D. Newell, MD, FAAP
Department of Pediatrics, Division of Dermatology
Children's Mercy Hospitals and Clinics
Associate Professor of Pediatrics—University of Missouri-Kansas City
Kansas City, MO

Jason G. Newland, MD, MEd, FAAP
Associate Professor of Pediatrics
Division of Infectious Diseases
Washington University in St. Louis School of Medicine
St Louis, MO

Ross E. Newman, DO, MPHE, FAAP
Department of Pediatrics
Division of General Pediatrics
Children's Mercy Hospitals and Clinics
Assistant Professor of Pediatrics
University of Missouri-Kansas City School of Medicine
Kansas City, MO

Laura E. Norton, MD, FAAP
Department of Pediatrics
Division of Infectious Diseases
Children's Mercy Hospitals and Clinics
Kansas City, MO

Catherine O'Keefe, DNP, APRN-NP
Associate Professor and NP Curriculum Coordinator
Creighton University, College of Nursing
Omaha, NE

Barbara Pahud, MD, MPH, FAAP
Department of Pediatrics
Division of Pediatric Infectious Diseases
University of Missouri-Kansas City
Children's Mercy Hospital
Kansas City, MO

Pia S. Pannaraj, MD, MPH
Department of Pediatrics
Molecular Microbiology and Immunology
Keck School of Medicine
University of Southern California
Division of Infectious Diseases
Children's Hospital Los Angeles
Los Angeles, CA

Laura M. Plencner, MD, FAAP
Children's Mercy Hospital
Division of Pediatric Hospital Medicine
Assistant Professor of Pediatrics, University of Missouri-Kansas City
Kansas City, Missouri

Krithiha Raghunathan, MD
Chief Resident
Department of Pediatrics
The Children's Hospital at Monmouth Medical Center
Long Branch, NJ

Sergio E. Recuenco, MD, MPH, DrPH
Rabies Program
National Center for Emerging and Zoonotic Infectious Diseases
Centers for Disease Control and Prevention
Atlanta, GA

Emmanuel Roilides, MD, PhD, FIDSA, FAAM
Professor of Pediatrics—Infectious Diseases
Head, Infectious Diseases Unit and Research Laboratory
3rd Department of Pediatrics
Aristotle University, Hippokration Hospital
Thessaloniki, Greece

José R. Romero, MD, FIDSA, FAAP
Department of Pediatrics
Director, Section of Infectious Diseases
University of Arkansas for Medical Sciences and Arkansas Children's Hospital
Director, Clinical Trials Research
Arkansas Children's Research Institute
Little Rock, AR

Roya Samuels, MD, FAAP
Hofstra Northwell School of Medicine
Steven and Alexandra Cohen Children's Medical Center of New York
Department of Pediatrics, Division of General Pediatrics
New Hyde Park, NY

Gordon E. Schutze, MD, FAAP
Professor of Pediatrics
Executive Vice Chairman
Martin I. Lorin, M.D., Endowed Chair in Medical Education
Department of Pediatrics
Baylor College of Medicine
Vice President International Programs
Baylor International Pediatric AIDS Initiative at Texas Children's Hospital
Houston, TX

Michelle Sewnarine, MD, FAAP
Fellow, Pediatric Infectious Diseases
Hofstra Northshore-LIJ School of Medicine
Steven and Alexandra Cohen Children's Medical Center of New York
New Hyde Park, NY

Eugene D. Shapiro, MD, FAAP
Departments of Pediatrics, Epidemiology, and Investigative Medicine
Divisions of General Pediatrics, Pediatric Infectious Diseases and Epidemiology
    of Microbial Diseases
Yale University School of Medicine and Graduate School of Arts and Sciences
New Haven, CT

Robert Sidbury, MD, MPH
Professor, Department of Pediatrics
Chief, Division of Dermatology
Seattle Children's Hospital
University of Washington School of Medicine
Seattle, WA

Kari A. Simonsen, MD, FAAP
Chief, Division of Pediatric Infectious Diseases
Department of Pediatrics
University of Nebraska Medical Center
Omaha, NE

Jessica Snowden, MD, FAAP
Division of Pediatric Infectious Diseases
University of Nebraska Medical Center
Omaha, NE

Kevin B. Spicer, MD, PhD, MPH
Department of Pediatrics
The Ohio State University College of Medicine
Section of Infectious Diseases
Nationwide Children's Hospital
Columbus, OH

Jeffrey R. Starke, MD, FAAP
Department of Pediatrics
Section of Infectious Diseases
Baylor College of Medicine
Houston, TX

Victoria A. Statler, MD, MSc, FAAP
Division of Pediatric Infectious Diseases
University of Louisville School of Medicine
Louisville, KY

Michelle Steinhardt, MD, MS, FAAP
Department of Pediatrics
Louisiana State University in New Orleans
New Orleans, LA

Mary R. Tanner, MD, FAAP
Fellow in Pediatric Infectious Diseases
St. Jude Children's Research Hospital
Le Bonheur Children's Hospital
Memphis, TN

Anna Katrina Tinio, MD
Chief Resident
Department of Pediatrics
The Children's Hospital at Monmouth Medical Center
Long Branch, NJ

John A. Vanchiere, MD, PhD, FAAP
Department of Pediatrics
Louisiana State University Health Sciences Center
Shreveport, LA

Renuka Verma, MD, FAAP
Pediatric Program Director
Section Chief, Pediatric Infectious Disease
The Children's Hospital at Monmouth Medical Center
Long Branch, NJ

Navjyot K. Vidwan, MD, MPH, FAAP
Division of Pediatric Infectious Diseases
University of Louisville School of Medicine
Louisville, KY

Jennifer Vodzak, MD, FAAP
Assistant Professor of Pediatrics
Drexel University College of Medicine
Department of Pediatrics, Section of Infectious Diseases
St. Christopher's Hospital for Children
Philadelphia, PA

Thomas J. Walsh, MD, PhD, FAAM, FIDSA
Transplantation-Oncology Infectious Diseases Program
Professor of Medicine, Pediatrics, Microbiology & Infectious Diseases
Henry Schueler Foundation Scholar
Investigator of the Save Our Sick Kids Foundation
Weill Cornell University Medical Center
New York Presbyterian Hospital
Hospital for Special Surgery
New York, NY

Gina Weddle, DNP, RN, CPNP-AC
Division of Infectious Diseases
Children's Mercy Hospital
Kansas City, MO

Julie Weiner, DO, FAAP
Division of Neonatology
The Children's Mercy Hospitals and Clinics
Associate Professor of Pediatrics
University of Missouri-Kansas City School of Medicine
Kansas City, MO

Kristi Williams, MD, FAAP
Department of Pediatrics
Division of General Academic Pediatrics
Children's Mercy Hospitals and Clinics
University of Missouri-Kansas City School of Medicine
Kansas City, MO

Charles F. Willson, MD, FAAP
Clinical Professor of Pediatrics
Brody School of Medicine at East Carolina University
Greenville, NC

Robert R. Wittler, MD, FAAP
Professor, Pediatric Infectious Diseases
Kansas University School of Medicine-Wichita
Wichita, KS

Joshua Wolf, MBBS, FRACP
Infectious Diseases Physician
St. Jude Children's Research Hospital
Memphis, TN

Albert C. Yan, MD, FAAP
Section Chief, Pediatric Dermatology
The Children's Hospital of Philadelphia
Associate Professor of Pediatrics and Dermatology
Perelman School of Medicine at the University of Pennsylvania
Philadelphia, PA

Diana L. Yu, PharmD, BCPS-AQ ID
Department of Pharmacy
Children's Mercy
Kansas City, MO

We are most appreciative for the "long-term" support and understanding from our families who have borne a great deal as we have toiled through this and many other projects.

To our loved ones—Barbara, Kimberly, Mitchell, and Greg (LGF) and Ann, Chas, Mary, Christian, Emily, Elisa, Erika, Aileen, and Kelsey (JDM).

Contents

Part 1
Infectious Diseases

Section 3
Viral Infections

Section 4
Fungal Infections

Section 5
Parasitic Infections

Part 2
Dermatology

Preface

Following the success of our first volume, it's even clearer to us as editors that the practice of pediatrics requires rapid access to evidence-based information to make timely diagnoses and offer accurate treatment for common conditions. This is our deliverable to you in *Succinct Pediatrics*.

This book is the second volume of *Succinct Pediatrics,* an ongoing series published by the American Academy of Pediatrics with plans to eventually cover the entire scope of pediatric medicine. This volume addresses the topics of infectious diseases and dermatology, and like volume 1, this book has the same straightforward design typified by short chapters supplemented with key figures and invaluable tables. It's our sincere hope that such a succinct approach will allow clinicians, be they a physician, physician assistant, nurse practitioner, or other qualified health care professional, an opportunity to deliver the highest quality of care to their patients in the most direct way possible.

As senior editors, we are fortunate to have wonderful associate editors who were able to select an excellent group of authors for the more than 250 chapters that will come to encompass the entire series. Those editors are Charles Willson, Jack Lorenz, Warren Seigel, James Stallworth, and Mary Anne Jackson. In *Succinct Pediatrics: Evaluation and Management for Infectious Diseases and Dermatologic Disorders,* the authors have provided discussions on 58 topics with key points and detailed therapies. We've also reproduced in this book Jeffrey Avner's excellent overview on the core knowledge needed for medical decision-making. Understanding medical decision-making is the foundation for making the right decisions at the right time for patients. Evidence-based levels of decision support (as appropriate) can be found throughout the book, permitting the clinician insight into the level of evidence for diagnostic tests as well as selection of different treatment modalities.

The first part of this book, Infectious Diseases, addresses 5 major areas: common infectious conditions, bacterial infections, viral infections, fungal infections, and parasitic infections. The second part, Dermatology, addresses 12 of the most common dermatologic problems seen in general pediatric practice. We are incredibly fortunate to have Mary Anne Jackson as the associate editor for both of these parts. Her expertise was superb in devising an excellent compendium of pediatric information.

We truly appreciate the wonderful guidance and assistance from the American Academy of Pediatrics. Our senior product development editor, Alain Park, was superb in helping score this key resource.

We sincerely hope you will find this volume of *Succinct Pediatrics* an indispensable handbook and guide to the evaluation and management of your patients.

Leonard G. Feld, MD, PhD, MMM, and John D. Mahan, MD

Core Knowledge for Medical Decision-making

Jeffrey R. Avner, MD

Key Points

- Rational medical decision-making requires knowledge of cognition, inherent biases, and disease prevalence and risk, and an understanding of pretest and posttest probabilities.

- Medical decision-making is influenced by clinical (ie, history and physical examination) and nonclinical (eg, patient, clinician, practice) factors.

- Clinicians need to learn and recognize the shortcomings and biases that may be part of their own decision-making.

- The hierarchy of study validity can provide a means of interpreting the level of evidence a study provides.

- Evidence-based medicine in the form of systematic reviews is a useful way of obtaining the best available data on a specific research question.

Overview

Medical decision-making is the cornerstone of diagnostic medicine. It is a complicated cognitive process by which a clinician sorts through a variety of clinical information to arrive at a likely diagnosis among many possibilities. This diagnostic impression then forms the basis of patient management with the ultimate goal of improved health.

However, any medical decision-making contains some inherent element of uncertainty. Furthermore, the ability of a clinician to obtain all necessary information and ensure its accuracy is time-consuming and often impractical in most clinical settings. Many turn to heuristics, an intuitive understanding of probabilities, to drive cognition and arrive at an "educated guess," one that is based on the recognition of specific patterns in clinical findings associated with a particular diagnosis and gleaned from years of experience. With this knowledge, the clinician can quickly sort through a limited set of historical and physical examination findings to support the decision. However, this type of "pattern recognition" is usually not data driven from the literature and therefore may contain bias, ultimately leading to many possible diagnostic errors (Box 1).

Box 1. Common Biases in Decision-making

Anchoring (Premature Closure)	Overly relying on a few initial clinical findings and failing to adjust diagnosis as new information is gathered. Non-supportive findings are devalued inappropriately.
Attribution Bias	Determining a diagnosis on the basis of incomplete evidence such as overemphasizing personality or behavioral characteristics
Availability Bias	Overestimating the likelihood of what comes to mind most easily, often a recent experience, therefore neglecting the true rate (prior probability) of the illness and overestimating the unusual or remarkable
Confirmation Bias	Tending to favor evidence that supports the considered diagnosis and devaluing or not seeking any evidence to the contrary
Diagnostic Momentum Error	Allowing the effect of a preexisting diagnostic label to constrain unbiased reasoning

Failure to appreciate the changing epidemiology of disease (eg, the decline in occult bacteremia prevalence after universal pneumococcal vaccination) may lead to an overestimation of illness. Not knowing accurate pretest probability or how to apply it can lead to inappropriate testing. Personal experience with patients with similar presenting findings also causes bias. For example, a clinician who has been sued for missing a particular diagnosis is likely to overestimate the prevalence of that diagnosis in the future. Alternatively, a clinician who has not seen a relatively rare event (eg, meningitis in a well-appearing 2-week-old febrile neonate) or particular diagnosis (eg, Lemierre syndrome) may underestimate the prevalence of or not even consider that illness. Furthermore, if symptoms supporting the educated guess are found early in decision-making, the clinician may settle on a diagnosis before gathering other important, and possibly conflicting, findings (see "Anchoring [Premature Closure]" in Box 1). Thus, rational medical decision-making requires knowledge of cognition, inherent biases, knowledge of disease prevalence and risk, and an understanding of pretest and posttest probabilities. Additionally, it is often helpful for clinicians to practice *metacognition*, a process to reflect on their decision-making approaches and resultant patient outcomes to ascertain why they may have missed a diagnosis or whether they should modify their management in the future. By becoming more aware of their cognitive process, clinicians may be able to reduce errors and increase efficiency in diagnosis.

Other strategies of medical decision-making are often used, each with particular advantages and disadvantages. An *algorithmic* approach is often favored in busy settings where rapid management or critical decisions must be made. Flowcharts or clinical pathways direct decision-making into a stepwise process based on preestablished criteria, allowing for rapid assessment and standardization of care. While clearly valuable for many situations (eg, advanced life support, head trauma), algorithms tend to be applied rigidly and limit independent thinking. Other decision-making approaches may focus on "ruling out the worst case" such that management overly focuses on rare but high-morbidity diagnoses or "making sure we don't miss it" by entertaining an exhaustive array of rare and perhaps esoteric diagnoses. These strategies generally overuse resources and testing.

In practice, clinicians generally use a combination of cognitive approaches adjusted for the practice setting, time limitation, available resources, and other factors. Furthermore, in the era of family-centered care, most management plans should take into account not just the clinician's clinical impression but also the patient's feelings about his health and the disease in question. Still, the basis of medical decision-making must lie in scientific reasoning, using the best available data and systematic observations to develop an effective approach to the patient and his symptoms. This requires the clinician to incorporate evidence-based medicine (EBM) into decision-making to derive the best answer to the clinical question. Evidence-based medicine focuses on clinically relevant research and takes into account the validity of study methodology, power of predictive markers, accuracy of diagnostic tests, and effectiveness and safety of treatment options to answer a specific clinical question concerning the individual patient. Although it is difficult for a clinician to find, analyze, and assimilate information from a multitude of journals, the development of systematic reviews, databases, and information systems allows for a rapid incorporation of EBM into clinical practice, aiding the clinician in keeping pace with new advances (Table 1).

Table 1. The Steps of Evidence-Based Medicine

Step	Action	Description
Step 1	Define the question.	Frame the need for specific information into an answerable clinical question.
Step 2	Find the evidence.	Systematically retrieve the best evidence to answer the question.
Step 3	Assess the evidence.	Critically evaluate the evidence for validity and application.
Step 4	Apply the evidence.	Integrate the evidence with clinical experience in the framework of patient-specific factors (biological and social) and patient values.
Step 5	Evaluate effectiveness.	Follow the patient's clinical course with regard to the desired outcome, and use it as a basis for similar strategies in the future.

Evaluation

In evaluation of a child, the clinician is continuously gathering new information to change the likelihood (or probability) of the child having a particular disease. Often this takes the form of Bayes theorem, in which new data are applied to a degree of uncertainty (prior probability) to yield a new, updated degree of certainty (posterior probability) (Figure 1).

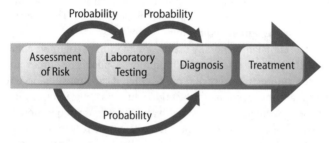

Figure 1. Clinician's thought process.

Because clinical research usually involves studies of groups of patients, the clinician must be able to apply those data to a specific patient who may not share characteristics with the study group. Thus, evaluation of any patient begins with the acquisition of factors that make the patient unique. In considering how likely a child is to have a particular disease, specific historical factors (eg, age, duration of symptoms, time of year), as well as physical examination findings (eg, clinical appearance, presence of fever, focal finding), allow the clinician to adjust the risk assessment by changing the pre-assessment probability. For example, risk of a urinary tract infection in a febrile 6-month-old may be 4% (pre-assessment probability). However, for a febrile uncircumcised boy with temperature above 39°C (102.2°F) for more than 24 hours and no other source on examination, that risk rises to 15% (post-assessment probability). For some patients, the increase in probability may lead the clinician to further hone risk assessment by ordering laboratory or radiologic testing. In other scenarios, the post-assessment probability alone might be sufficient to begin preliminary treatment and further management. For example, a febrile 2-year-old who is ill appearing and has petechiae on the extremities has a high probability of having a serious bacterial illness (eg, meningococcemia) just on risk assessment alone. For this patient, further testing may be done with the caveat that administration of empiric antibiotics should not be delayed. The clinician should not weigh the probability of having a disease in isolation but must also take into account the morbidity of a delay in diagnosis. In a sense, the clinician needs to weigh risks and benefits relative to the certainty of diagnosis to determine what level of probability testing or management should be initiated.

Testing

· · · · · · ·

Laboratory tests should always complement but not replace clinical judgment. Generally, testing is used in 2 ways. In screening, an asymptomatic patient is tested to determine her risk of a particular disease. In diagnostic testing, the patient already has a symptom and the test is used to help reduce ambiguity of the underlying diagnosis. After the patient is assessed, and if there is still sufficient uncertainty of diagnosis or resultant management strategy, the clinician should use laboratory testing to increase or decrease the patient-specific probability of disease. This is determined by characteristics inherent in the test as well as the manner in which the test is being used.

Some tests provide continuous results and a wide range of numeric values, with magnitude of the increments in value being significant and consistent. Continuous tests include those for white blood cell count, erythrocyte sedimentation rate, and C-reactive protein concentration. Because no single value will rule in or rule out a diagnosis, a selected cutoff is often used. However, this cutoff is somewhat arbitrary, because it only gives rise to increasing or decreasing the probability of disease. Other tests have dichotomous results such as positive or negative. A positive result (eg, a positive blood culture result) usually confirms or eliminates a disease from consideration. However, every test has its limitations, including false-positive and false-negative results.

Test results in the clinical arena are often used as predictors of disease. For example, the predictive value of a positive test is what percentage of patients with this positive test has the disease, while the negative predictive value is how many patients with a negative test do not have the disease. These predictive values are useful because clinicians often have the test result and seek to determine who has or does not have the disease. However, predictive values depend on incidence of the disease. Tests used to predict rare events (eg, bacteremia in a well-appearing febrile infant) will usually have low positive and high negative predictive values solely because the incidence of disease is so low. On the other hand, sensitivity (ie, what percentage of patients with the disease has a positive test result) is independent of incidence. Clinicians need to consider which testing characteristic is most relevant to the clinical situation being evaluated. This often depends on the risks and benefits of testing versus morbidity and mortality of missing the illness in the context of disease prevalence.

One of the best statistical approaches to decision-making is the use of likelihood ratios. A likelihood ratio provides an estimate of how much a test result will change the probability of the specific patient having a disease (percentage of ill children with a test result versus percentage of well children with a test result). The higher the likelihood ratio of a positive test result, the more effective the test will be in increasing the probability of disease (ie, it will lead to a higher posttest probability). Similarly, the lower the likelihood ratio (ie, below 1), the less likely the child has the disease. A likelihood ratio of 1 has no effect, likelihood ratios of 5 to 10 or 0.1 to 0.2 have moderate effect, and likelihood ratios of greater than 10 or less than 0.1 have large effect. These data allow the clinician to estimate the likelihood of the patient having or not having a disease. This must then be integrated into the clinician's medical decision-making by taking into account the risk and benefit of performing the test and its resultant effect on the probability of illness.

Management

Ultimately, the clinician's approach to the patient determines health outcome. In that regard, the clinician decides on a specific probability threshold above which management is indicated. Effectiveness of a particular outcome is best determined by prior studies looking at risk factors, interventions, and outcomes in a similar population, the strength of which usually depends on study design (Table 2).

Descriptive studies, such as case reports or case series, report on a particular occurrence or outcome. Because a case study describes only an event, it is difficult to show causation. While the cases may be instructive, care must be taken in generalizing the results. Explanatory studies have stronger, hypothesis-driven study designs. *Randomized controlled trials* have the highest level of scientific rigor. This type of design starts with a study group, randomizes subjects into intervention and control groups, and measures effect of an intervention on the outcome in each group, limiting systemic differences between the groups. A *cohort study* begins with a study population that is free of the outcome, classifies the group on the basis of presence or absence of the risk factor, and measures the outcome in each group. In this type of design, subjects already had the risk factor, rather than it being imposed on them. However, it is impossible to be sure that the groups are comparable in con-founding variables. A *case-control study* begins with a group of patients with a disease and a matched group of control patients without the disease and compares the presence of a risk factor. Although this study design is very common, especially if the outcome is rare, the retrospective design may not take into account other factors that can lead to the outcome. Finally, *cross-sectional studies* compare the presence of a risk factor in groups of patients with and without the disease at a single point in time. While this is also a common methodology, especially in epidemiologic investigation of a disease outbreak, it is a very weak method of establishing causality.

Because it is often difficult for the clinician to synthesize information from available studies, *systematic reviews* have become a useful means of summing up the best available data on a specific research question. After an exhaustive review of the literature, each study is screened for quality in a transparent manner to avoid bias and, if possible, the results are combined. These studies are generally readily available online (eg, The Cochrane Collaboration available at www.cochrane.org) and provide a practical means for clinicians to practice EBM.

Table 2. Hierarchy of Study Validity

Validity (Level of Evidence)	Study Type	Sampling	Advantages	Disadvantages	Statistics
Higher	Systematic reviews	Literature search with objective assessment of methodological quality	Provide an exhaustive summary of relevant literature	May vary in standards and guidelines used	Meta-analysis
	Randomized controlled trials	Prospective	Allow for determination of superiority or non-inferiority of an intervention; can use intent to treat design	Limit systematic differences between groups	Incidence, relative risk
	Cohort studies	Prospective or retrospective	Allow for determination of causality	Make it difficult to ensure that groups are comparable	Incidence, relative risk
	Case-control studies	Retrospective	Are inexpensive, efficient; are practical for rare disorders	Are prone to sampling and recall bias	Odds ratio
	Cross-sectional studies	Single occasion	Are inexpensive	Present no clear evidence of causality; are impractical for rare disorders	Prevalence, odds ratio
Lower	Case reports or series	Retrospective	Are inexpensive, efficient	Present no statistical validity	None

Modified from Perry-Parrish C, Dodge R. Validity hierarchy for study design and study type. *Pediatr Rev.* 2010;31(1):27–29.

Understanding different levels of design allows the stratification of evidence by quality (Box 2). This popular hierarchy permits a standard approach to quality and was selected as a method of assessing the evidence for this publication. However, the clinician is still required to assess not just the type of study design but also how well the study was conducted (internal validity) and adequacy of the conclusions. For example, a poorly conducted randomized controlled trial with an insufficient sample size may not be of better quality than a well-designed case-control study. Other categorizations may be useful to assess levels of certainty regarding net benefit (Table 3) and recommendations for practice (Table 4).

Box 2. Levels of Evidence Used in This Publication

Level I	Evidence obtained from at least one properly designed randomized controlled trial
Level II-1	Evidence obtained from well-designed controlled trials without randomization
Level II-2	Evidence obtained from well-designed cohort or case-control analytic studies, preferably from more than one center or research group
Level II-3	Evidence obtained from multiple time series with or without the intervention. Dramatic results in uncontrolled trials might also be regarded as this type of evidence.
Level III	Opinions of respected authorities, based on clinical experience, descriptive studies, or reports of expert committees

Adapted from Harris RP, Helfand M, Woolf SH, et al. Current methods of the US Preventive Services Task Force: a review of the process. *Am J Prev Med.* 2001;20(3 Suppl):21–35, with permission.

Cause results are generally reported as relative risk or odds ratios. These statistical tests are used to determine the probability of having a particular outcome based on presence (or absence) of a particular test result. *Relative risk* is risk of an outcome in an intervention group divided by risk of the same outcome in the control group and is used in prospective cohort studies to determine the probability of a specific outcome. *Odds ratio* is the odds of an outcome in an intervention group divided by the odds of the same outcome in the control group and is used in case-control, retrospective studies to determine the "odds" of having an outcome. If there is no difference between the groups, the relative risk is 1 or the odds ratio is 1. If the intervention lowers the risk, the value is less than 1, and if it increases the risk, the value is greater than 1. In an effort to incorporate factors related to an intervention in assessing effectiveness of that intervention to achieve a desired outcome, some studies report results in terms of the *number needed to treat* (NNT). This is the number of patients you need to treat to prevent one bad outcome or cause one good outcome. An NNT of 1 means that the treatment is effective in all patients (ie, as the NNT increases, effectiveness decreases). A high NNT needs to be weighed against morbidity of the outcome being studied. For example, if 8 children would have to be treated continuously with phenobarbital for 2 years to prevent 1 febrile seizure, the NNT is 8. The clinician can then decide if the consequence of treating these children justifies the prevention of one febrile seizure. A higher NNT may be acceptable in situations in which the outcome is, for example, bacterial meningitis because there are potentially devastating consequences and the clinician might be willing to accept treating many children unnecessarily to prevent even one case.

Table 3. US Preventive Services Task Force Levels of Certainty Regarding Net Benefit

Level of Certainty	Description
High	The available evidence usually includes consistent results from well-designed, well-conducted studies in representative primary care populations. These studies assess the effects of the preventive service on health outcomes. This conclusion is therefore unlikely to be strongly affected by the results of future studies.
Moderate	The available evidence is sufficient to determine the effects of the preventive service on health outcomes, but confidence in the estimate is constrained by such factors as • The number, size, or quality of individual studies • Inconsistency of findings across individual studies • Limited generalizability of findings to routine primary care practice • Lack of coherence in the chain of evidence As more information becomes available, the magnitude or direction of the observed effect could change, and this change may be large enough to alter the conclusion.
Low	The available evidence is insufficient to assess effects on health outcomes. Evidence is insufficient because of • The limited number or size of studies • Important flaws in study design or methods • Inconsistency of findings across individual studies • Gaps in the chain of evidence • Findings not generalizable to routine primary care practice • Lack of information on important health outcomes More information may allow estimation of effects on health outcomes.

From Agency for Healthcare Research and Quality, US Preventive Services Task Force. *The Guide to Clinical Preventive Services 2014: Recommendations of the U.S. Preventive Services Task Force.* http://www.ahrq.gov/professionals/clinicians-providers/guidelines-recommendations/guide. Accessed April 11, 2016.

With the availability of sophisticated health information systems, use of clinical decision-support tools is becoming a useful new technology to enhance care and reduce errors. Interactive computer software can be used by the clinician, in real time, to provide automated reasoning that takes into account the patient's clinical findings and the latest medical knowledge. By entering patient-specific information, preset rules of logic based on scientific evidence can help the clinician make a diagnosis or analyze patient data in a way that, in some ways, the clinician may not be able do on his own. To be sure, this technique cannot account for those nonclinical factors that may affect decision-making, but it may provide the clinician an efficient, inexpensive process to consider other diagnoses, reduce medical errors, and direct the most EBM approach.

Table 4. US Preventive Services Task Force Recommendation Definitions and Suggestions for Practice

Grade	Definition	Suggestions for Practice
A	The USPSTF recommends the service. There is high certainty that the net benefit is substantial.	Offer or provide this service.
B	The USPSTF recommends the service. There is high certainty that the net benefit is moderate, or there is moderate certainty that the net benefit is moderate to substantial.	Offer or provide this service.
C	The USPSTF recommends against routinely providing the service. There may be considerations that support providing the service in an individual patient. There is at least moderate certainty that the net benefit is small.	Offer or provide this service only if other considerations support the offering or providing of the service in an individual patient.
D	The USPSTF recommends against the service. There is moderate or high certainty that the service has no net benefit or that the harms outweigh the benefits.	Discourage the use of this service.
I Statement	The USPSTF concludes that the current evidence is insufficient to assess the balance of benefits and harms of the service. Evidence is lacking, of poor quality, or conflicting, and the balance of benefits and harms cannot be determined.	Read the clinical considerations section of USPSTF recommendation statement. If the service is offered, patients should understand the uncertainty about the balance of benefits and harms.

Abbreviation: USPSTF, US Preventive Services Task Force.
From Agency for Healthcare Research and Quality, US Preventive Services Task Force. *The Guide to Clinical Preventive Services 2014: Recommendations of the U.S. Preventive Services Task Force.* http://www.ahrq.gov/professionals/clinicians-providers/guidelines-recommendations/guide. Accessed April 11, 2016.

Ultimately, the clinician must decide how to apply the best evidence to the patient. As noted previously, this is a very complicated process that should take into account clinical decision-making but may also be affected by nonclinical influences, be they patient related (eg, socioeconomic status, ethnicity, attitudes, preferences), clinician related (eg, time constraints, professional interactions), or practice related (eg, organization, resource allocation, cost). These factors are often integrated into medical decision-making, consciously or subconsciously, and may have a positive influence (eg, increasing patient adherence) or negative influence (eg, creation of health disparities) on health outcome. It is essential that clinicians be aware of these nonclinical factors to account for a patient's specific interest, thereby optimizing management.

Suggested Reading
• • • • • • • • • • • • • • • • • •

Agency for Healthcare Research and Quality, US Preventive Services Task Force. *The Guide to Clinical Preventive Services 2014: Recommendations of the U.S. Preventive Services Task Force.* http://www.ahrq.gov/professionals/clinicians-providers/guidelines-recommendations/guide. Accessed April 11, 2016

Finnell SM, Carroll AE, Downs SM; American Academy of Pediatrics Subcommittee on Urinary Tract Infection. Diagnosis and management of an initial UTI in febrile infants and young children. *Pediatrics.* 2011;128(3):e749–e770

Hajjaj FM, Salek MS, Basra MK, Finlay AY. Non-clinical influences on clinical decision-making: a major challenge to evidence-based practice. *J R Soc Med.* 2010;103(5): 178–187

Harris RP, Helfand M, Woolf SH, et al. Current methods of the US Preventive Services Task Force: a review of the process. *Am J Prev Med.* 2001;20(3 Suppl):21–35

Kianifar HR, Akhondian J, Najafi-Sani M, Sadeghi R. Evidence based medicine in pediatric practice: brief review. *Iran J Pediatr.* 2010;20(3):261–268

MacKinnon RJ. Evidence based medicine methods (part 1): the basics. *Paediatr Anaesth.* 2007;17(10):918–923

MacKinnon RJ. Evidence based medicine methods (part 2): extension into the clinical area. *Paediatr Anaesth.* 2007;17(11):1021–1027

Onady GM. Evidence-based medicine: applying valid evidence. *Pediatr Rev.* 2009;30(8):317–322

Papier A. Decision support in dermatology and medicine: history and recent developments. *Semin Cutan Med Surg.* 2012;31(3):153–159

Perry-Parrish C, Dodge R. Research and statistics: validity hierarchy for study design and study type. *Pediatr Rev.* 2010;31(1):27–29

Raslich MA, Onady GM. Evidence-based medicine: critical appraisal of the literature (critical appraisal tools). *Pediatr Rev.* 2007;28(4):132–138

Sandhu H, Carpenter C, Freeman K, Nabors SG, Olson A. Clinical decision making: opening the black box of cognitive reasoning. *Ann Emerg Med.* 2006;48(6):713–719

PART

1

Infectious Diseases

CHAPTER 1

Acute Otitis Media and Acute Bacterial Rhinosinusitis

Christopher Harrison, MD

Key Points

- The diagnosis of acute otitis media is objective and relies specifically on physical findings. The diagnosis of acute bacterial rhinosinusitis (ABRS) is more subjective and relies heavily on history or evolution of symptoms.

- Acute otitis media cannot be diagnosed unless there is either a bulging tympanic membrane or otorrhea from a perforated tympanic membrane.

- Sinus opacity on a computed tomographic scan or magnetic resonance image is not sufficient in and of itself to diagnose ABRS because the finding is frequently detected with uncomplicated viral upper respiratory tract infections or in asymptomatic children.

- Radiologic imaging is not warranted or recommended for routine diagnosis or treatment of uncomplicated ABRS, but is useful in defining potential ABRS complications or underlying anatomic abnormalities that cause recurrent ABRS.

- All oral cephalosporins are less active against pneumococcus than high-dose amoxicillin and exhibit less than 50% activity against penicillin-resistant pneumococci.

- Cefdinir is not as active against either pneumococcus or non-typeable *Haemophilus influenzae* as cefuroxime axetil or cefpodoxime proxetil.

Otitis Media

Overview

Guidelines from the American Academy of Pediatrics (AAP) for management of otitis media and acute bacterial rhinosinusitis (ABRS) in children focus on specific diagnostic criteria that are relatively easy for clinicians to use. Watchful waiting has become not only acceptable but recommended for certain acute otitis media (AOM) presentations.

Causes and Differential Diagnosis
· ·

The 2 most common pathogens in AOM are pneumococcus and non-typeable *Haemophilus influenzae*. *Moraxella catarrhalis* and group A *Streptococcus* are also pathogens, but less frequently (Table 1-1). More than one pathogen can be detected in approximately 8% of AOM episodes. Rarely, *Staphylococcus aureus* may be isolated from middle ear fluid, usually when other head and neck infectious foci are evident or pressure-equalizing (PE) tubes are in place. *Candida* species have also been implicated in otorrhea with PE tubes in place, particularly after multiple courses of antibacterial drugs.

The major condition from which AOM must be distinguished is otitis media with effusion (OME). This is important because antibiotics are not indicated for OME, while antibiotics should be considered for AOM. Overdiagnosis of AOM when the condition is really OME is a common scenario for antibiotic overuse.

Otitis media with effusion is differentiated from AOM mostly by AOM having a bulging tympanic membrane (TM) while OME does not. The TM in OME is usually retracted but may sometimes be in a neutral position. Most OME occurs when pressure in the middle ear is lower than atmospheric yet middle ear fluid is also present. This occurs predominantly from 2 mechanisms, both due to eustachian tube dysfunction. The first is caused by the eustachian tube failing to equalize pressure while the normal physiologic daily process of

Table 1-1. Expected Pathogens in Acute Otitis Media (Percentage of Episodes With Pathogen), 2005–2012[a]

	Intermittent	Persistent/Recurrent
Pneumococcus		
Penicillin susceptible	33	10
Penicillin non-susceptible—intermediate	10	12
Penicillin non-susceptible—resistant	5	20
Non-typeable *Haemophilus influenzae*		
β-Lactamase producing	10	39
β-Lactamase nonproducing	38	17
Moraxella catarrhalis	5	9
Group A *Streptococcus*	5	0

[a] Percentage >100% total because approximately 8% of AOM episodes will have more than one pathogen.

Data from Harrison CJ, Woods C, Stout G, Martin B, Selvarangan R. Susceptibilities of *Haemophilus influenzae*, *Streptococcus pneumoniae*, including serotype 19A, and *Moraxella catarrhalis* paediatric isolates from 2005 to 2007 to commonly used antibiotics. *J Antimicrob Chemother*. 2009;63(3):511–519; Harrison CJ. The changing microbiology of acute otitis media. In: Collier AM, Hagmann M, Harrison C, Jacobs MR, Murillo J, eds. *Acute Otitis Media: Translating Science into Clinical Practice*. London: Royal Society of Medicine Press, Ltd; 2007; Harrison CJ and Swanson D, 2016, unpublished.

approximately 1 cm^3 of air in the middle ear is being absorbed by the mastoid bone. Mostly this is itself because of post-viral, smoke-induced, or allergic inflammation in the posterior nasopharynx and eustachian tube. The second mechanism is a residual from a prior AOM episode despite there no longer being viable bacteria. In this scenario, residual inflammation and retained bacterial antigens impede absorption or clearance of the residual effusion from the AOM. This inflammation, however, is not sufficient to increase middle ear pressure as is seen with AOM.

Less common conditions in the differential diagnosis of AOM are hemotympanum, traumatic hemorrhage into TM, or cerumen impaction. Hemotympanum is usually associated with basilar skull fracture and can produce bulging of the TM as well as opacity and color changes. Color change of the TM is often blue-purple or deep red (blood). Pneumatic otoscopy will reveal limited motion of the TM because of blood filling the middle ear cavity. Traumatic hemorrhage into the TM itself can occur with direct trauma (eg, insertion of cotton-tipped applicator too deep into external ear canal or post-barotrauma or an explosion causing pressure that overstretches the TM without rupturing it). The TM is rarely bulging with traumatic hemorrhage, but there can be an intense erythema. Pneumatic otoscopy will usually reveal near-normal movement, or possibly excessive movement if the middle ear ossicles have been disrupted. Cerumen impaction seems unlikely to be confused with AOM, but if the visible surface of the impaction is deep in the canal and has been molded to have a concave surface by cleaning attempts with cotton-tipped applicators, such a misdiagnosis has occurred.

Acute otitis media can be more common in patients with altered immune states (ie, less defenses) or anatomic conditions that impair eustachian tube function.

Immune-altered states associated with AOM are wide ranging. The simplest and most common is a temporary condition (ie, the immature immune capabilities of children <2 years). Immune systems of young children fail to recognize and respond to polysaccharide antigens in the capsules of pneumococci. Repeated AOM episodes can therefore occur from the same serotype because protective antibody is not produced. Recent use of pneumococcal conjugate vaccines (PCVs) has helped overcome this problem. Any congenital or acquired immunodeficiency that has a B-cell deficiency, with or without a T-cell deficiency, also makes a host more susceptible to AOM. Examples of this are X-linked agammaglobulinemia (also called Bruton agammaglobulinemia), common variable immunodeficiency, severe combined immunodeficiency, or uncontrolled HIV infection.

Anatomic predispositions to AOM include anomalies such as cleft palate, malformed or floppy eustachian tubes (eg, any young child or any with Down syndrome), or congenital absence of cilia. Mucosal-disrupting conditions also increase risk of AOM. Examples of this are viral upper respiratory tract infections (URTIs). Acute otitis media is more frequent in children attending day care or living in a household with more than 3 children, or after passive smoke exposure.

Clinical Features
• • • • • • • • • • • • • • •

Acute otitis media is an acute purulent inflammatory condition of the middle ear cavity. It has an expanding volume of purulent material that bulges an intact TM, or causes otorrhea if increased middle ear pressure perforates the TM. The presence of shiny mucous in otorrhea or in external ear canal secretions indicates a connection between the canal and middle ear via a TM perforation and differentiates otorrhea caused by a perforated TM from that caused purely by acute otitis externa. Pain from pressure on the tragus most often indicates otitis externa.

Other clinically associated symptoms/signs may include recent onset of otalgia or intense erythema/opacity of the TM. Fever, irritability, sleep disturbance, and reduced appetite and activity may also occur.

Acute otitis media usually occurs coincident with or following a viral URTI. Acute otitis media is most often exclusively caused by bacterial pathogens. Less often it is caused by both viral and bacterial pathogens in the middle ear effusion (MEE). Least often it is exclusively caused by viral pathogens in MEE. Acute otitis media should be classified as severe or non-severe to aid in treatment decisions (Box 1-1).

The criteria most recently accepted as diagnostic for AOM include a bulging TM with some increased opacity or intense erythema plus recent onset of symptoms, either otalgia or fever equal to or higher than 39°C (102.2°F).

Box 1-1. Acute Otitis Media Definitions

AOM: acute inflammatory MEE characterized by bulging of TM and visible TM changes, such as intense erythema and opacity

OME: mildly inflammatory MEE characterized by neutral or retracted TM, often with visible changes such as mild erythema, a meniscus, or bubbles in the MEE

Severe AOM: AOM with moderate/severe otalgia *or* otalgia lasting ≥48 h *or* concurrent fever ≥39°C (102.2°F)

Intermittent AOM: AOM episode with no recent AOM episode within 1 mo

Persistent AOM: ongoing symptoms or TM signs consistent with AOM despite management

Early treatment failure: persistent signs of AOM with persistent symptoms of otalgia or fever >48 h but <7 d into management

Late treatment failure: persistent signs of AOM after 7 d or a full course of prescribed therapy

Recurrent AOM: AOM episode <1 mo after a prior AOM episode that was confirmed or presumed to have resolved

Uncomplicated AOM: inflammatory process limited to middle ear with an intact TM in a host with presumed normal middle ear and facial anatomy and normal immune function

Abbreviations: AOM, acute otitis media; MEE, middle ear effusion; OME, otitis media with effusion; TM, tympanic membrane.

Clinical symptoms associated with AOM may be relatively minor or even absent particularly early in the course of AOM. Because viral URTIs often precede or accompany AOM, their signs may be difficult to differentiate from those of AOM. These include fever, irritability, decreased activity, or decreased appetite. Viral-induced symptoms also often make it difficult to determine whether the AOM is improving early in the course of management.

Otalgia is a reasonably specific symptom of AOM that is caused by traction on the annulus of the TM by increased middle ear pressure. However, "ear pain" can also be caused by intense paratonsillar inflammation due to pharyngotonsillitis or recent tonsillectomy. Likewise, otitis externa (also called swimmer's ear) can produce similar pain; but, in otitis externa the pain is intensified by compression of the tragus (the tragus sign, which is not seen in uncomplicated AOM). Ear tugging is considered by some to be a possible surrogate for otalgia. However, ear tugging may simply be a sign of overall infant irritability and thus is not highly specific.

Physical examination is paramount in diagnosing AOM. Bulging of the TM and presence of an inflammatory effusion are the essential findings. Without both bulging and an inflammatory effusion, the diagnosis is not AOM, regardless of the color of the TM. The clinician must have sufficient visualization of the TM to make a confident decision on the diagnosis. Therefore, cleaning cerumen or foreign material from the external ear canal is the first step toward a correct diagnosis.

Given that the major criterion, and sine qua non, of AOM on examination is bulging of the TM, assessing for its presence should be the primary goal during otoscopy. The portion of the TM that first shows bulging is the pars flaccida in the upper pole of the TM. This portion is composed of only 2 opposing membranes. Therefore, it is less rigid than the pars tensa, which has the same 2 membranes but also an intervening relatively stiff middle fibrous layer, sandwiched between the membranes.

Initially the pars flaccida will bulge and partially obscure the usually visible ossicle (the long process of the malleolus) (Figure 1-1). As the pressure and

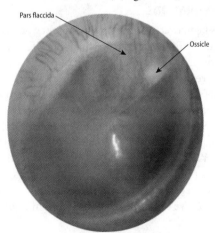

Figure 1-1. Normal tympanic membrane.

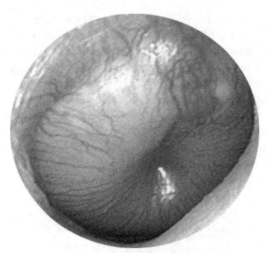

Figure 1-2. Completely bulging tympanic membrane (bagel ear).

volume of the purulent material in the middle ear increase, the pars tensa eventually bulges as well. At some point, the ossicle is completely obscured, resulting in no visible landmarks. Often the TM is then reminiscent of a donut or bagel (Figure 1-2).

Presence of an effusion is also considered essential. Effusions may be detected by reduced movement on insufflation of the external ear canal with a pneumatic otoscope. Opacity of the TM or a visible meniscus also adds credence to the presence of an MEE.

Evaluation

Laboratory Investigations

Tympanometry has been used to confirm the presence of an effusion but cannot distinguish the MEE of AOM from that of OME. Tympanometry involves applying constant low levels of sound to a sealed external ear canal and measuring reflected versus absorbed sound while varying the pressure in the canal from negative ($<$1 atm) to positive ($>$1 atm). This results in a linear readout for which the shape indicates whether an effusion is present.

A normal middle ear produces a tympanogram readout designated as an A curve, in which a peak occurs at zero pressure (the point at which most of the sound is absorbed). When sound is reflected and not absorbed (meaning the TM is less flexible than usual and is under positive or negative pressure), the linear readout runs closer to the baseline. The more sound that is reflected, the closer to baseline the curve drops. Three tympanogram results are consistent with an effusion.

The tympanogram of AOM is a relatively flat B curve (no true peak) close to the baseline. The flat curve indicates that nearly all the sound is being reflected back from the TM at all pressures, because the volume of MEE dampens any TM movement that would transmit sound through the ossicles (ie, prevents proper vibration of the TM).

At times, early AOM may have a C2 curve when the amount of effusion has yet to completely dampen TM mobility. The peak occurs, but it is generally of lower than normal amplitude and at a negative pressure. Less frequently, early AOM may have an App curve with a peak that is blunted because of decreased absorption of sound due to the evolving middle ear pus, but the peak is shifted to the positive pressure region. C2 curves are precursors to App curves that are in turn precursors to B curves as AOM evolves.

Radiology

There is no role for radiologic evaluation in management of uncomplicated AOM. When potential mastoid, temporal bone, or intracranial extensions of AOM become a concern, computed tomographic scans or magnetic resonance images are warranted. Discussion with the radiologist is recommended to ensure that the modality is appropriate for the desired results.

Management

Overall, neither topical nor systemic decongestants or antihistamines have been shown to be beneficial in increasing clinical cure for AOM.

Pain Management

The first step in management of AOM is to control pain as much as is safely feasible (Evidence Quality Grade B, Recommendation Strength: Strong per the AAP Guideline). Pain relief can take several forms with varying degrees of efficacy.

No data support homeopathic remedies, nor are there convincing data that application of heat, cold, or unmedicated oils provides benefit (Evidence Level II-1).

Topical agents containing anesthetics (eg, benzocaine, procaine, or lignocaine) seem to provide brief relief of pain in children older than 5 years. They may be of benefit for younger children, but data are inconclusive (Evidence Level I).

Orally administered acetaminophen, ibuprofen, naproxen, or codeine/codeine analogs have been shown to be modestly effective (Evidence Level I). Nonnarcotic agents are recommended for routine use. Potential narcotic use must take into account added cost and risks inherent with narcotics.

Spontaneous perforation relieves much of the pain, but the ragged edges may heal poorly. If pressure relief is desired, controlled release via tympanocentesis or myringotomy is preferred (Evidence Level II-2). This is quite effective but requires special training to prevent procedural complications. Thus, tympanocentesis is not routine in most practices.

Antimicrobial Treatment Decisions

The choice of initial antibiotics versus observation is outlined in Table 1-2. Various antibiotic recommendation options are outlined in Box 1-2.

Observation is reasonable because many children spontaneously improve (up to 50%, particularly if non-typeable *H influenzae* or *M catarrhalis* is the pathogen) within 48 to 72 hours and do not require antibiotics. Among the usual oto-pathogens, only pneumococcus is invasive. Invasive disease is more likely in younger children with high fevers and if they have not been fully immunized with pneumococcal 13-valent conjugate vaccine (PCV13). This is one rationale for the universal recommendation to prescribe antibiotics with high fever (severe AOM) in young children.

Some experts recommend giving families a "rescue" prescription for antibiotics when initially choosing observation (Evidence Level I). Data indicate that less than half the families need to use the rescue prescription. Parents are instructed to call the clinician to report worsening or failure to improve within 72 hours. In this case the prescription can be filled without a

Table 1-2. Consideration of Antibiotic Use for Acute Otitis Media

Recommended	Preferred	Optional[a]
Severe[b] AOM at any age	Unilateral non-severe AOM ≤24 mo of age	Unilateral non-severe AOM ≥24 mo of age
Bilateral AOM of any severity ≤24 mo of age		Non-severe AOM regardless of laterality ≥24 mo of age

Abbreviation: AOM, acute otitis media.

[a] When using careful observation plus pain management as a joint decision with parent or guardian, assured follow-up at 72 h is required. Children whose AOM worsens or fails to improve within 72 h of observation should be seen again and started on antibiotics.

[b] Severe AOM is an episode with moderate to severe otalgia, or otalgia lasting >48 h or with a concurrent fever >39°C (102.2°F). All other presentations are classified as non-severe.

Box 1-2. Antibiotic Recommendations/Preferences

Antibiotics are *recommended* for
- Severe AOM (bilateral or unilateral), any age (Evidence Level I)
- Bilateral non-severe AOM, <24 mo (Evidence Level I)

Antibiotics are *preferred* by some experts for
- Unilateral non-severe AOM, <24 mo. Antibiotics are initially preferred because of superior outcome compared to placebo (Evidence Level I).

Antibiotics are optional[a] and careful observation is reasonable for
- Unilateral non-severe AOM, <24 mo (Evidence Level I)
- Non-severe AOM (bilateral or unilateral), <24 mo (Evidence Level I)

Abbreviation: AOM, acute otitis media.

[a] When using careful observation plus pain management as a joint decision with parent or guardian, assured follow-up at 72 h is required. Children whose AOM worsens or fails to improve within 72 h of observation should be seen again and antibiotics reconsidered.

return office/clinic visit. The return call can be important so that the clinician can feel assured that a serious invasive complication, one that might require parenteral antibiotics or even hospitalization, has not occurred.

Specific Antibiotic Choices

When a decision has been made to prescribe antibiotics, the choice of antibiotic depends on the clinical presentation or frequency of AOM episodes and recent antibiotic use.

First-line Antibiotics

First-line antibiotics can be used for intermittent AOM in patients with no antibiotic use in the past month (Table 1-3).
• Amoxicillin at 90 mg/kg/day divided into 2 doses administered every 12 hours (Evidence Level I).

Table 1-3. Antibiotic Choices for Acute Otitis Media

Patient Allergy Categorization	Antimicrobial Choice[a]
First-line Choice at Initial Diagnosis or at Clinical Failure on 48–72 h of Observation	
Penicillin nonallergic	Amoxicillin—high dose (90 mg/kg/d divided in 2 doses)
Penicillin allergic—not type I	β-Lactamase stable oral 2nd- or 3rd-generation cephalosporin[b]
Penicillin allergic—type I	Trimethoprim/sulfamethoxazole, clindamycin, or azithromycin
Second-line Choice for Persistent AOM Either at 48–72 h of First-line Treatment or at End of Therapy, or Recurrent AOM <1 mo After Prior Antibiotic Use	
Penicillin nonallergic	Amoxicillin/clavulanate—high dose
Penicillin allergic—not type I	β-Lactamase stable oral cephalosporin[b] or IM ceftriaxone
Penicillin allergic—type I	Trimethoprim/sulfamethoxazole plus either clindamycin or azithromycin
AOM Due to Known Multidrug Highly Resistant Pneumococcus	
Susceptible to clindamycin	Clindamycin
Clindamycin resistant but ceftriaxone susceptible	Ceftriaxone (3 IM doses)
Clindamycin and ceftriaxone resistant	Levofloxacin or linezolid

Abbreviations: AOM, acute otitis media; IM, intramuscular.

[a] Oral cephalosporins are less efficacious than amoxicillin against pneumococcus and less effective than amoxicillin/clavulanate against both pneumococcus and non-typeable *Haemophilus influenzae*. Cephalexin is never recommended for AOM therapy. This is in contradistinction to ceftriaxone which is more active against both pneumococci and non-typeable *H influenzae* than amoxicillin.

[b] If a child is unable to retain oral antibiotics, parenteral ceftriaxone is a reasonable choice to start. Oral drug can be initiated when the vomiting has ceased to be an issue.

Modified from American Academy of Pediatrics Subcommittee on Management of Acute Otitis Media. Diagnosis and management of acute otitis media. *Pediatrics*. 2004;113(5):1451–1465.

- o *Expectation:* Better than 85% clinical resolution, with failures shared near evenly between highly penicillin-resistant pneumococci (minimal inhibitory concentration ≥2.0 mcg/mL) and β-lactamase–producing non-typeable *H influenzae*.
- If the AOM patient is penicillin allergic but not exhibiting type I allergy, use a β-lactamase-stable cephalosporin, either cefdinir or cefuroxime axetil at 30 mg/kg/day divided in 2 doses administered every 12 hours or cefpodoxime proxetil at 10 mg/kg/day divided in 2 doses every 12 hours (Evidence Level I). Cefdinir tastes better but has less clinical efficacy than amoxicillin (against pneumococcus) or its two cephalosporin alternatives (against non-typeable *H influenzae*), even at the "high dose" recommended here. This 30 mg/kg daily dose of cefdinir is not in the package insert but is based on pharmacokinetic data and expected susceptibility of likely oto-pathogens. Cefixime is the best oral cephalosporin for non-typeable *H influenzae* but is active against only highly penicillin-susceptible pneumococci, so it is currently not recommended as monotherapy in the AAP guidelines.
  - o *Expectation:* Between 75% and 85% clinical resolution for cefuroxime or cefpodoxime, with most failures due to pneumococci with intermediate or high penicillin resistance rather than non-typeable *H influenzae*. More non-typeable *H influenzae* and pneumococcal failures are expected with cefdinir than cefuroxime or cefpodoxime.
- If there is penicillin-caused anaphylaxis or confirmed type I allergy to both penicillin and cephalosporins, consider trimethoprim/sulfamethoxazole (TMP/SMX) plus either azithromycin or clindamycin (Evidence Level III). Trimethoprim/sulfamethoxazole dosing is 10 mg/kg/day divided in 2 doses based on the trimethoprim component. Azithromycin can be used at 10 mg/kg/day as a single dose for 3 days but has inferior coverage for pneumococcus and generally should not be used for bacterial respiratory tract infections. Clindamycin dosing is 30 to 40 mg/kg divided in 3 daily doses. Clindamycin has substantial taste issues and no gram-negative activity.

Second-line Antibiotics

Second-line antibiotics are for use with persistent/recurrent AOM particularly with receipt of amoxicillin in the past 30 days, clinical failure on amoxicillin, or concurrent purulent conjunctivitis (see Table 1-3). Purulent conjunctivitis nearly always indicates that the pathogen is non-typeable *H influenzae,* so a β-lactamase–stable drug is recommended. These drugs are also recommended for both early and late treatment failures of first-line drugs (see above).

- Amoxicillin/clavulanate at 90 mg/kg/day divided in 2 doses every 12 hours (Evidence Level I).
  - o *Expectation*: Approximately 90% clinical resolution, with failures mostly due to highly penicillin-resistant pneumococci and a few cases of β-lactamase–producing non-typeable *H influenzae*. β-Lactamase–negative ampicillin-resistant non-typeable *H influenzae* is very rare in the United States.

or

- β-Lactamase–stable oral cephalosporin (Evidence Level I).
  - *Expectation:* Between 65% and 80% clinical resolution, with most failures due to pneumococci with intermediate or high penicillin resistance for cefuroxime or cefpodoxime. More non-typeable *H influenzae* and pneumococcal failures are expected with cefdinir than cefuroxime. Note: Because no pneumococcal strain has ever produced β-lactamase, β-lactamase stability of a drug adds no extra activity against pneumococcus, but is important in extending activity against non-typeable *H influenzae and M catarrhalis.*

or

- Ceftriaxone intramuscularly at 50 mg/kg/dose (Evidence Level II-1). Up to 3 doses can be used, with second or third doses used when symptoms persist longer than 48 hours after the prior dose. No oral cephalosporin is fully equivalent to ceftriaxone.
  - *Expectation:* Approximately 90% resolution; failures mostly due to highly penicillin-resistant (ceftriaxone-resistant) pneumococci.

Third-line Antibiotics

When cause is known to be highly penicillin-resistant pneumococci or patient's second-line treatment of persistent/recurrent AOM has failed, creative choices are required and often not within standard US Food and Drug Administration (FDA)–approved indications or current guidelines.

Serotype 19A pneumococcus is the most frequent type with high-level multidrug resistance (MDR), but has recently become less frequent since full implementation of PCV13. The 19A strains are most often resistant to azithromycin and all oral cephalosporins. Almost 40% of cases are clindamycin resistant, and up to 30% are ceftriaxone resistant. Oral antibiotic choices are limited. Levofloxacin or linezolid is active against greater than 98% of these MDR pneumococci and can be used (Evidence Level II-1). Consultation with an infectious diseases expert can be useful when prescribing these off-label drugs that can have unusual adverse effects.

Otorrhea With Pressure-Equalizing Tube in Place

Topical antibiotics are usually sufficient to treat acute otorrhea (<7 days) associated with PE tubes. Most such episodes are caused by the same pathogens as AOM. However, *S aureus* (particularly methicillin-resistant *S aureus* [MRSA]) and *Candida* species can emerge with recurrent episodes.

Topical ofloxacin alone or ciprofloxacin with dexamethasone usually administered as 4 drops twice daily is effective in nearly 90% of episodes, reducing symptoms in less than 5 days when routine oto-pathogens are the cause (Evidence Level II-1). Both are superior to and produce less adverse effects than oral or other systemic antibiotics. If cultures of otorrhea that has been present less than 72 hours reveal staphylococci or *Candida* species, referral to an otolaryngologist is warranted because the PE tubes may need to be removed.

Chronic suppurative otitis media (CSOM) produces chronic recurring otorrhea. If a foul odor is present, one should suspect anaerobes and potential cholesteatoma. This warrants referral to an otolaryngologist. If no special odor is noted, pathogens include standard pathogens of AOM, but may also include MRSA, *Candida albicans,* gram-negative organisms that flourish in moist areas (eg, *Pseudomonas, Acinetobacter, Achromobacter, Enterobacter,* or occasionally *Aspergillus* or molds).

Often CSOM cultures will reveal multiple pathogens that may need to be addressed one at a time. *Pseudomonas* is normal flora for the external ear canal and cannot usually be eradicated; however, bacterial burden can be quantitatively reduced, which in turn can at least temporarily eliminate otorrhea. Consultation with an infectious diseases expert or otolaryngologist is usually warranted in cases of CSOM. Aural toilet (direct cleaning of the external ear canal with suction) is often a critical component to a successful outcome.

Follow-up

Even when antibiotics are initially prescribed, the option should be explained to the caregiver that if the child's symptoms worsen or fail to respond within 48 to 72 hours for AOM or 7 days for CSOM, a repeat visit will help determine if a change in therapy is needed.

Prevention

Prophylactic Antibiotics for AOM

Clinicians should not routinely prescribe prophylactic antibiotics to reduce the frequency of episodes of AOM in children with recurrent AOM (Evidence Level I). This approach increases antibiotic resistance in the nasopharynx of the recipient, and evidence indicates no real reduction in AOM episodes for the usual patient with recurrent AOM.

Surgical Approach

Tympanostomy tubes can be effective in reducing recurrent AOM and are a reasonable option when 3 AOM episodes occur within 6 months, or when 4 AOM episodes occur within 1 year with 1 episode in the preceding 6 months (Evidence Level I). Evidence is less supportive of adenoidectomy in preventing AOM. Tonsillectomy is not indicated for preventing AOM.

Vaccines

Pneumococcal conjugate vaccine administration to all children according to the recommended schedule of the Advisory Committee on Immunization Practices and AAP has had an overall effect of reducing AOM episodes. The current PCV13 includes the MDR 19A serotype, and its continued use appears to be reducing community prevalence of 19A. This, in turn, should lead to fewer AOM episodes caused by antibiotic-resistant strains, even if the overall reduction of AOM incidence is not significant compared to PCV7.

Annual influenza vaccine administered to all children according to the recommended schedule of the Advisory Committee on Immunization Practices and AAP is recommended with a likely effect on AOM only during influenza season (Evidence Level I). This has the effect of reducing the numbers of influenza cases in AOM-susceptible children for which influenza is the predisposing factor to AOM.

Social Strategies

Encouraging breastfeeding for at least 6 months is recommended because it likely reduces rates of viral URTIs and thereby AOM episodes. Avoiding pacifier use after 6 months of age, tobacco smoke exposure, and supine bottle-feeding (bottle propping) also likely reduces episodes of AOM (Evidence Level II-2).

Long-term Monitoring and Implications

In the 1980s, a standard of care was to follow up each AOM episode at 2-week intervals until the ear normalized. In part, this was because it was believed that significant developmental and hearing issues would occur if a child had even a unilateral ongoing MEE for longer than 3 months.

Because data revealed that such sequelae are not likely (Evidence Level I), the "2-week follow-up" for AOM is no longer recommended unless a child shows a pattern of frequent episodes of AOM. Then the objective is to confirm resolution of the AOM episode and counsel about potential tympanostomy tubes if AOM episodes are sufficiently frequent. Still, if a child has signs suggestive of hearing impairment and bilateral effusions longer than 3 months, referral to an otolaryngologist is warranted.

Perforation of the TM for longer than a week into treatment should trigger otolaryngological referral as well. Otorrhea with a pungent or foul smell may indicate a cholesteatoma, a potentially life-threatening condition, and is an indication for referral to an otolaryngologist.

Acute Bacterial Rhinosinusitis

Overview

There are millions of diagnoses of ABRS in pediatric patients annually. A form of sinusitis or rhinosinusitis occurs with every viral URTI. While not all cases of ABRS are secondary to viral URTIs, most are. Therefore, an important distinction that affects potential antibiotic treatment is whether a secondary bacterial

Box 1-3. Definitions of Acute Bacterial Rhinosinusitis

Persistent symptoms A: Nasal discharge (of any quality) or daytime cough (which may be worse at night), or both, persisting for >10 d without improvement. Recently, sleep disturbance via cough has been suggested as more specific than daytime cough.

Persistent symptoms B: Acutely worsening symptoms of nasal discharge or daytime cough (or sleep disturbance via cough), worsening after the sixth day of symptoms, *plus* either a new onset of fever (>38.1°C [100.6°F]) or substantial increase in nasal discharge or cough after having experienced transient improvement of symptoms.

Severe symptoms: Fever ≥39°C [102.2°F] *plus* purulent (thick, colored, and opaque) nasal discharge with both being present concurrently >3 d consecutively.

infection develops in addition to the instigating URTI. Three presentations are sufficient for the diagnosis of ABRS (Box 1-3).

Acute bacterial rhinosinusitis is usually a complication of a viral URTI or other upper respiratory tract inflammatory precondition in which rhinorrhea is a prominent sign/symptom. In a recent study in which more than 2,000 children 1 to 10 years of age with rhinorrhea were screened, 139 (6.5%) had ABRS, demonstrating that the risk of ABRS simply from presenting with URTI symptoms is low. Of those with ABRS, 89% presented with persistent symptoms (Persistent symptoms A, Box 1-3) as the diagnostic criteria, 8% had worsening symptoms (Persistent symptoms B, Box 1-3), and 3% had severe symptoms. Further, 43% were considered mild, while 57% were more than mild. A take-home message is that if ABRS is diagnosed in greater than 6.5% of children presenting with URTI symptoms, there is likely a modicum of overdiagnosis.

Causes and Differential Diagnosis

The pathogens are for the most part the same as for AOM (see Otitis Media, Causes and Differential Diagnosis section, and Table 1-1). Antimicrobial choices are therefore substantially the same (see Otitis Media, Antimicrobial Treatment Decisions section). Because cilia are damaged during ABRS, rhinorrhea and cough are prominent symptoms. The customary 6-week time frame to allow ciliary healing means that some rhinorrhea/cough may persist up to 6 weeks even in adequately treated ABRS episodes. This is the ABRS equivalent of OME after AOM, but in ABRS, noninfected secretions have a visible exit path through the nose (rhinorrhea), whereas in AOM/OME the eustachian tube dysfunction leads to MEE. Likewise, in AOM, residual draining secretions into the posterior pharynx are not visible.

Microbiology

As with AOM, the causative pathogens are primarily of pneumococcus and non-typeable *H influenzae,* comprising approximately 75% of detectable pathogens. Pneumococcus has generally been slightly more common than non-typeable *H influenzae* in pediatric ABRS. *Moraxella catarrhalis* is a traditional co-pathogen in approximately one-third of cases of pediatric ABRS. In the past 10 years there are increasing reports of *S aureus* with MRSA making up a proportion of sinusitis isolates in uncomplicated ABRS in adults. However, in children, *S aureus* is mostly associated with complicated ABRS. Therefore, initial empiric therapy of uncomplicated pediatric ABRS does not require coverage for *S aureus*.

Associations with other diseases, conditions, or exposures include
- Conditions with altered nasopharyngeal anatomy: nasal polyps, deviated septum, inadvertent or medical foreign bodies, tumors, choanal atresia, or abnormally developed sinus structures.
- Conditions with inflammation or altered secretions: cystic fibrosis, seasonal or environmental allergies, immotile cilia, recent viral infection, or intense exposure to dusts or irritating chemicals.
- Decreased defenses: immune disorders that affect antibody production, mostly B-cell problems (see Otitis Media, Causes and Differential Diagnosis section).
- Dental caries or apical dental abscesses have been associated with maxillary sinusitis.

Differential Diagnosis

Major conditions in the differential diagnosis include
- *Viral URTI.* Most viral URTIs are improving by day 6 or 7 and usually do not produce fever at that late date after onset of symptoms (Figure 1-3). Acquiring a second respiratory virus while in the midst of the first viral URTI can create a scenario indistinguishable from an episode of ABRS secondary to the initial viral URTI. These second viral URTIs may be acquired in reception rooms during visits to clinicians. Alternatively, they may be acquired from siblings or day care mates. Absence of facial pain and of cough that causes sleep disturbance has recently been shown to more likely indicate a viral URTI than ABRS despite rhinorrhea persisting for longer than 10 days.

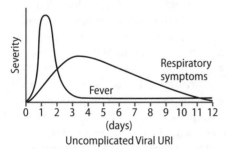

Figure 1-3. Graphic of typical uncomplicated viral URI.

Abbreviation: URI, upper respiratory infection.

From Chow AW, Benninger MS, Brook I, et al. IDSA clinical practice guideline for acute bacterial rhinosinusitis in children and adults. *Clin Infect Dis*. 2012;54(8):e72-e112, with permission.

- *Allergic rhinitis.* It may be difficult to establish that persistent rhinorrhea is not caused by allergies in the atopic child or adolescent. Fever should not occur with seasonal or environmental allergies alone, however. Facial pain is also not a classic symptom of allergies. Eosinophils in a nasal smear lend credence to allergies as the cause of ongoing rhinorrhea.
- *Periorbital cellulitis* can be preseptal and caused by breaks in the skin barrier of the face after insect bites or local trauma, rather than a complication of ABRS. When skin breaks are the portal, the pathogens are most likely *S aureus* or group A *Streptococcus.*

Clinical Features

Uncomplicated ABRS presents nearly always with some degree of persistent rhinorrhea. Cough is also a frequent symptom, including daytime cough. There is also often sleep disturbance because of cough. Fever is an inconsistent finding, as it is with AOM, and is not more frequent with ABRS than uncomplicated URTIs. A history or physical examination finding of facial pain has been associated with ABRS. However, such a history or finding on facial palpation can be difficult to elicit from preschool-aged children. In addition, pain fibers in swollen turbinates from a simple URTI can produce a sensation of facial pain that may be indistinguishable from the facial pain of ABRS.

Complicated ABRS can present with periorbital or orbital cellulitis, cavernous sinus thrombosis, Pott puffy tumor, brain abscess, or seizures. Fever is more frequent in complicated than uncomplicated ABRS, likely because of added infectious foci that comprise the complications. Concurrent rhinorrhea is not always present in these complications.

Three clinical presentations are recommended to distinguish ABRS from viral rhinosinusitis (URTI).

1. *Persisting.* Persistent symptoms or signs compatible with ABRS, lasting for longer than 10 days without evidence of clinical improvement (Evidence Level II-1). Note: Recent data in children with a persisting but mild symptom presentation suggest that the lack of certain signs or symptoms indicates uncomplicated viral URTI or an ABRS that may spontaneously clear. If symptoms are considered mild and there is no facial pain, sleep disturbance, or green rhinorrhea, this appears to parallel non-severe AOM, for which observation without antibiotics may be an option. These data were not available when the current Infectious Diseases Society of America (IDSA) guidelines were released. There is an option to observe in the guidelines, but absence of these 3 specific findings was not included in the discussion (see Acute Bacterial Rhinosinusitis, Management section). However, in the presence of mild persistent symptoms and the absence of the 3 signs/symptoms above, it seems reasonable to observe without antibiotics with the same caveats as with observation in the case of AOM (ie, there is assurance of follow-up and the parents are in agreement with withholding antibiotics).

2. *Double-sickening.* Worsening symptoms or signs with new onset of fever, headache, or increase in nasal discharge after a typical viral URTI that lasted 5 to 6 days and was initially improving (Evidence Level II-2).
3. *Acute severe.* Severe symptoms or signs of high fever ($\geq$39°C [102.2°F]) and purulent nasal discharge or facial pain lasting for at least 3 to 4 consecutive days at the beginning of illness (Evidence Level II-2).

Evaluation

Routine laboratory investigations, such as complete blood cell count, C-reactive protein, or nasal/middle meatus cultures, are not recommended and are not useful. Middle meatus cultures have been reasonably reliable for adults in identifying potential ABRS pathogens, but this is not so for children. Children are more frequently colonized with pneumococcus, non-typeable *H influenzae*, or *M catarrhalis* than adults. In addition, middle meatus cultures in children usually reveal multiple organisms. Faced with multiple potential pathogens, the clinician has no reliable means to decide which of the detected organisms is the true pathogen versus a colonizing organism.

Because uncomplicated pediatric ABRS is a clinical diagnosis and no simple, inexpensive, or reliable imaging study is currently available, imaging studies such as plain radiographs or computed tomography are not recommended for evaluation of uncomplicated ABRS. Positive findings are not infrequent in children with URTIs but without ABRS (approximately 50%). Magnetic resonance imaging is even less specific; 68% of children with URTI and even 42% of nonsymptomatic school-aged children have sinus opacities by MRI.

While normal imaging studies can be reasonably assuring that a patient with respiratory symptoms does not have ABRS, an abnormal radiographic study does not confirm ABRS but would add expense and radiation risk when clinical criteria should suffice.

Computed tomography or magnetic resonance imaging with contrast should be reserved for evaluation of a serious complication or if frequently recurrent ABRS raises concern that surgery is needed to correct abnormal anatomy in the nasopharynx or sinuses themselves.

Management

Adjunctive Therapy in Patients With ABRS

Intranasal saline irrigation with either physiologic or hypertonic saline solution is recommended as an adjunctive treatment only in adults with ABRS (Evidence Level II-3). Intranasal corticosteroids are recommended as an adjunct to antibiotics in the empiric treatment of ABRS, primarily in patients with a history of allergic rhinitis (Evidence Level II-3). Neither topical/oral decongestants nor antihistamines are recommended as adjunctive treatment with the presumption of improving cure rates in patients with ABRS (Evidence Level I).

Antimicrobials (Table 1-4)

The duration of therapy in children is recommended to be 10 to 14 days depending on the severity and rapidity of initial clinical response (Evidence Level II-1). Note: The ABRS guidelines use the term *second-line* therapy to define anything but standard dose amoxicillin/clavulanate therapy (the first-line drug in the guidelines), likely to simplify the algorithm (Figure 1-4). This author uses *first-line* to indicate the drug used initially in any given patient and *second-line* as those drugs used when first-line drugs fail.

Table 1-4. Antibiotic Choices for Children

Patient and Allergy Categorization	Antimicrobial Choice
Outpatient Mild to Moderate ABRS	
First-line Choice at Initial Diagnosis or at Clinical Failure on 48–72 h of Observation	
Penicillin nonallergic	Amoxicillin—high dose (90 mg/kg/d divided in 2 doses)
Penicillin allergic—not type I	β-Lactamase stable oral 2nd- or 3rd-generation cephalosporin[a]
Penicillin allergic—type I	Clindamycin ± trimethoprim/sulfamethoxazole
Second-line Choice for Persistent ABRS Either at 48–72 h of First-line Treatment or at End of Therapy, or Recurrent ABRS <1 mo After Prior Antibiotic Use	
Penicillin nonallergic	Amoxicillin/clavulanate—high dose
Penicillin allergic—not type I	IM ceftriaxone—3 doses IM[a] or levofloxacin
Penicillin allergic—type I	Trimethoprim/sulfamethoxazole plus either clindamycin or levofloxacin
Severe ABRS Requiring Hospitalization[b]	
Penicillin nonallergic	Ampicillin/sulbactam (200–400 mg/kg/d divided in 3 doses every 8 h)
Penicillin allergic—not type I	IV ceftriaxone (75 mg/kg/d) or levofloxacin[c]
Penicillin allergic—type I	Levofloxacin
ABRS Due to Known Multidrug Highly Resistant Pneumococcus	
Susceptible to clindamycin	Clindamycin
Clindamycin resistant but ceftriaxone susceptible	Ceftriaxone (3 IM doses)
Clindamycin and ceftriaxone resistant	Levofloxacin or linezolid

Abbreviations: ABRS, acute bacterial rhinosinusitis; IM, intramuscularly; IV, intravenous.

[a] Cephalexin is never recommended for ABRS therapy. Other oral cephalosporins are less efficacious than amoxicillin against pneumococcus and less effective than amoxicillin/clavulanate against both pneumococcus and non-typeable *Haemophilus influenzae*. This is in contradistinction to ceftriaxone, which is more active against both pneumococci and non-typeable *H influenzae* than amoxicillin.

[b] If *Staphylococcus aureus* is among considerations as being a pathogen or if patient is critically ill, vancomycin (60 mg/kg/d) divided every 6 h can be added.

[c] Cefotaxime (150 mg/kg/d) divided in 4 doses every 6 hours is an alternative.

Derived from Chow AW, Benninger MS, Brook I, et al. IDSA clinical practice guideline for acute bacterial rhinosinusitis in children and adults. *Clin Infect Dis*. 2012;54(8):e72–e112.

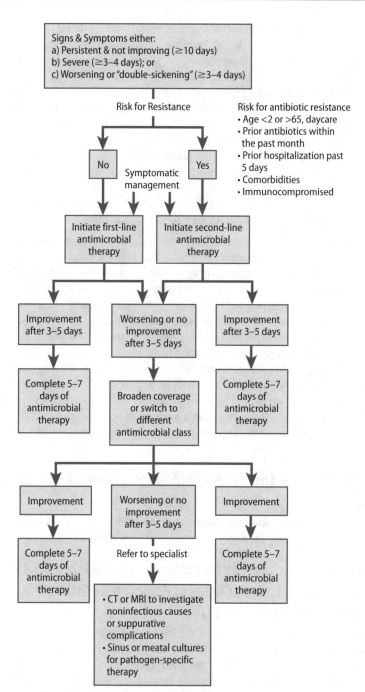

Figure 1-4. Algorithm for the management of acute bacterial rhinosinusitis from 2012 IDSA acute bacterial rhinosinusitis guideline.

From Chow AW, Benninger MS, Brook I, et al. IDSA clinical practice guideline for acute bacterial rhinosinusitis in children and adults. *Clin Infect Dis.* 2012;54(8):e72–e112, with permission.

- Per the current IDSA guidelines, antimicrobial empiric therapy is recommended as soon as the clinical diagnosis of ABRS is made. These guidelines use the terminology as *recommendation: strong, evidence: moderate.* Recent evidence indicates that up to 25% of children with mild symptoms plus meeting the definition of uncomplicated ABRS, as noted previously, still have URTIs and not ABRS and thus do not need antibiotics. Therefore, clinicians may choose to observe such patients without antibiotics for 3 to 5 days if symptoms are mild and follow-up is assured (Evidence Level II-1). This would be similar to the option used currently for AOM. Note: Periorbital or orbital cellulitis is often secondary to ethmoid sinusitis and requires antibiotic treatment.

Not Recommended for ABRS per IDSA Guidelines

Azithromycin is not recommended for empiric therapy because of high rates of resistance among non-typeable *H influenzae* and pneumococci.

Trimethoprim/sulfamethoxazole monotherapy is also not recommended for empiric therapy because of high rates of resistance among both pneumococci (up to 40%) and non-typeable *H influenzae* (30%–40%) by some in vitro reports. However, data from 2013 in our laboratory indicate that TMP/SMX resistance among non-typeable *H influenzae* decreased to 20%, although resistance among pneumococci remained high.

Single-drug empiric therapy with cefuroxime axetil, cefpodoxime proxetil, or cefdinir is not recommended for ABRS because of pneumococcal resistance rates up to 50% and up to 20% for non-typeable *H influenzae* with cefdinir at the time of guideline release. Note: Data again from our laboratory in 2015 indicate pneumococcal resistance rates of 34% for cefuroxime and 38% for cefdinir.

First-line Empiric Therapy for Mild Uncomplicated ABRS per IDSA Guidelines

Standard dose. Amoxicillin/clavulanate or amoxicillin may be considered for initial first-line therapy for uncomplicated ABRS (Evidence Level II-3).

First-line Empiric Therapy for Patients With Moderate ABRS in Areas With High Endemic Rates of Penicillin-Resistant Pneumococci or Increased Risk

High dose. Amoxicillin/clavulanate if the local prevalence of highly penicillin-resistant invasive pneumococci is greater than 10% (Evidence Level II-3).

High dose. Amoxicillin/clavulanate is also recommended for those with evidence of systemic toxicity (eg, fever of 39°C [102.2°F] or higher, or with threat of suppurative complications; attendance at day care, age: <2 years;

recent hospitalization; antibiotic use within the past month; or immunocompromising conditions [Evidence Level III]).

First-line Empiric Therapy of ABRS in Type I Penicillin-Allergic Outpatients (See Table 1-4.)

The IDSA guidelines recommend doxycycline as a first-line alternative in type I penicillin-allergic patients for empiric therapy of ABRS in children older than 8 years. It is greater than 85% active against respiratory pathogens, but has the potential teeth staining and bone issues that preclude its routine use at earlier ages (Evidence Level III).

The IDSA guidelines recommend levofloxacin as initial empiric therapy of children with type I penicillin allergy (Evidence Level II-2). However, this would result in a great deal of quinolone use in children, a phenomenon feared by those who care for adults and elderly patients, because resistant clones disseminate more rapidly in young children.

Consider clindamycin for pneumococci (approximately 80% activity; confirm with regional antibiogram) plus TMP/SMX for non-typeable *H influenzae* (70%–80% activity). Unless symptoms are severe or the patient is highly febrile, this combination should provide approximately 80% or greater clinical response (Evidence Level III).

Levofloxacin or linezolid (gram-positive pathogen coverage) plus an oral third-generation cephalosporin (cefixime, or cefpodoxime for gram-negative coverage) are reasonable for outpatient treatment in the patient with known resistant pneumococci plus non-typeable *H influenzae* (Evidence Level III). For most clinicians, prescribing a quinolone (not FDA approved for ABRS in children) or linezolid (very expensive and potentially causing bone marrow suppression starting in second week of therapy) is an unusual event. Consider discussion with an infectious diseases expert prior to prescribing these drugs.

For first-line empiric therapy of mild ABRS in penicillin non–type I allergic patients, see Table 1-4.

First-line Empiric Therapy for Toxic, Complicated, or Hospitalized ABRS Patients (See Table 1-4.)

Ceftriaxone plus either clindamycin or vancomycin (depending on rates of clindamycin-resistant methicillin-sensitive *S aureus* and MRSA, or the need for central nervous system penetration) is preferred (Evidence Level II-2). Because of the widely variable rates of *S aureus* in complicated ABRS, particularly in those with intracranial complications, some experts do not include coverage for *S aureus* in initial empiric therapy even in hospitalized patients. In severely ill patients, obtaining culture material from the suppurative complicating site or sinus itself can assist in specific antibiotic choices.

Second-line Empiric Therapy for Mild Uncomplicated ABRS (See Table 1-4.)

Therapeutic failure should be considered if the patient's symptoms have either not improved or worsened over a 3- to 5-day period. The goal with failures is to optimize therapy for penicillin-resistant pneumococci while providing a drug that is active against β-lactamase-producing *M catarrhalis* and non-typeable *H influenzae*.

Penicillin nonallergic outpatients. High-dose amoxicillin/clavulanate for those whose amoxicillin or standard-dose amoxicillin/clavulanate therapy fails.

Non–type I penicillin-allergic outpatients. Levofloxacin is the only mono-therapy that improves pneumococcal coverage while maintaining activity in the face of β-lactamase from non-typeable *H influenzae* and *M catarrhalis* for those in whom combination of an oral cephalosporin plus clindamycin fails. It provides greater than 99% activity against all 3 major pathogens. It is prudent to inform families that quinolones are not FDA approved for use in ABRS for children. For AOM, 3 intramuscular doses of 50 mg/kg of ceftriaxone at 24- to 48-hour intervals is recommended. However, there are no data or recommendations for short-course intramuscular ceftriaxone to treat ABRS.

Type I penicillin-allergic outpatients. Levofloxacin is also recommended for these patients. Alternatively, linezolid plus TMP/SMX could be considered but is not recommended in the IDSA guidelines (Evidence Level III). Linezolid provides 100% activity against pneumococcus and also greater than 95% activity against MRSA or methicillin-susceptible *S aureus* if that is considered necessary in a given patient. The TMP/SMX provides 75% to 80% activity against non-typeable *H influenzae*.

Patients Failing Second-line Empiric Therapy

For these patients, referral to an otolaryngologist for potential culture is warranted. These patients often require input from both the otolaryngologist and an infectious diseases specialist to achieve a good clinical outcome. If cultures reveal specific organisms, antimicrobials can be tailored to those pathogens.

Long-term Monitoring and Implications

Long-term monitoring of episodes of uncomplicated ABRS is not warranted. Monitoring of complicated ABRS should be focused on the complication and directed as such.

Because frequent or recalcitrant ABRS can be associated with cystic fibrosis, antibody deficiencies, ciliary abnormalities, or anatomic abnormalities, consideration for evaluations for these conditions may be warranted in those with excessive numbers of episodes.

Suggested Reading
• • • • • • • • • • • • • • • • • •

American Academy of Pediatrics Subcommittee on Management of Acute Otitis Media. Diagnosis and management of acute otitis media. *Pediatrics.* 2004;113(5):1451–1465

Chow AW, Benninger MS, Brook I, et al. IDSA clinical practice guideline for acute bacterial rhinosinusitis in children and adults. *Clin Infect Dis.* 2012;54(8):e72–e112

Dohar J, Giles W, Roland P, et al. Topical ciprofloxacin/dexamethasone superior to oral amoxicillin/clavulanic acid in acute otitis media with otorrhea through tympanostomy tubes. *Pediatrics.* 2006;118(3):e561–e569

Harrison CJ, Woods C, Stout G, Martin B, Selvarangan R. Susceptibilities of *Haemophilus influenzae, Streptococcus pneumoniae,* including serotype 19A, and *Moraxella catarrhalis* paediatric isolates from 2005 to 2007 to commonly used antibiotics. *J Antimicrob Chemother.* 2009;63(3):511–519

Macfadyen CA, Acuin JM, Gamble CL. Topical antibiotics without steroids for treating chronically discharging ears with underlying eardrum perforations. *Cochrane Database Syst Rev.* 2005;(4):CD004618

Shaikh N, Hoberman A, Kearney DH, et al. Signs and symptoms that differentiate acute sinusitis from viral upper respiratory tract infection. *Pediatr Infect Dis J.* 2013;32(10):1061–1065

Spiro DM, Tay KY, Arnold DH, Dziura JD, Baker MD, Shapiro ED. Wait-and-see prescription for the treatment of acute otitis media: a randomized controlled trial. *JAMA.* 2006;296(10):1235–1241

Wald ER. Acute otitis media and bacterial sinusitis. *Clin Infect Dis.* 2011;52(Suppl 4): S277–S283

Wald ER, Nash D, Eickhoff J. Effectiveness of amoxicillin/clavulanate potassium in the treatment of acute bacterial sinusitis in children. *Pediatrics.* 2009;124(1):9–15

CHAPTER 2

Central Venous Catheter–Associated Bloodstream Infections

Gina Weddle, DNP, RN, CPNP-AC

Key Points

- Catheter-related bloodstream infection (BSI) is the most common cause of health care–associated infections in pediatrics.

- Catheter removal should be considered particularly in the setting of severe sepsis, suppurative thrombophlebitis, endocarditis, BSIs that persist longer than 72 hours despite adequate therapy, recrudescent infection with the same organism, and infections due to *Staphylococcus aureus, Pseudomonas aeruginosa, Candida,* or mycobacteria.

- Prevention is the key to reduce catheter-related BSI.

Overview

Bloodstream infections (BSIs) are the most common health care–associated infections in pediatrics, with most being associated with intravascular catheters. Central venous catheters (CVCs) are frequently used in pediatrics for a variety of reasons, including medication administration, nutrition, and chemotherapy agents. Children with catheter-related BSI have longer hospital stays and higher death rates along with increased cost.

Causes and Differential Diagnosis

Infections can occur during insertion, manipulation, accessing by contaminated parenteral fluids, or translocation from the mouth or gastrointestinal tract. Infections can additionally involve the exit site, subcutaneous tissue, or bloodstream.

The most common organism associated with catheter-related BSI is coagulase-negative *Staphylococcus* (CoNS) (40%) followed by gram-negative organisms (25%), including *Enterobacter* species, *Pseudomonas aeruginosa, Klebsiella pneumoniae,* and *Escherichia coli. Staphylococcus aureus* and enterococci are the third most common organisms seen in catheter-related BSI.

Other skin-colonizing organisms reported include *Candida, Corynebacterium, Propionibacterium,* and *Bacillus.*

The major differential diagnosis rests with differentiating when a blood culture isolate is a contaminant (eg, one culture of a skin-colonizing organism). As of January 2015, the Centers for Disease Control and Prevention has identified a subcategory of catheter-related BSI in oncology patients with severe mucositis or mucosal barrier injury with oral flora noted on blood culture; therefore, these patients are no longer counted in the overall central catheter–associated BSI rates. New recommendations about identifying an additional subcategory regarding patients with intestinal insufficiency such as short bowel syndrome with suspected translocation of enteric bacteria are being discussed but currently are not in place.

Clinical Features

Clinical signs and symptoms are typical of any acute systemic illness, and fever is generally the symptom that heralds diagnosis. In young infants, including premature infants, fever is less often noted and hypothermia may be seen along with other nonspecific signs and symptoms. Criteria for reporting include one positive blood culture of a recognized pathogen with at least one of the following symptoms: fever, hypothermia or apnea if younger than 1 year, chills, or hypotension.

Exit site infection is suggested if the child has purulence at the catheter exit site. If the infection extends into the subcutaneous tissue, signs and symptoms of pain, induration, erythema, or exudate may be noted and tunnel infection may be diagnosed.

If there is a concurrent thrombus in association with infection, the patient is at risk for septic embolic complications. In patients with multiple positive blood culture results over time, endocarditis may be a complicating feature and may be suggested by onset of a new or changing heart murmur. In patients with persistently positive blood culture results, an evaluation to exclude endocardial involvement (eg, echocardiogram) should occur. A careful evaluation should look for signs and symptoms of clinical instability (ie, signs of shock) or embolic phenomena.

Evaluation

Bloodstream infection must be considered in any child with a CVC who has an acute febrile illness or inflammation or purulence around the exit site. Sensitivity and specificity of accurately diagnosing a BSI based on clinical symptoms is low for catheter-related BSI.

Blood cultures should be obtained prior to the initiation of antibiotic therapy and are required to make this diagnosis (Evidence Level II). Blood cultures are recommended both peripherally and centrally (Evidence Level III).

If a peripheral blood culture cannot be obtained, then 2 central blood cultures should be obtained (Evidence Level III).

Recognized pathogens include *S aureus, E coli, Pseudomonas, Klebsiella, Candida,* and *Enterococcus.* For common skin pathogens such as CoNS, viridians streptococci, or *Micrococcus,* 2 positive blood cultures are required.

Careful examination of the catheter site is necessary in all patients with fever and an indwelling CVC. If exudate is present at the exit site, this should be sent for Gram stain and culture (Evidence Level II) and an exit site infection should be diagnosed. Quantitative blood cultures are the most accurate way to identify a catheter-related BSI.

A diagnosis of catheter-related BSI is made when the same organism grows on 2 separate samples, or is determined from the differential time to positivity (Evidence Level II). For quantitative cultures the diagnosis of catheter-related BSI is made when there is a threefold greater colony count from the catheter blood culture when compared to the peripheral culture. For differential time to positivity, the growth from the catheter culture will grow 2 hours earlier than that from the peripherally obtained culture.

Additional testing that may be necessary includes ultrasound of the CVC site to exclude a concurrent thrombus and echocardiogram to evaluate for endocarditis in the patient with persistently positive blood culture results (>3 days after initiation of appropriate antibiotics in the patient who has had catheter removal). Transthoracic echocardiogram is sufficient for infants and children, but transesophageal echocardiogram should be considered in older patients (>10 years) or those with body weight greater than 40 kg.

Management

Physicians should define the indication and continued need for the CVC in patients with suspected catheter-related BSI. In cases where there is no longer a reasonable medical indication for the catheter, removal should be considered immediately.

Empiric therapy should be considered in a child who has a CVC when a BSI is being considered. The decision of which antibiotics depends on several factors, including the patient's underlying diagnosis; regional resistance patterns; risk factors for infection, including total parenteral nutrition; previous antibiotic exposure; and the severity of illness at presentation.

Exit site infection may be treated with catheter removal and local care. Tunnel infection (involvement of the subcutaneous tissue) requires systemic antibiotics, and removal of the catheter is recommended (Evidence Level I). In the patient with catheter-related BSI, the decision to attempt salvage of the catheter depends on the child's underlying disease and clinical appearance and whether the child has other vascular access options.

In the otherwise healthy child who is clinically stable, vancomycin may be instituted for empiric coverage following blood culture, because CoNS is the most common identified pathogen (Evidence Level II). Consider daptomycin or linezolid in patients who have increased vancomycin minimum inhibitory concentrations greater than 2 mcg/mL or in patients with a known isolate with a concentration greater than 2 mcg/mL (Evidence Level II). Concurrent coverage that includes gram-negative pathogens should be initiated along with vancomycin in the patient with an underlying health condition or in those who are clinically unstable at time of presentation.

For hematology/oncology patients with fever and neutropenia, assuming there is clinical stability and no findings related to the CVC (eg, erythema, tenderness), vancomycin is not necessary at outset and treatment should target gram-negative organisms, including *P aeruginosa* or multidrug-resistant organisms.

For patients who are seriously ill or known to be previously colonized with multidrug-resistant pathogens, vancomycin plus a fourth-generation cephalosporin, carbapenem, or β-lactam/β-lactamase combination of antibiotics should be considered according to local susceptibility patterns (Evidence Level II).

Candidemia should be suspected in patients who are receiving total parenteral nutrition, prolonged broad-spectrum antibiotic use, hematologic malignancy, bone marrow transplant, solid organ transplant, or femoral CVC placement (Evidence Level II). Antifungal empiric therapy can include either fluconazole for patients who have not previously received an azole or are not known to be colonized with a fluconazole-resistant *Candida* (ie, *Candida krusei* or *Candida glabrata*). For patients who previously received an azole or are colonized with a fluconazole-resistant *Candida,* echinocandins should be considered (Evidence Level III).

Limited data exist in pediatrics regarding catheter removal in the setting of a BSI because of difficulty in obtaining access. In adults, guidelines exist that recommend removal of short-term peripherally inserted catheters in the setting of a BSI (Evidence Level II). In pediatrics, evidence supports removal of the catheter in the setting of a tunnel or pocket infection (Evidence Level I).

Catheter removal should additionally be considered in the setting of severe sepsis, suppurative thrombophlebitis, endocarditis, BSIs that persist longer than 72 hours despite adequate therapy, recrudescent infection with the same organism, and infections due to *S aureus, P aeruginosa, Candida,* or mycobacteria (Evidence Level II).

Few data exist regarding the length of therapy in pediatrics, but adult guidelines are available to extrapolate. Length of therapy will depend on the organism that grows along with host factors, but counting should begin with the first day of negative culture results (Evidence Level III). Empiric therapy recommendations, along with minimal length of therapy, are listed in Table 2-1 for those with uncomplicated clinical course (Evidence Level II).

Antibiotic lock therapy has been used when attempting to salvage a catheter. Lock therapy is used in combination with systemic therapy and should not be used in the setting of an exit site or tunnel infection (Evidence Level II). Antibiotic lock therapy can be difficult because longer dwell times are required for effective therapy; therefore, the catheter cannot be used at that time.

Table 2-1. Antibiotic Choice and Length of Therapy

Organism	Preferred Empiric Antibiotic	Alternative Antibiotic	Length of Therapy, d
Gram-positive			
MSSA	Oxacillin/nafcillin	Cefazolin/vancomycin	Minimum: 14
MRSA	Vancomycin	Daptomycin	Minimum: 14
Methicillin-susceptible CoNS	Oxacillin/nafcillin	1st-generation cephalosporin	5–7 if catheter removed 10–14 if catheter in place
Methicillin-resistant CoNS	Vancomycin	Daptomycin	5–7 if catheter removed 10–14 if catheter in place
Enterococcus			
Ampicillin-susceptible	Ampicillin ± aminoglycoside	Vancomycin	7–14
Ampicillin-resistant	Vancomycin ± aminoglycoside	Linezolid/daptomycin	7–14
Vancomycin-resistant	Linezolid/daptomycin	Quinupristin/dalfopristin	7–14
Gram-negative			
Escherichia coli, ESBL-negative	3rd-generation cephalosporin	Ciprofloxacin/aztreonam	10–14
E coli, ESBL-positive	Carbapenem	Ciprofloxacin/aztreonam	10–14
Enterobacter/Serratia	4th-generation cephalosporin	Ciprofloxacin/carbapenem	10–14
Acinetobacter	Ampicillin/sulbactam	Carbapenem	10–14
Pseudomonas	4th-generation cephalosporin	Carbapenem/ciprofloxacin	10–14
Fungi			
Candida	Echinocandin/fluconazole	Liposomal amphotericin	14

Abbreviations: CoNS, coagulase-negative *Staphylococcus*; ESBL, extended-spectrum β-lactamase; MRSA, methicillin-resistant *Staphylococcus aureus*; MSSA, methicillin-susceptible *Staphylococcus aureus*.

The lock consists of a mixture of antibiotics with heparin with a total volume to be adequate to fill the catheter lumen (Table 2-2) (Evidence Level II). This mixture is placed and left in the catheter and ideally exchanged every 24 to 48 hours. When exchanging the lock, it should not be flushed through but withdrawn and discarded.

Preferred dwell time is 24 hours and should not exceed 48 hours (Evidence Level II).

Table 2-2. Antibiotic Concentrations for Lock Therapy

Antibiotic	Dosage, mg/mL	Heparin/Saline, IU/mL
Vancomycin	2.5	2,500 *or* 5,000
Vancomycin	2.0	10
Vancomycin	5.0	0 *or* 5,000
Ceftazidime	0.5	100
Cefazolin	5.0	2,500 *or* 5,000
Ciprofloxacin	0.2	5,000
Gentamicin	1.0	2,500
Ampicillin	10.0	10 *or* 5,000
Ethanol	70%	0

Ethanol locks have recently become available that provide broad antimicrobial spectrum by denaturation without a specific molecular target, thereby minimizing the potential for development of resistance. Ethanol locks have been used in the gastrointestinal patient population for both prevention and treatment of catheter-related BSI and have been found to be effective with low relapse rate (Evidence Level II). Concentrations of 70% ethanol are used with a priming volume to fill the catheter with a dwell time of 2 to 24 hours. Ethanol locks are compatible only with silicone catheters. Case reports have shown polyurethane catheters can crack or fracture, although a study in 2005 by Crnich, Halfmann, Crone, and Maki did not show a difference in catheter integrity when comparing polyurethane versus silicone catheters (Evidence Level III).

Long-term Monitoring and Implications

Prevention is the best way to reduce catheter-related BSI. Avoiding unnecessary catheter placement along with promptly discontinuing unnecessary catheters is key to avoiding a catheter-related BSI (Evidence Level I). Education and designated staff who have met established competency for placement of catheters have been shown to reduce the incidence of catheter-related BSI (Evidence Level I). In pediatrics, the preferred site for catheter placement includes upper extremities, lower extremities, scalp, or subclavian (Evidence

Level II). During catheter placement, strict adherence to aseptic skin technique along with sterile procedure with maximal barriers is a necessity to prevent subsequent infection (Evidence Level I).

Once the catheter is in place, a sterile dressing should be applied (Evidence Level I). Dressing changes should occur every 2 days for gauze dressings and every 7 days for transparent dressings, or as needed if the dressing becomes soiled or loose (Evidence Level II). Daily skin cleansing with a 2% chlorhexidine wash has been shown to reduce the rate of catheter-related BSI in the intensive care unit setting (Evidence Level II). Other strategies that can be used include minimizing manipulation/accessing of the catheter, adequate hand hygiene prior to manipulation, proper hub preparation prior to access, replacing end caps frequently, and covering all stopcocks within the catheter (Evidence Level II). The role for antibiotic impregnated catheters is not clear.

The Centers for Disease Control and Prevention instituted the National Healthcare Safety Network (NHSN) in 1970 as a way to track hospital-acquired infections. Adult institutions are required to report catheter-related BSI to NHSN. Although it is currently voluntary for free-standing children's hospitals to report catheter-related BSI to NHSN, mandatory reporting will likely occur in the future.

Suggested Reading

Acuña M, O'Ryan M, Cofré J, et al. Differential time to positivity and quantitative cultures for noninvasive diagnosis of catheter-related bloodstream infection in children. *Pediatr Infect Dis J.* 2008;27(8):681–685

Bleasdale SC, Trick WE, Gonzalez IM, Lyles RD, Hayden MK, Weinstein RA. Effectiveness of chlorhexidine bathing to reduce catheter-related bloodstream infections in medical intensive care unit patients. *Arch Intern Med.* 2007;167(19):2073–2079

Dannenber C, Bierbach U, Rothe A, Beer J, Körholz D. Ethanol-lock technique in the treatment of bloodstream infections in pediatric oncology patients with Broviac catheter. *J Pediatr Hematol Oncol.* 2003;25(8):616–621

Horan TC, Andrus M, Dudeck MA. CDC/NHSN surveillance definition of health care-associated infection and criteria for specific types of infections in the acute care setting. *Am J Infect Control.* 2008;36(5):309–332

Mermel LA, Allon M, Bouza E, et al. Clinical practice guideline for the diagnosis and management of intravascular catheter-related infections: 2009 update by the Infectious Diseases Society of America. *Clin Infect Dis.* 2009;49(1):1–45

O'Grady NP, Alexander M, Burns LA, et al. Guidelines for the prevention of intravascular catheter-related infections. *Am J Infect Control.* 2011;39(4 Suppl 1):S1–S34

Wheeler DS, Giaccone MJ, Hutchison N, et al. A hospital-wide quality-improvement collaborative to reduce catheter-associated bloodstream infections. *Pediatrics.* 2011;128(4):e995–e1007

CHAPTER 3

Gastroenteritis

Laura E. Norton, MD, and James Christopher Day, MD

Key Points

- Bacterial enteritis should be considered in the child with fever and bloody diarrhea.

- A thorough history, including diet, travel, and other exposure, as well as physical examination findings can aid in distinguishing between bacterial pathogens.

- Stool culture should be performed prior to initiation of antibiotics for bloody diarrhea.

- Initial management of suspected bacterial enteritis should focus on rehydration and in most cases can be accomplished with oral rehydration therapy.

- Uncomplicated salmonellosis does not require antibiotic treatment in the immunocompetent host. However, treatment should be considered in high-risk cases including children younger than 3 months and children with underlying gastrointestinal disorders, hemoglobinopathies, and immunosuppression.

- Management goals for children with bacterial enteritis should include return to an age-appropriate diet as soon as possible. Restrictive diets are not recommended during acute diarrheal episodes.

Overview

While rotavirus vaccine has reduced the rate of hospitalization for infectious diarrhea, bacterial, viral, and parasitic pathogens continue to account for substantial morbidity in children. Typical management includes maintaining or restoring hydration and nutrition during the acute illness. The need for antimicrobial therapy depends on factors specific to the pathogen, host, and nature of the illness.

Causes and Differential Diagnosis

Many infectious causes of diarrhea have been identified. Box 3-1 outlines common and some uncommon pathogens. Bloody stools are more typical of bacterial enteritis and less likely to be seen with illnesses caused by viruses or single-celled eukaryotic parasites.

In a child with diarrhea, the history obtained should include duration of symptoms, underlying medical conditions, and dietary exposures. Diarrhea with viral and bacterial pathogens is typically acute ($\leq$1 week), while diarrhea with parasitic infections can be acute or chronic. Antibiotic-associated diarrhea, like most infectious diarrhea, is typically acute. Diarrhea prolonged beyond 1 week should prompt consideration of both noninfectious and infectious etiologies.

The incubation period and duration of symptoms varies depending on the bacterial pathogen (Table 3-1). Liver disease and malignancy increase the risk of infection with *Plesiomonas*. Immunosuppression, certain immunodeficiencies, and hemoglobinopathies (in particular sickle cell disease) increase the risk for infection and complications with *Salmonella*.

Several bacterial causes of enteritis are associated with extraintestinal manifestations, but they are rarely the exclusive cause of such syndromes. Examples include

- Hemolytic uremic syndrome is typically secondary to *Escherichia coli* O157:H7 or other Shiga toxin–producing *E coli*. It has also been associated with pneumococcal infection as well as certain genetic mutations of the complement system; less commonly it is reported as drug associated (eg, cytotoxic drugs, oral contraceptives).

Box 3-1. Infectious Causes of Diarrhea

Bacteria	Viruses	Parasites
- *Aeromonas hydrophila* - *Bacillus cereus*[a] - *Campylobacter jejuni* and *Campylobacter coli* - *Clostridium difficile* - *Clostridium perfringens* - *Escherichia coli* - *Listeria monocytogenes* - *Plesiomonas shigelloides* - *Salmonella enteritidis* - *Shigella* spp - *Staphylococcus aureus*[a] - *Vibrio cholerae* - *Vibrio vulnificus* and *Vibrio parahaemolyticus* - *Yersinia enterocolitica*	- Adenovirus (enteric strains 40 and 41) - Astrovirus - Norovirus - Rotavirus - Sapovirus	- *Cryptosporidium parvum* - *Cyclospora cayetanensis* - *Cystoisospora belli* - *Entamoeba histolytica* - *Giardia intestinalis*

Abbreviation: spp, species.

[a] Symptoms generally caused by preformed toxin, not infection with the organism.

Table 3-1. Incubation Period, Duration, and Sources of Bacterial Pathogens Causing Diarrhea

Pathogen	Incubation Period	Symptoms Duration	Common Sources
Aeromonas hydrophila	1–2 d	0–2 wk	Meat, seafood, vegetables, water and soil
Bacillus cereus	Emetic: 30 min–6 h Diarrheal: 6–24 h	1–2 d	Fried rice
Campylobacter jejuni	2–5 d	2–7 d	Poultry, young dogs and cats
Clostridium difficile	2–3 d (median)	Varies	Antibiotic associated, hospitalization/health care
Clostridium perfringens	6–24 h	1 d	Meat, pork, vegetables, poultry
Escherichia coli	1–8 d	3–6 d	Ground beef, alfalfa sprouts, travel, petting zoos
Listeria monocytogenes	1 d–3 wk	2 d	Dairy, soft cheeses, raw produce, smoked fish
Plesiomonas shigelloides	1–2 d	0–2 wk	Oysters, seafood, aquarium water
Salmonella	6–72 h	2–7 d	Eggs, dairy, meat, reptiles
Shigella	1–7 d	2–7 d	Swimming pools
Staphylococcus aureus	30 min–8 h	1–2 d	Pastries, custards, salad dressing, deli meats and meat products
Vibrio cholerae	1–3 d	5–7 d	Shellfish, raw fish, water
Vibrio vulnificus and *Vibrio parahaemolyticus*	1–3 d	2–5 d	Raw oysters, sea water
Yersinia enterocolitica	0–6 d	>2 wk–months	Pork, chitterlings

- Guillain-Barré syndrome is associated with *Campylobacter* most commonly; it is also associated with Epstein-Barr virus, cytomegalovirus, *Mycoplasma pneumoniae,* and hepatitis A and B viruses.
- Seizures are commonly seen with *Shigella* infection.

Clinical Features

Common manifestations of bacterial enteritis include fever, vomiting, diarrhea, and abdominal pain. More complicated infection as well as extraintestinal manifestations can also be seen (Table 3-2).

Table 3-2. Intestinal and Extraintestinal Signs and Symptoms Associated With Common Enteric Pathogens

Pathogen	Stool	Vomiting	Abdominal Pain	Extraintestinal Manifestations	Complications
Campylobacter jejuni	Mucus, gross rectal bleeding	−	+	Guillain-Barré syndrome, reactive arthritis, erythema nodosum, mesenteric lymphadenitis, glomerulonephritis, hemolytic anemia, Reiter syndrome (the triad of arthritis, urethritis, and conjunctivitis)	Bacteremia, meningitis, cholecystitis, pancreatitis
Escherichia coli	Watery, then visible or occult blood	±	+	HUS (E coli O157:H7)	Hemorrhagic colitis
Salmonella	Watery or blood + mucus	+	+	Erythema nodosum, reactive arthritis, Reiter syndrome	Enteric fever, bacteremia, meningitis, osteomyelitis, myocarditis
Shigella	Watery ± painful bloody stool	−	+	High fever, seizure, HUS (Shigella dysenteriae 1), reactive arthritis (HLA-B27 associated), glomerulonephritis, Reiter syndrome	Perforation
Yersinia enterocolitica	Watery or blood + mucus	+	+	Erythema nodosum, glomerulonephritis, hemolytic anemia, reactive arthritis, Reiter syndrome	Perforation, intussusception, peritonitis, toxic megacolon, cholangitis, bacteremia

Abbreviation: HUS, hemolytic uremic syndrome.

Evaluation

Although not all children presenting with diarrhea require a stool culture, stool culture should be obtained when bacterial enteritis is suspected. Shiga toxin–producing *E coli* is always part of the differential diagnosis of bacterial enteritis.

In addition to culture for *Salmonella, Shigella, Yersinia,* and *Campylobacter,* specific testing should include culture for *E coli* O157:H7 plus an assay for Shiga toxin. Molecular methods such as multiplex polymerase chain reaction are coming into use; clinical interpretation of these very sensitive tests is not always straightforward.

Specific historical features suggesting bacterial enteritis include diarrhea plus

- Presence of bloody stools.
- Recent exposure to a known or suspected case of bacterial enteritis.
- Exposure during an outbreak/known day care exposure.
- Fevers, especially persistent or high fevers.
- Patient appears systemically ill.
- The infecting pathogen should generally be identified prior to initiation of antibiotics to reduce the risk of antimicrobial resistance, prevent unnecessary treatment, and avoid possible adverse effects of antibiotics. Antibiotic susceptibility testing should be performed on recovered organisms.

Management

Dehydration is the most common clinical concern in diarrheal illness. An assessment of hydration status is based on history and physical examination findings. Laboratory evaluation is frequently unnecessary, especially in mild or moderate dehydration.

Use of oral rehydration therapy as treatment for mild to moderate dehydration has been well demonstrated and is recommended as primary therapy (Evidence Level I). Parenteral fluids are usually required for severe dehydration.

Nutrition should also be a focus of management of bacterial enteritis. Malnutrition becomes a particular concern in chronic diarrhea and if there is underlying suboptimal nutrition. Management goals should include returning the child to an age-appropriate diet as soon as possible.

Clinicians and laboratories play an important role in outbreak detection and infection control. Procedures and requirements for reporting infections differ by location and are available through local and state health departments. Safe food handling practices and good hand hygiene are important in controlling spread of infection. Educational information about food safety practices is available through the Centers for Disease Control and Prevention.

Many cases of enteritis in immunocompetent children, including some cases of bacterial enteritis, are self-limited and do not require antimicrobial therapy. Table 3-3 details instances in which antibiotics should be considered in bacterial enteritis.

Table 3-3. Recommendations for Management of Bacterial Enteritis by Pathogen

Pathogen	Antibiotic Options, With Decision Based on Susceptibility Results
Aeromonas hydrophila	TMP/SMX, fluoroquinolone
Bacillus cereus	*Noninvasive disease:* supportive care *Invasive disease:* vancomycin or clindamycin
Campylobacter jejuni	Azithromycin shortens duration if early in course; fluoroquinolone.[a]
Clostridium difficile	Discontinue antibiotics; if ineffective oral metronidazole; oral vancomycin for severe, refractory, or multiple recurrent disease.
Clostridium perfringens	Supportive care
Escherichia coli	*STEC:* Most experts advise against antibiotic use; avoid antimotility drugs. *ETEC:* azithromycin or fluoroquinolone
Listeria monocytogenes	Supportive care
Plesiomonas shigelloides	TMP/SMX or fluoroquinolone
Salmonella	*Noninvasive disease:* supportive care *Invasive/high-risk[b]:* TMP/SMX, amoxicillin, fluoroquinolone,[a] or 3rd-generation cephalosporin
Shigella	*Severe/high-risk cases[c]:* TMP/SMX, fluoroquinolone,[a] ceftriaxone, azithromycin, or 3rd-generation cephalosporin
Staphylococcus aureus	Supportive
Vibrio cholerae	*Moderate to severe cases:* doxycycline, azithromycin, tetracycline, or fluoroquinolone[a]
Vibrio vulnificus and *Vibrio parahaemolyticus*	*Severe cases:* doxycycline, tetracycline, or cefotaxime
Yersinia enterocolitica	*Severe cases:* TMP/SMX, or doxycycline + aminoglycoside

Abbreviations: ETEC, enterotoxigenic *Escherichia coli*; STEC, Shiga toxin–producing *Escherichia coli*; TMP/SMX, trimethoprim/sulfamethoxazole.

[a] Fluoroquinolones are not US Food and Drug Administration approved for this indication in patients <18 y, but the American Academy of Pediatrics supports their use in suspected or documented cases of multidrug-resistant *Shigella, Salmonella, Vibrio cholerae,* and *Campylobacter jejuni.*

[b] High-risk includes underlying gastrointestinal disorders, hemoglobinopathies, immunosuppression, and children <3 mo.

[c] Treatment is often indicated to prevent spread of infection.

Suggested Reading

American Academy of Pediatrics Committee on Infectious Diseases. *Clostridium difficile* infection in infants and children. *Pediatrics.* 2013;131(1):196–200

Guerrant RL, Van Gilder T, Steiner TS, et al. Practice guidelines for the management of infectious diarrhea. *Clin Infect Dis.* 2001;32(3):331–351

King CK, Glass R, Bresee JS, Duggan C. Managing acute gastroenteritis among children: oral rehydration, maintenance, and nutritional therapy. *MMWR Recomm Rep.* 2003;52(RR-16):1–16

CHAPTER 4

Meningitis

Ross E. Newman, DO, MPHE, and Keith J. Mann, MD, MEd

Key Points

- Meningitis should be considered in all children with fever and sepsis-like syndrome; seizures or altered mental status, though nonspecific signs and symptoms, may be the only clinical markers in neonates.

- Cerebrospinal fluid (CSF) evaluation (ie, red and white blood cell counts, glucose and protein concentrations, Gram stain, and culture) should be used to confirm the diagnosis of meningitis. Blood culture is positive in most cases, but not all.

- Traumatically obtained CSF cannot be used to exclude the diagnosis of meningitis.

- Enteroviral meningitis is most common and can be diagnosed on the basis of CSF counts and polymerase chain reaction confirmation and has an excellent prognosis in those beyond 7 days of age.

- Prompt initiation of vancomycin and ceftriaxone or cefotaxime (ampicillin and cefotaxime for neonates) should be considered for all patients with suspected bacterial meningitis.

- The use of adjunct therapy (eg, corticosteroids) and anticipation of and careful monitoring for common complications (eg, seizures, syndrome of inappropriate antidiuretic hormone) should occur.

- All children with bacterial meningitis should have hearing screening at the end of the course of therapy and careful neurodevelopmental follow-up.

Overview

Meningitis is an inflammatory process involving tissues surrounding the brain and spinal cord. It is caused by a variety of infectious and noninfectious processes. Bacterial causes of meningitis are associated with significant morbidity and mortality, and this diagnosis is considered a medical emergency requiring immediate diagnostic and therapeutic interventions.

Causes and Differential Diagnosis

The most common pathogens vary by age of the patient, time of the year, and exposure to infected individuals. However, the etiology can be quite broad depending on underlying comorbid disease, travel, or exposure to developing countries or endemic areas. Patients with mechanical risk factors, such as traumatic dural tears, cochlear implants, or ventricular shunts, are at increased risk for meningitis. Those with immunodeficient states, such as HIV, asplenia, chronic renal disease, and sickle cell disease, may develop central nervous system (CNS) infection caused by unusual pathogens. While most cases of meningitis are the result of hematogenous seeding of the choroid plexus, for patients with a history of a recent infection including otitis media, sinusitis, and mastoiditis and in those with dural leak, direct spread to the meninges may occur.

Bacterial pathogens associated with meningitis are age specific and include group B *Streptococcus, Listeria monocytogenes,* and gram-negative pathogens (eg, *Escherichia coli, Citrobacter koseri, Chromobacter sakazakii, Serratia marcescens,* and *Salmonella* species) in the neonate and *Streptococcus pneumoniae* and *Neisseria meningitidis* in older infants and children. *Haemophilus influenzae* type b meningitis needs to be considered in unvaccinated patients or patients acquiring disease from the developing world, but is now rarely seen because of success of the universal vaccine program. Non-type b encapsulated strains may also cause meningitis and are more commonly encountered today than type b strains. Group A *Streptococcus* is a less commonly encountered cause of bacterial meningitis. A lymphocytic choriomeningitis is associated with early disseminated Lyme disease caused by *Borrelia burgdorferi;* a more subacute presentation is typical compared to enteroviral meningitis, and the diagnosis should be considered for those who reside in distinct geographic endemic regions (ie, New England, mid-Atlantic states, Wisconsin and Minnesota, and northern California). Nonpathogenic bacteria like *Staphylococcus epidermidis* that represent normal skin flora may cause meningitis in the setting of a neurocutaneous fistula.

Viral pathogens are the most common cause of meningitis in all age groups. Enterovirus is the predominant virus identified in cases in which an infectious pathogen is confirmed. Predictable summer–early fall outbreaks of such infections are usually caused by members of the Picornaviridae family and echoviruses.

Other viruses associated with CNS presentations include parechovirus; all members of the Herpesviridae family; arboviruses, including West Nile virus; influenza virus; and other less common viruses, including rabies virus and lymphocytic choriomeningitis virus. Rabies and the arboviruses more commonly produce meningoencephalitis. Herpes of the CNS is a risk in the neonate whose mother has primary genital herpes simplex virus (HSV) disease during pregnancy/delivery, but generally these neonates have an encephalitic CNS presentation. In the older patient, especially with HSV-2, a monophasic meningitis may occur and recurrent aseptic meningitis (termed *Mollaret meningitis*), as well as myelitis or radiculitis, may be seen.

Tuberculosis can cause subacute meningitis and should be considered in patients born in or who have traveled to high-risk countries or who have a family member with tuberculosis. Unusual causes of meningitis include *Baylisascaris procyonis* (raccoon roundworm) and fungal pathogens, including endemic mycoses and *Aspergillus* species.

Aseptic meningitis is the term used for situations in which patients have signs and symptoms of meningitis and compatible cerebrospinal fluid (CSF) findings but no etiology is uncovered by testing. Autoimmune diseases (eg, lupus), drug reactions (eg, trimethoprim/sulfamethoxazole), and malignancies (eg, leukemia, lymphoma) can cause aseptic meningitis. Tick-borne rickettsial infections (Rocky Mountain spotted fever and ehrlichiosis) can be associated with encephalopathy and pleocytosis, and testing may not acutely confirm this diagnosis.

Many diseases mimic meningitis, and these should be considered when formulating a differential diagnosis. Patients with fever and nuchal rigidity may have a retropharyngeal abscess, whereas the patient with febrile seizure may have *Human herpesvirus 6* infection.

Other considerations in the differential in a patient with classic symptoms for meningitis and pleocytosis should include an intracranial or epidural abscess, encephalitis, CNS trauma resulting in subarachnoid hemorrhage, and brain tumors. Neuroimaging and microbiologic examination of the CSF are often helpful in distinguishing these other entities.

Clinical Features

Classic signs and symptoms of meningitis include headache, fever, photophobia, and nuchal rigidity; however, it is extremely important to note that clinical features vary depending on age and infecting organism. Younger pediatric patients may not demonstrate classic symptoms, like nuchal rigidity (Table 4-1).

Especially in young infants, clinical manifestations of bacterial meningitis are variable and nonspecific, and clinicians should know that no single sign is pathognomonic. While fever may be a presenting sign, many patients in this age group have no fever or may present with hypothermia. When obtaining the history of present illness, parental reporting of lethargy, irritability, tremor or twitching, poor feeding, apnea, or vomiting should raise clinical concern for meningitis. Other findings in the age group that may indicate meningeal inflammation include paradoxic irritability with the infant appearing more irritable when held and most comfortable when left flat, extended, and motionless. A bulging fontanel may be noted. Additionally, any neonate presenting with a sepsis-like picture needs to be evaluated for meningitis.

The older the patients, the more likely they are to present with classic symptoms of meningitis, including headache, fever, photophobia, and nuchal rigidity. As with the neonatal population, presentation with a sepsis-like picture,

Table 4-1. Historical Features of the Child Who Has Central Nervous System Infection

Important Historical Information	Key Questions
Past medical history	• Recent illness • Chronic illness • Head/facial trauma
Past surgical history	• Asplenia • CNS shunts • Cochlear implants
Birth/perinatal history	• Maternal sexually transmitted infection • Chorioamnionitis • Prolonged rupture of membranes • Perinatal infection
Immunizations	Full review of vaccines, including dates of pneumococcal and meningococcal vaccines
Medications in past 6 mo	• Nonsteroidal anti-inflammatory drugs • Immunosuppressive agents • Recent IVIG • Antibiotics
Exposures	• Ill contacts • Child care • Vectors, including bites/contacts (ticks, mosquitos, cats, or bats) • Tuberculosis exposure (institutionalized contacts, contacts in jail, or homeless) • Travel (out of country or wooded area/camping)

Abbreviations: CNS, central nervous system; IVIG, intravenous immune globulin.

including multiorgan involvement, necessitates consideration of pathogens that also infect the meninges.

Physical examination findings should look for classic signs of meningeal irritation that can be elicited with testing for Kernig and Brudzinski signs. Kerning sign is positive when a patient lying supine whose thigh is flexed at a right angle to the trunk has pain with knee extension. Brudzinski sign is positive when the patient flexes the knees or lower extremities on passive flexion of the neck. Importantly, negative Kernig or Brudzinski signs do not rule out meningitis, especially in the younger patient population. Other physical examination findings to consider include cranial nerve palsies in patients with Lyme disease–caused meningitis and skin manifestations like purpura that may be classic for meningococcal infection.

Patients with viral meningitis have clinical signs and symptoms that are similar to bacterial meningitis but are typically less severe. In some cases, the diagnosis of viral meningitis is suggested when the patient with fever, stiff neck, and lymphocytic pleocytosis feels and looks remarkably better immediately following lumbar puncture (LP).

Evaluation
· · · · · · · · · ·

Most evaluations in the patient with suspected meningitis include a complete blood cell count (CBC), serum electrolyte concentrations, and cultures from blood and CSF and other potential sites as clinically suggested. It is important to note that the serum white blood cell (WBC) count is generally normal in the setting of meningitis, and a normal value should not be used to exclude the diagnosis. Lumbar puncture for CSF evaluation and culture is the mainstay of diagnosis and should be obtained from all patients with concern for meningitis. Contraindications for LP include signs concerning increased intracranial pressure, such as focal neurologic deficits, and a computed tomographic (CT) scan of the head should be performed first to evaluate for underlying lesions, including mass, hemorrhage, or midline shift, noting that a normal CT head scan finding does not necessarily exclude increased intracranial pressure. Other contraindications include uncorrected coagulopathy, skin infection over LP site, and an unstable patient with cardiopulmonary compromise. For this patient population, treatment with broad-spectrum antibiotics should not be delayed while waiting on CSF testing.

Cerebrospinal fluid evaluation. Cerebrospinal fluid evaluation should include measurement of pressure, red and white blood cell counts with differential, glucose concentration, and protein measurements, as well as Gram stain and culture. Other testing including viral identification by polymerase chain reaction (PCR) or serology can be considered in the appropriate clinical scenario.

Interpretation of CSF in neonate. To properly interpret CSF results, the age of the patient is extremely important because normal values vary by age. In a 2010 study of over 1,000 neonates and infants including nearly 400 who did not have a confirmed CSF infection or other risk for pleocytosis, those 28 days or younger had on average a WBC count of 3/mcL (95th percentile: 19/mcL) and those 28 to 56 days had 2/mcL (95th percentile: 9/mcL) in CSF. This can be clinically interpreted that the youngest patients can have a CSF WBC count up to 19/mcL and be within reference range. This same database provides information on age-specific CSF protein concentrations, noting the 95th percentile for protein by age categories as ages 0 to 14 days, 132 mg/dL; ages 15 to 28 days, 100 mg/dL; ages 29 to 42 days, 89 mg/dL; and ages 43 to 56 days, 83 mg/dL. Cerebrospinal fluid glucose values should always be compared with the serum glucose, and the ratio of serum to CSF glucose should normally be 75%; in viral meningitis, 40% to 75%; and in bacterial and tuberculosis meningitis, less than 40%.

Interpretation of CSF in the older child. In infants and children older than 3 months, CSF WBC count greater than 6/mcL is considered abnormal and meningitis should be considered. Cerebrospinal glucose concentration less than 40 mg/dL with a ratio of serum to CSF glucose is less than 40%, and CSF protein greater than 45 mg/dL is abnormal.

Laboratory features characteristic of bacterial meningitis. Bacterial meningitis is typically characterized by pleocytosis with a polymorphic nuclear cell predominance. Increased CSF WBC count, typically greater than 1,000/mcL, is highly suggestive with a classic elevated CSF protein concentration (>100–150 mg/dL) and decreased CSF glucose concentration (often <20%). Blood cultures are often positive for the same offending organism, especially in younger patients/neonates. The criterion standard is isolation of a bacterial pathogen from the CSF via culture or by visualization on Gram stain.

Laboratory features characteristic of viral meningitis. Viral meningitis is typically characterized by a lower pleocytosis compared to bacterial, with WBC count often greater than 10 to 500/mcL with a lymphocyte predominance, although a polymorphic nuclear cell predominance can be seen early in the course of infection and higher CSF counts can be seen in young infants. Glucose and protein concentrations are typically normal, and Gram stain will remain negative. Assumed viral meningitis is supported by classic CSF findings with negative cultures and confirmed by identification of a virus with PCR (culture may also grow enterovirus but it is less sensitive). Neonatal HSV-CNS disease should be considered in neonates between 3 and 21 days of age (up to 4–6 weeks) especially if the presentation includes seizures, vesicular skin lesions, and liver dysfunction or coagulopathy. When HSV is considered, viral surface cultures of the eye, oral/nasal mucosa, and rectum are important to obtain and PCR for HSV should be obtained from the blood and CSF. It is important to note that a negative HSV PCR from CSF does not exclude neonatal skin/eye/mucous membrane disease, nor is it always positive in the setting of disseminated disease.

Interpretation of a bloody tap. Interpretation of CSF results is difficult in the setting of a traumatic LP, or bloody tap. The WBC count cannot reliably be identified as originating from the CSF, and serum concentrations of protein and glucose are different than normal CSF concentrations. Formulas attempting to correct the CSF WBC count for the exposure of serum red blood cells and WBCs (one common example includes subtracting 1 WBC for every red blood cell count of 1,000/mcL) are not recommended and should not guide clinical care. Culture and Gram stain results are the only reliable laboratory indicator in this setting. Patients with a bloody tap should be treated for meningitis until culture results are known or a repeat LP can be performed.

Interpretation of CSF when the patient has had antecedent antibiotic treatment. Sterilization of the CSF can occur quickly after administration of either oral or intravenous (IV)/intramuscular antibiotics. With certain pathogens, specifically *N meningitidis*, this can occur as quickly as 1 hour after the first dose. For patients treated with antibiotics prior to obtaining CSF, all standard studies, including culture, should be obtained. Negative culture results are no longer clinically reliable; however, all other CSF evaluation, including red and white blood cell counts and protein and glucose concentrations, can be interpreted normally. For patients with classic laboratory finding of meningitis and a negative culture following pretreatment, discussion with an infectious diseases specialist is recommended.

Blood tests. The most important serum blood test to obtain is a standard blood culture. Additional serum blood tests to consider include CBC with differential, serum electrolytes, glucose, and in some cases inflammatory markers. The CBC will not be diagnostic for meningitis, but abnormalities may focus the differential diagnosis with findings such as leukopenia and thrombocytopenia seen in meningococcal meningitis (or in those with rickettsial infection). Electrolytes will aid in evaluation of meningitic complications, such as syndrome of inappropriate antidiuretic hormone (SIADH), which is commonly present in bacterial meningitis but less often in meningitis caused by other infections. Inflammatory markers, specifically C-reactive protein, are not a diagnostic indicator for meningitis but may be clinically useful to trend response to therapy.

Neuroimaging. Neuroimaging is not indicated for all patients with meningitis and can be suggestive but is not diagnostic for meningitis. Patients presenting with findings concerning for increased intracranial pressure should have neuroimaging, usually with a contrasted CT of the head, prior to obtaining CSF to evaluate for abnormalities that may result in herniation if an LP is performed. Other considerations for neuroimaging, either CT or magnetic resonance imaging, are to evaluate for complications, specifically looking for abscess development or increased ventricular size. For patients with persistent fever, seizures (especially occurring >72 hours into therapy), focal neurologic deficits, continued positive CSF culture results, or continued elevation of CSF WBC count despite treatment or patients with recurrent meningitis, neuroimaging is recommended. In the neonatal population, some practices recommend magnetic resonance imaging near the end of the treatment course to evaluate for complications for the infection.

Follow-up CSF evaluation. A repeat CSF evaluation should be performed after 48 to 72 hours of treatment for all infants with gram-negative meningitis and for those with multidrug-resistant pneumococcal meningitis. It should be considered for those who have been treated with corticosteroids, in any neonate with confirmed bacterial meningitis, and in any patient who does not clinically respond to therapy within 72 hours. A repeat CSF evaluation should also be performed within 2 to 4 days in those in whom a bloody tap precludes initial evaluation of CSF and in infants with confirmed HSV-CNS disease at the end of course of therapy (ie, 21 days).

Management

Important elements of management to consider are immediate treatment of cardiorespiratory compromise if present; prompt initiation of appropriate antimicrobial therapy with attention to the correct dosing; and attention to and potential prevention of anticipated complications (ie, SIADH, seizures). Admission to a pediatric intensive care unit should be considered for patients with cardiorespiratory compromise (ie, respiratory distress or shock), a Glasgow Coma Scale score of less than 8, or signs and symptoms of increased intracranial pressure or focal neurologic deficits. Some experts recommend that any baby younger than 1 year with bacterial meningitis be cared for initially in a pediatric intensive care unit, even if apparently clinically stable on admission.

Any patient with clinical symptoms or laboratory evaluation concerning for meningitis, either bacterial or viral, should be treated with IV antibiotic therapy until definitive testing determines the underlying etiology. Treatment is initiated with empiric antibiotics that have adequate CSF penetration for presumed bacterial processes. Initial antibiotic choices vary, based on age of patient, to cover the most likely bacterial organisms. Therapy can eventually be narrowed on the basis of results of cultures and clinical response to treatment (Figure 4-1).

Antibiotic therapy should not be delayed when CNS infection is suspected because prompt recognition of meningitis and administration of antibiotics results in decreased morbidity and mortality. If an LP cannot be performed or is contraindicated, a blood culture should be obtained and antibiotics started immediately, with the consideration of CSF evaluation when clinically safe.

A variety of antibiotic therapies are proposed and vary by reference considered and clinician preference. However, all therapy options are based on the most common infectious pathogens in the patient's age range.

Drug of choice in neonate. A combination of ampicillin (300 mg/kg/day divided every 6 hours) and cefotaxime (200–300 mg/kg/day divided every 6 hours) is adequate empiric therapy for suspected meningitis. Alternative use of ampicillin and gentamicin is commonly used, but gentamicin does not penetrate the meninges and should not be used if gram-negative infection is considered. With increasing resistance patterns of S pneumoniae, vancomycin (60 mg/kg/day divided every 6 hours) is recommended to be added for patients with clinical suspicion of this pathogen based on evaluation of the Gram stained smear of CSF. In general, for any patient with concerning CSF analysis or clinical picture, empiric addition of vancomycin pending culture results and sensitivities is prudent.

Herpes simplex virus–CNS disease should be considered in the infant in the first month of life if suggested by clinical appearance and CSF findings. Acyclovir (60 mg/kg/day every 8 hours) is recommended in addition to antibiotics until clarity in etiology is established. Some clinicians advocate for the use of acyclovir in all patients younger than 30 days presenting with fever and treated with antibiotics for sepsis-like illness, while others suggest its use in patients with concerning risk factors (ie, pleocytosis, seizures, vesicular rash).

Drug of choice in older children. Empiric coverage with a third-generation cephalosporin (ceftriaxone 100 mg/kg/day given once daily or divided twice daily or cefotaxime 200–300 mg/kg/day divided every 6 hours) plus vancomycin (60 mg/kg/day divided every 6 hours) is recommended for suspected meningitis. A vancomycin level of 15 mcg/mL should be targeted for those with pneumococcal meningitis for which cephalosporin resistance is confirmed. Clindamycin has poor penetration into the CSF and is not appropriate therapy for bacterial meningitis.

The choice of antibiotics for patients with a history of anaphylaxis to penicillins or cephalosporins should be discussed with an infectious diseases

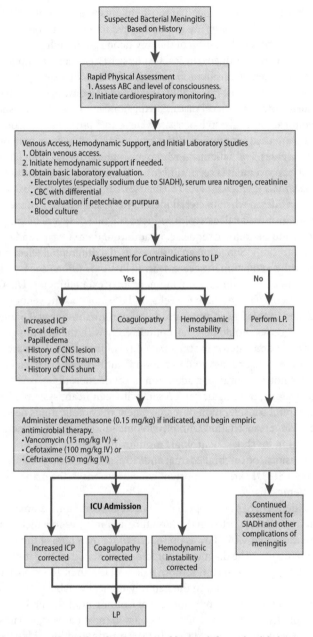

Figure 4-1. Algorithm for suspected bacterial meningitis in infants older than 1 month.

Meningitis suspected clinically or by cerebrospinal fluid findings.

Abbreviations: ABC, airway, breathing, and circulation; CBC, complete blood cell count; CNS, central nervous system; DIC, disseminated intravascular coagulation; ICP, intracranial pressure; ICU, intensive care unit; IV, intravenously; LP, lumbar puncture; SIADH, syndrome of inappropriate diuretic hormone.

specialist. It is important to note that most patients with a history of non-anaphylactic penicillin allergy are not confirmed to be allergic on testing.

Duration of therapy. Duration of therapy depends on multiple factors, including organism identified, clinical response to treatment, complications, and age of the patient. Consultation with an infectious diseases specialist is likely to be helpful in most cases. Shorter courses of 7 days are considered appropriate for meningococcal disease, while longer 14-day courses should be considered for *Listeria,* group B *Streptococcus*, and *S pneumoniae.* Courses of at least 21 days are used for gram-negative organisms and in cases of neonatal HSV-CNS diseases. For patients in whom an enterovirus has been identified and clinical improvement is seen, antibiotics therapy can be discontinued.

Corticosteroids (Evidence Level I). The use of adjunctive corticosteroids should be considered when bacterial meningitis is suspected. In a meta-analysis across all age groups, corticosteroids reduced the rate of severe hearing loss, any hearing loss, and neurologic sequelae. In addition, there was a trend towards a decrease in mortality. Subgroup analysis revealed a differential effect based on organism, with a reduction in severe hearing loss in *H influenzae* type b meningitis and a reduced mortality in pneumococcal meningitis. Data are limited in patients younger than 6 weeks, and dexamethasone is not routinely recommended in this age group. A dosage of dexamethasone at 0.6 mg/kg/day divided into 4 doses should be given concurrently with the first dose of antibiotics and administered for the first 4 days of treatment. Data are not available to support corticosteroid initiation if antibiotics have been given for longer than 4 hours prior to consideration of corticosteroids.

Supportive care. Meningitis can present with significant systemic complications, and careful consideration of management of complications needs to be prioritized. Fluid resuscitation with physiologic saline solution or lactated Ringer injection for shock; neurologic monitoring for development of seizures, subdural effusions, or cerebral edema; and clinical monitoring of fluid balance for those with SIADH are all important considerations in the management of pediatric meningitis.

The incidence of SIADH in pediatric bacterial meningitis is unknown with widely varying rates reported in the literature, but in cases in which vasopressin levels were measured, SIADH was present in more than 80% of those with bacterial meningitis. The diagnosis should be considered in all patients with bacterial meningitis *plus* serum sodium values of less than 135 mg/dL or in the patient with low urine output. In the hemodynamically stable patient, moderate fluid restriction (80% of normal) and use of isotonic fluid should be considered. Resolution of SIADH occurs in 48 to 72 hours in most patients, so laboratory monitoring should be continued serially over this time and fluid restriction can be discontinued as the patient clinically improves and serum sodium values normalize.

Seizures occur in 20% to 30% of children with bacterial meningitis. Generalized seizures typically occur on presentation or in the first 72 hours of illness and reflect irritation to the meninges. Focal seizures often occur after the third day of illness and should alert the clinician to a vascular or infectious complication of bacterial meningitis. Late-onset seizures are associated with long-term neurologic sequelae.

Long-term Monitoring and Implications

Bacterial meningitis has a death rate as high as 10% with neurologic morbidity the most common sequela among survivors. Hearing loss is a common concern and is most often seen in patients with pneumococcal or meningococcal meningitis; all patients with bacterial meningitis from any etiology should have a hearing screening performed prior to hospital discharge. Developmental delay requires long-term evaluation with developmental screening performed at all post-hospitalization visits and referral to subspecialty evaluation promptly made when appropriate. Other complications include intellectual deficits, hydrocephalus, spasticity, blindness, late-onset seizures, and cerebral palsy. Risk for sequelae is related to the severity of illness on initial presentation to a clinician; however, all cases of bacterial meningitis have potential for significant morbidity. Patients with seizures greater than 72 hours after presentation are at high risk for neurologic sequelae.

Patients beyond the first week of life with enteroviral meningitis generally do not have sequelae, and full recovery is typical. Fewer data are available to predict outcome in infants with parechoviral disease. Sequelae for infants with neonatal HSV-CNS disease may occur in as many as 70%; acyclovir in oral suppressive dosing *after* completion of the treatment course of IV acyclovir therapy has been shown to improve outcomes.

Suggested Reading

American Academy of Pediatrics. Meningococcal infections. In: Kimberlin DW, Brady MT, Jackson MA, Long SS, eds. *Red Book: 2015 Report of the Committee on Infectious Diseases.* 30th ed. Elk Grove Village, IL: American Academy of Pediatrics; 2015:547–558

Brouwer MC, McIntyre P, Prasad K, van de Beek D. Corticosteroids for acute bacterial meningitis. *Cochrane Database Syst Rev.* 2015;(9):CD004405

Chávez-Bueno S, McCracken GH Jr. Bacterial meningitis in children. *Pediatr Clin North Am.* 2005;52(3):795–810

Kestenbaum LA, Ebberson J, Zorc JJ, Hodinka RL, Shah SS. Defining cerebrospinal fluid white blood cell count reference values in neonates and young infants. *Pediatrics.* 2010;125(2):257–264

Mann K, Jackson MA. Meningitis. *Pediatr Rev.* 2008;29(12):417–429

Shah SS, Ebberson J, Kestenbaum LA, Hodinka RL, Zorc JJ. Age-specific reference values for cerebrospinal fluid protein concentration in neonates and young infants. *J Hosp Med.* 2011;6(1):22–27

Tunkel AR, Hartman BJ, Kaplan SL, et al. Practice guidelines for the management of bacterial meningitis. *Clin Infect Dis.* 2004;39(9):1267–1284

CHAPTER 5

Osteomyelitis and Septic Arthritis

Angela L. Myers, MD, MPH

Key Points

- Osteoarticular infections are most commonly encountered in the young and school-aged child but also occur in neonates and patients with underlying chronic disease processes.

- *Staphylococcus aureus* is the most common bacterial pathogen in the setting of bone and joint infection. However, age- and special circumstance–related differences should be considered in the appropriate setting.

- Empiric therapy of osteomyelitis and septic arthritis should target *S aureus*, and the addition of *Kingella kingae* coverage should be given in the child younger than 3 years. Local antibiogram data should be considered when planning antimicrobial therapy.

- Therapy is typically initiated parenterally in the hospitalized patient and transitioned to oral agents when the patient has clear evidence of clinical and laboratory improvement, assurance of medication adherence, and ideally an identified pathogen enabling targeted therapy.

- Length of therapy is 4 to 6 weeks for acute osteomyelitis and 3 to 4 weeks for septic arthritis.

Overview

Osteomyelitis and septic arthritis are caused by bacterial infections of the bone and joint, respectively. Bone and joint infections in children primarily occur from hematogenous seeding, but infections related to penetrating trauma, surgery, and implantable devices and contiguous infection may also occur. The most common organism for bone and joint infection overall is *Staphylococcus aureus*, although other organisms play a more prominent role in different age groups and clinical scenarios.

Causes and Differential Diagnosis

Osteomyelitis and septic arthritis are most commonly caused by hematogenous seeding from a primary bacteremia. Less common causes include traumatic injury with environmental wound contamination, penetrating trauma, chronic deep decubitus ulcer, and internal and external hardware. Additionally, extension of infection from the epiphysis into joint space may also occur, and is more common in children younger than 18 months of age (up to 75% in neonates) because of presence of bridging vessels from the epiphysis to physis.

   Staphylococcus aureus is the most frequent pathogen identified in the setting of osteomyelitis and septic arthritis, but other pathogens play a role in different age groups and clinical settings (Table 5-1). Dependent on local epidemiology, both methicillin-susceptible *S aureus* and methicillin-resistant *S aureus* (MRSA) are commonly seen. *Streptococcus pyogenes, Kingella kingae,* and *Streptococcus pneumoniae* are other relatively commonly encountered organisms. Although *S pneumoniae* has become a less frequent pathogen with widespread immunization, it continues to be seen occasionally in young children. Some data suggest that *K kingae* is the most frequent cause of osteomyelitis and septic arthritis in the toddler age group, between 15 months and 3 years of age. Nasal colonization is close to 30% in those who attend day care in this age group. Infection with *K kingae* is often preceded with a viral upper respiratory tract infection and is presumably the portal of entry for hematogenous spread.

   Osteomyelitis and septic arthritis in the neonate is a different disease entity than in the older child. Neonates are more likely to have polymicrobial infection or multifocal infection (20%–50%) and to develop permanent sequelae

Table 5-1. Age- and Special Circumstance–Related Common Bacterial Pathogens in Osteomyelitis and Septic Arthritis

Patient Age/Circumstance	Organism
Neonate (≤28 d)	• *Streptococcus agalactiae* (also called GBS) • *Escherichia coli* and other enteric gram-negative organisms • *Staphylococcus aureus* • Coagulase-negative staphylococci • *Candida* spp
Toddler (15 mo–3 y)	• *S aureus* • *Kingella kingae* • *Streptococcus pyogenes* • *Streptococcus pneumoniae*
Child (>3 y)	• *S aureus* • *S pyogenes*
Hardware associated	• *S aureus* • Coagulase-negative staphylococci • *Propionibacterium acnes*
Hemoglobinopathy	• *S aureus* • *Salmonella* spp • Enteric gram-negative organisms • *S pneumoniae* • *Haemophilus influenzae* type B

Abbreviations: GBS, group B *Streptococcus;* spp, species.

after treatment (up to 50%). In addition to bacteremia, the risk factors for neonatal disease include prematurity, indwelling catheters, fetal scalp electrodes, and repeated heel sticks. The causative pathogens are somewhat different than for older children as well, with *Streptococcus agalactiae* (also called group B *Streptococcus*), enteric gram-negative organisms (eg, *Escherichia coli*), and *Candida* species of clinical importance in addition to *S aureus*. *Neisseria gonorrhoeae* is also a known cause of neonatal osteomyelitis and septic arthritis.

Neisseria gonorrhoeae may also cause septic arthritis in adolescents with an associated sexually transmitted infection. It is more common in girls than boys and considered a feature of disseminated infection that usually stems from cervicitis. The knee is the joint most commonly affected, with shoulder and hip being involved uncommonly. Culture of all sites of infection should be obtained, including joint fluid. However, joint fluid cultures are less frequently positive than with other etiologies of septic arthritis. The treatment course is 7 days of a parenteral third-generation cephalosporin. Joint sequelae from this infection are rare.

Mycobacterium tuberculosis is an uncommon cause of osteomyelitis and septic arthritis, and osteoarticular disease accounts for approximately 1% of disease manifestations in patients infected with this organism. This infection differs from the other more common bacteria by its ability to remain dormant or cause low-grade symptomatology for years. Low-grade fevers and weight loss are more common features in addition to pain and swelling at the site of infection compared with other more common pathogens. Lower thoracic vertebrae are the most common bones involved in this infection (as seen in Pott disease) followed by the long bones and hands and feet. Multifocal disease is more common than with typical osteomyelitis (up to 15%).

Salmonella species and other gram-negative enteric organisms are typically uncommon pathogens, but increase in frequency in the setting of hemoglobinopathies (eg, sickle cell disease), which is thought to be related to enteric translocation of bacteria. Soil pathogens, such as *Pseudomonas aeruginosa*, *Nocardia* species, nontuberculous *Mycobacteria* species, and fungal organisms (eg, *Aspergillus* species), play a role in soil-contaminated wounds, penetrating injuries, and occasionally the immunocompromised host. Patients with chronic decubitus ulcers are also at risk for bone infection with environmental pathogens, and in the setting of sacral ulcer, gram-negative enteric and anaerobic organisms are frequent pathogens. *Actinomyces* species are a well-recognized cause of mandibular osteomyelitis (ie, lumpy bumpy jaw syndrome), related to tooth extraction, caries, oral surgery, or oral trauma.

Although not typically a pathogen in the healthy host, coagulase-negative staphylococci and *Propionobacterium acnes* may be the causative agent in the setting of spinal hardware, prosthetic joint, or external fixators. Oral anaerobes from humans (*Eikenella corrodens*), cats (*Pasturella multocida*), or dogs (*Capnocytophaga* species) may cause bone or joint infection in the setting of a penetrating bite wound. Other anaerobic organisms, such as *Fusobacterium necrophorum, Bacteroides fragilis, Peptostreptococcus,* and *Clostridium* species, are rare causes of bone and joint infection. Additionally, *Bartonella henselae* (ie, cat-scratch disease) is a rare cause of granulomatous bone infection in patients with a history of kitten or cat exposure, even without a recognized scratch event.

The differential diagnosis of acute osteomyelitis and septic arthritis is large and includes oncologic processes such as leukemia, osteosarcoma, Ewing sarcoma and other primitive neuroectodermal tumors, and neuroblastoma. Non-oncologic possibilities include Gaucher disease, polyarteritis nodosa, serum sickness, and, extremely rarely, scurvy. Central nervous system disease, birth trauma with neuropathy, and violent trauma should also be considered in the differential for neonates with pseudoparalysis.

Chronic recurrent multifocal osteomyelitis (CRMO) is a noninfectious form of bone inflammation, presenting in a similar fashion to bacterial infection. The median age of onset is slightly older at 10 years (versus 5 years for bacterial osteomyelitis), with girls being more often affected than boys. Chronic recurrent multifocal osteomyelitis may present with SAPHO (synovitis, acne, pustulosis, hyperostosis, and osteitis) syndrome, helping to distinguish from bacterial infection. It is currently estimated that approximately 25% of individuals with CRMO have an associated inflammatory disorder, the most common of which are plantar-palmar pustulosis, psoriasis, and Crohn disease. Unusual bones are more commonly affected in CRMO (eg, clavicle), and multiple bones may be affected simultaneously. Whole body magnetic resonance imaging (MRI), bone scan, and skeletal survey are useful tools to evaluate for silent lesions at noncontiguous sites.

Clinical Features

Common clinical features of bone and joint infection include fever, pain, edema, erythema, and decreased range of motion of the affected area. Point tenderness over the metaphysis is also typically noted in bone infections, while severely limited range of motion is a more common feature of septic arthritis. Referred pain is common in both osteomyelitis (eg, abdominal pain in vertebral osteomyelitis) and septic arthritis (eg, knee pain in septic hip) and can make determining the focus of infection difficult.

Other subtle differences on physical examination may provide diagnostic clues when the site of infection is not readily obvious on clinical examination. Infection in the upper extremity leads to a decrease in voluntary movement and sometimes complete refusal to use the extremity. Neonates and young infants may present with pseudoparalysis in the affected arm that resembles Erb-Duchenne paralysis, with internal rotation of the shoulder and forearm pronation (ie, waiter's tip appearance). Infection in the lower extremity often leads to a refusal to bear weight in that extremity. Nonambulatory infants may keep their leg in flexion and external rotation when held upright on examination, or may exhibit only asymmetric movements. Spinal osteomyelitis may be suspected by an inability to bend forward toward the toes. Other nonspecific presenting symptoms may include anorexia, malaise, and vomiting.

Long bones of the appendicular skeleton are the most commonly affected (75%–90%) in the setting of osteomyelitis, with multifocal disease occurring in 5% of cases outside the neonatal period. In the setting of osteomyelitis, it is imperative to carefully examine the adjacent joint for evidence of concomitant septic arthritis, because up to 30% of joints surrounding the affected bone may be affected. The knee is the most commonly affected joint in the setting of septic arthritis, followed by the hip and then ankle. Polyarticular infection is uncommon (<10%), but occurs with *Neisseria meningitidis, N gonorrhoeae,* and *Salmonella* species. Concomitant cellulitis or myositis may also be present in the setting of bone and joint infection and can make it difficult to determine whether there is an underlying osteomyelitis or septic arthritis based on clinical examination findings.

Vertebral osteomyelitis presents in a nonspecific manner, which often leads to a delay in diagnosis. Infants may present with sepsis, while older children generally have concerns of abdominal, leg, chest, or back pain. Point tenderness should be present over the infected area, and surrounding soft-tissue swelling may be seen. A loss of the normal curvature may also be seen on clinical examination. Neurologic deficits related to spinal cord compression may be present at diagnosis and occur in up to 20% of cases.

Pelvic osteomyelitis accounts for 6% to 9% of bone infections and is similar to vertebral infection in that it often presents with symptoms that are non-localizing, which may lead to delayed diagnosis. The ilium and ischium are the 2 most common bones involved, and pain in the hip, leg, and buttock are often seen. Septic hip is oftentimes considered in this setting; however, in converse to septic arthritis, movement of the hip joint is less restricted, pain is elicited with pelvic girdle rocking, and point tenderness over the affected bone is commonly seen in pelvic osteomyelitis.

Evaluation

Bacteremia is present in approximately 50% of cases of osteomyelitis and slightly less prominent in septic arthritis (40%). Bacteria may also be identified from bone aspirate, or synovial fluid, in 60% of infections. *K kingae* is a fastidious organism whose growth is enhanced by inoculation of aspiration specimens into a blood culture bottle. Polymerase chain reaction testing is also available for *K kingae,* with a high degree of sensitivity. All culture specimens should be kept for at least a week to optimize growth.

Cell counts within the joint fluid should be analyzed in addition to obtaining specimens for culture. A cloudy appearance of the fluid is typically seen on gross examination. A white blood cell (WBC) count of greater than 50,000/mcL with a neutrophil predominance in the synovial fluid is indicative of bacterial infection even in the absence of a positive culture. Conversely, a synovial fluid that grows a pathogenic bacterium is considered diagnostic confirmation of septic arthritis, even in the setting of a low synovial WBC count.

Inflammatory markers, such as C-reactive protein level and erythrocyte sedimentation rate, are elevated in greater than 90% of infections. Although these markers are not specific for bone or joint infection, they are useful monitoring tools, and when negative provide good evidence that osteoarticular infection is not present (Evidence Level III). C-reactive protein level should peak on the second day and typically normalizes after 1 week of appropriate therapy. Erythrocyte sedimentation rate tends to peak a little later (3–5 days) and lowers more slowly with normalization at 3–5 weeks. Failure of one or both of these markers to lower with pathogen-targeted therapy should raise the clinician's suspicion of infectious complication, such as subperiosteal abscess, infarction, or other sequestered focus. The WBC count may be elevated or normal, and the platelet count may become elevated after the first week of symptomatology.

Magnetic resonance imaging is the diagnostic modality of choice early in the course of disease, with a sensitivity nearing 100% (Evidence Level II). Marrow changes related to infection appear low in signal intensity on T1 images and high on T2. Gadolinium enhancement helps delineate abscesses and soft-tissue involvement, which is especially useful in certain clinical situations when it is difficult to distinguish between type of infection on physical examination, or the presence of more than one type is suspected. The extent of cartilage destruction in the joint, as well as periarticular abscesses, is also well-defined by MRI. Finally, MRI may have utility in differentiating between acute infection and a more chronic process.

Technetium phosphate radionuclide scans (ie, bone scans) and computed tomography scans have largely been replaced by MRI for evaluation of osteoarticular infection. Bone scan has the ability to show abnormalities in both the affected bone and joint prior to appearance on plain radiograph. Increased uptake in the metaphysis is indicative of osteomyelitis, while increased uptake on both sides of a joint indicates articular infection. Diaphyseal enhancement is more consistent with tumor, trauma, or bone infarction. The sensitivity is between 80% and 100% and most useful in the setting of suspected multifocal infection.

Plain radiograph may show abnormalities such as periosteal elevation, a lytic lesion, and new bone formation in as few as 10 days into the course of infection. In the setting of articular infection, plain radiograph may reveal a widening of the joint space and displacement of fat planes surrounding the joint. Sclerosis of the bone may be seen when infection has been present for longer than 1 month. Plain radiography is a less expensive diagnostic method but carries the drawback of being less sensitive than MRI, and bone demineralization of 50% must be present for a lytic lesion to be apparent. In patients who have undergone multiple previous radiographies or other radiation exposures, reducing further exposure should also be a consideration.

Management

Treatment of osteomyelitis and septic arthritis should include surgical washout or debridement in the setting of osteomyelitis associated with soft-tissue abscess, subperiosteal abscess, necrotic bone, presence of foreign body, or contaminated wound and in the setting of septic joint (Evidence Level II). Surgical debridement is imperative in the setting of septic hip, but arthrocentesis may be sufficient for infection in other joints. Surgical management not only aids in delineating an organism and thus optimal antimicrobial therapy but also allows for improved antimicrobial penetration into the bone or joint, and serves to hasten clinical recovery.

Antimicrobial therapy should be empirically initiated to provide coverage for the typical pathogens according to age and mechanism of infection. In addition, local susceptibility patterns should be taken into consideration when choosing therapy. In the hospitalized patient, parenteral therapy is typically initiated, including anti-staphylococcal penicillins (eg, oxacillin), first-generation cephalosporins (eg, cefazolin), or clindamycin. Common dosing regimens are detailed in Table 5-2. All of these agents possess good bone penetration and provide good *S aureus* coverage. Clindamycin has the added advantage of providing coverage for MRSA. However, it should not be used in the setting of known inducible resistance. Further, in some communities the resistance rate to clindamycin is rising for both methicillin-susceptible *S aureus*

Table 5-2. Common Parenteral and Enteral Antimicrobial Dosing for Osteomyelitis and Septic Arthritis

Parenteral Medication	Dosing	Monitoring Parameters
β-Lactam Antibiotics		
Oxacillin	• 200 mg/kg/d divided every 4–6 h (maximum: 12 g/d) (children and neonates >2.0 kg) • 100 mg/kg/d every 12 h (<7 d and <2.0 kg) • 150 mg/kg/d every 8 h (>2.0 kg and <1 wk or <2.0 kg and >1 wk)	• CBC and hepatic and renal function periodically for prolonged therapy
Ampicillin/ sulbactam	• 200 mg/kg/d divided every 4–6 h (>1 y) (maximum: 12 g/d) • 150 mg/kg/d divided every 6 h (children >1 mo)	
Cefazolin	• 100 mg/kg/every 8 h (maximum: 6 g/d) • 25 mg/kg every 12 h (≤7 d or ≤2.0 kg) • 25 mg/kg every 8 h (8–28 d of age and >2.0 kg)	

Continued

Table 5-2 *(cont)*

Parenteral Medication	Dosing	Monitoring Parameters
Lincosamide		
Clindamycin	• 40 mg/kg/d divided every 6 h (maximum: 4.8 g/d)	• CBC and renal function periodically for prolonged therapy
Miscellaneous		
Vancomycin	• 15 mg/kg/dose every 6 h (Adjust on the basis of trough level.)	• Vancomycin troughs in patients receiving therapy >48 h or in the setting of renal dysfunction • Serum creatinine and urine output
Linezolid	• 10 mg/kg/dose every 8 h (children <5 y) • 10 mg/kg/dose every 12 h (neonates <34 wk in the first week of life and children 5–11 y; maximum dose: 600 mg/dose) • 600 mg every 12 h (≥12 y)	• CBC in patients requiring linezolid therapy >2 wk • Lactic acid weekly and for clinical signs of acidosis • Vision testing in patients receiving therapy >3 mo or with visual changes
Daptomycin	• 6–10 mg/kg/dose once daily (Limited information exists.)	• Baseline and weekly creatine kinase during daptomycin therapy • Renal function monitoring
RIF	• 5–10 mg/kg/dose every 12 h (maximum: 600 mg/d)	• CBC and liver function periodically for prolonged therapy
Enteral Medication	**Dosing**	**Monitoring Parameters**
β-Lactam Antibiotics		
Amoxicillin/ clavulanate	• 90–100 mg/kg/d divided every 8 h	
Cephalexin	• 100 mg/kg/d divided every 6 h	• CBC and renal function periodically for prolonged therapy
Lincosamide		
Clindamycin	• 10 mg/kg/dose every 8 h (maximum: 1.8 g/d)	• CBC and renal function periodically for prolonged therapy
Miscellaneous		
Linezolid	• 10 mg/kg/dose every 8 h (children <5 y) • 10 mg/kg/dose every 12 h (neonates <34 wk in the first week of life and children 5–11 y; maximum dose: 600 mg/dose) • 600 mg every 12 h (12 y)	• CBC in patients requiring linezolid therapy >2 wk • Lactic acid weekly and for clinical signs of acidosis • Vision testing in patients receiving therapy >3 mo or with visual changes
RIF	• 5–10 mg/kg/dose every 12 h (maximum: 600 mg/d)	• CBC and liver function periodically for prolonged therapy

Abbreviations: CBC, complete blood cell count; RIF, rifampin.

and MRSA, decreasing the utility of this therapy. Currently, it is recommended that vancomycin be considered as initial therapy in communities with clindamycin resistance rates greater than 10% to 15% (Evidence Level II). Additionally, vancomycin should be used as empiric therapy in patients who present with toxic shock syndrome or sepsis (Evidence Level III). It is recommended that vancomycin dosing should be adjusted to achieve a target trough level between 15 and 20 mcg/mL in this setting (Evidence Level III).

Clinical response to vancomycin should be monitored and continued if adequate response is seen when the minimum inhibitory concentration is 2 mcg/mL or less (susceptible according to Clinical Laboratory Standards Institute break point) (Evidence Level III). An alternative therapy should be used in the setting of minimum inhibitory concentration greater than 2 mcg/mL (Evidence Level III). Alternatives to vancomycin and clindamycin may include daptomycin or linezolid in the setting of MRSA infection (Evidence Level III). Daptomycin may have further benefit when added to standard therapy for invasive MRSA infection in the presence of osteomyelitis. The addition of rifampin (RIF) may also be considered in patients with refractory or concomitant endovascular disease or in the setting of hardware infection (Evidence Level III).

Fluoroquinolones are not recommended routinely for children with bone and joint infections but are sometimes necessary in the setting of infection related to soil-contaminated wound or sacral decubitus ulcer. Gentamicin or a third-generation cephalosporin (eg, cefotaxime) should be a part of the empiric therapy regimen in neonates. Additionally, a third-generation cephalosporin should be used in the setting of *N meningitidis* or *N gonorrhoeae* articular infection.

Disease caused by *M tuberculosis* is treated with surgical debridement when an abscess is present or stabilization surgery in the setting of spinal instability. Isolation of the patient's organism or the organism from the epidemiologic source is critical in determining the optimal therapeutic regimen. Therapy includes 4 antibiotics for the first 2 months of therapy, followed by a prolonged (7–10 months) 2-drug regimen with isoniazid and RIF in patients whose isolates are susceptible.

Therapy length is not often determined at diagnosis but is determined over time involving multiple factors, including response to therapy, surgical intervention, extent of disease, specific pathogen, and chronicity of infection. The Infectious Diseases Society of America guidelines for adult osteomyelitis recommend 8 weeks of antimicrobial therapy in the setting of MRSA infection (Evidence Level II). Three to 4 weeks of therapy is recommended for septic arthritis caused by MRSA (Evidence Level II). The guideline further recommends 4 to 6 weeks of therapy for osteomyelitis and 3 to 4 weeks for septic arthritis in children, which may be longer if contiguous osteomyelitis is present (occurs in 75% of neonates and 30% in older children). Transition to oral therapy is acceptable once definite clinical improvement is shown and the clinician has a sufficient level of confidence for medication adherence (Evidence Level II). In specific patients with subacute or chronic infection, some experts will prescribe the entire therapeutic course using an oral agent (Evidence Level III).

Long-term Monitoring and Implications

Most children with acute hematogenous osteomyelitis or septic arthritis have no long-term clinical sequelae from infection. However, 10% to 25% of children with articular infection will develop long-term sequelae, including decreased joint mobility, chronic dislocation, and avascular necrosis of the femoral head. Presence of concomitant osteomyelitis increases the risk to 50%. Risk factors for development of sequelae because of septic arthritis are listed in Box 5-1.

Box 5-1. Risk Factors for Permanent Sequelae Following Septic Arthritis

- Infant <6 mo
- Adjacent bone infection
- Hip or shoulder infection
- ≥4 d delay in joint decompression and antibiotic therapy
- Prolonged time to synovial fluid sterilization
- Infection with *Staphylococcus aureus* or a gram-negative bacillus

Adverse effects related to prolonged antimicrobial therapy may also occur, and patients should be monitored clinically and with laboratory testing specific to the antibiotic in use. Laboratory monitoring may provide early clues of a developing adverse effect and is important for defining the duration of therapy (see Table 5-2).

A subset of patients with *S aureus* disease from a Panton-Valentine leukocidin-producing strain are more likely to develop more severe disease and phlebothrombosis as a complication. Involvement of a hematologist is important in this setting to initiate and manage anticoagulation therapy and provide guidance regarding testing for an underlying hypercoagulable state. In addition, Panton-Valentine leukocidin-producing strains may increase the risk of developing chronic infection.

Acute osteomyelitis develops into chronic infection in less than 5% of cases, and this is more often associated with non-hematogenous osteomyelitis (eg, hardware-associated infection). The patient may have a prolonged asymptomatic period followed by recrudescence of pain, edema, and sinus tract formation that does not improve, or only partially improves with prolonged antimicrobial therapy. Polymicrobial infection is often present in such cases, making surgical debridement for culture and to remove necrotic bone and tissue the key to management. Skin grafts and muscle flaps are used to enhance blood flow in some traumatic wounds and in wounds with impaired sensation (eg, decubitus ulcers). Antibiotic-impregnated beads or cement material is sometimes placed at the time of debridement to enhance antibiotic delivery to the area and promote stability of the bone. Additionally, intraarticular antibiotics have been used in the setting of infected joint prosthesis.

Treatment of an infected joint prosthesis somewhat depends on timing of onset related to surgery, length of symptoms prior to diagnosis, and the surgical approach to address the infected hardware. Rifampin in addition to initial parenteral therapy followed by a transition to long-term enteral therapy is recommended (Evidence Level II). Similarly, for spinal implant infections that occur early after implantation, parenteral therapy plus RIF followed by long-term enteral therapy is recommended. However, in the setting of late spinal hardware infection (>30 days after implant placement), it is ideal to remove the hardware if the spine has fused (Evidence Level II).

Suggested Reading

Ardura MI, Mejías A, Katz KS, Revell P, McCracken GH Jr, Sánchez PJ. Daptomycin therapy for invasive gram-positive bacterial infections in children. *Pediatr Infect Dis J*. 2007;26(12):1128–1132

Carillo-Marquez MA, Hulten KG, Hammerman W, Mason EO, Kaplan SL. USA300 is the predominant genotype causing *Staphylococcus aureus* septic arthritis in children. *Pediatr Infect Dis J*. 2009;28(12):1076–1080

Ceroni D, Cherkaoui A, Ferey S, Kaelin A, Schrenzel J. *Kingella kingae* osteoarticular infections in young children: clinical features and contribution of a new specific real-time PCR assay to the diagnosis. *J Pediatr Orthop*. 2010;30(3):301–304

Chamber JB, Forsythe DA, Bertrand SL, Iwinski HJ, Steflik DE. Retrospective review of osteoarticular infections in a pediatric sickle cell age group. *J Pediatr Orthop*. 2000;20(5):682–685

Chometon S, Benito Y, Charker M, et al. Specific real-time polymerase chain reaction places *Kingella kingae* as the most common cause of osteoarticular infections in young children. *Pediatr Infect Dis J*. 2007;26(5):377–381

Ferguson PJ, Sandu M. Current understanding of the pathogenesis and management of chronic recurrent multifocal osteomyelitis. *Curr Rheumatol Rep*. 2012;14(2):130–141

Liu C, Bayer A, Cosgrove SE, et al. Clinical practice guidelines for the Infectious Diseases Society of America for the treatment of methicillin-resistant *Staphylococcus aureus* infections in adults and children. *Clin Infect Dis*. 2011;52(3):e18–e85

Long SS, Pickering LK, Prober CG. *Principles and Practice of Pediatric Infectious Diseases*. 4th ed. Philadelphia, PA: Saunders; 2008

CHAPTER 6

Pneumonia and Empyema

Krow Ampofo, MB, ChB

Key Points

- Community-acquired pneumonia in children is generally caused by respiratory viruses (eg, respiratory syncytial virus, influenza virus, rhinovirus, metapneumovirus) or bacterial pathogens (eg, *Streptococcus pneumoniae, Staphylococcus aureus,* and group A *Streptococcus*); coinfection (viral-viral or viral-bacterial) is common.

- A chest radiograph should be reserved for younger infants, those with respiratory distress or recurrent pneumonia, or those with failed outpatient amoxicillin therapy.

- If chest radiograph shows lobar infiltrate or moderate-large pleural effusion, this favors the diagnosis of bacterial pneumonia.

- For clinically stable, hospitalized children with pneumonia, ampicillin or a third-generation cephalosporin should be used for empiric coverage, with the addition of vancomycin in those with suspected staphylococcal pneumonia or who are seriously ill.

- Antiviral therapy should be used for hospitalized children with suspected influenza.

- Pneumonia with empyema (loculated pleural effusion) should be managed with antibiotics and pleural drainage with fibrinolysis or video-assisted thoracoscopic surgery.

Overview

Pneumonia is a clinical condition that results from inflammation of the lower respiratory tract and alveoli caused most commonly by respiratory viruses or bacteria. When inflammation is a result of an infection acquired in the community, it is referred to as *community-acquired pneumonia* (CAP). Community-acquired pneumonia may be classified on the basis of the microbiologic pathogen detected or radiographic appearance on chest radiograph.

Causes and Differential Diagnosis

A number of respiratory viruses, bacteria, and atypical organisms cause CAP in children. The most common pathogens vary by age (Table 6-1). Using different microbiologic methods (eg, culture, polymerase chain reaction [PCR], and serology), a respiratory virus can be detected in 45% to 77% of children and a potential bacterial etiology in 2% to 60% of children with CAP, especially those who are hospitalized. Coinfection (viral-viral and bacterial-viral) is relatively common and detected in up to 22% to 33% of children hospitalized with CAP.

Neonates (<3 Weeks)

Pneumonia in neonates and young infants may be early-onset (within 7 days of life) or late-onset (after 7 days of life). Young infants with pneumonia can present with early-onset pneumonia alone or as part of the spectrum of early-onset sepsis, most commonly with group B *Streptococcus, Listeria monocytogenes,* and *Escherichia coli* following aspiration of infected amniotic fluid or genital secretions during birth. *Chlamydia trachomatis, Bordetella pertussis, Mycoplasma hominis,* and *Ureaplasma urealyticum,* as well as the bacteria causing early-onset pneumonia, should be considered in all young infants presenting after 7 days of life. Congenitally and perinatally acquired infection with herpes simplex virus, cytomegalovirus, and *Treponema pallidum* can cause pneumonia in young infants.

Infants, Children, and Adolescents

Respiratory viruses are by far the most common cause of CAP in children, with the highest rates among children younger than 5 years. The rate of viral pneumonia decreases with increasing age. Polymerase chain reaction testing has improved detection of previously known viral respiratory tract infections, such as respiratory syncytial virus (RSV), influenza virus, parainfluenza virus (PIV), adenovirus, and rhinovirus, and led to the discovery of previously unrecognized respiratory viruses, including *Human metapneumovirus* (HMPV), human coronavirus (HCoV), and human bocavirus (HBoV). Of the respiratory viruses isolated, RSV, rhinovirus, HMPV, and influenza virus are the most common.

Bacteria are the second most common cause of CAP in children. Conjugate vaccines have decreased the frequency of some bacterial causes of CAP. *Haemophilus influenzae* type b vaccine in the United States has significantly decreased CAP caused by *H influenzae* type b in children, which is now infrequent. *Streptococcus pneumoniae*, especially non–pneumococcal 7-valent conjugate vaccine serotypes, were the most common cause of typical bacterial CAP outside the neonatal period. Since the transition to the pneumococcal 13-valent conjugate vaccine containing antigens against some of the emerging *S pneumoniae* serotypes, there has been a further decrease in CAP caused by *S pneumoniae*. Recently, methicillin-susceptible *Staphylococcus aureus* (MSSA), methicillin-resistant *S aureus* (MRSA), and group A *Streptococcus* have

Table 6-1. Microbial Causes of Community-Acquired Pneumonia in Childhood

Age	Etiologic Agents	Clinical Features
Birth–3 wk	Group B *Streptococcus*	Part of early- or late-onset sepsis; usually severe
	Gram-negative enteric bacilli	Frequently nosocomial; occurs infrequently within 1 wk of birth
	Cytomegalovirus	Part of systemic cytomegalovirus infection
	Listeria monocytogenes	Part of early-onset sepsis
	HSV	Part of disseminated infection
	Treponema pallidum	Part of congenital syndrome
	Mycoplasma hominis or *Ureaplasma urealyticum*	From maternal genital infection; afebrile pneumonia
3 wk–3 mo	*Chlamydia trachomatis*	From maternal genital infection; afebrile, subacute, interstitial pneumonia
	RSV	Peak incidence at 2–7 mo of age; usually wheezing illness (bronchiolitis/pneumonia)
	HPIV-3	Similar to RSV, but in slightly older infants and not epidemic in the winter
	Streptococcus pneumoniae	The most common cause of bacterial pneumonia
	Bordetella pertussis	Primarily causes bronchitis (Secondary bacterial pneumonia and pulmonary hypertension can complicate severe cases.)
3 mo–5 y	RSV, PIV, influenza virus, HMPV, adenovirus, rhinovirus, HCoV, and HBoV	Most common causes of pneumonia
	S pneumoniae	Most likely cause of lobar pneumonia (Incidence has decreased after PCV7 vaccine use.)
	Haemophilus influenzae	Type b uncommon with vaccine use (Nontypeable stains cause pneumonia in immunocompromised hosts and developing countries.)
	Staphylococcus aureus	Uncommon, although community-acquired MRSA is becoming more prevalent
	Mycoplasma pneumoniae	Causes pneumonia primarily in children >4 y
	Mycobacterium tuberculosis	Major concern in areas of high prevalence, children with HIV, and refugees
5–15 y	*M pneumoniae*	Major cause of pneumonia; radiographic appearance variable
	Chlamydophila pneumoniae	Controversial, but probably an important cause in older children in this age group

Abbreviations: HBoV, human bocavirus; HCoV, human coronavirus; HMPV, *Human metapneumovirus;* HPIV, *Human parainfluenzavirus;* HSV, herpes simplex virus; MRSA, methicillin-acquired *Staphylococcus aureus;* PCV7, pneumococcal 7-valent conjugate vaccine; PIV, parainfluenza virus; RSV, respiratory syncytial virus.

Adapted from Mani CS, Murray DL. Acute pneumonia and its complications. In: Long SS, Pickering LK, Prober CG, eds. *Principles and Practice of Pediatric Infectious Diseases.* 4th ed. Philadelphia, PA: Saunders; 2012, with permission from Elsevier.

increasingly been identified as causes of severe CAP. Methicillin-resistant *S aureus* was a major cause of mortality during the 2009 pandemic influenza outbreak and continues to be a major cause of CAP during seasonal influenza. In general, CAP caused by bacteria occurs in all pediatric age groups and is a major cause of pneumonia in older children. Hospitalization with bacterial CAP occurs throughout the year but is diagnosed more frequently during the winter and spring months, when respiratory viral activity is increased.

Interaction of respiratory viruses and bacteria in the development of CAP has increasingly been appreciated, most commonly with a preceding history of viral CAP followed by a superimposed bacterial infection. Presentation is biphasic, with typical influenza-like illness that begins to resolve over several days followed by acute deterioration with the development of chest pain and new infiltrates, and bacteriologic evidence of infection.

Atypical bacterial pathogens have been isolated from 3% to 30% of children with CAP, with *Chlamydophila pneumoniae* frequently isolated from young children and *Mycoplasma pneumoniae* in older children. Focal outbreaks caused by *M pneumoniae* occur, and community-wide outbreaks have been reported to occur every 2 to 4 years. *Chlamydia trachomatis, M hominis,* and *U urealyticum* also cause pneumonia in newborns and young infants.

Other pathogens cause CAP in children, albeit less frequently (Table 6-2). Infection by *Mycobacterium tuberculosis* should be considered, especially in refugee children and those with exposure to adults at high risk for tuberculosis (TB). Endemic fungi (eg, *Blastomyces, Histoplasma, Cryptococcus,* and *Coccidioides*) infrequently cause CAP but should be considered in children who reside in locales where these endemic fungi are prevalent.

Table 6-2. Rare Microorganisms Causing Pediatric Community-Acquired Pneumonia or Occurring in Specialized Populations

Microorganism	Comment	Diagnostic Methods
Viruses		
Varicella-zoster virus	Potential complication after primary chickenpox infection. Often severe and associated with secondary bacterial infection.	Culture, DFA, and PCR test on the respiratory tract secretions
Measles virus	Measles. Pneumonia is a frequent complication.	Acute and convalescent serology; culture of respiratory tract secretions
Hantavirus	Hantavirus pulmonary syndrome. Rodent exposure.	Acute and convalescent serology; PCR test on the respiratory tract secretions
Bacteria		
Bordetella pertussis	Pneumonia is an uncommon manifestation. Bacterial coinfection may be severe, especially in infants.	PCR test, culture, or DFA of respiratory tract secretions
Group B *Streptococcus*	Neonatal pneumonia and sepsis.	Culture of respiratory tract secretions and blood

Continued

Table 6-2 (cont)

Microorganism	Comment	Diagnostic Methods
Listeria monocytogenes	Neonatal pneumonia and sepsis.	Culture of respiratory tract secretions and blood
Gram-negative enteric bacilli	Neonatal pneumonia and sepsis. Potential pathogens in aspiration pneumonia.	Culture of respiratory tract secretions and blood
Chlamydia trachomatis	Cause of afebrile pneumonia in young infants (<3 mo).	PCR test on the respiratory tract secretions
Anaerobes (oral flora)	Potential pathogens in aspiration pneumonia.	Culture of respiratory tract secretions and blood
Legionella pneumophila	Legionnaires' disease. Rare in children but associated with community outbreaks. Exposure to contaminated artificial freshwater systems.	Culture or DFA of respiratory tract secretions; antigen test on urine (type 1 only)
Coxiella burnetii	Q fever. Exposure to wild and domesticated herbivores or unpasteurized dairy (eg, cattle, sheep, goats). Also, potential bioterrorism agent.	Culture and PCR test on the respiratory tract secretions or blood; acute and convalescent serology
Chlamydophila psittaci	Psittacosis. Bird (eg, pet birds, pigeons) exposure.	Acute and convalescent serology
Francisella tularensis	Tularemia. Rabbit exposure.	Gram stain, culture, and PCR test on the respiratory tract secretions; acute and convalescent serology
Yersinia pestis	Pneumonic plague. Rodent flea exposure.	Gram stain, culture, and PCR test on the respiratory tract secretions; acute and convalescent serology
Bacillus anthracis	Anthrax. Inhalational anthrax. Wild and domesticated herbivore (eg, cattle, sheep, goats) exposure. Also, potential bioterrorism agent.	Gram stain, culture, and PCR test on lower respiratory tract secretions; acute and convalescent serology
Leptospira interrogans	Leptospirosis. Exposure to urine of wild and domestic animals carrying the bacterium.	Acute and convalescent serology
Mycobacterium tuberculosis	Rare in US children. Usually associated with high-risk exposures.	Culture of respiratory tract secretions or gastric aspirates
Brucella abortus	Brucellosis. Exposure to wild and domesticated animals or unpasteurized dairy (eg, cattle, sheep, pigs, goats, deer, dogs).	Acute and convalescent serology; culture of respiratory tract secretions or gastric aspirates
Burkholderia pseudomallei	Melioidosis. Travel to rural areas of Southeast Asia.	Culture of respiratory tract secretions; acute and convalescent serology

Continued

Table 6-2 *(cont)*

Microorganism	Comment	Diagnostic Methods
Fungi		
Histoplasma capsulatum	Histoplasmosis. Exposure to bird or bat droppings (eg, poultry/bird roosts, caves). Endemic to eastern and central United States.	Culture of respiratory tract secretions; urinary antigen test; serum immunodiffusion antibody test; serum *Histoplasma* complement fixation antibody test
Blastomyces dermatitidis	Blastomycosis. Environmental exposure to fungal spores (wooded areas). Endemic to southeastern and Midwestern United States.	Culture of respiratory tract secretions; serum immunodiffusion antibody test
Cryptococcus neoformans	Cryptococcosis. Exposure to soil contaminated with bird droppings. Significant pathogen nearly exclusively among immunocompromised hosts.	Culture of respiratory tract secretions; cryptococcal capsular antigen in serum, urinary, or bronchoalveolar lavage specimens
Coccidioides immitis	Primary coccidioidomycosis (also called valley fever). Environmental exposure to fungal spores (dry, dusty environments). Endemic to southwestern United States.	Culture of respiratory tract secretions; serum immunodiffusion antibody test

Abbreviations: DFA, direct fluorescence assay; PCR, polymerase chain reaction.

Adapted from Williams DJ, Shah SS. Community-acquired pneumonia in the conjugate vaccine era. *J Pediatr Infect Dis Soc.* 2012;1(4):314–328, by permission of Oxford University Press.

Other noninfectious disorders may present with signs and symptoms similar to CAP. A detailed history and physical examination can help distinguish noninfectious mimics of CAP (Box 6-1).

Box 6-1. Differential Diagnosis of Pediatric Community-Acquired Pneumonia

- Cardiac
  - o Pulmonary edema from congestive heart failure
  - o Vascular ring
- Pulmonary
  - o Bronchiolitis/bronchitis
  - o Reactive airway disease/asthma
  - o Atelectasis (eg, mucous plug, foreign body)
  - o Aspiration
  - o Lung abscess
  - o Parapneumonic effusion
  - o Congenital lung malformations
  - o Pulmonary embolism
  - o Bronchiectasis
  - o Cystic fibrosis
  - o Tuberculosis
- Drugs
  - o Nitrofurantoin, bleomycin, cytotoxic drugs, opiates
- Other
  - o Sepsis and ARDS
  - o Vasculitic syndromes
  - o Radiotherapy
  - o Smoke inhalation
  - o Lipoid pneumonias

Abbreviation: ARDS, acute respiratory distress syndrome.

Clinical Features
• • • • • • • • • • • • • • • •

The triad of acute fever, rapid or labored breathing, and cough is reported to be a classic presentation of CAP in children. Other common clinical symptoms include hypoxia, chest and abdominal pain, physical signs of tachypnea, and retraction, with auscultation findings of rales and decreased breath sounds (Table 6-3). However, these signs and symptoms are nonspecific, especially in young children in whom bronchiolitis and CAP are common. The likelihood of CAP is heightened with more signs and symptoms (Evidence Level II-3). Gradual onset, preceding nasal congestion, cough, and bilateral wheezing, is suggestive of viral pneumonia and more commonly associated with atypical bacteria than traditional bacterial infections. High temperature, rigors, and chest and abdominal pain, along with rales and bronchial breath sounds, are significantly more common on presentation in patients with bacterial or mixed infection. However, significant overlap limits the utility of these clinical signs and symptoms. In a small proportion of children, high fever (>39°C [102.2°F]) alone may be the only symptom associated with CAP. Neonates and young infants with CAP may present with apneic spells and lower respiratory tract symptoms but without fever. A staccato-like cough in an infant older than 3 weeks is suggestive of infection with *C trachomatis;* conjunctivitis may be present. Clinical symptoms caused by *M pneumoniae* and *C pneumoniae* infections in older children are similar to other CAP, but other constitutional symptoms of malaise, severe sore throat, and headache are common.

Table 6-3. Common Symptoms and Signs of Community-Acquired Pneumonia in Children

Symptoms	Signs
Fever[a]	Lower respiratory tract signs
Cough	• Tachypnea, grunting, suprasternal, intercostal, and
Apnea[b]	subcostal retractions
Labored breathing	• Splinting of the chest wall with pleurisy
Poor feeding[b]	Percussion
Vomiting	• Dull with CAP and stony dull with pleural effusion
Irritability[b]	Auscultation
Lethargy	• Louder breath sounds with CAP and diminished or
Abdominal pain[c,d]	absent with pleural effusion
Pleuritic chest pain[c,d]	• Rales/crackles/crepitations
Meningism[c-e]	

Abbreviation: CAP, community-acquired pneumonia.

[a] May be absent in young infants.

[b] Common in children <3 mo.

[c] Common in children >3 mo and <5 y.

[d] Common in children >5 y.

[e] May be present in older children with upper lobar pneumonia.

Complications

Complications associated with CAP include bacteremia, parapneumonic effusion, empyema, necrotizing pneumonia, lung abscesses, and, rarely, pneumococcal hemolytic uremic syndrome. These complications are associated with significant morbidity (eg, prolonged hospital stay, intensive care unit admission) but infrequent mortality.

Parapneumonic Effusion and Empyema

Parapneumonic effusions develop when excess fluid accumulates in the pleural cavity during CAP. It is one of the most common complications associated with CAP. Parapneumonic effusion or empyema is thought to be present in 1% of all patients with CAP and up to 40% of children hospitalized with CAP. Effusions and empyema are associated with significant morbidity and some mortality.

The pleural fluid is initially sterile with a low white blood cell (WBC) count. With time, bacteria invade the fluid and WBC count increases in the pleural fluid. This progression results in empyema, defined as the presence of grossly purulent fluid in the pleural cavity or positive bacterial culture of pleural fluid.

Incidence of parapneumonic effusion and empyema increased in the United States coincident with the widespread use of pneumococcal 7-valent conjugate vaccine, but has decreased since the transition to the pneumococcal 13-valent conjugate vaccine. Because of prior antibiotic therapy before pleural fluid drainage, a pathogen is detected by blood or pleural fluid culture in less than 30% of cases. *Streptococcus pneumoniae*, MSSA, MRSA, and group A *Streptococcus* are the most common bacteria isolated from US children with empyema. Testing of culture-negative pleural fluid by PCR-based technology has increased pathogen identification. *Streptococcus pneumoniae* is the most common bacteria detected by PCR of the pleural fluid (Evidence Level II-3). Additionally, PCR testing has occasionally detected respiratory viruses, *M pneumoniae*, and fusobacterium in the pleural fluid of children with parapneumonic effusion and empyema. Overall, *S pneumoniae* remains the most common cause of empyema and accounts for much of the increase in the burden of empyema. Community-acquired MRSA has also recently emerged as an important cause of empyema in some parts of the United States.

Most children with parapneumonic effusion or empyema present with signs and symptoms of CAP. These complications should be considered in any child with CAP and persistent fever despite adequate antibiotic treatment (Evidence Level III), pleuritic chest, diminished breath sounds, stony dullness to percussion, and persistently elevated erythrocyte sedimentation rate or C-reactive protein concentration. Fluid in the pleural cavity can be identified by a chest radiograph (blunting of the costophrenic angle), ultrasound, or computer tomography, as described next.

Evaluation
· · · · · · · · · ·

Determining the microbiologic etiology of CAP is essential to guide the specific treatment and management of CAP. However, identification of the causative pathogen may be challenging. Reasons for this difficulty include scarcity of samples obtained from the lower respiratory tract, antibiotic therapy before presentation, and lack of sensitive diagnostic methods that distinguish between colonizing respiratory viruses and bacteria and those responsible for the illness. Even in research studies, no pathogen can be identified in 14% to 23% of pediatric CAP cases, suggesting the need for improved diagnostics and possibility of unrecognized pathogens.

Respiratory Viral Pathogens

Antigen detection testing of respiratory specimens is quick and useful in some clinical settings. Rapid antigen testing for RSV and influenza virus are specific but exhibit variable sensitivity. Direct fluorescent assay performed in the laboratory rapidly detects RSV, influenza virus, PIV, adenovirus, and HMPV. Sensitivity of DFA is highest for RSV (>95%) and lowest for adenovirus (approximately 65%–70%). Polymerase chain reaction testing has increased the detection of previously known (RSV, influenza A and B viruses, PIV, adenovirus, rhinovirus, and HMPV) and emerging (enterovirus, HBoV, and HCoV) respiratory viruses in children with CAP. However, the role of newly discovered respiratory viruses (HBoV and HCoV) in CAP is unclear. A positive respiratory viral test can guide decision-making, including the need for further diagnostics, antibiotic therapy, and isolation in hospitalized children (Evidence Level II-1). A positive influenza test should be used to guide the initiation of antiviral therapy in hospitalized and nonhospitalized children (Evidence Level II-1).

Culture-Based Testing

Although culture of blood or lung tissue remains the criterion standard for identifying bacterial pathogens responsible for CAP, yield of blood culture is low and lung tissue is generally not readily available. Blood cultures are positive in less than 10% of children hospitalized with CAP, but isolation rates are higher (approximately 30%) in children with CAP complicated by parapneumonic effusion and empyema (Evidence Level II-3). Blood culture should not be routinely performed in nonhospitalized children with CAP who are non-toxic and fully vaccinated (Evidence Level II-2) but should be performed on all children hospitalized with presumed bacterial CAP and children with no clinical improvement despite therapy (Evidence Level II-2). Pleural fluid, when available, should also be submitted for Gram stain and bacterial culture to identify likely bacteria commonly responsible for parapneumonic effusion and empyema (Evidence Level II-1).

Obtainment of respiratory specimens, such as expectorated sputum, should be attempted in children 8 years and older with severe disease or failure of outpatient therapy. Sputa with 10 or fewer epithelial cells and 25 or more polymorphonuclear leukocytes under low power are considered to be appropriate for culture. For children admitted to intensive care with CAP, respiratory samples collected from the endotracheal tube using a suction catheter, standard protected specimen brush, or bronchoalveolar lavage should be sent for Gram stain, bacterial culture, and respiratory viral testing (Evidence Level III).

Other Testing

Testing is recommended in children with a high likelihood of *M pneumoniae* and *C pneumoniae* infection, especially in older children (Evidence Level II-3). Measurements of serologic responses to *M pneumoniae* and *C pneumoniae* are available. However, in the setting of acute CAP, serologic testing is unreliable. Polymerase chain reaction testing for *M pneumoniae* and *C pneumoniae* in respiratory specimens is more sensitive. Neonates with a clinical suspicion of pneumonia and staccato-like cough should be tested for *C trachomatis* by PCR (Evidence Level III). For children with signs and symptoms consistent with pertussis, testing of nasopharyngeal and oropharyngeal samples for *B pertussis* by PCR should be performed (Evidence Level II-3).

When TB is of concern, a tuberculin test or the interferon-γ release assay (IGRA) in children older than 5 years and adults should be performed on the patient and close family members and contacts. Results of a chest radiograph will differentiate latent TB (tuberculin test or IGRA positive and a normal chest radiograph) from active pulmonary TB disease (tuberculin test or IGRA positive and an abnormal chest radiograph). Because of variable resistance, every attempt should be made to obtain specimens (sputum, bronchoalveolar lavage, or gastric aspirate) for acid-fast bacilli staining and culture (Evidence Level II-2) from children with clinical suspicion of active pulmonary TB.

Antigen testing of urine for pneumococcal antigen has been useful in detecting pneumococcal pneumonia in adults. However, nasopharyngeal colonization with *S pneumoniae* leads to high rates of false-positive tests in children, and urinary antigen assays cannot be recommended in the pediatric patient (Evidence Level II-2).

Pleural Fluid Evaluation

Pleural fluid, when present, should be submitted for Gram stain and bacterial culture to identify likely bacteria commonly responsible for parapneumonic effusion and empyema. White blood cell count with differential, pH, glucose, protein, and lactate dehydrogenase are useful in distinguishing a transudative from an exudative effusion, and to differentiate among bacterial, fungal, mycobacterial, and other causes of effusion or empyema (Evidence Level II-3). If cultures are negative, PCR or antigen testing of pleural fluid may be useful to detect *S pneumoniae* or *S aureus* (Evidence Level II-3). Testing by species-specific PCR should be performed if available to further increase pathogen identification (Evidence Level II-3).

Complete Blood Cell Count

Complete blood cell count with WBC and differential should be performed in hospitalized children with moderate to severe CAP (Evidence Level II-3). However, WBC count alone is a poor predictor of bacterial pneumonia, as the degree of elevation does not reliably distinguish bacterial from viral infection (Evidence Level II-2). A WBC count less than 15,000/mcL suggests a nonbacterial etiology. Nonetheless, neutropenic and severely ill children may have a low count. A WBC count greater than 15,000/mcL is suggestive of bacterial disease, but has been reported in CAP caused by *M pneumoniae* and infections with some respiratory viruses (eg, adenovirus). Anemia or thrombocytopenia may raise suspicions for hemolytic uremic syndrome, which may occur with pneumococcal pneumonia.

Acute Phase Proteins

Acute phase proteins, such as erythrocyte sedimentation rate, C-reactive protein, and procalcitonin, do not reliably distinguish bacterial from viral infections and should not be used as the only diagnostic test (Evidence Level II-2). Although procalcitonin concentration is consistently higher in children with bacterial pneumonia, moderate elevations do not distinguish nonserious bacterial from viral pneumonia in children. However, low values may be helpful in distinguishing viral from bacterial pneumonia associated with bacteremia (Evidence Level II-2). Declining values of C-reactive protein or procalcitonin may correlate with improvement in clinical symptoms and thus have the potential to serve as objective measures of disease resolution (Evidence Level II-3).

Imaging Studies

For clinically stable children with the classic signs and symptoms of CAP, a confirmatory chest radiograph is not required (Evidence Level II-2). However, it should be obtained in babies younger than 12 months with lower respiratory tract signs and symptoms (with the exception of those with routine bronchiolitis), children with failing initial antibiotic therapy, severely ill or hospitalized children, and children with a history of recurrent pneumonia (Evidence Level II-3). A supine anteroposterior chest view (young children) or upright posteroanterior chest view (>4 years) is recommended. An upright lateral view is useful for the evaluation of retrocardiac pneumonia, which may be obscured by the heart. When there is clinical suspicion of CAP with a pleural effusion, a lateral decubitus view should be performed (affected side down). A chest ultrasound or computed tomography is useful in defining anatomy of the pleural cavity in cases of suspected complicated parapneumonic effusion (Evidence Level II-2).

Chest radiographic features and suggestive CAP etiologies are summarized in Table 6-4. However, while suggestive, none of these features reliably differentiate among a bacterial, atypical bacterial, and viral pneumonia. Chest radiographs in children with CAP can appear normal early in the course of pneumonia in dehydrated or neutropenic children.

A lobar infiltrate is suggestive of CAP caused by bacteria. Lobar pneumonia is generally caused by *S pneumoniae,* but may also be seen with MSSA, MRSA, *M pneumoniae,* and even viral pneumonia. A consolidative lobar infiltrate in the presence of a large pleural effusion or parenchymal necrosis is highly suggestive of bacterial etiology. Lung pneumatoceles, cavitation, and necrotizing processes are suggestive of bacterial infection. Round solitary consolidative pneumonias are seen in young children. Round pneumonias are commonly associated with *S pneumoniae,* but are seen with other streptococci, staphylococci, *H influenzae,* and *M pneumoniae.*

Interstitial pneumonia or diffuse bilateral interstitial inflammatory infiltrates are typically associated with viral pneumonia, *M pneumoniae,* and *Pneumocystis jiroveci.* Bronchopneumonia has been described in the setting of *M pneumoniae* and viral respiratory tract infections. Typical bacteria are not commonly associated with these patterns.

Enlarged mediastinal or hilar lymphadenopathy with or without calcification on chest radiograph is suggestive of TB, histoplasmosis, or *M pneumoniae* infection with compatible exposure history.

Chest radiograph features of CAP lag behind clinical resolution by 3 to 6 weeks, with persistent and residual abnormalities observed in 10% to 30% of children. Serial imaging is not useful in a patient who is improving clinically (Evidence Level II-3), but should be considered for those with lobar collapse, complicated pneumonia, recurrent pneumonia, foreign body aspiration, and round pneumonia (Evidence Level III).

Table 6-4. Radiographic Features of Pneumonia

	Bacteria	Respiratory Virus	Atypical Bacteria	Endemic Fungi	Tuberculosis	*Pneumocystis jiroveci*
Lobar						
Single	++	−	+	−	++	−
Multiple	+	+	+	−	−	−
Alveolar	++	++	+	−	−	+
Interstitial	−	++	++	−	−	++
Nodular	+	+	+	++	−	−
Hilar lymphadenopathy	+	+	+	++	++	−
Effusion	++	+	+	−	+	−
Hyperinflated lungs	−	++	−	−	−	−

Minus sign (−) indicates infrequent manifestation, plus sign (+) indicates occasional manifestation, and double plus sign (++) indicates frequent manifestation.

Management

Most children with CAP who present to medical care have mild disease and are treated without the need for hospitalization. These children should be monitored and reevaluated if there is no clinical response to therapy after 48 hours or clinical deterioration occurs (Evidence Level II-2). Children younger than 3 months or with respiratory distress (Box 6-2) should be hospitalized (Evidence Level II-1).

Box 6-2. Criteria for Respiratory Distress in Children With Community-Acquired Pneumonia

- Tachypnea, respiratory rate, breaths/min[a]
  - o 0–2 mo: >60
  - o 2–12 mo: >50
  - o 1–5 y: >40
  - o >5 y: >20
- Dyspnea
- Retractions (suprasternal, intercostal, or subcostal)
- Grunting
- Nasal flaring
- Apnea
- Altered mental status
- Sustained pulse oximetry measurement of <90% on room air

[a] Adapted from World Health Organization criteria.

Adapted from Bradley JS, Byington CL, Shah SS, et al. The management of community-acquired pneumonia in infants and children older than 3 months of age: clinical practice guidelines by the Pediatric Infectious Diseases Society and the Infectious Diseases Society of America. *Clin Infect Dis.* 2011;53(7):e34–e76, by permission of Oxford University Press.

Antimicrobials

Respiratory viruses are the most common cause of CAP in children. Antibiotics are not indicated in the management of CAP caused by respiratory viruses (Evidence Level II-1). With the exception of infection with influenza virus, most hospitalized CAPs caused by respiratory viruses are managed with supportive therapy and do not require antibiotic therapy. Children hospitalized with influenza-associated pneumonia should be treated with antivirals (Evidence Level II-1). Antimicrobials recommended for the treatment of CAP are shown in Table 6-5.

Antibiotics should be administered if the history, physical examination, laboratory data and chest radiographic findings and values are suggestive of bacterial infection or coinfection (Evidence Level II-1). The initial choice of antibiotics is often empiric and depends on age of the child, immunization status, likely pathogen and resistance patterns, route of administration, tolerability of the antimicrobial, and cost.

In the pneumococcal conjugate vaccine era, *S pneumoniae* remains the most common cause of bacterial CAP in all children. In children who are

Table 6-5. Empiric Antimicrobial Strategies for Pediatric Community-Acquired Pneumonia

Population		Bacterial Pneumonia	Atypical Pneumonia	Influenza Pneumonia
Outpatient				
Neonates–3 mo		Outpatient therapy not recommended		
3 mo–5 y	Preferred	Amoxicillin	Azithromycin	Oseltamivir
	Alternatives	Amoxicillin/clavulanate Levofloxacin for children with serious penicillin allergy	Clarithromycin Erythromycin	None
5–17 y	Preferred	Amoxicillin	Azithromycin	Oseltamivir
	Alternatives	Amoxicillin/clavulanate Levofloxacin for children with serious penicillin allergy	Clarithromycin Erythromycin Doxycycline if >7 y	Zanamivir if ≥7 y
Inpatient				
Neonates	Preferred	Ampicillin + gentamicin	Azithromycin	No US FDA-approved antivirals for children <1 y. Oseltamivir dosing recommendations are available at www.cdc.gov.
	Alternatives	Ampicillin + cefotaxime	Erythromycin	
1–3 mo	Preferred	Cefotaxime or ceftriaxone (if child is >1 mo)	Azithromycin if *Chlamydia trachomatis* or *Bordetella pertussis* is suspected	No FDA-approved antivirals for children <1 y. Oseltamivir dosing recommendations are available at www.cdc.gov.
	Alternatives	None	Erythromycin	

3 mo–17 y, fully immunized, or local epidemiology that indicates low prevalence of penicillin-nonsusceptible *Streptococcus pneumoniae*	Preferred	Ampicillin or penicillin G	Azithromycin	Oseltamivir
	Alternatives	Ceftriaxone or cefotaxime Anti-staphylococcal coverage for suspected *Staphylococcus aureus*,[a] including clindamycin or vancomycin in MRSA-prevalent regions Levofloxacin for children with serious penicillin allergy	Clarithromycin Erythromycin Doxycycline if >7 y Levofloxacin for those who have reached skeletal maturity	Zanamivir if ≥7 y
3 mo–17 y, not fully immunized, or local epidemiology that indicates moderate to high prevalence of penicillin-nonsusceptible *S pneumoniae*	Preferred	Ceftriaxone or cefotaxime	Azithromycin	Oseltamivir
	Alternatives	Levofloxacin Antistaphylococcal coverage for suspected *S aureus*, including clindamycin or vancomycin in MRSA-prevalent regions	Clarithromycin Erythromycin Doxycycline if >7 y Levofloxacin for those who have reached skeletal maturity	Zanamivir if ≥7 y

Abbreviations: FDA, Food and Drug Administration; MRSA, methicillin-resistant *Staphylococcus aureus*.

[a] *Staphylococcus aureus* should be considered in the setting of intensive care unit admission, pneumatocele, or pulmonary abscess.

Adapted from Williams DJ, Shah SS. Community-acquired pneumonia in the conjugate vaccine era. *J Pediatr Infect Dis.* 2012;1(4):314–328, by permission of Oxford University Press.

appropriately immunized, amoxicillin is the recommended first-line antimicrobial therapy for nonhospitalized children, and ampicillin or penicillin G for
hospitalized children (Evidence Level II-3). A third-generation parenteral
cephalosporin (eg, ceftriaxone or cefotaxime) is recommended for children
who are not fully immunized, in regions where the prevalence of high-level
penicillin resistance is high among invasive *S pneumoniae* (Evidence Level II-3),
or for infants and children with life-threatening infection, including those with
parapneumonic effusion or empyema (Evidence Level II-1). Clindamycin or
vancomycin should be added to β-lactam antibiotic therapy if clinical, laboratory, or imaging characteristics are consistent with infection caused by *S aureus*
until MRSA can be excluded (clindamycin should be considered only if local
antibiogram shows <10% resistance for *S aureus*) or in children with shock,
overwhelming pneumonia, pneumatocele, or lung abscess (Evidence
Level II-3).

A macrolide should be considered for a child with CAP when *M pneumoniae* or *C pneumoniae* is suspected (ie, >5 years) (Evidence Level II-3).

Among young infants, therapy with ampicillin and gentamicin or a third-
generation cephalosporin is appropriate for pneumonia because the pathogens
are similar to those of sepsis (Evidence Level II-3). A macrolide (azithromycin
in babies <1 month) is recommended for *C trachomatis* or *B pertussis* infection
(Evidence Level III).

For children with parapneumonic effusion or empyema, initial antibiotic
choice should be based on the most common causes of CAP according to
regional epidemiology. Antibiotic treatment of parapneumonic effusion and
empyema is similar to that for CAP without effusion. Empiric therapy with a
third-generation cephalosporin and clindamycin is recommended. The
addition of vancomycin or linezolid should be considered in children admitted
to intensive care and in locales with high rates of community-acquired MRSA.

The decision to drain pleural fluid depends on the size of the pleural effusion
and degree of the respiratory distress (Evidence Level II-3). Small effusions can
initially be managed with antibiotics alone and monitored for disease progression (Evidence Level II-3). Moderate-sized and free-flowing effusions should be
drained by chest thoracostomy tube without fibrinolytic agents (Evidence Level
II-3). Moderate- to large-sized effusions, loculated effusions, or empyema
should be drained by chest thoracostomy tube with fibrinolytic agents or
video-assisted thoracoscopic surgery (Evidence Level II-2). Figure 6-1 summarizes the indications and modalities of pleural fluid drainage.

Long-term Monitoring

High immunization rates and ready access to medical care in the United States
result in low CAP-associated pediatric mortality. Most children with uncomplicated CAP recover without sequelae. Some patients, especially premature
infants and children with chronic lung, neuromuscular, or cardiovascular

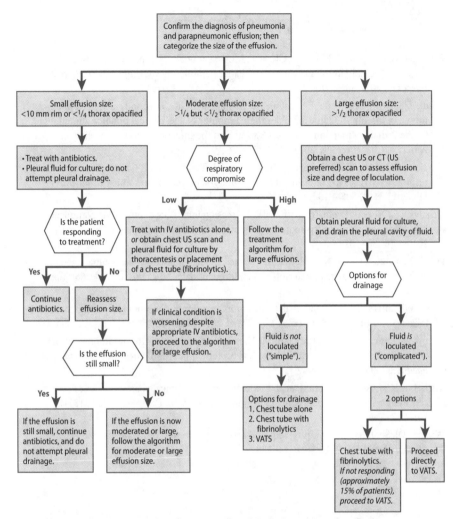

Figure 6-1. Management of pneumonia with parapneumonic effusion.
Abbreviations: CT, computed tomography; IV, intravenous; US, ultrasound; VATS, video-assisted thoracoscopic surgery.
Adapted from Bradley JS, Byington CL, Shah SS, et al. The management of community-acquired pneumonia in infants and children older than 3 months of age: clinical practice guidelines by the Pediatric Infectious Diseases Society and the Infectious Diseases Society of America. *Clin Infect Dis.* 2011;53(7):e34–e76, by permission of Oxford University Press.

diseases, frequently develop complications, which include parapneumonic effusion, empyema, necrotizing pneumonia, lung abscess, and pneumatocele formation. Children with parapneumonic effusion and empyema who have had pleural fluid drainage recover without any long-term consequences. Pneumatoceles that develop as a result of lung abscess or necrotizing pneumonia typically resolve within 6 to 8 weeks.

Suggested Reading

Blaschke AJ, Heyrend C, Byington CL, et al. Molecular analysis improves pathogen identification and epidemiologic study of pediatric parapneumonic empyema. *Pediatr Infect Dis.* 2011;30(4):289–294

Bradley JS, Byington CL, Shah SS, et al. The management of community-acquired pneumonia in infants and children older than 3 months of age: clinical practice guidelines by the Pediatric Infectious Diseases Society and the Infectious Diseases Society of America. *Clin Infect Dis.* 2011;53(7):e25–e76

García-García ML, Calvo C, Pozo F, Villadangos PA, Pérez-Brena P, Casas I. Spectrum of respiratory viruses in children with community-acquired pneumonia. *Pediatr Infect Dis.* 2012;31(8):808–813

Grijalva CG, Nuorti JP, Zhu Y, Griffin MR. Increasing incidence of empyema complicating childhood community-acquired pneumonia in the United States. *Clin Infect Dis.* 2010;50(6):805–813

Harris M, Clark J, Coote N, et al. British Thoracic Society guidelines for the management of community-acquired pneumonia in children: update 2011. *Thorax.* 2011;66(Suppl 2):ii1–ii23

Jain S, Williams DJ, Arnold SR, et al. Community-acquired pneumonia requiring hospitalization among U.S. children. *N Engl J Med.* 2015;372(9):835–845

Korppi M, Don M, Valent F, Canciani M. The value of clinical features in differentiating between viral, pneumococcal and atypical bacterial pneumonia in children. *Acta Paediatr.* 2008;97(7):943–947

Michelow IC, Olsen K, Lozano J, et al. Epidemiology and clinical characteristics of community-acquired pneumonia in hospitalized children. *Pediatrics.* 2004;113(4): 701–707

William DJ, Shah SS. Community-acquired pneumonia in the conjugate vaccine era. *J Pediatr Infect Dis.* 2012;1(4):314–328

CHAPTER 7

Skin and Soft-Tissue Infections

Joan E. Giovanni, MD, and Jason G. Newland, MD, MEd

Key Points

- Abscess, impetigo, cellulitis, and erysipelas are common skin and soft-tissue infections seen in the pediatric population and frequently seen in the acute care setting.

- Skin and soft-tissue infections have overlapping features and are largely diagnosed according to their historical and clinical presentations.

- Many skin and soft-tissue infections are caused by disruption in the skin barrier in healthy children as well as those with underlying medical/dermatologic conditions.

- Most abscesses can be treated with local care and incision and drainage without need for adjuvant antibiotics, although recurrences are common.

- Consider other etiologies, including gram-negative pathogens and nontuberculous mycobacteria, depending on clinical scenario (eg, water or soil-contaminated wound).

- Ecthyma gangrenosum is diagnosed most commonly in the child with known malignancy. If this diagnosis is made in a previously well child, consider neutrophil defect or leukemia.

- Treatment in usual cases with oral antibiotics in the outpatient setting should target *Staphylococcus aureus* (methicillin-resistant and methicillin-susceptible) and *Streptococcus pyogenes* infections.

- In the ill-appearing child with soft-tissue infection, hospitalization and treatment with clindamycin and cefepime (inclusion of vancomycin in unstable child) while awaiting cultures is recommended. Surgical debridement should not be delayed if fasciitis is suspected.

- Preventive measures against skin and soft-tissue infections should be discussed with children and caregivers, including skin care, personal/hand hygiene, and environmental cleaning.

Overview
· · · · · · · · ·

Skin and soft-tissue infections are common in the pediatric population and frequently encountered in the acute care setting. Most cases occur in healthy children without known risk factors. Breaks in the skin, whether caused by a dermatologic condition, like eczema, or by varicellar trauma, are a potential site of entry. Other risk factors include close contacts with abscesses, poor general health, poor personal hygiene, obesity, tight clothing, neutrophil dysfunction, lymphedema, blood dyscrasias, and diabetes mellitus.

Distinguishing among these infections is important because management and treatment options vary among the conditions. Clinicians should be able to differentiate the commonly encountered skin and soft-tissue infections in the primary care setting, including abscess, impetigo, erysipelas, and cellulitis, and be able to promptly diagnose more virulent or atypical soft-tissue infections, like necrotizing fasciitis and ecthyma gangrenosum.

Causes and Differential Diagnosis
· ·

Most skin and soft-tissue infections are caused by bacteria that colonize the skin. *Staphylococcus aureus* and *Streptococcus pyogenes* (also known as group A *Streptococcus*) account for the majority. While methicillin-resistant *S aureus* (MRSA) is often thought to be the main cause of skin abscesses, methicillin-susceptible *S aureus* can also cause these infections. *Aeromonas hydrophila* (water injury), *Vibrio vulnificus* (contaminated seawater or injury from contaminated shellfish), and *Edwardsiella tarda* (catfish spine) may also cause cutaneous infection, depending on the clinical scenario. Bites from humans and animals may also be implicated in skin and soft-tissue infections.

Rarely, uncommon infectious pathogens, including those caused by nontuberculous mycobacteria, may cause a superficial skin infection. *Mycobacterium marinum* has been associated with water contact, and other nontuberculous mycobacteria have been associated with contaminated tattoo inks and water used for pedicures. *Pseudomonas aeruginosa* has been implicated in hot tub exposure and typically causes a folliculitis.

While ecthyma gangrenosum, a less commonly encountered cutaneous infectious process, can occur in immunocompetent children, it typically occurs in those with neutrophil disorders or underlying malignancy. In addition to *S aureus* and *Streptococcus pyogenes,* unusual pathogens include *Chromobacterium violaceum, P aeruginosa,* unusual gram-negative pathogens, and fungal agents, including *Aspergillus, Mucor,* and *Fusarium.*

The differential diagnosis for skin and soft-tissue infections includes hidradenitis suppurativa, sporotrichosis, leishmaniasis, and tularemia. The differential diagnosis of impetigo includes contact dermatitis, seborrhea, cutaneous herpes simplex virus infection, scabies, bacterial folliculitis, excoriated insect bites, bullous pemphigoid, and Stevens-Johnsons syndrome.

Ecthyma gangrenosum can be confused with the lesions of cutaneous anthrax (contaminated animal meat or carcasses) or orf infection (generally sheep- or goat-associated).

Rarely, autoimmune-mediated panniculitis may mimic a soft-tissue infection, and cutaneous manifestations of familial Mediterranean fever, an autoinflammatory syndrome, can mimic erysipelas. Lastly, infections that occur in deeper soft tissues or cases of osteomyelitis with subperiosteal abscess formation can produce superficial soft-tissue inflammation that may be mistaken for cellulitis. Circumferential swelling is usually noted in such cases, and the margins of the "cellulitis" are indistinct.

Clinical Features

Children with skin abscesses typically present with a painful nodule that may be erythematous and indurated, often with an overlying pustule. Well-formed abscesses typically have a central region of fluctuance or may exhibit spontaneous purulent drainage. Systemic signs of toxicity are less common in children with skin abscesses, although fever may be present.

A skin abscess is a collection of pus in the dermis and deeper skin tissues. A furuncle, commonly termed a *boil*, involves an infected hair follicle that extends from the dermis into the subcutaneous tissue. A carbuncle is a deeper infection of several inflamed follicles that combine to form an interconnecting abscess.

Impetigo is a superficial infection of the epidermis and can also be referred to as *pyoderma* or *impetigo contagiosa*. Primary impetigo is caused by minor breaks in the skin. Secondary impetigo arises because of underlying dermatologic skin disorders and traumatic injury in the skin. This condition is most commonly found in younger children. Two types of impetigo exist: nonbullous and bullous. Nonbullous impetigo is more common, with superficial small vesicles or pustules that rupture, resulting in erosions, followed by a golden-yellow crust over approximately a 1-week period. Bullous impetigo consists of vesicles and bullae containing clear yellow fluid without surrounding erythema, and frequently involves the trunk or intertriginous areas.

Cellulitis is an infectious inflammatory process of the skin that affects the dermis and subcutaneous tissue. It is typically a superficial process, and when no associated break in skin is noted, *S pyogenes* should be suspected. It is important to differentiate simple cellulitis from a deeper necrotizing process (eg, fasciitis), which progresses rapidly and requires prompt surgical intervention.

Erysipelas is a distinct form of cellulitis that is confined to the upper dermis and superficial lymphatics and predominantly caused by *S pyogenes*. Clinically, erysipelas is distinguished from other forms of skin infections by a raised border and clear line of demarcation from uninvolved skin. Superficial vesiculation that is described as "peau de orange," or orange peel, in appearance is a typical associated feature. Erysipelas is commonly associated with an abrupt onset, and generally children have systemic symptoms, such as fevers, chills, and malaise. Children tend to have involvement of a lower extremity in contrast to adults.

Ecthyma gangrenosum is a local cutaneous process that manifests as a deep ulcerative process with central necrosis.

Necrotizing fasciitis is sometimes mistaken initially for simple cellulitis. However, a hallmark of infection is that the child presents with severe pain that is out of proportion to the cutaneous findings. The skin is tender and faintly red, but borders of the process are indistinct. The central portion of the involved site is anesthetic, and bullae with frank necrosis rapidly evolve. The child generally appears toxic, and multiorgan dysfunction may occur.

Evaluation

Diagnosis of a skin abscess is usually accomplished with history and physical examination alone. However, adjunctive modalities for the diagnosis of skin abscess include fine-needle aspiration biopsy or limited bedside ultrasonography.

The diagnosis of impetigo is clinical and based on the history and physical examination. Routine cultures, especially of intact skin, are not recommended. Cultures may be helpful only in cases that fail to respond to empiric therapy. Treatment of impetigo includes topical or oral antibiotic therapy with agents that are effective against S aureus and S pyogenes. For mild nonbullous impetigo, topical treatment with mupirocin applied on the lesions and to the nares 3 times daily is recommended (Evidence Levels I and II-2). Cephalexin or clindamycin is a recommended oral antibiotic treatment for bullous impetigo in children. Additionally, hand washing and other preventive measures are helpful in decreasing transmission to close contacts.

The diagnosis of cellulitis is typically based on clinical and historical features. In cases of mild infections, blood or wound cultures are not routinely recommended (Evidence Level II-2). Blood or wound cultures should be considered in children who require hospital admission, have rapidly progressing symptoms, or have large areas of skin involvement (Evidence Level III). Use of bedside ultrasonography can assist with distinguishing between abscess and cellulitis, and magnetic resonance imaging may be indicated in severe infections to differentiate between cellulitis, osteomyelitis, pyomyositis, or necrotizing fasciitis.

Necrotizing fasciitis should be considered when pain is out of proportion to the physical examination findings in a child with a soft-tissue infection. Faint erythema is usually noted, and borders of the involved skin are usually indistinct in contrast to cellulitis and erysipelas. The central portion often becomes bluish and eventually forms bullae before becoming frankly necrotic. Magnetic resonance imaging can demonstrate fascial involvement but should not be pursued, because this will result in a delay in diagnosis. Prompt surgical exploration is the diagnostic intervention of choice.

The diagnosis of ecthyma is generally made on clinical grounds on the basis of appearance of the lesion. Additional workup should be done to identify an underlying neutrophil defect. Ecthyma may be the heralding manifestation of childhood leukemia or occur in a child with a known malignancy.

Management

Drainage is the primary treatment of skin abscesses in children. Smaller lesions may drain spontaneously after application of warm compresses or the use of anesthetic creams. Larger abscesses are treated with incision and drainage. Wound cultures, including susceptibility testing, are recommended to help guide antibiotic therapy and disease surveillance, especially in the era of MRSA (Evidence Level III). Routine blood cultures are not recommended in children with abscesses unless systemic signs of infection are present (Evidence Level III).

Some pediatric studies suggest that incision and drainage alone may be sufficient therapy for an abscess and that adjuvant antibiotics may not be indicated in healthy, well-appearing children with abscesses less than 5 cm in diameter without associated cellulitis (Evidence Level I). Figure 7-1, based on these studies, describes the current recommendations for management of an abscess.

Empiric antibiotic therapy should be targeted toward the treatment of *S aureus*. Depending on the local rate of MRSA, empiric therapy with an anti-MRSA drug may be indicated. Oral agents commonly used for empiric antibiotic therapy include cephalexin, clindamycin (if clindamycin resistance in the community is low), and trimethoprim/sulfamethoxazole (if *S pyogenes* is not suspected). Doxycycline can also be considered in older children (>8 years) in whom *S pyogenes* is not suspected. Although abscess recurrence can be common in some children, the role of antibiotics in abscess recurrence, spread, or progression has not been well studied in children. Finally, children and families need to be provided education on prevention measures that include keeping wounds covered, frequent hand washing, avoiding sharing personal items, and maintenance of a clean environment.

Initial empiric antimicrobial therapy for mild cases of cellulitis in the outpatient setting is targeted to treat *S aureus* (MRSA and methicillin-susceptible) and *S pyogenes* infections (especially common in those without antecedent skin trauma). Depending on the local antibiotic susceptibility pattern, empiric therapy could include clindamycin or cephalexin. Trimethoprim/sulfamethoxazole is not recommended in cellulitis because of its lack of activity against *S pyogenes*.

Therapy for simple pediatric skin or soft-tissue infection is usually recommended for 7 to 10 days, and individualized according to clinical response.

Amoxicillin or penicillin is the appropriate empiric therapy for erysipelas, because these antimicrobials are the first-line therapies in treating *S pyogenes* infections.

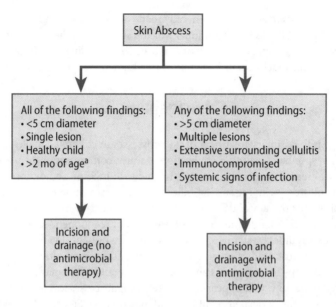

Figure 7-1. Skin abscess management.
a No published trials on lower limits of patient age. Expert recommendation.

Surgical debridement is mandatory when necrotizing fasciitis is suspected. Antibiotic therapy should initially target both gram-positive and gram-negative organisms; vancomycin plus clindamycin and cefepime represents good empiric coverage. Treatment should also target pain control and anticipate the complications that rapidly evolve in the patient with necrotizing fasciitis, including shock, multiorgan dysfunction, and need for blood product support in the setting of multiple debridement procedures.

Table 7-1 summarizes the clinical features, common pathogens, diagnosis, and management of the skin and soft-tissue infections previously described.

Table 7-1. Overview of Common Skin and Soft-Tissue Infections in the Outpatient Setting

Type of Skin and Soft-Tissue Infection	Clinical Features	Common Pathogens	Diagnosis	Treatment Options
Abscess (furuncle, carbuncle)	• Painful erythematous indurated nodule ± o Fluctuance o Drainage o Associated cellulitis • Fever maybe present • Signs of systemic toxicity rare	Staphylococcus. aureus (MRSA and MSSA)	• History and physical examination ± fine-needle aspiration biopsy or ultrasonography, when indicated	• Local care (warm compresses) • Incision and drainage ± clindamycin or cephalexin
Impetigo (nonbullous and bullous)	*Nonbullous:* small vesicles or pustules → rupture → crusted yellow lesions *Bullous:* vesicles and bullae with clear yellow fluid	• S aureus (less commonly MRSA) • Streptococcus pyogenes	• History and physical examination • Routine skin cultures not recommended	*Mild/localized:* topical mupirocin *Moderate/diffuse:* clindamycin or cephalexin
Cellulitis	• Skin erythema, edema, and warmth • Progresses over days	• S aureus (MRSA and MSSA) • S pyogenes	• History and physical examination • Radiographic evaluation (US, MRI) for severe cases	Clindamycin or cephalexin
Erysipelas	• Skin erythema, edema, and warmth • Raised • Clear demarcation from uninvolved skin • Abrupt onset • Often signs of systemic toxicity	S pyogenes (also known as GAS)	History and physical examination	Penicillin or amoxicillin
Ecthyma	Local deep ulcer with necrotic center	• Pseudomonas aeruginosa • Other gram-negative pathogens • S aureus • Aspergillus • Fusarium	• History and physical examination • Biopsy	Targeting S aureus and P aeruginosa: vancomycin + cefepime or meropenem; addition of antifungals for patient with known malignancy and neutropenia
Necrotizing fasciitis	Toxic-appearing child; pain out of proportion to soft-tissue findings	• S pyogenes • S aureus • Can be polymicrobial	Clinical; prompt surgical consultation (Do not delay by ordering imaging studies.)	• Surgical debridement • Vancomycin and cefepime • Pain control • Anticipation of shock and multiorgan involvement

Abbreviations: GAS, group A Streptococcus; MRI, magnetic resonance imaging; MRSA, methicillin-resistant Staphylococcus aureus; MSSA, methicillin-susceptible Staphylococcus aureus; US, ultrasound.

Suggested Reading
· · · · · · · · · · · · · · · · · ·

Duong M, Markwell S, Peter J, Barenkamp S. Randomized, controlled trial of antibiotics in the management of community-acquired skin abscesses in the pediatric patient. *Ann Emerg Med.* 2010;55(5):401–407

George A, Rubin G. A systematic review and meta-analysis of treatments for impetigo. *Br J Gen Pract.* 2003;53(491):480–487

Iverson K, Haritos D, Thomas R, Kannikeswaran N. The effect of bedside ultrasound on diagnosis and management of soft tissue infections in a pediatric ED. *Am J Emerg Med.* 2012;30(8):1347–1351

Lee MC, Rios AM, Aten MF, et al. Management and outcome of children with skin and soft tissue abscesses caused by community-acquired methicillin-resistant *Staphylococcus aureus. Pediatr Infect Dis J.* 2004;23(2):123–127

Liu C, Brayer A, Cosgrove SE, et al. Clinical practice guidelines by the Infectious Diseases Society of America for the treatment of methicillin-resistant *Staphylococcus aureus* infections in adults and children. *Clin Infect Dis.* 2011;52(3):e18–e55

Stevens DL, Bisno AL, Chambers HF, et al. Practice guidelines for the diagnosis and management of skin and soft-tissue infections. *Clin Infect Dis.* 2005;41(10):1373–1406

Stryjewski ME, Chambers HF. Skin and soft-tissue infections caused by community-acquired methicillin-resistant *Staphylococcus aureus. Clin Infect Dis.* 2008;46(Suppl 5): S368–S377

Swartz MN. Clinical practice. Cellulitis. *N Engl J Med.* 2004;350(9):904–912

PART

1

Infectious Diseases

CHAPTER 8

Anaerobic Infections

Mary R. Tanner, MD, and Jason G. Newland, MD, MEd

Key Points

- Anaerobes are common components of normal microbial flora.
- Anaerobic infections should be suspected when suggested by infection site, clinical picture, or microbiologic studies.
- Diagnostic considerations include specialized collection, transport, and culture techniques for anaerobes.
- Treatment depends on the type of infection, location, and suspected etiologic agents.

Overview

Anaerobes are important and sometimes under-recognized pathogens in the pediatric population. Anaerobic bacteria are defined by their requirement for a low- or no-oxygen state to replicate and are typically recognized as normal colonizing flora of skin and other mucosal surfaces. In clinical practice, anaerobes are frequently identified in mixed cultures with aerobic bacteria, and are often found as coinfecting pathogens in clinical conditions, such as bowel perforation or sinusitis.

Cause and Differential Diagnosis

Anaerobic organisms colonize the upper respiratory tract and mouth, as well as gastrointestinal (GI) tract, female genitourinary system, and surface of the skin. In the GI tract, which is highly populated by aerobic organisms, anaerobes still account for 95% to 99% of the normal flora. Box 8-1 shows some of the more common organisms by site of colonization.

Box 8-1. Selected Anaerobes/Microaerophiles by Typical Sites of Significant Colonization

Oral/Upper Respiratory Tract	Gastrointestinal	Genitourinary	Skin
• *Streptococcus* spp • *Fusobacterium* spp • *Prevotella* spp • *Bacteroides* spp	• *Bacteroides* spp • *Peptostreptococcus* spp • *Clostridium* spp • *Bifidobacterium* spp	• *Lactobacillus* spp • *Prevotella* spp • *Peptostreptococcus* spp • *Bacteroides* spp	• *Propionibacterium* spp • *Peptostreptococcus* spp

Abbreviation: spp, species.

Anaerobes are frequently involved in polymicrobial infections related to sites where they form a significant part of the normal flora. Examples include odontogenic infections, pneumonia associated with aspiration of oral contents, peritonitis associated with ruptured viscous, infections associated with human or animal bites, and abscesses or necrotizing infections of the skin, brain, lung, or female genital tract.

Because definitive diagnosis often requires culture of suspected infected sites, the exclusion of specimen contamination by endogenous flora is essential. Diagnosis depends on appropriate culture with use of proper media, transport, and storage conditions. When anaerobic infections are considered, the differential diagnosis depends on the site of involvement, mechanism of injury, and underlying host factors. Other diagnostic possibilities sometimes include infections caused by other pathogens, malignancies, foreign body reactions, vascular diseases, and inflammatory processes (eg, colitis). Because certain underlying conditions increase the risk of anaerobic infection (eg, leukemia with neutropenic colitis and perforation), a primary process with secondary infection should also be considered.

Clinical Features

Anaerobic infections can present with a variety of clinical pictures. The following situations should prompt consideration of possible anaerobic pathogens:

- The infection is in a location commonly associated with anaerobes.
- A patient's infection is failing to resolve with appropriate empiric therapy targeting aerobic bacteria.
- A culture from an evidently infected site fails to grow a pathogen.
- The Gram stain indicates mixed bacterial flora.
- A wound exhibits gas formation or a putrid odor.
- Findings are suggestive of a clostridial syndrome.

The level of clinical suspicion for an anaerobic infection must be based on the patient's specific findings and risk factors.

Central Nervous System Infections

Anaerobes are frequently isolated from brain abscesses and subdural empyemas. They are less likely to be the cause of classic meningitis, so isolation of anaerobes from the cerebrospinal fluid should prompt consideration of an occult parameningeal abscess or complicated meningitis. Brain abscesses, especially solitary lesions, are often caused by spread from a contiguous site and can be a complication of head and neck infections like otitis media and sinusitis. In contrast, hematogenous spread of bacteria often causes multiple brain lesions, classically along the distribution of the middle cerebral artery. Presence of a ventriculoperitoneal shunt increases the risk of GI anaerobes as potential pathogens, particularly in the setting of peritonitis.

Head and Neck Infections

Anaerobes thrive as normal flora of the mouth and upper respiratory tract, so they should always be considered as possible pathogens in head and neck infections. They are implicated in most odontogenic infections, including dental abscesses and perimandibular space infections.

Because of their ubiquitous presence in the mouth, it is critical to include coverage for anaerobes in the treatment of potentially life-threatening head and neck infections. Ludwig angina, for example, is an aggressive cellulitis involving the floor of the mouth. Without effective treatment, it can rapidly progress to cause airway compromise. It is usually secondary to a dental infection and is generally polymicrobial.

Classic Lemierre syndrome or jugular vein suppurative thrombophlebitis occurs most commonly in the adolescent patient who presents with sore throat, neck pain, and a septic syndrome. *Fusobacterium necrophorum* is the anaerobic bacterium frequently implicated in this syndrome. Septic emboli are common and may result in abscesses in the lungs or other organs.

Actinomycosis is caused by *Actinomyces* species bacteria, most typically *Actinomyces israelii*. *Actinomyces* species are part of normal human flora but can cause infection when tissue injury or breach of the mucosa allows them access to structures beyond their colonization sites. Infection spreads from the site of origin without regard for normal tissue planes. Localized pain and induration may progress to abscesses and firm ("woody") nodular or mass-like lesions, which may develop draining sinus tracts and fistulae. Cervicofacial infection, most frequently along the mandible, is the most common clinical manifestation. Thoracic and abdominal infections are the two other most common anatomic sites. *Actinomyces* species infections may also be identified in the pelvis, liver, heart, testicles, brain, skin, and other anatomic sites.

With regard to oropharyngeal abscesses, such as infections of the submandibular, parapharyngeal, retropharyngeal, and peritonsillar spaces, clinical findings depend on the site of infection. Common features include pain, fever, asymmetry on examination, or limitation in range of motion of the neck. Predominant organisms depend on the site of origin. Many infections are polymicrobial, and anaerobes are the sole isolates in some patients. Anaerobes are also potential pathogens in chronic otitis media and sinusitis.

Pulmonary Infections

Anaerobic lower respiratory tract infections are usually the sequelae of an aspiration event. Consequently, pathogens are most often flora of the upper airway or GI tract. In the acute setting, symptoms follow the usual pneumonia pattern with fever, cough, and respiratory distress. Generally, symptomatology cannot distinguish between aspiration and community-acquired pneumonia, so empiric coverage for anaerobes should be considered in any patient with risk factors for aspiration. Lung abscess formation 1 to 2 weeks after an aspiration event is a well-described complication of anaerobic pulmonary infection.

Thoracic actinomycosis may be caused by aspiration of oropharyngeal secretions, extension from cervicofacial infection, or esophageal disruption. Pneumonia is a common manifestation, which may be complicated by abscesses, empyema, or pleurodermal sinuses. Other possible manifestations include single or multiple pulmonary or mediastinal masses. (See Head and Neck Infections section for additional discussion of actinomycosis.)

Intra-abdominal Infections

Anaerobes are a significant part of normal flora in the intestinal tract, and their presence should be considered any time an infection is related to a breach of the natural GI barriers. Anaerobic coverage should be included in any case of bowel perforation, whether surgical or due to a pathologic process.

In addition to their role in peritonitis and intra-abdominal abscesses, anaerobes can cause intraluminal pathology. *Clostridium perfringens* causes acute self-limiting gastroenteritis when spores are ingested, usually from improperly prepared meat. *Clostridium difficile* is another potential GI pathogen. It can exist in the GI tract as normal flora, but under certain circumstances, toxigenic strains can produce colitis. The most commonly recognized trigger is antibiotic therapy that causes alteration in the usual colonic microflora.

Less commonly, other *Clostridium* species can cause severe systemic reactions from ingestion of spores or toxins. *Clostridium botulinum* produces a neurotoxin that can cause weakness, paralysis, cranial neuropathies, and autonomic changes. Botulism can be caused by ingestion of the thermolabile toxin (foodborne type), ingestion of spores that then produce toxin in the GI tract (infant or adult intestinal colonization type), or contamination of a wound by the bacteria (wound type). The most common type in pediatrics is infant botulism. The characteristic presentation is an infant with descending or global hypotonia (ie, the "floppy baby") and constipation. Alterations in cranial nerve function occur early, but symptoms have usually progressed before medical recognition. Wound and foodborne botulisms are more common in older age groups. Rare cases of older children and adults with infant botulism have been described, usually in the setting of preexisting GI tract pathology. Foodborne botulism often begins with prodromal symptoms, including abdominal pain, diarrhea, and vomiting. Symptomatic disease is characterized by cranial nerve palsies and symmetric descending flaccid paralysis, but degree of symptomatology can vary significantly between cases.

Abdominal actinomycosis may occur secondary to trauma or intestinal perforation. Infection of the appendix or ileocecal region may produce symptoms similar to appendicitis. Additional manifestations may include intra-abdominal masses, abscesses, and peritoneal-dermal sinuses. (See Head and Neck Infections section for additional discussion of actinomycosis.)

Genitourinary Infections

Anaerobes are normal flora in the female genital tract and second only to sexually transmitted organisms in terms of potential pathogens in this area. Coverage for anaerobes should be considered in empiric treatment regimens for infections of the female genital tract.

Actinomycosis can also present as a pelvic infection, and in some cases has been linked to use of intrauterine contraceptive devices (IUDs). Some described manifestations include pelvic inflammatory disease, abscesses, and masses that may be mistaken for gynecologic malignancies. (See Head and Neck Infections section for additional discussion of actinomycosis.)

Skin and Soft-Tissue Infections

Anaerobes thrive in the low-oxygen environment of injured tissue and are frequent pathogens in skin and soft-tissue infections, especially in wounds that are below the waist, deep, or chronic. They are potential pathogens in any skin infection but particularly characteristic of bite wounds, diabetic foot ulcers, decubitus ulcers, postsurgical wounds, and infections adjacent to mucosal surfaces. Anaerobes have been implicated in necrotizing forms of cellulitis, fasciitis, and myositis. One classically described anaerobic infection is gas gangrene or myonecrosis. Traumatic gas gangrene is most often caused by *C perfringens*, although other *Clostridium* species have also been identified. Myonecrosis is characterized by pain, skin discoloration, bulla, gas formation in tissues, and a putrid odor. Major risk factors include wounds contaminated with soil or stool, foreign bodies, tissue ischemia, and immune system dysfunction.

Another clostridial syndrome, tetanus, is caused when *Clostridium tetani* spores gain access to injured tissue. The tetanospasmin they produce causes increased muscle tone/rigidity, painful spasms, and autonomic instability. The clinical picture may evolve from localized spasms into generalized symptoms. The usual source of entry is a contaminated wound, but in the case of neonatal tetanus, entry can result from infection of the umbilical stump.

Botulism can result from *C botulinum* infection of wounds. Risk factors include traumatic injuries and use of illicit injection drugs, and disease is characterized by cranial nerve palsies and symmetric descending flaccid paralysis. Prodromal symptoms are usually absent in wound botulism, and unlike other botulism syndromes, fever and leukocytosis may be present.

Evaluation

Microbiologic identification of anaerobes requires appropriate specimen collection, transport, and incubation techniques. Aspirates and biopsies are the preferred collection methods because swabs allow exposure of the specimen to air. Samples should be transported in anaerobic transport tubes. Anaerobic cultures require selective laboratory techniques and sometimes must be requested separately from standard aerobic cultures. Many laboratories also require a special request for susceptibility testing of these organisms. Mass spectrometry bacterial identification methods, where available, may provide more rapid identification of certain anaerobic species.

Histopathology may be useful in evaluation of suspected actinomycosis. Microscopic evaluation of discharge from *Actinomyces* species infections sometimes reveals characteristic "sulfur granules"—dense aggregates of bacterial filaments mixed with cellular debris. Actinomycetes appear as beaded, branched, gram-positive bacilli under microscopic evaluation. They are acid-fast negative, in contrast to *Nocardia* species bacteria, which are variably acid-fast positive. *Actinomyces* species can be species to identify in culture, and recovery can be complicated by previous antibiotic use and other issues. The microbiology laboratory should be informed when a diagnosis of actinomycosis is being considered. Diagnosis may also be made via immunofluorescent stains, 16s rRNA sequencing, and organism-specific polymerase chain reaction. *Actinomyces* species frequently present as part of a polymicrobial infection, and isolation of *Aggregatibacter actinomycetemcomitans* may predict the presence of actinomycetes, though *A actinomycetemcomitans* also functions as an independent pathogen.

Table 8-1 outlines evaluations specific to clostridial syndromes.

Management

General treatment considerations include wound care as indicated, drainage of abscesses when required, and selection of appropriate antimicrobial therapy (Table 8-2). Because of the challenges and delays inherent in isolating anaerobes from conventional culture techniques, decisions to provide antibiotic coverage for anaerobes must often be based on clinical suspicion of anaerobic involvement. Anaerobes are a heterogeneous group of bacteria, and susceptibility patterns may vary widely between organisms. For example, many anaerobes are penicillin susceptible, but in some species resistance is common. Some common antibiotics with generally broad anaerobic coverage include β-lactamase–β-lactam combination antibiotics, clindamycin, metronidazole, and

Table 8-1. Evaluation of Suspected Clostridial Syndromes

Suspected Syndrome	Diagnostic Tests
Botulism	Infant • Serum assays for botulinum toxin are often negative. • Definitive diagnosis is via isolation of *Clostridium botulinum* organisms or toxin from stool. Stool should be sent for specialized culture and toxin neutralization bioassay. • Sample should be obtained in timely fashion; enema may be used if necessary. Sample containers should not contain fixatives. • Tests performed by specialized laboratories. Contact state health department or regional CDC office. • Treatment should not be delayed for test results. Foodborne • Serum assay for toxin should be performed. Toxin identification may also be performed on stool or suspected food. • Test performed by specialized laboratories. Contact state health department or regional CDC office. Wound • Diagnosis is via isolation of *C botulinum* organisms or toxin from wound sample. • Serum toxin assays may be negative even in confirmed infection. Stool studies are not indicated. In all types, presumptive diagnosis based on clinical presentation is crucial because results from confirmatory testing may be delayed. EMG studies can be used as part of the initial evaluation, but are not required for the diagnosis.
Tetanus	Diagnosed clinically from presentation, history, and exclusion of other causes of spasms. Culture of *Clostridium tetani* can be difficult, and negative cultures do not exclude diagnosis.
Myonecrosis	The presumptive diagnosis is clinical. Definitive diagnosis is via identification of organism in culture, usually obtained through samples from surgical debridement/exploration of wound. Blood cultures should also be performed.
Clostridium difficile colitis	To distinguish colonization from true pathology, *C difficile* testing should take place only in patients with characteristic symptoms, and usually only in patients older than a year of age (because of high rates of colonization in younger children). Diagnosis is based off clinical picture and either of the following findings: • A stool test positive for *C difficile* toxins. Specific tests vary by institution. • Endoscopic findings of pseudomembranous colitis.

Abbreviations: CDC, Centers for Disease Control and Prevention; EMG, electromyogram.

Derived from American Academy of Pediatrics. *Red Book: 2015 Report of the Committee on Infectious Diseases.* Kimberlin DW, Brady MT, Jackson MA, Long SS, eds. 30th ed. Elk Grove Village, IL: American Academy of Pediatrics; 2015.

Table 8-2. Overview of Possible Empiric Antibiotic Regimens for Selected Clinical Syndromes in Immunocompetent Hosts[a]

Anatomic Location	Suspected Pathogens	Empiric Antibiotic Considerations
CNS		
Brain abscess Subdural empyema	Differs by primary infection site	Metronidazole is the preferred anti-anaerobic agent for brain abscesses and should be used in combination with a 3rd- or 4th-generation cephalosporin and vancomycin. Clindamycin and β-lactam–β-lactamase combinations should be avoided because they do not attain reliable CSF concentrations. Carbapenems (meropenem or imipenem) are an alternative choice and can be used in combination with vancomycin for initial empiric therapy.
Head/Neck		
Oropharyngeal abscesses	*Streptococcus* species, oral anaerobes, *Staphylococcus aureus*, gram-negative bacilli	*Peritonsillar:* ampicillin-sulbactam *or* clindamycin *Pharyngeal:* ampicillin-sulbactam *or* ceftriaxone + either clindamycin or metronidazole Add vancomycin depending on severity and risk factors for MRSA.
Ludwig angina	*Streptococcus* species, oral anaerobes, *Staphylococcus aureus*, gram-negative bacilli	Broad-spectrum empiric therapy is indicated pending pathogen identification. Possible regimens include ceftriaxone + metronidazole + vancomycin or carbapenem (ie, meropenem or imipenem) + vancomycin *or* β-lactam–β-lactamase inhibitor + vancomycin.
Jugular vein suppurative thrombophlebitis (Lemierre syndrome)	*Fusobacterium* species, other oral anaerobes, *Streptococcus* species, *S aureus*, gram-negative bacilli	Broad-spectrum empiric therapy is indicated pending pathogen identification. Possible regimens include ceftriaxone + metronidazole + vancomycin or carbapenem (ie, meropenem or imipenem) + vancomycin *or* β-lactam–β-lactamase inhibitor + vancomycin. The first two regimens are preferred if CNS involvement is suspected.
Chronic sinusitis	Oral anaerobes, gram-negative bacilli, *S aureus*	Amoxicillin-clavulanate Clindamycin is recommended for penicillin-allergic patients or if MRSA is suspected.
Dental abscess	Oral streptococci (eg, viridans, mutans), oral anaerobes	*IV:* ampicillin-sulbactam *or* clindamycin *or* penicillin G + metronidazole *Oral:* clindamycin *or* amoxicillin-clavulanate

Lung		
Aspiration pneumonia	Vary by patient age and clinical scenario	*IV:* clindamycin *or* ampicillin-sulbactam *Oral:* clindamycin *or* amoxicillin-clavulanate
Abdomen		
Complicated intra-abdominal infections (Non-biliary)	Enteric anaerobes, *Enterococcus* species, gram-positive aerobic cocci, or gram-negative bacilli	*Possible regimens include* *Single agents:* piperacillin-tazobactam *or* carbapenem (meropenem, ertapenem, or imipenem–cilastatin) *Combination therapy:* 3rd- or 4th-generation cephalosporin (ceftriaxone, cefotaxime, ceftazidime, or cefepime) + metronidazole *or* aminoglycoside (gentamicin or tobramycin) + metronidazole + ampicillin *Health care–associated:* Include agent expected to be active against *Enterococcus faecalis* (ampicillin, piperacillin-tazobactam, vancomycin). Consider adding vancomycin for MRSA depending on disease severity and risk factors. Consider adding empiric antifungal for *Candida* species if significant risk factors (eg, recent abdominal surgery, anastomotic leaks, necrotizing pancreatitis, neonates with necrotizing enterocolitis). *Community-acquired, severe disease:* Consider including agent expected to be active against *E faecalis* (ampicillin, piperacillin–tazobactam, vancomycin).
Clostridium difficile colitis	*C. difficile*	*Non-severe disease:* Oral metronidazole. Oral vancomycin if metronidazole contraindicated or refractory disease. *Severe disease:* Oral vancomycin ± IV metronidazole. Rectal vancomycin + IV metronidazole if oral route contraindicated. *Recurrent disease:* Metronidazole may be used for first relapse but avoid repeated courses. Use tapered or pulse regimens of oral vancomycin for recurrent disease. IV vancomycin is ineffective. Discontinue precipitating antibiotic therapy or narrow spectrum if possible. Avoid antiperistaltic medications.

Continued

Table 8-2 *(cont)*

Anatomic Location	Suspected Pathogens	Empiric Antibiotic Considerations
Botulism	*Clostridium botulinum*	*Supportive care:* General supportive care, including intubation/mechanical ventilation if signs of impending respiratory failure. *Antitoxin* • Human-derived botulinum immune globulin: For use in children <1 y. Administer as soon as possible in the course of infant botulism. • Equine serum heptavalent botulism antitoxin: Used for children >1 y and adults. Indicated if index of suspicion is high and disease progressing. Can cause sensitization and anaphylaxis. • Suspected botulism is a nationally notifiable disease and should be reported immediately. Consultation with the CDC or state health department is usually required to obtain antitoxin. *Antibiotics:* Antibiotics are not recommended for infant or GI botulism. Used after antitoxin in wound botulism. Recommended: Penicillin G or metronidazole. Wound infections are often polymicrobial, so additional coverage may be required. Aminoglycosides are contraindicated.
Skin/Soft Tissue		
Gas gangrene	*Clostridium* species	*Wound care:* Surgical debridement and removal of foreign bodies are critical to recovery. Efficacy of hyperbaric oxygen therapy remains unproven. *Antibiotics:* IV penicillin G + clindamycin (Clindamycin alone may be used in penicillin-allergic patients.)
Tetanus	*Clostridium tetani*	*Supportive care:* Intubation for airway protection because of potential laryngospasm is required for generalized tetanus. Respiratory support, spasm control, nutrition, and cardiovascular monitoring are crucial to care. *Wound care:* Debridement and wound care are critical. Antimicrobials will not eradicate bacteria in necrotic tissue. *Toxin neutralization:* TIG. Infiltration of part of the dose locally around the wound is usually recommended. Tetanus immunization is indicated. *Antibiotics:* Oral or IV metronidazole is preferred.

Abbreviations: CDC, Centers for Disease Control and Prevention; CSF, cerebrospinal fluid; CNS, central nervous system; GI, gastrointestinal; IV, intravenous; MRSA, methicillin-resistant *Staphylococcus aureus*; TIG, tetanus immune globulin.

[a] Immunocompromised patients require consideration of additional pathogens, and in many cases, broader empiric antimicrobial coverage.

carbapenems. However, it is important to note that susceptibility patterns may shift over time and attention should be paid to updates in antimicrobial recommendations. For example, increasing clindamycin resistance among *Bacteroides fragilis* has led to the recommendation to use metronidazole or another anti-anaerobic agent for infections involving intestinal flora.

Recommended medical therapy for actinomycosis typically begins with intravenous penicillin G or ampicillin for 4 to 6 weeks, followed by an extended course of high-dose oral penicillin (up to 2 g/day for adults), usually for a total of 6 to 12 months. In the initial phase of treatment, additional or broader-spectrum antimicrobial agents are sometimes required to treat co-pathogens. Oral antibiotic therapy for the entire therapeutic course has been demonstrated to be effective in some cases of cervicofacial actinomycosis. Amoxicillin may be used as an alternative to oral penicillin. For penicillin-intolerant patients, alternatives include clindamycin, erythromycin, and doxycycline. Other antimicrobial agents that appear active in vitro include ceftriaxone, clarithromycin, linezolid, piperacillin-tazobactam, and meropenem, though susceptibilities may vary by *Actinomyces* species for some agents. Several of these agents have been used as part of successful treatment regimens described in case reports. Antibiotics considered to have poor or absent activity against *Actinomyces* species include cephalexin, oxacillin and dicloxacillin, fluoroquinolones, metronidazole, aminoglycosides, and aztreonam. In addition to medical management, surgical drainage, debridement, or excision of lesions is often required. Treatment of pelvic actinomycosis associated with an IUD should include IUD removal.

Suggested Reading

American Academy of Pediatrics. *Actinomycosis*; *Bacteroides* and *Prevotella* infections; Clostridial infections; *Fusobacterium* infections; Tetanus. In: Kimberlin DW, Brady MT, Jackson MA, Long SS, eds. *Red Book: 2015 Report of the Committee on Infectious Diseases.* 30th ed. Elk Grove Village, IL: American Academy of Pediatrics; 2015

American Academy of Pediatrics Committee on Infectious Diseases. *Clostridium difficile* infection in infants and children. *Pediatrics.* 2013;131(1):196–200

Brook I. Spectrum and treatment of anaerobic infections. *J Infect Chemother.* 2016;22:1–13

Kuppalii K, Livorsi D, Talati NJ, Osborn M. Lemierre's syndrome due to *Fusobacterium necrophorum. Lancet Infect Dis.* 2012;12(10):808–815

Lin HW, O'Neill A, Cunningham MJ. Ludwig's angina in the pediatric population. *Clin Pediatr (Phila).* 2009;48(6):583–587

Solomkin JS, Mazuski JE, Bradley JS, et al. Diagnosis and management of complicated intra-abdominal infection in adults and children: guidelines by the Surgical Infection Society and the Infectious Diseases Society of America. *Clin Infect Dis.* 2010;50(2):133–164

CHAPTER 9

Brucella

Kimberly C. Martin, DO, MPH, and José R. Romero, MD

Key Points

- The most common mode of transmission of brucellosis in the United States is ingestion of imported unpasteurized milk or cheese products.
- Brucellosis should be considered in all returning travelers being evaluated for a fever of unknown origin.
- Fever and nonspecific concerns are the most common symptoms of acute brucellosis.
- All patients with brucellar infections will require antimicrobial therapy with multiple antibiotics to effectively treat the disease.
- A specialist in pediatric infectious diseases should be consulted in all cases of suspected or confirmed brucellosis in children.

Overview

Brucellosis is transmittable to humans through the ingestion of infected meat, through unpasteurized milk or cheese products, or via contact with secretions from infected animals. Most cases diagnosed in the United States occur in travelers to endemic countries or are secondary to foodborne transmission from imported unpasteurized milk products. Consequently, most cases of brucellosis diagnosed in the United States are geographically clustered in states bordering Mexico. Confirmed infection with a *Brucella* species requires antimicrobial therapy in all patients because of its propensity to result in chronic infection.

Causes and Differential Diagnosis

The genus *Brucella* contains 6 species, 4 of which are known to cause disease in humans (*Brucella abortus, Brucella melitensis, Brucella suis,* and *Brucella canis*).

The differential diagnosis of patients with fever of unknown origin should include brucellosis, particularly if the patient has the appropriate risk factors, such as travel to an endemic region or consumption of unpasteurized dairy products. All patients being evaluated for prolonged fevers of unknown origin should be questioned regarding their dietary habits, specifically the consumption of unpasteurized milk and milk-based products (eg, fresh cheeses) and their animal source (cow or goat). In the returning traveler, patients should also be queried regarding any animal contact. Patients should be further questioned regarding personal and parental occupation along with hobbies that may lead to animal contact.

Other infectious diseases to be considered in the differential diagnosis in a patient with appropriate exposures include malaria, typhoid fever, chikungunya, tuberculosis, and visceral leishmaniasis. In addition, conditions such as juvenile idiopathic arthritis and oncologic processes should be considered.

Clinical Features

Clinical presentations of brucellosis range from subclinical to chronic and recurrent disease. The initial presentation of the disease is typically nonspecific in nature, consisting of fever, malaise, lethargy, and anorexia. Symptoms usually begin approximately 2 to 4 weeks after exposure and can be acute or subtle in nature. In addition to the nonspecific concerns listed previously, the most common localized symptom of the disease in children is osteoarticular involvement, usually of the large peripheral joints. While monoarthritis is more common, polyarthritis involving 2 or more joints has been reported. Although sacroiliitis is commonly associated with brucellosis in adults, it is rare in children.

The central nervous system (CNS) is also commonly involved in cases of brucellosis. Even without direct infection of the CNS, children frequently report headache and exhibit inattentiveness. Additionally, disturbances of mood, such as depression, have occasionally been noted. Meningitis is the most common of the neurologic complications. Other CNS presentations include encephalitis, myelitis, neuritis, and brain abscess.

Uveitis is the most common ocular complication. In addition, endophthalmitis, optic neuritis, and chorioretinitis have also been reported.

Hematologic derangements, such as anemia, leukopenia, and thrombocytopenia, are frequently observed in children and resolve with antibiotic therapy. Severe hematologic manifestations are much less commonly reported.

Other organ systems involved in brucellar infection include the respiratory, gastrointestinal, and genitourinary tracts. Cough is often present in children with brucellosis, although complications such as pneumonia, pulmonary nodules, and empyema are very uncommon. Gastrointestinal symptoms, such as nausea, vomiting, abdominal pain, and anorexia with associated weight loss, are often seen. Splenomegaly and hepatitis are rarely observed. Orchitis and epididymitis are common genitourinary complications that are difficult to diagnose and may initially be misdiagnosed as due to a malignancy.

Cardiac manifestations of brucellosis are much less commonly seen than the conditions listed previously. Endocarditis, myocarditis, and pericarditis, in association with rare severe valvular disease requiring cardiac surgery, have been reported with brucellar infections. Cutaneous manifestations include contact dermatitis, generalized urticaria, and inoculation abscesses among the varied skin eruptions seen in patients infected with *Brucella*.

Evaluation

Definitive diagnosis of brucellosis is based on isolation of the organism through culture. Blood, bone marrow, and fluids such as synovial and cerebrospinal fluids should be cultured for the presence of the organism. Laboratory personnel should be alerted to the possibility of a brucellar infection so that cultures can be incubated for a minimum of 4 weeks and to allow for the institution of appropriate laboratory precautions.

In cases of brucellar meningitis, analysis of the cerebrospinal fluid reveals a lymphocytic pleocytosis with elevated protein and normal or low glucose concentrations.

In addition to culture, serologic testing can confirm the diagnosis. The serum agglutination test is considered to be the criterion standard. The assay can detect antibodies to *B abortus, B suis,* and *B melitensis.* A fourfold rise or greater in titers of paired sera, taken 2 weeks apart, confirms the diagnosis in patients exhibiting compatible signs and symptoms. While a single titer is not considered diagnostic, in patients with acute infection who live in non-endemic areas, a titer of 1:160 or greater within 2 to 4 weeks of illness onset is seen.

It is of note that elevated IgG titers may be seen in acute or chronic infection and cases of relapse. IgM antibodies may persist for years following the primary infection.

Enzyme immunoassay for the detection of antibodies to *Brucella* appears to be the most sensitive laboratory method. However, it is currently not standardized across all commercial laboratories.

Management

Treatment of brucellosis depends on the clinical stage of infection (ie, acute or chronic) and in certain cases its extent. Because of a high relapse rate associated with monotherapy, combination treatment is always used in pediatric and adult patients. Table 9-1 lists the currently recommended therapy for acute brucellosis in pediatric patients by age. In addition, therapies for meningitis, endocarditis, and osteomyelitis caused by *Brucella* are presented.

Although no specific follow-up is required for patients diagnosed with brucellosis, given the prolonged length of time that antimicrobials are prescribed, all patients should be followed closely during treatment to augment adherence and monitor for untoward effects of the treatment. Patients treated with long-term trimethoprim/sulfamethoxazole should be evaluated routinely

Table 9-1. Antimicrobial Therapy for Acute Brucellosis in Pediatric Patients: Evidence Level I (Acute *Brucella* Disease) and Evidence Level III Data (Complicated *Brucella* Disease)

Condition	Antimicrobial Agent	Dose	Adult Maximum	Route	Minimum Duration of Treatment
Acute brucellosis (age <8 y)	TMP/SMX + Rifampin	TMP, 10 mg/kg/d, and SMX, 50 mg/kg/d, divided twice daily 15–20 mg/kg/d divided twice daily	TMP, 480 mg/d, and SMX, 2.4 g/d 600–900 mg/d daily or divided twice daily	Orally Orally	4–6 wk 6 wk
Acute brucellosis (age >8 y)	Doxycycline + Rifampin	2–4 mg/kg/d divided twice daily 15–20 mg/kg/d divided twice daily	200 mg/d 600–900 mg/d daily or divided twice daily	Orally Orally	6 wk 6 wk
Meningitis and endocarditis (age <8 y)	TMP/SMX + Rifampin + Gentamicin	TMP, 10 mg/kg/d, and SMX, 50 mg/kg/d, divided twice daily 15–20 mg/kg/d divided twice daily 5 mg/kg/d as single daily dose	TMP, 480 mg/d, and SMX, 2.4 g/d 600–900 mg/d daily or divided twice daily	Orally Orally IM or IV	4–6 mo 4–6 mo 7–14 d
Osteomyelitis (age <8 y)	Same as meningitis and endocarditis				6 wk
Meningitis and endocarditis (age >8 y)	Doxycycline + Rifampin + Gentamicin	2–4 mg/kg/d divided twice daily 15–20 mg/kg/d divided twice daily 5 mg/kg/d as single daily dose	200 mg/d 600–900 mg/d daily or divided twice daily	Orally Orally IM or IV	4–6 mo 4–6 mo 7–14 d
Osteomyelitis (age >8 y)	Same as meningitis and endocarditis				6 wk

Abbreviations: IM, intramuscularly; IV, intravenously; SMX, sulfamethoxazole; TMP, trimethoprim.

for bone marrow suppression. Those receiving gentamicin should be closely monitored for potential ototoxicity and nephrotoxicity. Patients treated with doxycycline should be cautioned against prolonged sun exposure and use sunscreen for all outdoor activities. Patients should always be advised to take medications, especially doxycycline, with an adequate volume of liquid so as to prevent the development of erosive pill esophagitis.

Despite appropriate therapy, some patients will continue to have nonspecific concerns, such as prolonged fatigue. Prolongation of the antimicrobial course has not been shown to improve these symptoms. In very rare cases, chronic brucellar infection may emanate from a persistent focus, such as a deep tissue abscess or osteomyelitis. High resolution radiologic imaging and surgical consultation may be helpful in evaluating and treating an occult infection.

Suggested Reading

American Academy of Pediatrics. Brucellosis. In: Kimberlin DW, Brady MT, Jackson MA, Long SS, eds. *Red Book: 2015 Report of the Committee on Infectious Diseases.* 30th ed. Elk Grove Village, IL: American Academy of Pediatrics; 2015:268–270

Shaalan MA, Memish ZA, Al Mahmoud SA, et al. Brucellosis in children: clinical observation in 115 cases. *Int J Infect Dis.* 2002;6(3):182–186

Shen MW. Diagnostic and therapeutic challenges of childhood brucellosis in a nonendemic country. *Pediatrics.* 2008;121(5):e1178–e1183

Solera J. Update on brucellosis: therapeutic challenges. *Int J Antimicrob Agents.* 2010;36(Suppl 1):S18–S20

CHAPTER 10

Cat-Scratch Disease

Kevin B. Spicer, MD, PhD, MPH

Key Points

- Cat-scratch disease should be considered in any child with subacute focal lymphadenopathy and suspected cat or dog contact.

- Regional lymph node involvement of axillary or epitrochlear nodes is typically seen, but disease may also involve cervical or inguinal nodes depending on the body area inoculated by cat scratch.

- Remember to consider *Bartonella henselae* in the differential diagnosis for conjunctivitis with preauricular lymphadenopathy, prolonged fever/fever of unknown origin, hepatosplenic disease with microabscesses identified on ultrasound or computed tomographic scan, encephalitis/encephalopathy, and neuroretinitis.

- Mild disease can be treated symptomatically and with reassurance.

- Fluctuant, suppurative nodes can be symptomatically treated with needle aspiration, which may need to be repeated; incision and drainage or excisional biopsy is not recommended.

- Consultation with an infectious diseases specialist is recommended in the context of moderate to severe disease and for disease in the immunocompromised host.

Overview

Cat-scratch disease, in its most common form, is a self-limited, focal, subacute lymphadenopathy generally associated with known cat contact (Box 10-1). Kittens are more commonly implicated in development of the disease than older cats. The lymphadenopathy is most often unilateral and more typically involves the axillary region in response to cat scratch on the distal arms or hands, but lymphadenopathy may be seen in other regions (eg, inguinal, cervical) as well. The affected node is generally not erythematous or tender, but can become red, tender, and fluctuant in about 10% of cases. Although typically associated with cats, the condition has been seen in association with dog contact and dogs can be symptomatically infected.

Box 10-1. Clinical Manifestations of Cat-Scratch Disease (*Bartonella henselae* Infection)

Common
- Focal lymphadenopathy

Uncommon
- Conjunctivitis with preauricular lymphadenopathy
- Neuroretinitis
- Prolonged fever or FUO

Rare
- Aseptic meningitis
- Encephalopathy/encephalitis
- Endocarditis
- Erythema nodosum
- Glomerulonephritis
- Hepatosplenic disease with microabscesses
- Osteomyelitis
- Thrombocytopenic purpura

Abbreviation: FUO, fever of unknown origin.

Causes and Differential Diagnosis

Cat-scratch disease is caused by *Bartonella henselae,* a slow-growing, gram-negative bacillus, which is an organism found in a significant proportion of cats (especially kittens) and spread cat to cat by cat flea (*Ctenocephalides felis*) feces. Infected cats undergo an asymptomatic bacteremia, and *B henselae* infects the salivary glands. Infection is spread from direct contact with saliva or a scratch after paws are licked. Differential diagnosis includes other causes of lymphadenopathy/lymphadenitis, including bacterial lymphadenitis, mycobacterial disease, viral illness, parasitic disease, and neoplasm.

Clinical Features

In the typical form of the disease, regional lymphadenopathy proximal to the site of a cat scratch is the prominent finding. The lymphadenopathy is generally subacute, evolving slowly over 1 to 2 weeks. Most nodes resolve spontaneously, but about 10% may become progressively tender, erythematous, and fluctuant. In about two-thirds of patients, a distal papular/nodular lesion may be identified at the site of the original scratch. This lesion will follow the precipitating scratch in 1 to 2 weeks, with the lymphadenopathy noted subsequently, generally within 2 to 3 weeks of occurrence of the distal papule/nodule. Low-grade fever and mild systemic symptoms occur in approximately 30% of patients. Less common manifestations, which often occur without associated lymphadenitis or a recognized cat scratch, include prolonged high fever with no obvious focus of infection, conjunctivitis with preauricular lymphadenopathy, aseptic meningitis, encephalitis, hepatosplenic microabscesses associated with prolonged high fever, neuroretinitis, erythema nodosum, and osteomyelitis. In the immunocompromised host, rare vasoproliferative disorders may be seen. Bacillary angiomatosis involves skin and subcutaneous tissues, while bacillary peliosis affects solid organs with reticuloendothelial components. Disseminated disease can occur in the immunocompromised host.

Diagnosis

Diagnosis of cat-scratch disease is based on supportive history (eg, cat contact), consistent signs and symptoms, and laboratory investigations (Box 10-2). Laboratory support is provided primarily by *B henselae* serology (indirect fluorescence assay or enzyme immunoassay), with titers of IgG 1:64 or greater consistent with acute infection and titers 1:256 or greater strongly suggestive of acute infection. A fourfold increase from acute to convalescent titers (obtained 2 weeks after acute) is confirmatory. Corroborating support may also be supplied by positive IgM antibody, although this may not be seen and is not required for diagnosis in the context of consistent history, examination, and supportive IgG antibody results. Polymerase chain reaction testing of a needle aspirate from infected lymph nodes or other samples may also provide definitive support for

---

Box 10-2. Criteria for Diagnosis of Cat-Scratch Disease

Definitive Diagnosis

1. *Bartonella henselae* serology (EIA or indirect fluorescence assay) with IgG ≥1:256 or positive IgM

or

2. Fourfold rise in acute to convalescent IgG titers

or

3. Positive PCR confirmation for *B henselae*

or

4. Biopsy specimen with non-caseating granulomas and a positive Warthin-Starry silver stain

Supportive Criteria

1. Contact with cat or cat flea[a]
2. *B henselae* serology (EIA or indirect fluorescence assay) with IgG ≥1:64
3. Microabscesses noted on ultrasound or CT scan of liver or spleen
4. Culture of node aspirate negative for other organism
5. Negative serologies for other potential causes

Abbreviations: CT, computed tomographic; EIA, enzyme immunoassay; PCR, polymerase chain reaction.

[a] Clinical manifestations and positive serology have also been noted after dog and dog flea contact on rare occasions.

the diagnosis. The pathology of biopsied tissue shows granulomas, and organisms may also be identified through visualization via use of the Warthin-Starry silver stain. Culture of the organism is possible but difficult and therefore lacking in sensitivity and rarely available in commercial laboratories.

Management

The management of cat-scratch disease is summarized in Box 10-3.

In the immunocompetent individual with focal lymphadenopathy, treatment is generally considered unnecessary. Most cases will spontaneously resolve within 8 to 16 weeks. A single randomized clinical trial (Evidence Level I) compared azithromycin with placebo and found more rapid improvement with azithromycin, but long-term results were similar. Case series (Evidence Level II-2) have reported successful use of tetracyclines, trimethoprim/sulfamethoxazole, rifampin, ciprofloxacin, and aminoglycosides. In a retrospective review of a number of antibiotics, rifampin demonstrated the greatest clinical effectiveness. In vitro studies have found effective use of a broad range of antimicrobials, but this does not necessarily suggest clinical effectiveness of these drugs. For example, β-lactam antibiotics appear to be clinically ineffective although they demonstrate in vitro activity. For invasive disease, or disease in an immunocompromised host, a combination of rifampin plus

Box 10-3. Management of Cat-Scratch Disease

Mild Disease (eg, focal lymphadenopathy with no, or only minor, associated symptoms)
- Reassurance and symptomatic treatment (eg, analgesics)

or
- Azithromycin at 10 mg/kg on day 1 (maximum dose: 500 mg); then 5 mg/kg/d (maximum dose: 250 mg) for an additional 4 d (Evidence Level I [or strong recommendation, moderate quality evidence])[a]

plus
- Needle aspiration of suppurative lymphadenitis (Evidence Level III [or strong recommendation, moderate quality evidence])

Moderate Disease
- Rifampin at 20 mg/kg/d given in 2 divided doses (maximum dose: 300 mg) for 10–14 d

plus 1 of the following:
- Azithromycin (dose as above but for 10–14 d)

or
- Ciprofloxacin at 20–30 mg/kg/d given in 2 divided doses (maximum dose: 500 mg) for 2–3 wk (for patients >17 y)

or
- TMP/SMX at 8–10 mg/kg/d (TMP component) given in 2 divided doses (maximum dose: 160 mg TMP or one DS tablet) for 2–3 wk (Evidence Level III [or weak recommendation, moderate quality evidence])

Continued

Box 10-3 *(cont)*

Neuroretinitis and CNS Disease
- Rifampin at 20 mg/kg/d given in 2 divided doses (maximum dose: 300 mg)

plus
- Doxycycline at 2.2 mg/kg/dose every 12 h (maximum dose: 100 mg)

For children <9 y, may substitute for doxycycline
- Azithromycin

or
- TMP/SMX (dosed as above) (Evidence Level III [or weak recommendation, moderate quality evidence])

Severe Disease (prolonged fever with or without hepatosplenic disease)[b]
- Rifampin 20 mg/kg/d given in 2 divided doses (maximum dose: 300 mg) for 10–14 d

plus
- Gentamicin (loading dose: 2 mg/kg, then 1.5 mg/kg every 8 h dosed on the basis of normal renal function and adjusted with monitoring) for 10–14 d

or
- Azithromycin (dosed as above) for 10–14 d (Evidence Level III [or weak recommendation, moderate quality evidence])

Endocarditis[b]
When culture-negative endocarditis is suspected to be caused by *Bartonella* infection, initiate
- Ceftriaxone (2 g IV/IM once daily for 6 wk)

plus
- Gentamicin (1 mg/kg IV every 8 h for 14 d
- With or without doxycycline (See dosing above for 6 wk.)

For proven *Bartonella* endocarditis, use doxycycline plus gentamicin (if gentamicin cannot be used, rifampin may be substituted) for a total of 6 wk, though optimal duration of therapy is not known and consultation with an infectious diseases expert should be obtained.

Abbreviations: CNS, central nervous system; DS, double strength; IM, intramuscularly; IV, intravenously; TMP/SMX, trimethoprim/sulfamethoxazole.

[a] Strength of recommendation and quality of evidence.

[b] Consultation with an infectious diseases specialist is strongly recommended.

either azithromycin or gentamicin should be considered (Evidence Level III). Only aminoglycosides have been found to be bactericidal to *B henselae* in laboratory models.

Up to 10% of affected nodes may become suppurative. Needle aspiration of fluctuant, suppurative nodes may provide pain relief, but may need to be repeated because of re-accumulation of fluid. Aggressive incision and drainage is not recommended because of concern for formation of sinus tract and chronic drainage. Excisional biopsy is generally unnecessary.

Favorable, and apparently complete, response is seen in the immunocompetent host, with or without treatment. Those with invasive disease or immunocompromise typically have good response to treatment, with minimal residual effects and no need for specific long-term monitoring.

Suggested Reading

Chen TC, Lin WR, Lu PL, Lin CY, Chen YH. Cat scratch disease from a domestic dog. *J Formos Med Assoc.* 2007;106(2 Suppl):S65–S68

Florin TA, Zaoutis TE, Zaoutis LB. Beyond cat scratch disease: widening spectrum of *Bartonella henselae* infection. *Pediatrics.* 2008;121(5):e1413–e1425

Margileth AM. Recent advances in diagnosis and treatment of cat scratch disease. *Curr Infect Dis Rep.* 2000;2(2):141–146

Rolain JM, Brouqui P, Koehler JE, Maguina C, Dolan MJ, Raoult D. Recommendations for treatment of human infections caused by *Bartonella* species. *Antimicrob Agents Chemother.* 2004;48(6):1921–1933

Schutze GE. Diagnosis and treatment of *Bartonella henselae* infections. *Pediatr Infect Dis J.* 2000;19(12):1185–1187

CHAPTER 11

Cholera

Jason B. Harris, MD, MPH

Key Points

- Cholera is generally diagnosed by its characteristic presentation: painless, voluminous watery diarrhea (rice-water stools); it can be confirmed by isolation of the organism.

- Treatment is focused on correcting hydration and electrolyte disturbances.

- Azithromycin or doxycycline is generally considered for those with moderate-severe illness, and antimotility agents should not be used.

- Safe water and sanitation are the key to prevention; an effective vaccine is not yet available.

Overview

Cholera is an acute secretory diarrhea caused by the bacterium *Vibrio cholerae*. Severe cholera is associated with massive fluid and electrolyte losses in the stool and rapid onset of hypovolemic shock. Appropriate fluid management reduces the mortality of severe cholera from greater than 10% to less than 0.5%. Antibiotics are a useful adjunctive therapy in the treatment of cholera.

Causes and Differential Diagnosis

Etiologic Agent

Cholera is caused by infection with cholera toxin–producing strains of the gram-negative bacterium *Vibrio cholerae*. Infection is acquired by ingestion of contaminated water or food, such as raw or undercooked shellfish, raw or partially dried fish, or moist grains or vegetables held at ambient temperatures. *Vibrio cholerae* is a facultative pathogen and can survive indefinitely in estuarine environments without human hosts.

Vibrio cholerae

Vibrio cholerae is unique among waterborne bacterial infections in its ability to cause global pandemics of disease. *Vibrio cholerae* O1 (El Tor biotype) is the predominant cause of cholera globally.

Differential Diagnosis

Asymptomatic infection or mild illness is more common after infection than severe cholera. Mild illness caused by *V cholerae* is indistinguishable from many other causes of infectious gastroenteritis. These include common etiologies of childhood gastroenteritis, such as enterotoxigenic *Escherichia coli* in older children and rotavirus in infants.

Severe cholera is more distinctive, because the loss of fluid and electrolytes is faster than typically seen in other causes of infectious gastroenteritis. Cholera should be considered in any case of severe watery diarrhea and vomiting that leads to rapid onset of dehydration. Geographic considerations are also important, because cholera is endemic in more than 50 countries and occurs primarily in resource-limited areas with inadequate access to safe water and sanitation, although very rare cases of cholera may also occur in the United States and other developed countries because of contaminated seafood. Even in areas where cholera has not previously been known to present, it should be suspected any time an adult or child 5 years or older develops acute watery diarrhea, which leads rapidly to severe dehydration or death. This is because other causes of infectious gastroenteritis seldom cause such rapid dehydration in older children and adults.

Clinical Features
· · · · · · · · · · · · · · · ·

Acute watery diarrhea is the major manifestation of cholera. In severe cholera, stools are passed frequently (more than 1 stool/hour) and have a characteristic rice-water appearance. *Rice water* refers to the appearance of water in which rice has been rinsed; such stools are predominantly white or slightly brown-tinged liquid and contain flecks of particulate matter. Vomiting is common, especially around the onset of illness. Stools are usually painless, but some mild abdominal cramping and distention may occur. Fever is usually absent or low-grade; high-grade fevers suggest an alternate or potential concomitant illness. Persistent diarrhea (>14 days) or diarrhea with stools containing blood also suggests an alternate (non-cholera) diagnosis.

The most common complication of severe cholera is life-threatening dehydration. Mortality from inadequately treated severe cholera may exceed 50% in some settings. The process is rapid, owing to the large volume of fluid loss in the stool; most deaths occur within 24 hours of the onset of symptoms.

Other complications of cholera include hypoglycemia, which is more common in young children and infants with cholera. Hypokalemia, often first manifesting as muscle weakness, is a significant cause of mortality in the post-rehydration phase of cholera. Metabolic acidosis is a complication of cholera and manifested by rapid or deep and labored (Kussmaul sign) breathing. Although stool losses are usually isotonic in cholera, hypo-natremia and hypernatremia may occur before or after oral rehydration therapy (ORT).

Evaluation

In resource-limited settings, the diagnosis of cholera is most often made on the basis of clinical suspicion that takes into account the local epidemiology of diarrheal illness. Where microbiology facilities are available, the diagnosis of *V cholerae* infection can be confirmed by isolation of the organism from stool on selective media. In the United States this is not a routine culture; therefore, contact the laboratory and ask for appropriate handling. Additionally, the state health department and the Centers for Disease Control and Prevention need to be notified. Isolation of the organism is the criterion standard for diagnosis and allows for antimicrobial sensitivity testing, which is important if the local patterns of antimicrobial resistance are unknown.

A classic rapid test for cholera uses darkfield microscopy, looking for the presence of motile *Vibrios,* whose "shooting star" movement is immediately stopped by *V cholerae*–specific antibodies. Compared to culture and darkfield microscopy, newer generation rapid lateral flow (eg, dipstick) assays have been produced that can be used even by inexperienced clinicians in resource-limited settings. One commercially available test, Crystal VC (Span Diagnostics), has a 97% sensitivity and 75% specificity compared with polymerase chain reaction.

While measurements of serum glucose and electrolytes may be helpful in complicated cases, these tests are often not available, nor are they routinely required in most cases, assuming an appropriate rehydration strategy is employed.

Management

Rehydration

Rehydration (Table 11-1) is the key to successful management of cholera or suspected cholera. However, the standards for rehydration in severe cholera differ substantially from the approach to children with gastroenteritis in developed countries owing to the more rapid loss of fluid in the stool and proportionally greater electrolyte losses than seen in non-cholera gastroenteritis. The most common errors in caring for patients with cholera are to underestimate the speed and volume of fluids required.

Approach to rehydration is guided by an assessment of the clinical signs and symptoms of dehydration using the World Health Organization (WHO) criteria (Figure 11-1). In addition, there are several general aspects involving the rehydration of cholera patients that bear mention.

- The goal of rehydration in all patients with cholera is to correct the entire initial fluid deficit quickly, within 3 hours after presentation (Evidence Level II-3).
- Correction of the initial fluid deficit must be performed in conjunction with the simultaneous replacement of ongoing losses; otherwise, patients

Table 11-1. Composition of Therapeutic Fluids for Cholera

		Sodium	Potassium	Chloride	Bicarbonate	Carbohydrate	Comment
				mmol/L			
IV therapy	Lactated Ringer injection	130	4	109	28	... (278 if 5% dextrose available)	Lactated Ringer injection is commonly available. Optimal infusions for cholera (cholera saline or Dhaka solution) contain more potassium, bicarbonate, and dextrose but may not be available.
	Physiologic saline solution	154	0	154	0	...	
	"Cholera saline solution"	133	13	154	48	140	
ORT	ORS (WHO)	75	20	65	10 (citrate)	75 g (glucose)	Standard ORS (WHO 2002 formulation) uses glucose as a carbohydrate source. Rice-based formulations are preferred if available.
	Rice-based ORS (eg, CeraORS 75)	75	20	65	10 (citrate)	27 g (rice syrup solids)	

Abbreviations: IV, intravenous; ORS, oral rehydration salts; ORT, oral rehydration therapy; WHO, World Health Organization.

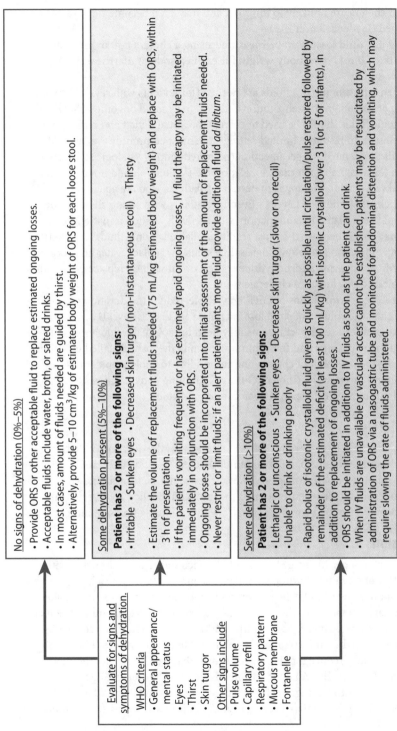

Evaluate for signs and symptoms of dehydration.

WHO criteria
- General appearance/mental status
- Eyes
- Thirst
- Skin turgor

Other signs include
- Pulse volume
- Capillary refill
- Respiratory pattern
- Mucous membrane
- Fontanelle

No signs of dehydration (0%–5%)
- Provide ORS or other acceptable fluid to replace estimated ongoing losses.
- Acceptable fluids include water, broth, or salted drinks.
- In most cases, amount of fluids needed are guided by thirst.
- Alternatively, provide 5–10 cm³/kg of estimated body weight of ORS for each loose stool.

Some dehydration present (5%–10%)
Patient has 2 or more of the following signs:
- Irritable • Sunken eyes • Decreased skin turgor (non-instantaneous recoil) • Thirsty

- Estimate the volume of replacement fluids needed (75 mL/kg estimated body weight) and replace with ORS, within 3 h of presentation.
- If the patient is vomiting frequently or has extremely rapid ongoing losses, IV fluid therapy may be initiated immediately in conjunction with ORS.
- Ongoing losses should be incorporated into initial assessment of the amount of replacement fluids needed.
- Never restrict or limit fluids; if an alert patient wants more fluid, provide additional fluid *ad libitum*.

Severe dehydration (>10%)
Patient has 2 or more of the following signs:
- Lethargic or unconscious • Sunken eyes • Decreased skin turgor (slow or no recoil)
- Unable to drink or drinking poorly

- Rapid bolus of isotonic crystalloid fluid given as quickly as possible until circulation/pulse restored followed by remainder of the estimated deficit (at least 100 mL/kg) with isotonic crystalloid over 3 h (or 5 for infants), in addition to replacement of ongoing losses.
- ORS should be initiated in addition to IV fluids as soon as the patient can drink.
- When IV fluids are unavailable or vascular access cannot be established, patients may be resuscitated by administration of ORS via a nasogastric tube and monitored for abdominal distention and vomiting, which may require slowing the rate of fluids administered.

Figure 11-1. Approach to rehydration in cholera.

Abbreviations: IV, intravenous; ORS, oral rehydration salts.

Adapted from World Health Organization. *The Treatment of Diarrhea: A Manual for Physicians and Other Senior Health Workers*. 4th revision. Geneva, Switzerland: World Health Organization; 2005. http://whqlibdoc.who.int/publications/2005/9241593180.pdf. Accessed August 22, 2016.

with cholera are unlikely to improve, and may even become more dehydrated (Evidence Level II-3).
- Ongoing fluid losses can be measured using a cholera cot, or estimated at 10 to 20 mL/kg of body weight for each episode of diarrheal stool or vomiting.
- When intravenous (IV) fluids are needed (for patients with severe dehydration or some signs of dehydration and extremely rapid ongoing losses), only isotonic fluids should be used to correct the initial deficit and replace ongoing losses. In resource-limited settings, the most commonly available IV fluids are lactated Ringer injection (preferred) and physiologic saline solution (an acceptable alternative). Hypotonic IV fluids should not be used.
- Oral rehydration therapy is preferred for patients who are able to drink sufficiently (Evidence Level I). Even for patients with severe cholera, ORT should be initiated in conjunction with IV fluids as soon as patients can drink. This is because the most readily available isotonic fluids (lactated Ringer injection and physiologic saline solution) replace water and sodium but do not provide a carbohydrate source, or sufficiently replace potassium or bicarbonate losses in choleraic stool.
- Rice-based formulations of ORT, if available, reduce the duration of diarrhea and the volume of stool lost in cholera (Evidence Level I).
- In an outbreak setting, clinicians may need to rapidly develop approaches to treat many patients and the community simultaneously. Detailed guidelines for the management of cholera and responding to cholera epidemics can be found through the Cholera Outbreak Training and Shigellosis Program, and through World Health Organization guidelines.

Antibiotics

Appropriate antibiotic therapy (Table 11-2) shortens the duration of diarrhea and reduces the volume of stool output by up to 50% (Evidence Level I). Therapy should be based on local antibiotic resistance patterns if known. Antibiotics should be given as soon as the initial fluid deficit is corrected and the patient has stopped vomiting (ideally, within 4 hours of presentation).

Nutrition

For nursing infants, breastfeeding should be encouraged in conjunction with oral rehydration salts. Children should be encouraged to resume a high-energy diet as soon as their fluid deficit is corrected and they can tolerate oral intake. These interventions may help prevent subsequent malnutrition and also reduce the risk of hypokalemia. Zinc supplementation has been found to reduce the duration of diarrhea and volume of stool in children with cholera (Evidence Level I) and may reduce the risk of subsequent diarrhea for several months (Evidence Level I). The WHO recommends zinc for children younger than 5 years with diarrhea (10 mg/day for babies <6 months and 20 mg/day for 10 days for children 6 months–5 years of age). Children with diarrhea in resource-

Table 11-2. Antibiotics for Suspected Cholera (Evidence Levels I and II-2)

Class	Antibiotic	Pediatric Dose[a]	Adult Dose	Comment
Tetracyclines	Tetracycline	12.5 mg/kg 4 times daily for 3 d	500 mg 4 times daily for 3 d	Resistance common in some areas. Not recommended for pregnant women and children <8 y because of risk of irreversible tooth discoloration.
	Doxycycline	4–6 mg/kg for 1 dose	300 mg for 1 dose	
Fluoroquinolones	Ciprofloxacin	15 mg/kg twice daily for 3 d	500 mg twice daily for 3 d	Decreased suscepti-bility to fluoroquin-olones is common. Concerns remain over potential toxicity in children.
Macrolides	Erythromycin	12.5 mg/kg 4 times daily for 3 d	250 mg 4 times daily for 3 d	Azithromycin is pre-ferred for children. Resistance reported but rare.
	Azithromycin	20 mg/kg for 1 dose	1 g for 1 dose	

[a] Not to exceed adult dose.

limited countries with a high incidence of vitamin A deficiency should also receive high-dose vitamin A supplementation.

Other Therapies

Antimotility agents (loperamide, diphenoxylate/atropine, and tincture of opium) and antiemetics (chlorpromazine, prochlorperazine, promethazine, and metoclopramide) are not recommended for the treatment of cholera and may have adverse effects that interfere with optimal rehydration (Evidence Level III).

Control and Prevention

Safe water and sanitation prevent cholera, but an estimated 1 billion people lack access to these and remain at risk of cholera. At the individual household level, boiled water, hand washing, and safe food preparation may decrease the risk of cholera transmission. In an outbreak, important public health measures involve not only safe water and sanitation but also creation of cholera treatment centers, as well as decentralized treatment centers, where oral rehydration salts are provided along with education (known as oral rehydration points).

Three commercially available, WHO prequalified, oral cholera vaccines are currently available. Dukoral (Crucell, Sweden AB), a monovalent vaccine against *V cholerae* O1, has been tested in several areas of endemic cholera, is licensed in more than 60 countries, and provides 60% protection for up to 2 years in older children and adults, but is less effective in young children. A bivalent (O1 and O139) vaccine, available as either Shanchol (Shantha Biotechnics) or Euvichol (EuBiologics, Korea), demonstrated 67% protective efficacy in a large recent field trial in Kolkata and is currently produced at a much lower cost than Dukoral. These vaccines are included in a global cholera vaccine stockpile. A live attenuated vaccine, Vaxchora (PaxVax, USA), is available in the United States and is approved for travelers, 18 years or older with a high risk of cholera exposure.

Long-term Monitoring

Patients presenting with cholera should be monitored until all signs of dehydration have resolved, and they have urinated and are able to compensate for ongoing fluid losses with adequate oral fluid intake (Evidence Level III). Patients presenting with cholera should also be assessed for comorbid conditions that commonly occur in conjunction with cholera, such as malnutrition, malaria, and pneumonia, which may require additional treatment, monitoring, and follow-up (Evidence Level III).

Suggested Reading

Chin CS, Sorenson J, Harris JB, et al. The origin of the Haitian cholera outbreak strain. *N Engl J Med.* 2011;364(1):33–42

The Cholera Outbreak Training and Shigellosis Program Web site. http://www.cotsprogram.com. Accessed March 28, 2016

Cholera vaccines: WHO position paper. *Wkly Epidemiol Rec.* 2010;85(13):117–128

Harris JB, LaRocque RC, Qadri F, Ryan ET, Calderwood SB. Cholera. *Lancet.* 2012;379(9835):2466–2476

Ivers LC, Farmer P, Almazor CP, Léandre F. Five complementary interventions to slow cholera: Haiti. *Lancet.* 2010;376(9758):2048–2051

Mutreja A, Kim DW, Thomson NR, et al. Evidence for several waves of global transmission in the seventh cholera pandemic. *Nature.* 2011;477(7365):462–465

Saha D, Karim MM, Khan WA, Ahmed S, Salam MA, Bennish ML. Single-dose azithromycin for the treatment of cholera in adults. *N Engl J Med.* 2006:354(23):2452–2462

Global Task Force on Cholera Control. *First Steps for Managing an Outbreak of Acute Diarrhea.* Geneva, Switzerland: World Health Organization; 2010. http://www.who. int/cholera/publications/en. Accessed March 28, 2016

CHAPTER 12

Diphtheria

Claudia Espinosa, MD, MSc, and Kristina Bryant, MD

Key Points

- While diphtheria may occasionally occur in immunized or partially immunized individuals, immunization prevents severe disease.

- Transmission is usually via respiratory droplets or contact with infected skin lesions and fomites.

- The characteristic lesion of pharyngeal/tonsillar diphtheria is an adherent, greenish gray membrane.

- Most sequelae are related to the effects of diphtheria toxin.

- When diphtheria is suspected, treatment with antitoxin and antibiotics should be instituted empirically.

- Cases of toxigenic *Corynebacterium diphtheriae* disease must be reported to public health authorities.

Overview

Diphtheria is an acute toxin-mediated disease usually caused by *Corynebacterium diphtheriae*. Diphtheria-like infections caused by *Corynebacterium ulcerans* have been increasingly reported in industrialized countries, while *Corynebacterium pseudotuberculosis* is a rarely identified cause of disease. Both *C ulcerans* and *C pseudotuberculosis* are a zoonosis, most commonly transmitted by contact with animals or raw dairy products.

Disease manifestations are related to the elaboration of an exotoxin. Absorption of toxin into the bloodstream results in systemic manifestations of diphtheria and damage to remote organs, most commonly myocardial and peripheral nerves. Proteinuria and thrombocytopenia may also occur.

Causes and Differential Diagnosis

Disease manifestations may be modified by prior immunization. Initially, the sore throat associated with respiratory diphtheria may be indistinguishable from other causes of respiratory/pharyngeal disease, including group A

Table 12-1. Differentiating Diphtheria From Other Common Causes of Pharyngitis

Characteristics	Diphtheria	Group A *Streptococcus*	Epstein-Barr Virus
Incubation period, d	2–7	2–5	30–50
Onset of symptoms	Gradual	Acute	Gradual
Fever	Low-grade (38°C [100.4°F])	High	High
Nasal discharge	Serosanguineous/ purulent	No	No
Pharyngeal exudate	Gray and white changing to dark	White coating	White coating Petechiae after 5th d of illness
Lymphadenopathy	Cervical, subman-dibular, and anterior bull neck (sign of severe illness)	Enlarged tender anterior lymph nodes	Generalized Anterior and posterior cervical common

Streptococcus, infectious mononucleosis caused by Epstein-Barr virus or cytomegalovirus (Table 12-1), or *Arcanobacterium hemolyticum*. The bluish white exudates of early pharyngeal or tonsillar diphtheria could be confused with oral candidiasis. Cutaneous diphtheria can resemble skin lesions caused by other pathogens, including *Staphylococcus aureus* and group A *Streptococcus*.

Clinical Features

Diphtheria may involve any mucous membrane. Symptoms depend on location of the infection and time elapsed to the start of therapy because bacterial concentration and toxin production both increase over time.

Diphtheria most commonly involves the respiratory tract. Anterior nasal disease is characterized by mucopurulent nasal discharge that may become bloody. Early disease can be confused with a common cold or foreign body. A white membrane on the nasal septum is a distinguishing feature. Because there is poor systemic absorption of toxin from this area, disease is typically mild.

Initial symptoms of pharyngeal or tonsillar disease include sore throat and malaise. A patchy white exudate on the tonsils, posterior pharynx, and uvula can mimic pharyngitis caused by other organisms. However, this exudate ultimately evolves into the characteristic pseudomembrane of diphtheria, becoming gray with patches of green and black necrosis. This may spread into the nose, larynx, or tracheobronchial tree, leading to suffocation. Impending respiratory compromise should be suspected if hoarseness is noticed. Massive cervical lymphadenopathy and soft-tissue neck edema can occur, leading to a bull neck. Depending on the concentration of toxin, other symptoms such as tachycardia, pallor, stupor, cardiovascular collapse, and coma may occur. Fever, however, is usually mild, even with severe illness.

Cutaneous diphtheria is generally less severe than respiratory diphtheria, and toxigenic sequelae are uncommon. Characteristic lesions include chronic non-healing sores or shallow ulcers with a dirty gray-brown base membrane. The presenting lesion, ecthyma diphtheriticum, begins as a vesicle or pustule filled with straw-colored fluid and progresses to a punched-out ulcer. The lesions are initially painful but become anesthetic after the pseudomembrane falls off and a hemorrhagic base appears. The surrounding tissue may have blisters or bullae. Cutaneous diphtheria may also manifest as dry, scaly lesions. Commonly involved sites include legs, feet, and hands, but the conjunctivae, eye, ear, and vagina may be affected. Lesions often appear at the site of previous skin lesions. Coinfections with other bacteria, particularly *S aureus,* occur.

Cutaneous disease is more transmissible than respiratory tract disease, and those with skin lesions may serve as a reservoir for the spread of respiratory diphtheria. Cutaneous diphtheria is increasingly caused by non-toxigenic forms of *C diphtheriae.*

Corynebacterium diphtheriae occasionally causes other localized and systemic infections, including bacteremia, septic arthritis, osteomyelitis, hepatic or splenic abscess, and endocarditis. While endocarditis is most often caused by non-toxigenic strains, disease with toxigenic strains has also been reported. Most children with *C diphtheriae* endocarditis have underlying structural heart disease and a history of prior immunization with diphtheria toxoid–containing vaccine. Concurrent signs of respiratory or cutaneous diphtheria are often absent.

Most long-term sequelae of diphtheria are related to diphtheria toxin. Myocarditis with heart failure may manifest during the acute phase of diphtheria or convalescence. At autopsy, hearts are described as dilated, pale, and flabby with extensive areas of hyaline degeneration and necrosis in the myocardium. Fluorescent antibody staining demonstrates toxin within myocardial fibers.

Approximately 20% of patients with respiratory diphtheria develop polyneuritis, but neuropathy is even more common in severe disease. Initially, this may manifest as paralysis of the soft palate and posterior pharyngeal wall. Cranial neuropathies involving oculomotor and ciliary paralysis occur. Peripheral neuritis may develop 10 days to 3 months after the onset of respiratory disease. Both motor and sensory nerves of the neck, trunk, and upper extremities may be affected, resulting in a glove and stocking neuropathy.

In developed countries, the case fatality rate associated with respiratory diphtheria ranges from 5% to 10%. The mortality associated with systemic infections, including bacteremia and endocarditis, may be as high 50%. Long-term sequelae from cutaneous diphtheria are rare.

Diagnosis

Diagnosis of diphtheria requires a high index of suspicion because microbiology laboratories may not routinely look for diphtheria in throat or wound specimens. When pseudomembranes are present, specimens for culture should be obtained from under the membrane because this is where bacteria are concentrated. Culture and microscopic examination of the membrane itself can also be useful. Laboratory personnel should be notified when diphtheria is suspected so that specimens can be plated on cystine-tellurite blood agar or modified Tinsdale agar.

Organisms are nonmotile gram-positive bacilli with club-shaped swellings at each end.

Corynebacterium diphtheriae isolates recovered from a patient with suspected diphtheria should be tested for toxin production; isolates should also be sent to the Centers for Disease Control and Prevention through the state health department. Polymerase chain reaction testing is now available to confirm the presence of the toxin gene.

Management

Intravenous diphtheria antitoxin and antibiotic therapy are the mainstays of treatment for diphtheria. A presumptive clinical diagnosis should prompt administration of antitoxin, even before culture confirmation. In the United States, antitoxin is available from the Centers for Disease Control and Prevention under an Investigational New Drug protocol. The dose varies by site of infection, duration of illness, and presence of toxic effects (Table 12-2). All patients should undergo sensitivity tests for reactions to horse serum before treatment with the antitoxin.

Antimicrobial therapy halts toxin production, eliminates *C diphtheriae,* and reduces the potential for transmission but is not a substitute for treatment with antitoxin. Effective antimicrobial therapy for respiratory disease consists of a

Table 12-2. Dose of Equine Antitoxin Recommended for Treatment of Diphtheria

Disease Manifestations	Antitoxin Dose, U
Pharyngeal/laryngeal disease ≤2 d′ duration	20,000–40,000
Nasopharyngeal	40,000–60,000
Extensive disease of ≥3 d′ duration	80,000–120,000
Diffuse swelling of the neck	80,000–120,000
Cutaneous disease[a]	20,000–40,000

[a] Recommended by some experts because of potential for toxic sequelae but value unproven.

14-day course of erythromycin (oral or intravenous), penicillin G (intramuscular or intravenous), or procaine penicillin (intramuscular). Ten days of therapy is considered sufficient for cutaneous disease. Beginning 24 hours after completion of therapy, eradication of *C diphtheriae* should be confirmed by 2 consecutive negative cultures obtained 24 hours apart. Because disease does not necessarily confer lifelong immunity, a diphtheria toxoid–containing vaccine should be administered during convalescence.

Guidelines for treatment of infective endocarditis do not address treatment of disease caused by *C diphtheriae*. Experts generally recommend 4 to 6 weeks of therapy with a β-lactam antibiotic, such as penicillin or ceftriaxone. Some experts advocate combination therapy with an aminoglycoside.

Close contacts of those with suspected diphtheria, especially household members and those who have been exposed to oral secretions, should be screened for nasal and pharyngeal carriage and treated prophylactically with either a 10-day course of oral erythromycin or a single intramuscular dose of benzathine G penicillin (600,000 U for children <30.0 kg and 1.2 million U for children >30.0 kg and adults). Intramuscular penicillin is preferred when surveillance of close contacts cannot be performed. Those proven to be carriers should undergo follow-up testing to document eradication of the organism. Persistent recovery of *C diphtheriae* mandates an additional 10-day course of erythromycin and repeat cultures. Unimmunized or partially immunized contacts, or those whose immunization status is unknown, should immediately receive a dose of a diphtheria toxoid–containing vaccine and complete the recommended immunization series. Fully immunized contacts should receive a booster dose of vaccine if more than 5 years have elapsed since the last dose of diphtheria toxoid–containing vaccine.

Five doses of diphtheria and tetanus toxoids and acellular pertussis vaccine are recommended for children 2 months to 6 years of age. As long as the fourth dose is administered before the fourth birthday, a fifth dose is recommended at 4 to 6 years. More than 95% of infants develop protective antibody against diphtheria after 4 doses of vaccine, and clinical efficacy is estimated at 97%.

A single dose of tetanus toxoid, reduced diphtheria toxoid, and acellular pertussis is recommended at age 11 to 12 years, with booster doses of tetanus and diphtheria toxoids given every 10 years thereafter.

All suspected and proven cases of respiratory diphtheria should be promptly reported to public health authorities. Cutaneous diphtheria associated with non-toxigenic strains of *C diphtheriae* is no longer a reportable disease in the United States.

Hospitalized patients with diphtheria should be treated with standard and droplet precautions until 2 cultures collected from the nose and throat 24 hours after completion of antimicrobial therapy are negative for *C diphtheriae*. Contact precautions are recommended for patients with cutaneous diphtheria until 2 cultures obtained from the skin lesion are negative. Cultures should be obtained 24 hours apart beginning 24 hours after completion of antimicrobial therapy.

Suggested Reading

Dewinter LM, Bernard KA, Romney MG. Human clinical isolates of *Corynebacterium diphtheriae* and *Corynebacterium ulcerans* collected in Canada from 1999 to 2003 but not fitting reporting criteria for cases of diphtheria. *J Clin Microbiol.* 2005;43(7):3447–3449

Efstratious A, George RC. Laboratory guidelines for the diagnosis of infections caused by *Corynebacterium diphtheriae* and *C ulcerans. Commun Dis Public Health.* 1999;2:250–257

Muttaiyah S, Best EJ, Freeman JT, Taylor SL, Morris AJ, Roberts SA. *Corynebacterium diphtheriae* endocarditis: a case series and review of the treatment approach. *Int J Infect Dis.* 2011;15(9):e584–e588

Tejpratap SP, Tiwari MD. Diphtheria. In: *VPD Surveillance Manual.* 5th ed. Atlanta, GA: Centers for Disease Control and Prevention; 2011:1–9. http://www.cdc.gov/vaccines/pubs/surv-manual/chpt01-dip.pdf. Accessed March 23, 2016

Quick ML, Sutter RW, Kobaidze K, et al. Risk factors for diphtheria: a prospective case-control study in the Republic of Georgia, 1995-1996. *J Infec Dis.* 2000;181(Suppl 1):S121–S129

Wagner KS, White JM, Neal S, et al. Screening for *Corynebacterium diphtheriae* and *Corynebacterium ulcerans* in patients with upper respiratory tract infections, 2007-2008: a multicentre European study. *Clin Microbiol Infect.* 2011;17(4):519–525

CHAPTER 13

Group A Streptococcal Infections

Angela L. Myers, MD, MPH

Key Points

- Group A *Streptococcus* (GAS) is a common cause of pharyngotonsillitis in school-aged children and a less common, but important, cause of invasive infection in children.

- Appropriate laboratory testing should be performed to diagnose GAS infection when clinical suspicion warrants.

- Penicillin or amoxicillin are preferred for treatment of GAS infection; macrolides should be reserved for penicillin-allergic patients with a history of anaphylaxis.

- Sequelae of GAS infection are rare with appropriate initial treatment of the infection.

Overview

Group A *Streptococcus* (GAS), *Streptococcus pyogenes,* is a gram-positive coccus that most commonly causes streptococcal pharyngotonsillitis as well as skin and soft-tissue infection. Penicillin is the treatment of choice, and resistance has never been encountered. Suppurative complications, including peritonsillar or retropharyngeal abscess, otitis media, mastoiditis, sinusitis, and suppurative adenitis, may complicate upper respiratory tract infection. Invasive disease is well described; bacteremia, pneumonia, osteomyelitis, toxic shock syndrome (TSS), necrotizing fasciitis, and endocarditis may be associated with significant morbidity. Antibiotic therapy not only treats focal sites of infection but also is effective to prevent acute rheumatic fever and may be beneficial in preventing secondary spread of nephritogenic strains causing acute glomerulonephritis.

Causes and Differential Diagnosis

More than 120 distinct serotypes of GAS cause a myriad of infections that somewhat depend on age of the child (Box 13-1). Pharyngitis is the most common manifestation of streptococcal infection in the school-aged child, and is the only commonly occurring cause of bacterial pharyngitis for which therapy is indicated. In the young child (ie, <3 years), streptococcal pharyngitis is rare (Evidence Level I). However, streptococcosis, a respiratory tract infection characterized by serous rhinitis, fever, anorexia, and irritability, may occur in this age group.

Although pharyngitis is the most common presentation of streptococcal infection, much overlap exists between streptococcal pharyngitis and pharyngitis from alternate etiologies, including other bacterial and viral agents (Table 13-1). Overall, viral etiologies are more common than bacterial pathogens, with adenovirus, influenza, and mononucleosis syndromes possessing characteristics that may mimic GAS. Group C *Streptococcus* is an endemic bacterium and thought to be a frequent cause of pharyngitis in college-aged individuals and adults. *Fusobacterium necrophorum* is a well-described but uncommon cause of bacterial pharyngeal infection, usually in adolescents, and may be complicated by metastatic foci resulting from associated suppurative jugular vein thrombophlebitis (so-called Lemierre syndrome).

Group A *Streptococcus* may also cause invasive infection, including bacteremia, pneumonia, skin and soft-tissue infection, and bone and joint infection (Box 13-1). Invasive infection may be severe and occur with associated TSS or necrotizing fasciitis. In the setting of TSS, an identifiable focus of local infection may not be identified, although history of mild trauma is often present in the setting of necrotizing fasciitis. Features of GAS TSS and necrotizing fasciitis overlap significantly with other infectious entities. Toxic shock syndrome

---

Box 13-1. Manifestations of Group A Streptococcal Infections

- Omphalitis (neonatal; ≤1 mo)
- Streptococcosis (toddler; 1–3 y)
- Pharyngitis (>3 y)
- Otitis media/mastoiditis/sinusitis
- Pyoderma/impetigo
- Erysipelas
- Peritonsillar/retropharyngeal abscess
- Perianal cellulitis
- Pneumonia
- Osteomyelitis/septic arthritis/myositis
- Wound infection
- Bacteremia
- Necrotizing fasciitis
- Endocarditis/pericarditis
- Vaginitis (prepubertal)
- Puerperal sepsis (postpartum/abortion)

Table 13-1. Infectious Etiologies With Overlapping Features of Streptococcal Pharyngitis

Organism	Clinical Manifestations
Viruses	
Adenovirus	Pharyngoconjunctival fever
EBV	Mononucleosis
CMV	Mononucleosis-like syndrome
Influenza virus	Influenza
Parainfluenza virus	Croup, common cold
Rhinovirus	Common cold
HCoV	Common cold
Coxsackievirus	Herpangina, hand-foot-and-mouth disease
HSV	Gingivostomatitis
HIV	Acute HIV infection syndrome
Bacteria	
Group C and G *Streptococcus*	Pharyngotonsillitis
Arcanobacterium haemolyticum	Pharyngitis, scarlatiniform rash
Fusobacterium necrophorum	Lemierre syndrome, peritonsillar abscess
Mixed anaerobes	Vincent angina
Neisseria gonorrhoeae	Pharyngitis
Treponema pallidum	Secondary syphilis
Francisella tularensis	Oropharyngeal tularemia
Corynebacterium diphtheriae	Diphtheria
Yersinia enterocolitica	Pharyngitis, enterocolitis
Yersinia pestis	Plague
Atypical Bacterial Pathogens	
Mycoplasma pneumoniae	Pneumonia, bronchitis
Chlamydophila pneumoniae	Pneumonia, bronchitis
Chlamydophila psittaci	Psittacosis

Abbreviations: CMV, cytomegalovirus; EBV, Epstein-Barr virus; HCoV, human coronavirus; HSV, herpes simplex virus.

is difficult to distinguish clinically since there is much overlap with *Staphylococcus aureus* infection. Definitive diagnosis of GAS TSS requires isolation of the organism along with clinical features of shock and organ dysfunction (Box 13-2). Similarly, necrotizing fasciitis may be caused by *Clostridium* species, mixed enteric gram-negative and anaerobic organisms, *S aureus*, and other *Streptococcus* species.

Box 13-2. Streptococcal Toxic Shock Syndrome (*Streptococcus pyogenes*) 2010 Case Definition[a]

- Hypotension defined by a systolic blood pressure ≤90 mm Hg for adults or less than the fifth percentile by age for children aged younger than 16 years.
- Multi-organ involvement characterized by 2 or more of the following:
  - o Renal impairment: creatinine ≥2 mg/dL (≥177 μmol/L) for adults or greater than or equal to twice the upper limit of normal for age. In patients with pre-existing renal disease, a greater than twofold elevation over the baseline level.
  - o Coagulopathy: platelets ≤100,000/mm³ (≤100 3 10⁶/L) or disseminated intravascular coagulation, defined by prolonged clotting times, low fibrinogen level, and the presence of fibrin degradation products.
  - o Liver involvement: alanine aminotransferase, aspartate aminotransferase, or total bilirubin levels greater than or equal to twice the upper limit of normal for the patient's age. In patients with pre-existing liver disease, a greater than twofold increase over the baseline level.
  - o Acute respiratory distress syndrome: defined by acute onset of diffuse pulmonary infiltrates and hypoxemia in the absence of cardiac failure or by evidence of diffuse capillary leak manifested by acute onset of generalized edema, or pleural or peritoneal effusions with hypoalbuminemia.
  - o A generalized erythematous macular rash that may desquamate.
  - o Soft-tissue necrosis, including necrotizing fasciitis or myositis, or gangrene.

[a]Clinical manifestations do not need to be detected within the first 48 hours of hospitalization or illness, as specified in the 1996 case definition. The specification of the 48 hour time constraint was for purposes of assessing whether the case was considered nosocomial, not whether it was a case or not.

From Centers for Disease Control and Prevention. Streptococcal toxic shock syndrome (STSS) (*Streptococcus pyogenes*) 2010 case definition. http://wwwn.cdc.gov/nndss/conditions/streptococcal-toxic-shock-syndrome/case-definition/2010. Accessed February 3, 2016.

Clinical Features

Clinical features of GAS pharyngeal infection are generally seen in the school-aged child and include fever, sore throat, and tender cervical lymphadenopathy without associated viral respiratory tract features (Table 13-2). Presence of viral signs or symptoms effectively rules out streptococcal pharyngitis, obviating the need for testing. However, clinical features consistent with GAS infection are insufficient to confirm a diagnosis and testing is always indicated in the setting of high clinical suspicion (Evidence Level I). Peritonsillar abscess (ie, quinsy) and retropharyngeal abscess are suppurative sequelae of streptococcal pharyngitis that typically occur in the older child and adolescent. Peritonsillar abscess is characterized by fever, severe sore throat and odynophagia with peritonsillar swelling, uvular deviation to the contralateral side, muffled voice, trismus, drooling, and cervical lymphadenopathy. Retropharyngeal abscess manifests

Table 13-2. Clinical and Epidemiologic Features of Streptococcal Pharyngitis and Viral Respiratory Tract Infections

Streptococcal Pharyngitis	
Clinical	Fever (+) Sudden onset of sore throat (+) Tonsillar exudates or swelling (+) Tender cervical lymphadenopathy (+) Nausea, vomiting, or abdominal pain (±) Palatal petechiae (±)
Epidemiologic	Winter or spring presentation History of exposure to streptococcal pharyngitis
Viral Respiratory Tract Infections	
Clinical	Fever (±) Cough (±) Congestion (±) Coryza (±) Conjunctivitis (±) Diarrhea (±) Hoarseness (±) Ulcerative stomatitis (±) Viral exanthema (±)
Epidemiologic	Off-peak season presentation Close contact with recent viral respiratory tract symptoms

Plus sign (+) indicates features that are typically present, and plus or minus sign (±) indicates features that may or may not be present.

with fever, sore throat, dysphagia, odynophagia, neck pain and swelling, decreased neck mobility (extension), and torticollis. Trismus and drooling are less common features.

Acute otitis media and mastoiditis are typically seen in children younger than 5 years, and are similar in appearance to these infections caused by other organisms with fever, otalgia, abnormal findings on otoscopy, and posterior auricular swelling along with erythema and pain in the setting of mastoiditis. Streptococcosis is also seen in the toddler age group and manifests as serous rhinorrhea with nasal excoriations followed by fever, malaise, and anorexia.

Skin and soft-tissue infections, including pyoderma, cellulitis, wound infections, and myositis, are similar in appearance to infections caused by *S aureus* and may occur at any age from birth (eg, omphalitis) through adulthood. Clinical signs and symptoms include erythema, warmth and tenderness of the site, and possible fluctuance in the setting of abscess formation. Erysipelas has a distinct appearance, however, with an edematous plaque and slightly raised, well-demarcated borders because of lymphatic involvement compared with cellulitis caused by *S aureus*. Streptococcal perianal cellulitis peaks at 3 to 5 years of age and is characterized by superficial, well-demarcated erythema around the anus and surrounding skin. Vulvar, vaginal, and penile involvement with erythema and discharge may occur in prepubertal girls and boys, respectively.

Features of invasive disease depend on the location of infection, although bacteremia and TSS may occur without associated focal infection. Pneumonia caused by GAS is often severe, leading to a complicated process with pleural effusions, empyema, lung abscess, and necrotizing pneumonia. Bone and joint infections are similar in presentation to infections caused by other organisms and include erythema, edema, warmth, pain, and refusal to use the affected limb. Toxic shock syndrome and necrotizing fasciitis are caused by toxin-producing strains of GAS and are most often seen in adolescence. Diagnostic criteria of streptococcal TSS are outlined in Box 13-2. Fasciitis is a clinical emergency but oftentimes difficult to recognize early in the course because patients may appear relatively well at presentation. The hallmark of this infection is patient-reported pain that is out of proportion to findings on examination. Edema and induration of the affected area may be seen in the first 24 hours followed by rapid blistering and bleb formation with subsequent tissue necrosis.

Evaluation

Clinical signs and symptoms of GAS pharyngeal infection may mimic many other infectious etiologies. Most notable are viral pathogens such as adenovirus, Epstein-Barr virus, and influenza. Several clinical scoring systems have been developed to predict the likelihood of streptococcal pharyngitis in children and adults with sore throat. They are based on clinical findings including fever, tonsillar swelling or exudate, enlarged and tender cervical lymphadenopathy, and absence of cough and other viral symptoms. In addition, age is included in some systems, providing 1 point to those between 3 and 15 years of age. The probability of streptococcal infection ranges from less than 2.5% with zero findings to greater than 50% with 4 to 5 clinical features. Clinical signs and symptoms alone are inadequate in determining infection, and a scoring system should be used only to determine whether testing is indicated or not (Evidence Level I).

Testing for streptococcal pharyngitis is not routinely indicated in children younger than 3 years because of the rarity of acute rheumatic fever in this age group, absence of classic symptomatology, and low incidence of streptococcal pharyngitis overall (Evidence Level I).

When a test is warranted, the most rapid method is a rapid antigen detection test (RADT) from a direct throat swab. Back-up throat culture should be performed in the setting of a negative RADT because of low sensitivity of the test and relatively higher likelihood (20%–30%) of streptococcal infection in children (Evidence Level I).

Presence of GAS on RADT or culture testing does not distinguish between infection and pharyngeal colonization. Selective testing of those in whom clinical and epidemiologic features are consistent with infection is thus important in making the correct diagnosis. Testing patients with clear viral symptoms or lack of features consistent with streptococcal pharyngitis results in unnecessary antibiotic use, contributing to adverse drug events and rising resistance rates in some antimicrobials (Evidence Level I).

In the setting of suspected GAS invasive disease, testing should be targeted to the site of infection. Positive blood culture results are necessary to diagnose bacteremia and endocarditis, but may also be of benefit in the setting of pneumonia, osteomyelitis, necrotizing fasciitis, and TSS. A positive culture result from a normally sterile site is required for a definite diagnosis of TSS; GAS is found on blood culture in greater than 50% of cases (in contrast to staphylococcal-associated TSS in which a positive culture result is generally unseen). Culture results of focal sites of infection such as pleural fluid or wound are often positive as well and remain positive for several days after effective therapy has been initiated. Therefore, it is prudent to obtain cultures in the setting of invasive infection even if drainage or debridement is delayed by several days (Evidence Level II).

Diagnostic studies are generally not indicated in the presence of high clinical suspicion of necrotizing fasciitis. This disease process is a surgical emergency, and irrigation and debridement should not be delayed to obtain radiologic imaging (Evidence Level I). In this setting, tissue should be sent for culture and pathologist review, which is key to defining the etiologic agent and demonstrating the extent of disease.

A rise in antibody titers to streptolysin O, deoxyribonuclease B, and other streptococcal enzymes may be seen 3 to 6 weeks after acute infection. While these serve as useful aids in the diagnosis of nonsuppurative sequelae such as rheumatic fever and glomerulonephritis, they are not of diagnostic benefit during acute infection (Evidence Level I).

Management

The antibiotic of choice for GAS infection is penicillin, because resistance has never been documented in any clinical isolate (Evidence Level I). Duration of treatment depends on the clinical syndrome with 10 days being the typical course for bacterial eradication. Equivalent alternatives to penicillin include amoxicillin (Evidence Level I). Therapeutic dosing is listed in Table 13-3. Prompt treatment is important for decreasing disease transmission and individual morbidity and preventing suppurative and nonsuppurative sequelae.

Patients with penicillin allergy without a history of anaphylaxis may receive a narrow spectrum (first-generation) cephalosporin for 10 days (Evidence Level I). Intramuscular penicillin may be used for the child in whom adherence to therapy is of concern. Long-acting penicillin G benzathine is effective but

Table 13-3. Weight-Based Treatment of Streptococcal Infections

Weight, kg	Recommended Therapy	Penicillin Hypersensitivity (not type I)	Penicillin Hypersensitivity (type I)
<27.0	• Penicillin V (oral): 250 mg 2–3 times daily for 10 d • Amoxicillin (oral): 50 mg/kg once daily for 10 d *or* 25 mg/kg/dose twice daily for 10 d • Penicillin G benzathine (IM): 600,000 U (375 mg) one time	• Cephalexin (oral): 20 mg/kg/dose twice daily for 10 d • Cefadroxil (oral): 30 mg/kg/dose once daily for 10 d	• Clindamycin (oral): 10 mg/kg/dose 3 times daily for 10 d • Azithromycin (oral): 12 mg/kg once daily for 5 d • Clarithromycin (oral): 7.5 mg/kg/dose twice daily for 10 d
≥27.0	• Penicillin V (oral): 250 mg 4 times daily *or* 500 mg twice daily for 10 d • Amoxicillin (oral): 50 mg/kg (maximum: 1,000 mg) once daily for 10 d *or* 25 mg/kg/dose (maximum: 500 mg/dose) twice daily for 10 d • Penicillin G benzathine (IM): 1.2 million U (750 mg) one time • Penicillin G procaine 300,000 U (187.5 mg) + penicillin G benzathine (IM): 900,000 U (562.5 mg) one time	• Cephalexin (oral): 20 mg/kg/dose twice daily for 10 d (maximum: 500 mg/dose) • Cefadroxil (oral): 30 mg/kg/dose once daily for 10 d (maximum: 1 g/d)	• Clindamycin (oral): 10 mg/kg/dose 3 times daily for 10 d (maximum: 300 mg/dose) • Azithromycin (oral): 12 mg/kg once daily for 5 d (maximum: 500 mg) • Clarithromycin (oral): 7.5 mg/kg/dose twice daily for 10 d

Abbreviation: IM, intramuscular.

associated with significant pain on injection. A fixed dose combination product that includes penicillin G procaine (CR Bicillin) is associated with less pain but not recommended for those greater than 60 kg (treatment failure related to inadequate penicillin dosing). Clindamycin is a reasonable alternative in patients with immediate or type I hypersensitivity to penicillin (Evidence Level I). Macrolides such as azithromycin for 5 days or clarithromycin for a 10-day course are also alternatives (Evidence Level I). However, GAS resistance to macrolides has increased in the last decade, with pockets of resistance between 6% and 12% in various geographic areas across the United States. Although less common, resistance to clindamycin may also be seen (2%–3%), and this may be most important to recognize when treating invasive infection for which susceptibility should be confirmed. Antibiotics that do not provide adequate therapy for GAS infection include sulfonamides (eg, trimethoprim/sulfamethoxazole), tetracyclines, and fluoroquinolones (Evidence Level I).

In addition to supportive therapies, irrigation, drainage, or debridement is an essential part of treating invasive infections. Some strains of GAS possess enzymes with the ability to cause widespread tissue necrosis in a short period of time. Hemodynamic monitoring and fluid resuscitation along with surgical intervention should not be delayed for radiologic testing.

Long-term Monitoring and Implications

Treatment is recommended for GAS pharyngeal infections to prevent suppurative and nonsuppurative sequelae. Nonsuppurative sequelae primarily include acute rheumatic fever and glomerulonephritis. Acute rheumatic fever is rare (<3: 100,000 population) and follows untreated pharyngeal infection. The true incidence of glomerulonephritis is unknown, but it is the most common cause of nephritis and acute renal insufficiency in preschool- and school-aged children that may follow either pharyngeal or skin infection. Poststreptococcal arthritis was originally described in patients with arthritis following streptococcal pharyngeal infection without concomitant carditis. It occurs in a bimodal age distribution and is thought to be increasing in prevalence, while acute rheumatic fever has decreased in developed countries.

The prognosis for acute glomerulonephritis is quite good, with greater than 95% recovering fully without sequelae. Less than 5% may continue to have abnormalities on urinalysis for up to 15 years after the acute period. Antibiotic therapy may eliminate the nephrogenic strain, but does not alter the clinical course of disease in acute glomerulonephritis. Treatment largely consists of supportive measures because anti-inflammatory medications have not been shown to hasten recovery.

Poststreptococcal reactive arthritis manifests as a nonmigratory polyarthritis that is not improved by use of nonsteroidal medications. The arthritis can occur in any joint, persist for several months, and be recurrent. Some experts advocate penicillin prophylaxis for 3 to 12 months in the setting of poststreptococcal arthritis with monitoring for development of valvular heart disease for several months. If carditis develops, a diagnosis of acute rheumatic fever should be made and prophylaxis should be continued.

Suggested Reading

Gerber MA, Baltimore RS, Eaton CB, et al. Prevention of rheumatic fever and diagnosis and treatment of acute streptococcal pharyngitis. *Circulation.* 2009;119(11): 1541–1551

Green MD, Beall B, Marcon MJ, et al. Multicentre surveillance of the prevalence and molecular epidemiology of macrolide resistance among pharyngeal isolates of group A streptococci in the USA. *J Antimicrob Chemother.* 2006;57(6):1240–1243

McIsaac WJ, Kellner, Aufricht P, Vanjaka A, Low DE. Empirical validation of guidelines for the management of pharyngitis in children and adults. *JAMA.* 2004;291(13):1587–1595

Shaikh N, Swaminathan N, Hooper EG. Accuracy and precision of the signs and symptoms of streptococcal pharyngitis in children: a systematic review. *J Pediatr.* 2012;160(3):487–493

Shulman S, Bisno AL, Clegg HW, et al. Clinical practice guidelines for the diagnosis and management of group A streptococcal pharyngitis: 2012 update by the Infectious Diseases Society of America. *Clin Infect Dis.* 2012;55(10):e86–e102

van der Helm-van Mil AH. Acute rheumatic fever and poststreptococcal reactive arthritis reconsidered. *Curr Opin Rheumatol.* 2010;22(4):437–442

Wessels MR. Streptococcal pharyngitis. *N Engl J Med.* 2011;364(7):648–655

CHAPTER 14

Group B Streptococcal Infections

Pia S. Pannaraj, MD, MPH

Key Points

- Group B *Streptococcus* is the predominant cause of neonatal sepsis and meningitis and occurs following maternal colonization and vertical transmission. Early-onset (0–6 days of age) infection most commonly presents as a systemic infection, and late-onset infection (7–89 days) as bacteremia or meningitis.

- The use of intrapartum antibiotic prophylaxis has resulted in an 80% reduction in early-onset infection but has not appreciably changed the incidence of late-onset infection.

- Cultures of blood, cerebrospinal fluid, and any other focal site of infection are recommended to establish the diagnosis.

- Ampicillin plus gentamicin remains the combination of choice for empiric treatment of presumptive invasive group B streptococcal infection.

- The combination of ampicillin and cefotaxime should be considered in empiric treatment of life-threatening early-onset infection (to cover potential of ampicillin-resistant gram-negative agents) or if meningitis is suggested by cerebrospinal fluid evaluation.

- Prognosis still remains guarded in certain subsets of infected patients. Severe neurologic sequelae are reported in approximately 20% with meningitis; only 51% demonstrate normal age-appropriate development.

Overview

Group B streptococcal (GBS) infection remains a leading cause of neonatal sepsis and meningitis in the United States despite widespread use of intrapartum antibiotic prophylaxis (IAP). Maternal colonization is the primary risk factor for neonatal infection. Additional risk factors include delivery at less than 37 weeks' gestation, prolonged rupture of membranes for 18 hours or longer, intrapartum fever, amnionitis, GBS bacteriuria during current pregnancy, or prior delivery of an infant with invasive GBS infection. Vertical transmission occurs by ascending route following rupture of membranes or contact with the organism in the birth canal during childbirth. After delivery, person-to-person transmission can occur in the nursery or from colonized family members.

Causes and Differential Diagnosis

Group B streptococci are facultative gram-positive diplococci that colonize the genital and gastrointestinal tracts of 18% to 35% of pregnant women.

Signs and symptoms of early-onset GBS infection are clinically indistinguishable from neonatal sepsis caused by other bacterial pathogens, such as *Escherichia coli,* and other enteric organisms or viral pathogens, such as herpes simplex virus or enterovirus. Group B streptococcal infection tends to appear earlier in the first day of life compared to typical *E coli* infection onset on the second or third day of life. Respiratory distress in early-onset infection may be confused with noninfectious causes, such as transient tachypnea of the neonate, persistent fetal circulation, congenital heart disease, pneumothorax, genetic metabolic diseases, and respiratory distress syndrome.

The differential diagnosis of late-onset infection depends on the focus of infection. Meningitis in infants of this age is also caused rarely by *Streptococcus pneumoniae, Neisseria meningitidis, Listeria monocytogenes, Haemophilus influenzae* (type b and non-typable), and viruses. Group B streptococcal osteomyelitis characteristically presents with a paucity of signs and the history that signs have been present since birth, thereby leading to confusion with Erb-Duchenne paralysis and neuromuscular disorders. *Staphylococcus aureus* should be considered in acute presentations of bone or joint infections.

Clinical Features

Group B *Streptococcus* causes systemic and focal infections in young infants. Clinical presentation varies depending on the infant's chronologic age at onset of infection (Table 14-1). Early-onset GBS infection usually occurs within the first 24 hours of life (range: 0–6 days). Infants present with signs of systemic infection, respiratory distress, apnea, shock, pneumonia, and, less commonly, meningitis. Late-onset infection typically occurs at 3 to 4 weeks of age (range: 7–89 days). Bacteremia without a focus and meningitis are the 2 most common manifestations of late-onset infection. Focal infections, including osteomyelitis, septic arthritis, necrotizing fasciitis, pneumonia, adenitis, and cellulitis, occur less often. Late, late-onset infections occur in infants older than 3 months who were born very prematurely or those with immunodeficiencies. Clinical manifestations are similar to those of typical late-onset infection.

Evaluation

Evaluation for suspected GBS infection includes
- Complete blood cell count with differential
- Blood culture
- Urinalysis with urine culture

Table 14-1. Features of Group B Streptococcal Infection in Neonates and Infants

Feature	Early-Onset Infection	Late-Onset Infection	Late, Late-Onset Infection
Age at onset	≤6 d; mean: 8 h; median: 1 h	7–89 d; mean: 36 d; median: 27 d	≥90 d
Neonates and infants affected	Premature infants or infants birthed after maternal obstetric complications	Term and preterm infants equally affected	Premature infants <32 wk' gestation or infants with immunodeficiency
Clinical presentation	Acute respiratory distress, apnea, and hypotension common	Fever, irritability, nonspecific signs, and occasionally fulminant	Fever, irritability, and nonspecific signs
Manifestations	Bacteremia (40%–55%), pneumonia (30%–45%), or meningitis (6%–15%)	Bacteremia without a focus (55%–67%), meningitis (26%–35%), osteoarthritis (approximately 5%), or cellulitis/adenitis (approximately 2%)	Bacteremia without a focus or focal infections as in late-onset disease
Case fatality rate, %	5–15	2–6	<5

- Chest radiograph (if respiratory signs are present)
- Lumbar puncture for cerebrospinal fluid (CSF) cell count, protein and glucose concentrations, Gram stain, and culture
- Urinary culture by sterile collection method (if the infant is ≥7 days)

The diagnosis of GBS infection is confirmed by isolation of the bacteria from normally sterile body sites, including blood, CSF, pleural fluid, joint fluid, bone aspiration, or soft tissue. Rapid antigen testing is available for CSF but should not be used as a substitute for bacterial culture. Rapid testing in body fluids other than CSF is not recommended because of poor specificity.

Management

Empiric Therapy

Antimicrobial therapy is based on in vitro susceptibility testing and response to therapy in observational studies (Evidence Level II-3). Initial empiric therapy of suspected sepsis should include broad coverage for organisms known to cause early- and late-onset infections in neonates (GBS and other streptococci, gram-negative enteric organisms, and, rarely, *L monocytogenes*). Ampicillin plus an aminoglycoside is the initial empiric regimen of choice (Table 14-2). In the era of IAP, up to 40% of early-onset sepsis cases are caused by

Table 14-2. Treatment of Group B Streptococcal Infections in Neonates and Infants

Focus of Infection	Antibiotic	Daily Dose	Duration
Suspected meningitis (initial empiric therapy)	Ampicillin + gentamicin	300–400 mg/kg (<7 d, 200–300 mg/kg) 7.5 mg/kg	Until CSF is sterile
Suspected sepsis[a] (initial empiric therapy)	Ampicillin + gentamicin	150–200 mg/kg	Until bloodstream is sterile
Meningitis	Penicillin G	450,000–500,000 U/kg (<7 d, 250,000–450,000 U/kg)	14 d minimum[b]
Bacteremia	Penicillin G	200,000 U/kg	10 d
Arthritis	Penicillin G	200,000–300,000 U/kg	2–3 wk
Osteomyelitis	Penicillin G	200,000–300,000 U/kg	3–4 wk
Endocarditis	Penicillin G	400,000 U/kg	4 wk[c]

Abbreviation: CSF, cerebrospinal fluid.

[a] Assumes that lumbar puncture has been performed and the CSF has no abnormalities.

[b] Should be extended to 21 d or longer if ventriculitis, cerebritis, subdural empyema, or other suppurative complications occur.

[c] In combination with low-dose gentamicin for the first 14 d.

ampicillin-resistant gram-negative organisms; addition of a third-generation cephalosporin may be warranted in severely ill neonates. For suspected late-onset infection, the usual initial therapy includes intravenous ampicillin in combination with cefotaxime or ceftriaxone. Empiric treatment depends on the clinical setting (hospital- versus community-acquired illness) and local bacterial resistance patterns. For example, vancomycin should be considered empirically for an infant with a central venous catheter. Ampicillin or penicillin G should be added to the regimen of infants receiving empiric vancomycin until GBS meningitis has been excluded because vancomycin is inhibitory rather than bactericidal against GBS in vitro (Evidence Level II-3).

Definitive Therapy

When GBS has been identified in cultures as the cause of infection, penicillin G alone should be used to complete therapy if the patient has improved clinically and repeat cultures are sterile (Evidence Level II-3). For meningitis, some experts recommend a second lumbar puncture at 24 to 48 hours after initiation of therapy to document sterilization and assist in management and prognosis (Evidence Level III). If CSF cultures remain positive, a complicated course can be expected. An increasing protein concentration suggests an intracranial complication, such as infarction or ventricular obstruction. Diagnostic imaging studies are indicated if response to therapy is unclear, neurologic abnormalities persist, or focal neurologic deficits occur. Recommendations concerning the optimal dose and duration have varied, but they should be dictated by the focus and severity of infection (see Table 14-2).

Supportive Care

Ventilatory support, careful management of fluids and electrolytes, prompt recognition and treatment of shock, and seizure control are important supportive management.

Sibling of Infected Infants

Siblings of an index case who are the product of a multiple pregnancy (eg, twins, triplets) have increased risk for development of early- and late-onset GBS infection. Therefore, siblings should be observed carefully and evaluated and treated empirically if signs of illness occur.

Prevention

The Centers for Disease Control and Prevention and American Academy of Pediatrics published revised guidelines for the prevention of perinatal GBS infection in 2010. All pregnant women should be screened at 35 to 37 weeks' gestation for rectovaginal colonization (Evidence Level II-2). Indications for IAP are shown in Table 14-3. Algorithms for screening and IAP for women presenting in preterm labor or with preterm premature rupture of membranes can be found in the 2010 Centers for Disease and Control Prevention revised guidelines.

Intrapartum antibiotic prophylaxis should begin at hospital admission for delivery or at rupture of membranes and continue until delivery. Antibiotics are administered intravenously. Penicillin G (5 million U initially, then 2.5 to 3 million U every 4 hours) is the preferred agent (Evidence Level I). Ampicillin (2 g initially, then 1 g every 4 hours) is the alternative. For penicillin-allergic women without a history of anaphylaxis, respiratory distress, angioedema, or urticaria, cefazolin (2 g initially, then 1 g every 8 hours) should be given (Evidence Level II-3). Women at high risk of anaphylaxis should receive clindamycin (900 mg every 8 hours) if their GBS isolate is known to be susceptible (Evidence Level III). If clindamycin susceptibility has not been performed, vancomycin (1 g every 12 hours) should be administered (Evidence Level III). Efficacy of clindamycin or vancomycin has not been established.

Treatment of an infant born to a mother given IAP depends on the clinical findings at birth, the antibiotic regimen, and timing of doses administered to the mother (Figure 14-1). Any neonate with signs of sepsis needs evaluation and empiric treatment for sepsis (Evidence Level II-2). Adequate IAP is defined as at least 4 hours of intravenous penicillin, ampicillin, or cefazolin. If the infant appears healthy and has a mother who received adequate IAP, neither diagnostic evaluation nor empiric antimicrobial therapy is required. Observation in the hospital is recommended for at least 48 hours; however, such infants may be discharged home as early as 24 hours after delivery if

Table 14-3. Indications and Non-indications for Maternal Intrapartum Prophylaxis to Prevent Early-Onset Group B Streptococcal Infection

Intrapartum GBS Prophylaxis Indicated	Intrapartum GBS Prophylaxis Not Indicated
Previous infant with invasive GBS infection	Colonization with GBS during previous pregnancy
GBS bacteriuria during any trimester of current pregnancy[a]	GBS bacteriuria during previous pregnancy
Positive GBS rectovaginal screening culture within preceding 5 wk[a]	Negative GBS rectovaginal screening culture, regardless of intrapartum risk factors
Unknown GBS status at onset of labor and any of the following indications: • Delivery at <37 wk' gestation • Prolonged rupture of membranes for ≥18 h • Intrapartum temperature 38°C (≥100.4°F)[b] • Intrapartum NAAT positive for GBS[c]	Cesarean delivery performed before onset of labor on a woman with intact amniotic membranes, regardless of GBS colonization status or gestational age

Abbreviations: GBS, group B streptococcal; NAAT, nucleic acid amplification test.

[a] Intrapartum chemoprophylaxis is not indicated in this circumstance if a cesarean delivery is performed before onset of labor on a woman with intact membranes.

[b] If amnionitis is suspected, broad-spectrum antibiotic therapy that includes an agent active against GBS should replace GBS prophylaxis.

[c] Group B streptococcal NAAT is optional and may not be available in all settings. If intrapartum NAAT is negative for GBS but any other above intrapartum risk factor is present, intrapartum GBS prophylaxis is indicated.

Adapted from Verani JR, McGee L, Schrag SJ; Division of Bacterial Diseases, National Center for Immunization and Respiratory Diseases, Centers for Disease Control and Prevention. Prevention of perinatal group B streptococcal disease—revised guidelines from CDC, 2010. *MMWR Recomm Rep.* 2010;59(RR-10):1–26.

other discharge criteria have been met, medical care is easily accessible, and a person able to adhere to instructions for home observation will be present (Evidence Level III). Healthy-appearing neonates who are born at least 37 weeks' gestation to a mother with an indication for IAP but who received inadequate IAP should be observed at least 48 hours. Healthy-appearing infants born to a mother with suspected chorioamnionitis should undergo a limited laboratory evaluation (complete blood cell count and blood culture) and receive antibiotic therapy pending culture results (Evidence Level II-2). An infant born at less than 37 weeks' gestation or following prolonged membrane rupture for 18 hours or greater duration to a mother with inadequate IAP should undergo limited laboratory evaluation and observation in the hospital for 48 hours without therapy (Evidence Level III). If the subsequent clinical course or laboratory results suggest infection, full diagnostic evaluation and therapy is initiated.

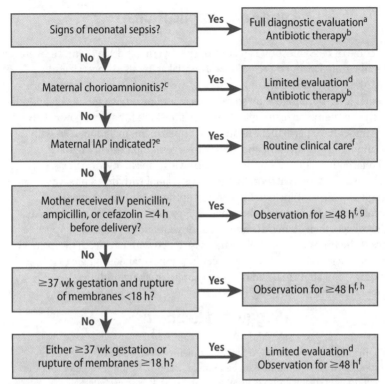

Figure 14-1. Evaluation and management algorithm for secondary prevention of early-onset group B streptococcal infection among neonates.

Abbreviation: IAP, intrapartum antibiotic prophylaxis; IV, intravenous.

a Includes complete blood cell count with differential, blood culture, and chest radiograph if respiratory abnormalities are present. When signs of sepsis are present, a lumbar puncture, if feasible, should be performed.

b Antibiotic therapy should be directed toward common causes of neonatal sepsis, including ampicillin for group B *Streptococcus* and coverage for *Escherichia coli* and other gram-negative pathogens, and should take into account local resistance patterns.

c Consultation with obstetricians is important to determine the level of clinical suspicion for chorioamnionitis. Chorioamnionitis is diagnosed clinically, and some of the signs are nonspecific.

d Includes complete blood cell count with differential and blood culture.

e See Table 14-3 for indications for maternal intrapartum prophylaxis.

f If signs of sepsis develop, a full diagnostic evaluation should be conducted and antibiotic therapy initiated.

g A healthy-appearing infant who was ≥37 wk' gestation at delivery and whose mother received ≥4 h of appropriate IAP before delivery may be discharged home after 24 h if other discharge criteria have been met, a person able to adhere fully to instructions for home observation will be present, and access to medical care is readily available. If any one of these conditions is not met, the infant should be observed in the hospital for at least 48 h and until criteria for discharge are achieved.

h Some experts recommend a complete blood cell count with differential at 6–12 h.

Adapted from Verani JR, McGee L, Schrag SJ; Division of Bacterial Diseases, National Center for Immunization and Respiratory Diseases, Centers for Disease Control and Prevention. Prevention of perinatal group B streptococcal disease—revised guidelines from CDC, 2010. *MMWR Recomm Rep.* 2010;59(RR-10):1–26.

Long-term Implications

The outcome of GBS infection is related to the severity and site of infection at initial evaluation. Death rate remains substantial at 2% to 8% overall and exceeds 20% in neonates born at less than 37 weeks' gestation. A contemporary multicenter long-term follow-up study of term and near term infants diagnosed with early- or late-onset meningitis found that 56% are functioning normally. The remainder have permanent neurologic impairment, including 25% with mild to moderate impairment and 19% with severe impairment of global mental retardation, cortical blindness, hearing loss, spasticity, or paresis. Clinical features on presentation that were associated with death or severe neurologic impairment included lethargy, respiratory distress, coma or semicoma, bulging fontanel, leukopenia, CSF protein greater than 300 mg/dL, CSF glucose less than 20 mg/dL, and need for ventilator or pressor support. Features at the time of hospital discharge associated with late death or severe impairment included failed hearing screening, abnormal neurologic examination findings, and abnormal end of therapy brain imaging findings.

Suggested Reading

Baker CJ, Byington CL, Polin RA; American Academy of Pediatrics Committee on Infectious Diseases, Committee on Fetus and Newborn. Recommendations for the prevention of perinatal group B streptococcal (GBS) disease. *Pediatrics.* 2011;128(3):611–616

Centers for Disease Control and Prevention. Trends in perinatal group B streptococcal disease—United States, 2000-2006. *MMWR Morb Mortal Wkly Rep.* 2009;58(5): 109–112

Jordan HT, Farley MM, Craig A, et al. Revisiting the need for vaccine prevention of late-onset neonatal group B streptococcal disease: a multistate, population-based analysis. *Pediatr Infect Dis J.* 2008;27(12):1057–1064

Libster R, Edwards KM, Levent F, et al. Long-term outcomes of group B streptococcal meningitis. *Pediatrics.* 2012;130(1):e8–e15

Stoll BJ, Hansen NI, Sánchez PJ, et al. Early onset neonatal sepsis: the burden of group B streptococcal and *E. coli* disease continues. *Pediatrics.* 2011;127(5):817–826

Verani JR, McGee L, Schrag SJ; Division of Bacterial Diseases, National Center for Immunization and Respiratory Diseases, Centers for Disease Control and Prevention. Prevention of perinatal group B streptococcal disease—revised guidelines from CDC, 2010. *MMWR Recomm Rep.* 2010;59(RR-10):1–36

CHAPTER 15

Helicobacter pylori Infections

Kari Neemann, MD; Catherine O'Keefe, DNP, APRN-NP;
and Archana Chatterjee, MD, PhD

Key Points

- *Helicobacter pylori* infection causes nodular gastritis and peptic ulcer disease; disease increases the risk of gastric cancer.

- Acquisition occurs in the first 5 years of life and is especially high in children from resource-limited countries that have high rates of gastric cancer.

- Diagnosis is established by endoscopy and culture of gastric mucosa and urease testing; noninvasive studies including breath tests (>3 years) or stool antigen testing can be used.

- Screening and, if positive, treatment should be prescribed in those with histologically proven gastritis, peptic ulcer disease, gastric mucosa-associated lymphoid tissue-type lymphoma, or gastric cancer; patients with a first-degree relative with gastric cancer or who are at high risk for gastric cancer (resource-limited countries with high risk for gastric cancer); and those with unexplained iron deficiency anemia.

- Effective treatment includes triple combinations that include a proton pump inhibitor *plus* clarithromycin *plus* amoxicillin or metronidazole; documentation of eradication may be performed following treatment.

Overview

Helicobacter pylori is a gram-negative bacterium that colonizes the surface of the gastric mucosa and can cause gastroduodenal inflammation. *Helicobacter pylori* infection causes dysregulation of local acid secretion, resulting in hypochlorhydria and gastroduodenal inflammation. Nodular gastritis is the most common finding on endoscopic evaluation.

Successful treatment and eradication of *H pylori* has potential to decrease the subsequent risk of gastric cancer (Evidence Level I). However, insufficient evidence supports widespread screening of asymptomatic children (Evidence Level III).

Causes and Differential Diagnosis

Helicobacter pylori infection is most frequently associated with poor sanitation, crowded living conditions, and infections within the family. The mechanism of acquiring the infection is unclear. Sources of infection can be person to person, waterborne, or via contaminated medical equipment. Transmission is most often through the stool-oral route.

Differential diagnoses to consider include gastroesophageal reflux, gastric ulcer disease secondary to chemical irritation from aspirin, nonsteroidal anti-inflammatory drugs or steroid therapy, and functional abdominal pain.

Clinical Features

Many children with *H pylori* infection are asymptomatic. However, more typically symptoms are consistent with peptic ulcer disease (PUD) and include epigastric pain, nausea, vomiting, hematemesis, and guaiac-positive stools.

Evaluation

Abdominal pain in a child without other known causes in whom PUD is suspected should prompt evaluation for *H pylori* infection. Infection is not associated with abdominal pain outside the realm of PUD, and *H pylori* eradication is not correlated with improvement in gastroesophageal reflux disease symptoms.

An evaluation for *H pylori* infection should occur in asymptomatic patients whose first-degree relatives have a diagnosis of gastric cancer, children who are at high risk for gastric cancer (eg, those whose parents were born in regions with high incidence of gastric cancer), or children with unexplained iron deficiency anemia.

Invasive Tests

Invasive tests require gastric tissue for the identification of *H pylori* and include culture, histopathology, rapid urease test, polymerase chain reaction, and fluorescence in situ hybridization.

The criterion standard for diagnosis of *H pylori* infection is a positive culture obtained at the time of endoscopy, which is considered to be 100% specific, although sensitivity is lower (Box 15-1). Clinicians should wait at least 2 weeks after stopping proton pump inhibitor (PPI) therapy and 4 weeks after stopping antibiotic therapy to perform any biopsy-based and noninvasive tests (Evidence Level II-2). When available, culture should be pursued with antibiotic susceptibility testing to help guide second-line therapy in the situation when the initial regimen for an *H pylori*–infected child fails. Diagnosis is confirmed by either a positive culture or concordance of 2 additional invasive tests (histopathology and rapid urease test) (Box 15-1). Rationale for the recommendation to perform more than 1 diagnostic test is based on the sensitivity results of invasive tests, which range from 66% to 100% for histology and 75% to 100% for rapid urease tests in published series from children (Evidence Level II-3). One exception to this rule is the presence of a bleeding peptic ulcer, in which case only 1 positive biopsy-based test is sufficient to make the diagnosis. If the results of histology and rapid urease test are discordant, a noninvasive test should be applied (Evidence Level II-3).

Box 15-1. Criteria for Diagnosis of *Helicobacter pylori* Infection

Positive tissue culture

or

Positive histopathology *plus* positive rapid urease test

or

Positive histopathology or positive rapid urease test *plus* positive noninvasive test (^{13}C-urease breath test or stool antigen test)

or

Positive histopathology or positive rapid urease test *plus* bleeding peptic ulcer

---

Noninvasive Tests

Noninvasive methods for detection of *H pylori* include serology, varying methods for detection of urease production, detection of salivary antibody, stool culture, stool antigen, polymerase chain reaction, and urine ammonia production. The ^{13}C-urease breath test is thought to have a high accuracy and can be used both for pretreatment diagnosis and posttreatment follow-up. *Helicobacter pylori* antigen testing in the stool by enzyme immunoassay is a more convenient way to assess for active infection and proof of cure in children of all ages, with higher accuracy based on monoclonal enzyme immunoassay tests. Serology has a role in epidemiologic surveys but no role in the clinical setting.

Management

Who Should Be Treated?

Eradication of *H pylori*–positive PUD has been shown to reduce the likelihood of recurrence in both adults and children; therefore, in this situation, treatment should always be recommended (Evidence Level II-1). The finding of *H pylori*–associated gastritis in the absence of PUD poses a clinical dilemma, because no strong evidence supports a causal relationship between *H pylori*–associated gastritis and abdominal symptoms. In adults there has been some evidence that eradication of *H pylori* nonulcer dyspepsia may prevent the development of PUD; therefore, therapy should be considered in the pediatric population as well (Evidence Level III). Asymptomatic *H pylori*–infected children with first-degree relatives with gastric cancer are recommended treatment, but otherwise therapy should be based on clinical judgment (Evidence Level III).

Treatment Regimens

The goal of therapy in *H pylori* infection is to induce eradication with the first-line therapy. If resistance to clarithromycin in the community is greater than 20%, it is recommended to obtain susceptibility testing prior to starting therapy. First-line eradication regimens are based on triple therapy, with the combination of 2 antibiotics and a PPI as outlined in Box 15-2, with a duration of 7 to 14 days.

Box 15-2. First-line Treatment Recommendations[a]

PPI (1–2 mg/kg/d) + amoxicillin (50 mg/kg/d) + metronidazole (20 mg/kg/d)

or

PPI (1–2 mg/kg/d) + amoxicillin (50 mg/kg/d) + clarithromycin (20 mg/kg/d)

or

Bismuth salts (bismuth subsalicylate or subnitrate at 8 mg/kg/d) + amoxicillin (50 mg/kg/d) + metronidazole (20 mg/kg/d)

or

PPI (1–2 mg/kg/d) + amoxicillin (50 mg/kg/d) for 5 d; then PPI (1–2 mg/kg/d) + clarithromycin (20 mg/kg/d) + metronidazole (20 mg/kg/d) for 5 d

Abbreviation: PPI, proton pump inhibitor.

[a] Maximum daily dose for amoxicillin: 2,000 mg/d; for metronidazole: 1,000 mg/d; and for clarithromycin: 1,000 mg/d. Administer divided twice a day for 7–14 d.

Adapted from Koletzko S, Jones NL, Goodman KJ, et al. Evidence-based guidelines from ESPGHAN and NASPGHAN for *Helicobacter pylori* infection in children. *J Pediatr Gastroenterol Nutr.* 2011;53(2):230–243, with permission from Wolters Kluwer.

An alternative regimen, with the goal of decreasing clarithromycin resistance, is given in a sequential method. Sequential therapy involves dual therapy with amoxicillin and a PPI for 5 days with the goal of decreasing the bacterial load, followed by 5 days of triple therapy (a PPI with clarithromycin and metronidazole/tinidazole). At this time both standard triple therapy and sequential therapy are viable first-line treatments (Evidence Level I).

Long-term Monitoring

Four to 8 weeks following completion of first-line treatment, a noninvasive test for eradication of *H pylori* may be performed (Evidence Level III). The absence of symptoms does not confirm the eradication. Reliable tests include the ^{13}C-urease breath test and a monoclonal enzyme-linked immunosorbent assay for detection of *H pylori* antigen in stool. However, stool antigen may remain positive for up to 90 days following treatment. Figure 15-1 outlines the steps to

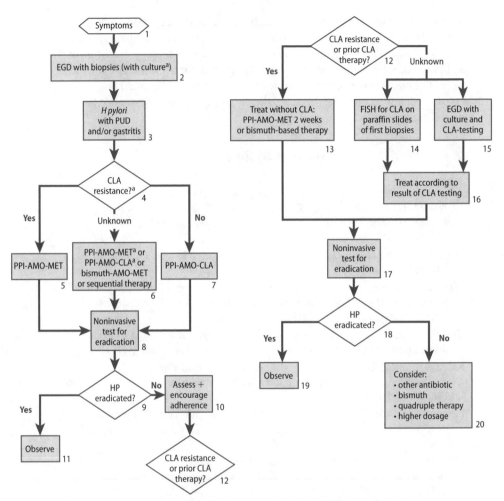

Figure 15-1. Treatment for *Helicobacter pylori* infections in pediatric patients.

Abbreviations: AMO, amoxicillin; CLA, clarithromycin; EGD, esophagogastroduodenoscopy; FISH, fluorescence in situ hybridization; HP, *Helicobacter pylori;* MET, metronidazole; PPI, proton pump inhibitor; PUD, peptic ulcer disease.

[a] In areas or populations with a primary clarithromycin-resistance rate of >20% or unknown background antibiotic-resistance rates, culture and susceptibility testing should be performed and the treatment should be chosen accordingly.

[b] If susceptibility testing has not been performed or has failed, antibiotics should be chosen according to the background of the child.

From Koletzko S, Jones NL, Goodman KJ, et al. Evidence-based guidelines from ESPGHAN and NASPGHAN for *Helicobacter pylori* infection in children. *J Pediatr Gastroenterol Nutr.* 2011;53(2): 230 –243, with permission from Wolters Kluwer.

take if initial eradication is not achieved. If culture and susceptibility testing is not available and retreatment is needed, either a longer course of therapy of 2 to 4 weeks or second-line agents should be used. Quadruple therapy consisting of PPI plus amoxicillin plus metronidazole plus bismuth or triple therapy consisting of PPI plus levofloxacin (or moxifloxacin) plus amoxicillin could be considered. For second-line therapies, the duration is generally extended to 14 days (Evidence Level I).

Suggested Reading

American Academy of Pediatrics. *Helicobacter pylori* infections. In: Kimberlin DW, Brady MT, Jackson MA, Long SS, eds. *Red Book: 2015 Report of the Committee on Infectious Diseases.* 30th ed. Elk Grove Village, IL: American Academy of Pediatrics; 2015

Ertem D. Clinical practice: *Helicobacter pylori* infection in childhood. *Eur J Pediatr.* 2013;172(11):1427–1437

Francavilla R, Lionetti E, Castellaneta SP, et al. Improved efficacy of 10-day sequential treatment for *Helicobacter pylori* eradication in children: a randomized trial. *Gastroenterology.* 2005;129(5):1414–1419

Guarner J, Kalach N, Elitsur Y, Koletzko S. *Helicobacter pylori* diagnostic tests in children: review of the literature from 1999 to 2009. *Eur J Pediatr.* 2010;169(1):15–25

Koletzko S, Jones NL, Goodman KJ, et al. Evidence-based guidelines from ESPGHAN and NASPGHAN for *Helicobacter pylori* infection in children. *J Pediatr Gastroenterol Nutr.* 2011;53(2):230–243

Levine A, Milo T, Broide E, et al. Influence of *Helicobacter pylori* eradication on gastroesophageal reflux symptoms and epigastric pain in children and adolescents. *Pediatrics.* 2004;113(1 Pt 1):54–58

Malfertheiner P, Megraud F, O'Morain C, et al. Current concepts in the management of *Helicobacter pylori* infection: the Maastricht III Consensus Report. *Gut.* 2007;56(6):772–781

Moayyedi P, Soo S, Deeks J, et al. Eradication of *Helicobacter pylori* for non-ulcer dyspepsia. *Cochrane Database Syst Rev.* 2006;(2):CD002096

CHAPTER 16

Listeria monocytogenes Infections

Jodi Jackson, MD, and Julie Weiner, DO

Key Points

- *Listeria monocytogenes* is a cause of sepsis and meningitis in the neonate, pregnant women, older adults, and those who are immunocompromised.

- Ampicillin plus gentamicin is the treatment of choice; cephalosporins are not active against *L monocytogenes*.

- Trimethoprim/sulfamethoxazole may be considered in non-neonates who have a history of anaphylaxis to penicillin.

- Clinicians should consider the diagnosis of invasive listerial infection if a gram-positive rod is noted on cerebrospinal fluid Gram stain or a diphtheroid grows from blood or cerebrospinal fluid, because laboratory misidentification may occur.

- For those at risk for listeriosis, dietary restrictions (eg, avoidance of unpasteurized milk products, soft cheeses, deli meats) and meticulous food preparation (heating, food preparation, and cleanup) should be ensured.

Overview

First described in 1926 and associated with human disease in 1929, *Listeria monocytogenes* is a well-recognized cause of foodborne disease outbreaks. Invasive infection has been described in neonates, pregnant women, elderly persons, and those with impaired cell-mediated immunity.

Causes and Differential Diagnosis

Listeria monocytogenes is a short, non-branching gram-positive rod, the morphology of which may cause confusion because it is similar to that of nonpathogenic diphtheroids and some streptococci. The organism can be recovered from blood, cerebrospinal fluid (CSF), meconium, gastric washings, placental and fetal tissue, amniotic fluid, and sites associated with disseminated disease, including joints and pleural and pericardial fluids.

Clinical manifestations overlap closely with other infections, and a broad differential is required. Neonatal disease resembles any other form of early sepsis or meningitis and can present similarly to group B *Streptococcus, Escherichia coli,* severe cytomegalovirus, rubella, or toxoplasmosis. Pneumonia often has nonspecific radiographic features, but can resemble respiratory distress syndrome with patchy bronchopneumonic infiltrates.

In the non-neonate, the patient presents with febrile illness and differential diagnosis includes other bacterial causes of sepsis and meningitis, such as *Neisseria meningitidis* and *Streptococcus pneumoniae.* When *L monocytogenes* infection occurs in the immunocompromised host, disseminated disease and neurologic presentations are common and may raise concern for common bacterial as well as opportunistic pathogens, including fungi (eg, *Cryptococcus,* endemic mycotic agents, *Aspergillus*) and viruses (eg, cytomegalovirus, herpes simplex virus).

Listeria monocytogenes should be considered in the setting of an outbreak of febrile gastroenteritis when routine cultures do not identify a pathogen. Box 16-1 shows clinical settings in which listeriosis should be considered strongly as part of the differential diagnosis.

Box 16-1. When to Consider the Diagnosis of Listeriosis

- Early-onset neonatal sepsis
- Late-onset neonatal meningitis
- Subacute meningitis in the immunocompromised host
- Subcortical brain abscess
- Foodborne outbreak of gastroenteritis when testing fails to identify a pathogen

Clinical Features

Disease presentation and severity vary by age and patient population.

Infection in Pregnancy

Listeriosis during pregnancy is usually acquired from ingestion of foodborne source. Although disease in pregnant women is usually mild (fever, aches, chills, back pain, and gastrointestinal symptoms), it can be devastating to the fetus if intrauterine or perinatal infection occurs. Premature labor and spontaneous abortion are common.

Bloodstream infection in pregnancy may present clinically as a mild acute febrile illness, often with related myalgia, arthralgia, headache, and backache. Illness usually occurs in the third trimester. Untreated systemic infection in pregnancy is usually self-limited; however, when amnionitis occurs, it can result in spontaneous abortion, fetal death, preterm delivery, and neonatal illness or death. It is extremely rare to have central nervous system (CNS) infection during pregnancy in the absence of other risk factors.

Neonatal Infection

Neonatal infection is the most common clinical form of human listeriosis and can be divided into 2 clinical groups: early-onset versus late-onset.

Maternal listerial infection may cause premature delivery. Likewise, premature infants are at higher risk than term infants to manifest early-onset disease. Early-onset disease may occur up to 7 days of age, but usually cases present by day 3 of life. Most often, evidence of disease is present at delivery, and there is history of a proceeding maternal illness (eg, malaise, myalgia), suggesting in utero acquisition of infection. Frequently, the presentation of early-onset neonatal infection is not easily discernable from that of more common pathogens (ie, group B *Streptococcus, E coli,* herpes simplex virus, enteroviruses). However, occasionally purulent conjunctivitis and an erythematous rash with small, pale papules may be distinguishing features.

Disease may be heralded by meconium staining, cyanosis, apnea, and respiratory distress. Pneumonia may be evident. Granulomatosis infantiseptica is a severe disseminated form of listerial neonatal infection that presents with microabscesses and granulomas mostly seen in the liver and spleen. Neonates affected in this way are usually stillborn or die within a few hours of birth. A heavy load of bacteria may be seen on the Gram stain of meconium in patients presenting in this manner.

Neonatal disease is considered late-onset when occurring in infants older than 7 days. There may be overlap between early and late disease, although the clinical patterns are usually distinct. Later occurrence of the disease suggests it is acquired from vaginal colonization during the process of neonatal delivery. However, cases have been reported after cesarean delivery, and nosocomial acquisition of infection is probable, specifically in some reported outbreaks.

The most common form of late-onset *L monocytogenes* infection is meningitis, occurring in 94% of late-onset cases and clinically similar in presentation to other forms of bacterial meningitis. Often, infants do not appear excessively ill and usually present with fever and irritability. Other less common forms of late-onset disease include colitis with diarrhea and sepsis without meningitis.

Non-neonatal Disease

After the neonatal period, bacteremia is most commonly seen in immunocompromised patients. Although a prodromal illness with nausea and diarrhea can occur, fever and myalgia are the most common clinical concerns. Complications can include disseminated intravascular coagulation, adult respiratory distress syndrome, and rhabdomyolysis with acute renal failure.

Listerial CNS infections are common in high-risk individuals, but may occur uncommonly in otherwise healthy individuals. Clinically, meningitis caused by *L monocytogenes* is similar in presentation to other common causes of meningitis. Many patients with meningitis experience altered consciousness, seizures, or movement disorders or have features of meningoencephalitis. *Listeria monocytogenes* is the most common cause of bacterial meningitis in patients with lymphoma, those with organ transplants, or those receiving corticosteroid immunosuppressive therapy for any reason and second to *S pneumoniae* as a cause of meningitis in adults older than 50 years.

Encephalitis (also known as rhombencephalitis) is a rare but serious form of listeriosis that involves the brainstem. In contrast to other listerial CNS infections, it usually occurs in healthy older children and adults. This manifestation generally has a biphasic presentation with fever, headache, nausea, and vomiting lasting a couple of days, followed by the abrupt onset of asymmetric cranial nerve deficits, cerebellar signs, and hemiparesis or hemisensory deficits, or both. Respiratory failure and nuchal rigidity is common, developing in 40% to 50% of cases.

Brain abscesses may occur in individuals who are not at known risk for listerial infection. Presentation of subcortical abscesses located in the thalamus, pons, and medulla is distinctive to listerial infection in that these are unusual sites for abscesses caused by other bacteria.

Rarely, patients with *L monocytogenes* infection have endocarditis (usually seen in adult population).

Rare localized focal infections have been reported. Bacteremia can lead to hepatic infection, cholecystitis, peritonitis, splenic abscess, pleuropulmonary infection, septic arthritis, osteomyelitis, pericarditis, myocarditis, arteritis, and endophthalmitis. These localized infections tend to occur in those known to be at risk for listeriosis.

Listerial gastroenteritis most often occurs approximately 24 hours after the ingestion of a large load of bacteria, but can range between 6 hours and 10 days after exposure. Illness usually lasts 1 to 3 days, but can last up to 7 days. The disease often presents as fever, watery diarrhea, nausea, headache, and pains in joints and muscles. Many patients who develop invasive disease have a history of a prior gastrointestinal illness with fever.

In the largest known foodborne outbreak reported, 1,566 mostly school-aged children became ill after eating caterer-provided cafeteria food at 2 schools. About a quarter required hospitalization for treatment.

Evaluation

Listeria monocytogenes grows readily in blood culture and may also grow from conjunctivae, external ear fluid, nose, throat, meconium, amniotic fluid, placenta, and occasionally CSF cultures. Evaluation of the meconium may provide early diagnosis with Gram stain. The lung and gut often have the largest concentrations of bacteria recovered.

Other laboratory studies that may be helpful include complete blood cell count, C-reactive protein, and CSF, which may show pleocytosis, hypoglycorrhachia, and elevated protein concentration. Leukocytosis with immature cells or neutropenia, thrombocytopenia, and anemia may be noted.

Radiographic features are nonspecific and may range from peribronchial to widespread infiltrations. The radiographic evaluation in long-standing infection may differ from acute infection in that the chest radiograph may show a coarser, mottled, or nodular appearance. In severe cases, oxygen exchange is affected to a greater degree than ventilation and prolonged hypoxia may occur after adequate ventilation is established.

In severe fatal neonatal disease, military granulomatosis with microabscesses in the liver, spleen, CNS, lung, and bowel may be seen at autopsy.

For patients with CNS manifestations, magnetic resonance imaging is superior to computed tomography for showing parenchymal brain involvement, especially in the brainstem.

Management

Currently, no controlled trials have established drug of choice or duration of therapy for listeriosis; however, ampicillin is generally considered the drug of choice and should be used in conjunction with gentamicin, which provides synergy. A treatment course of a minimum of 2 weeks is suggested for bacteremia and no fewer than 3 weeks for meningitis.

Trimethoprim/sulfamethoxazole is the best alternative if ampicillin cannot be used. However, it is contraindicated in babies younger than 2 months. Other alternatives include quinolones, linezolid, and rifampin.

Cephalosporins are not active against *L monocytogenes,* and vancomycin is not recommended because treatment failures have been reported.

Treatment is not warranted in non–pregnancy-related gastroenteritis because the illness is self-limited.

Long-term Implications

When listerial infection is acquired during pregnancy, fetal mortality rates are probably high, although the relative risk of intrauterine death is unknown. Early treatment of maternal disease seems to have a beneficial effect on outcomes for the fetus and neonate. There is no suggestion that *Listeria* is associated with repeat fetal loss.

Most neonatal survivors from early-onset infection do not seem to have sequelae. Long-term morbidities are related to the associated factors and complications, such as prematurity, pneumonia, or sepsis.

Major sequelae of neonatal late-onset listerial meningitis are hydrocephalus and impaired neurologic function.

For non-neonatal listerial infections,

- The outcome of other listerial diseases depends on the associated underlying disease and accessibility to adequate care.

- Meningitis in older infants has a relatively good prognosis.
- Brainstem encephalitis and abscesses have a high death rate, with serious sequelae in survivors.
- Listerial endocarditis is associated with a high rate of septic complications and mortality.

There are specific recommendations concerning "high-risk foods" that should be avoided during pregnancy and in individuals at a higher risk for invasive disease. These foods include raw meat, unwashed vegetables, unpasteurized milk, soft cheeses, and delicatessen meats.

Intrapartum prophylactic antibiotic therapy is not recommended for mothers with a history of perinatal listeriosis. There is no known risk of repeat neonatal infection.

There is no vaccine. Trimethoprim/sulfamethoxazole given as pneumocystis pneumonia prophylaxis to recipients of organ transplants or individuals with HIV infection has been shown to be effective in preventing listerial infections.

Suggested Reading

American Academy of Pediatrics. *Listeria monocytogenes* infections (listeriosis). In: Kimberlin DW, Brady MT, Jackson MA, Long SS, eds. *Red Book: 2015 Report of the Committee on Infectious Diseases.* 30th ed. Elk Grove Village, IL: American Academy of Pediatrics; 2015

Centers for Disease Control and Prevention. Multistate outbreak of listeriosis associated with Jensen Farms cantaloupe—United States, August-September 2011. *MMWR Morb Mortal Wkly Rep.* 2011;60(39);1357–1360

Centers for Disease Control and Prevention. Outbreak of invasive listeriosis associated with the consumption of hog head cheese—Louisiana, 2010. *MMWR Morb Mortal Wkly Rep.* 2011;60(13):401–405

Cherubin CE, Appleman MD, Heseltine PN, Khayr W, Stratton CW. Epidemiological spectrum and current treatment of listeriosis. *Rev Infect Dis.* 1991;13(6):1108–1114

Posfay-Barbe KM, Wald ER. Listeriosis. *Pediatr Rev.* 2004;25(5):151–159

Posfay-Barbe KM, Wald ER. Listeriosis. *Semin Fetal Neonatal Med.* 2009;14(4):228–233

CHAPTER 17

Lyme Disease

Eugene D. Shapiro, MD

Key Points

- Classical disease is divided into 3 stages: early localized, early disseminated, and late disease.

- Erythema migrans is the characteristic presentation seen in most children, and clinical diagnosis alone is sufficient to initiate therapy in children who have been exposed in endemic regions.

- Endemic regions in the United States include New England, mid-Atlantic states, upper Midwest (Wisconsin and Michigan), and less often northern California.

- Immunoglobulin G antibody is used for diagnostic testing in the setting of early disseminated disease without rash or late Lyme disease; 2-tier testing has excellent sensitivity, 80% to 90% in patients with either early disseminated neurologic or cardiac disease and nearly 100% in patients with Lyme arthritis.

- Doxycycline is the drug of choice for children older than 8 years with early localized disease (amoxicillin for younger children); ceftriaxone is reserved for those with symptomatic heart block and central nervous system infection.

Overview

Lyme disease, caused by the tick-transmitted spirochete *Borrelia burgdorferi*, is the most common vector-borne infection in the United States. A large majority of children with Lyme disease (85%–90%) will have a cutaneous manifestation, either a single erythema migrans rash or, if there is dissemination (spirochetemia), multiple erythema migrans. Extracutaneous manifestations of early disseminated Lyme disease include cranial nerve (especially facial nerve) palsy or, less commonly, lymphocytic choriomeningitis or carditis that, rarely, may progress to complete heart block. The common manifestation of late Lyme disease is Lyme arthritis, typically affecting a knee. Antimicrobial treatment of Lyme disease is extremely effective against both cutaneous and extracutaneous manifestations. Most children with Lyme disease are treated successfully without long-term sequelae. Although children occasionally have lingering, nonspecific symptoms, such as fatigue or arthralgia, after treatment, these symptoms almost always resolve spontaneously over time. No scientific evidence supports the diagnosis of so-called chronic Lyme disease. There is substantial evidence that the risks and costs of unusually prolonged anti-microbial therapy are significant, while there is no evidence of benefit. The same tick that transmits *B burgdorferi* can also transmit the agents that cause babesiosis and human granulocytic anaplasmosis, which also should be considered in children with Lyme disease with either unusually severe symptoms or an atypically poor response to treatment. Cases of congenital Lyme disease have not been documented, and Lyme disease has not been transmitted via breastfeeding.

Causes and Differential Diagnosis

Lyme disease in the Unites States is caused by *B burgdorferi*. Different strains of the bacteria, some of which are more neurotropic, cause Lyme disease in Europe and Asia. The differential diagnosis of erythema migrans is shown in Table 17-1.

Erythema migrans can also be caused by southern tick-associated rash illness, the cause of which is unknown (it may not be an infection), which is associated with the bite of *Amblyomma americanum* (the lone star tick). It has a benign course without dissemination or extracutaneous manifestations. No diagnostic tests are available.

Early disseminated Lyme disease occurs when *B burgdorferi* enters the bloodstream and disseminates to various sites. Multiple erythema migrans is the most common manifestation. Others include cranial nerve palsy (most commonly facial nerve palsy), for which the differential diagnosis includes idiopathic (ie, Bell) palsy, lymphoma, and acoustic neuroma; lymphocytic choriomeningitis, for which the differential diagnosis includes viral causes of meningitis, including enteroviral meningitis (uncommonly, a radiculoneuropathy may develop [it may be a polyneuropathy] that may be painful and must be distinguished from compressive lesions, such as tumors); and carditis, which usually manifests as heart block and rarely may progress to complete heart block, for which differential diagnosis includes other causes of carditis, such as viral myocarditis, autoimmune disorders, and rheumatic fever. The typical manifestation of late disseminated disease is Lyme arthritis, which is usually subacute and can mimic other causes of subacute arthritis, such as juvenile inflammatory arthritis, HLA-B27 arthritis, dermatomyositis, psoriatic arthritis, and others, including traumatic injury. Lyme arthritis also may sometimes mimic acute bacterial arthritis.

Table 17-1. Differential Diagnosis of Early Lyme Disease (Erythema Migrans)

Condition	Characteristics
Single erythema migrans	Erythematous macule or papule at site of tick bite (though tick often not seen) and enlarges relatively rapidly from 5–30 cm or more. Typically flat and circular. Usually uniformly erythematous or with heightened central erythema and may have central clearing with bull's-eye appearance. Without treatment, persists for average of 3–4 wk. Often on head or neck in young children. May be in groin, axilla, trunk, or extremities. Similar lesion can be caused by southern tick-associated rash illness.
Nummular eczema	Usually smaller and less erythematous than erythema migrans. Does not enlarge rapidly, pruritic, well demarcated, and skin may be thickened or weepy.
Ringworm	Margin of rash raised with scale on the edges and central clearing is typical. Pruritic.
Granuloma annulare	Small (2–5 cm), circular, and with erythematous papules and clear center. Develops over weeks. Often on dorsum of extremities.
Cellulitis	Often at site of trauma to skin. Warm. Enlarges rapidly, rarely circular, and may be tender and associated with fever.
Insect bite	Often raised papule with central punctum. Pruritic. Usually smaller than erythema migrans and rarely continues to enlarge.
Spider bite	Necrotic with central eschar. Often very painful.
Hypersensitivity to tick bite	Small and does not expand like erythema migrans. Typically present at time tick bite is recognized and uniformly erythematous.
Multiple erythema migrans	Multiple erythematous circular rashes, often with central clearing, at different sites, due to spread of bacteria via the bloodstream. Often associated with fever, myalgia, arthralgia, fatigue, and headache.
Erythema multiforme	Multiple diffuse lesions often quite small, associated cause (eg, drug, infection) may be apparent, and mucosa, palms, and soles may be involved.
Urticaria	Pruritic, raised, and may appear and disappear rapidly.

Clinical Features

Early Lyme Disease

Localized Disease

The most common manifestation of Lyme disease (about two-thirds of cases) is single erythema migrans. Single erythema migrans typically begins as an erythematous macule or papule at the site at which the tick injects *B burgdorferi* into the skin and then expands in a circular or oval pattern.

Although it can appear as a classic target lesion with central clearing, most often (about two-thirds of the time) the rash is uniformly erythematous, sometimes with enhanced central erythema or, occasionally, with a center that is vesicular or even somewhat necrotic. The rash usually appears 7 to 14 days (range: 3–32 days) after the tick bite (which is often not recognized). The rash is often asymptomatic but can be warm or slightly painful. Nonspecific systemic symptoms, such as myalgia, arthralgia, headache, malaise, and, less commonly, fever, may accompany the rash. Untreated, the rash "migrates" or gradually expands to an average diameter of 15 cm (although lesions >30 cm can occur) and persists for an average of 3 to 4 weeks. Lesions can occur anywhere on the body but are particularly common in the groin, belt line, or axilla and, especially in young children, on the head or neck.

Disseminated Disease

Multiple erythema migrans, a manifestation in 15% to 23% of cases of Lyme disease, occurs when *B burgdorferi* disseminates via the bloodstream to multiple sites in the skin, usually manifesting as smaller lesions with central clearing that can be present at many sites, especially on the extremities and trunk. These are often accompanied by fever, myalgia, headache, and fatigue; conjunctivitis and lymphadenopathy can also develop.

Dissemination can also lead to early neurologic Lyme disease. The most common manifestation, cranial nerve palsy, especially palsy of the facial nerve, is relatively common in children and may be the only manifestation of Lyme disease. The palsy usually lasts from 2 to 8 weeks and resolves completely, although sensitive neurologic testing may reveal mild, inapparent, residual weakness. Rarely, palsy resolves partially or not at all. Lymphocytic choriomeningitis may also occur. Although only a concomitant erythema migrans rash can definitively distinguish Lyme meningitis from aseptic meningitis clinically, papilledema is a relatively common feature of Lyme meningitis (20%–40% of cases). The associated increased intracranial pressure can mimic pseudotumor cerebri in its presentation and may pose a risk of compression of the optic nerve or other cranial nerves. Radicular pain with motor and sensory abnormalities of peripheral nerves (eg, radiculitis or myeloradiculitis) has been reported in children in the United States, although it is rare.

Carditis, which can involve any portion of the heart but usually presents as heart block, is another complication of early disseminated Lyme disease. Because mild carditis is usually asymptomatic and children with Lyme disease are often not screened for evidence of carditis, the actual frequency of any degree of carditis in children is unknown. Lyme carditis can present as syncope with complete heart block, the circumstance in which this complication usually comes to clinical attention (<1% of cases of Lyme disease in children).

Late Disease

Arthritis, the usual manifestation of late Lyme disease, occurs in 6% to 8% of children with Lyme disease. Most patients with Lyme arthritis have no history of erythema migrans since if recognized and treated at that stage, arthritis rarely occurs. It is an oligoarthritis with the knee being involved 90% or more of the time. Presentation of the arthritis varies widely, most often subacute in onset, although at times it can mimic an acute bacterial arthritis. Often a large volume of fluid is in the joint, although inflammation, pain, and limitation of motion are usually modest and typically less marked than in most other bacterial arthritides. However, sometimes Lyme arthritis may present like septic arthritis, with an inflamed, very painful joint. With treatment, the arthritis usually improves slowly in the first week, with complete resolution in 2 to 6 weeks. In 5% to 20% of treated patients, the arthritis persists or recurs, although it usually resolves with re-treatment. Very rarely in children, signs of synovitis persist, although even in these unusual cases, the arthritis usually ultimately resolves without long-term sequelae to the joint. Although the mechanism for this chronic arthritis is controversial, it is clear it is not caused by persistence of viable bacteria. In virtually all untreated patients, arthritis recurs, often in other joints. Lyme encephalomyelitis has been reported in adults, although it is extremely rare. In children, late central nervous system disease is exceptionally rare. If suspected, referral to a specialist is indicated.

Congenital and Neonatal Lyme Disease

There are no well-documented cases of congenital Lyme disease despite extensive investigations to try to identify it. In addition, Lyme disease cannot be transmitted via human milk.

Evaluation

Usual diagnostic tests for Lyme disease are shown in Table 17-2.

Diagnosis of erythema migrans (early Lyme disease) is based on the clinical history, distinctive character of the rash, and history of potential exposure to ticks in an area endemic for Lyme disease. Erythema migrans typically occurs in the late spring and summer. Single erythema migrans appears at the site of the tick bite (although the responsible tick is often not seen). Use of antibody tests to document infection with *B burgdorferi* in patients with only erythema migrans is generally not recommended in clinical practice because recommended 2-tier serologic testing has poor sensitivity early after infection. In patients with erythema migrans without evidence of dissemination during the acute phase, only some have a positive result, and even in the convalescent phase after antimicrobial treatment, a substantial proportion of patients never develop a positive result. Although a somewhat higher proportion of patients with erythema migrans and evidence of dissemination will have a positive result, up to 40% will still have a negative result. Culture of a biopsy of the erythema migrans skin lesion, especially when combined with polymerase chain reaction test for bacteria in the culture, is quite sensitive but impractical in clinical practice because it requires an invasive procedure as well as special

Table 17-2. Usual Diagnostic Tests for Lyme Disease in Children

Condition	Diagnostic Tests[a]
Early Localized Lyme Disease	
Single erythema migrans	Clinical diagnosis; serologic results often negative
Early Disseminated Lyme Disease	
Multiple erythema migrans	Clinical diagnosis; serologic results potentially negative but may be positive
Neurologic disease	
Cranial nerve (often VII nerve) palsy	Serology
Meningitis	Serology; lumbar puncture with tests for opening pressure, cell count, glucose, and protein plus antibody tests of CSF, eye examination for papilledema
Heart disease	
Carditis	Serology
Late Disseminated Lyme Disease	
Arthritis	Serology (arthrocentesis with culture also if condition presents like acute septic arthritis)

Abbreviation: CSF, cerebrospinal fluid.

[a] Serology consists of 2-tier testing; a quantitative test, such as an enzyme immunoassay; and, if result is positive or equivocal, a Western immunoblot to confirm specificity of the result.

media and equipment, and the bacteria grow slowly, so results may not be known for weeks.

Diagnostic testing for Lyme disease in clinical settings in children who do not have erythema migrans has largely depended on tests for antibodies against *B burgdorferi*. The standard has been 2-tier testing, which consists of a quantitative test, such as an enzyme-linked immunosorbent assay (ELISA), against a whole-cell sonicate of *B burgdorferi*, and if the result is positive (significantly elevated) or equivocal, a Western immunoblot is done to confirm specificity of the positive result. Although ELISA for antibodies against the C6 peptide has sensitivity comparable to or better than the standard ELISA, specificity of 2-stage testing is superior. There is some evidence that the C6 ELISA may be useful alone or as a confirmatory second tier test. Tests are usually done for IgM and IgG antibodies against *B burgdorferi*. However, the specificity of IgM results tends to be poor (even of immunoblots). Diagnosis of Lyme disease rarely should be made on the basis of results of IgM tests alone in persons who have had symptoms/signs of Lyme disease for 4 weeks or longer. Specificity of immunoblots for either IgG or IgM antibody diminishes if they are done without a positive or equivocal first-tier quantitative test result and should not be performed alone. Unlike for erythema migrans, sensitivity of 2-tier testing for later stages of Lyme disease is good: 80% to 90% in patients with either early disseminated neurologic or cardiac disease and nearly 100% for IgG antibody results in patients with Lyme arthritis.

Children with Lyme meningitis often have a somewhat more indolent onset than is typical for viral meningitis and are more likely to be afebrile. Presence of facial nerve palsy, erythema migrans, or papilledema may be helpful signs that suggest Lyme meningitis. Cerebrospinal fluid (CSF) typically reveals a lymphocytic choriomeningitis with a moderate number (average: about 150) and large preponderance (often ≥90%) of lymphocytes, moderately elevated protein concentration, and relatively normal glucose concentration. Evaluation for Lyme meningitis should ideally include tests for concentrations of both specific antibodies against *B burgdorferi* and total immunoglobulin (ie, IgM, IgG) in both CSF and serum. Production of specific antibody in CSF (relative concentrations that exceed that in serum) may be determined by the ratio of concentrations in CSF of isotype-specific antibody against *B burgdorferi*/total antibody isotype in CSF divided by the same ratio in serum. A ratio greater than 1 suggests local infection with intrathecal production of antibody to *B burgdorferi*. However, the sensitivity of this test is uncertain and a negative result does not definitively rule out Lyme meningitis. Occasionally, magnetic resonance imaging of the brain may be useful in defining a demyelinating process and perhaps in differentiating parenchymal disease from Lyme meningitis. Polymerase chain reaction test has poor sensitivity in CSF and is subject to contamination (and thus false-positive results) in some laboratories. Measuring opening pressure on the lumbar puncture and ophthalmologic examination (or, if not possible, imaging of the brain, if indicated) to assess whether there is increased intracranial pressure is important.

Lumbar puncture in children with isolated facial or other cranial nerve palsy suspected to be caused by Lyme disease is not indicated routinely, since such patients respond well to oral treatment even if there is a pleocytosis. However, if there are clinical signs of meningitis (eg, nuchal rigidity, severe headache), a lumbar puncture for CSF evaluation is indicated.

Children with Lyme carditis typically have heart block on electrocardiogram and may present with syncope if there is complete heart block. Serologic testing is used to confirm the diagnosis if erythema migrans is not present.

Children with Lyme arthritis may present with a wide spectrum of manifestations. Most will be afebrile and have arthritis of a knee that is often subacute in its manifestations with only mild to moderate tenderness and limitation of motion, sometimes despite large effusions. However, in some children the presentation can mimic acute bacterial arthritis with fever and an acutely inflamed and tender joint. Arthrocentesis should not be routine, since it rarely is helpful or necessary in children with a subacute presentation, but arthrocentesis is mandatory in patients who present with acute signs that are consistent with a possible septic arthritis, since it is important to determine the bacterial cause for appropriate treatment. Two-tier IgG serology is positive in virtually all patients with Lyme arthritis. White blood cell counts in synovial fluid of patients with typical Lyme arthritis usually range from 15,000 to 50,000/mcL, but sometimes can be 100,000/mcL or more with a preponderance of neutrophils, requiring culture of joint fluid (negative in Lyme arthritis) and serum tests for IgG antibodies to *B burgdorferi* to make an accurate diagnosis. Antibody tests of synovial fluid are not useful (many false-positive results). Polymerase chain reaction test of synovial fluid may be useful in select cases in which the diagnosis is in question. A positive result simply means that a component of the bacteria, depending on polymerase chain reaction target, is present (which may persist for some time after treatment with antimicrobials has killed the bacteria). It does not necessarily indicate the presence of live organisms.

Coinfections

Ixodes scapularis ticks can also transmit *Babesia microti,* the usual cause of babesiosis, and *Anaplasma phagocytophilum,* the cause of human granulocytic anaplasmosis (formerly termed *human granulocytic ehrlichiosis*). These may be transmitted by the same bite that transmits *B burgdorferi.* Consequently, these possible coinfections, though they occur in only some cases of Lyme disease, should be considered in patients with symptoms, signs, or test results that are atypical or unusually severe (eg, very high or prolonged fever, leukopenia, thrombocytopenia, or anemia) or who do not respond as expected to treatment. In addition, these ticks can also transmit *Borrelia miyamotoi,* an organism in the relapsing fever group of Borrelia, and deer-tick (Powassan) virus, which can cause severe encephalitis.

Management

Recommended treatment for children with Lyme disease is shown in Table 17-3. Patients with Lyme disease sometimes develop a Jarisch-Herxheimer–like reaction (ie, increased temperature, myalgia, arthralgia, and chills) during the first 24 to 48 hours of treatment because of the effects of lysis of the bacteria. Antimicrobial treatment should be continued if this occurs, since the reaction resolves spontaneously in 24 to 48 hours. Nonsteroidal anti-inflammatory drugs may provide symptomatic relief.

Single and Multiple Erythema Migrans

As outlined in the Table 17-3, treatment with a 14- to 21-day regimen of orally administered antimicrobials is recommended for erythema migrans and highly effective. The preferred drugs are doxycycline (children ≥8 years; a large trial in adults indicated that 10 days is sufficient treatment) or amoxicillin. Cefuroxime is the preferred alternative drug. Although macrolides (azithromycin, clarithromycin, or erythromycin) have been used to treat early Lyme disease, they may not be quite as effective as the 3 preferred drugs and should be used only if there are contraindications to all of those antimicrobials (Evidence Level II [in adults]; III [in children]). Doses for children are azithromycin (10 mg/kg/day, maximum: 500 mg/dose, administered once a day for 7–10 days), clarithromycin (15 mg/kg/day, maximum: 500 mg/dose, administered in divided doses

Table 17-3. Treatment of Lyme Disease in Children

Condition and Level of Evidence	Drug[a]	Dosage	Duration	Comments
Erythema migrans[b] Evidence Level I (for adults); II-2 (for children)	Doxycycline (patients ≥8 y)	4 mg/kg/d (up to 100 mg/dose) divided 2 times/d	14 d (range: 10–21 d)	Do not use in children <8 y or pregnant or lactating women. Caution about exposure to sun since photosensitivity rash in 15%–30%. Good penetration into CNS. Take with food and fluids to minimize nausea and GI irritation. Also effective against human granulocytic anaplasmosis.
	Amoxicillin	50 mg/kg/d (up to 500 mg/dose) divided 3 times/d	14 d (range: 14–21 d)	Not effective against human granulocytic anaplasmosis.
	Cefuroxime axetil	30 mg/kg/d (up to 500 mg/dose) divided 2 times/d	14 d (range: 14–21 d)	Not effective against human granulocytic anaplasmosis.
Neurologic disease Meningitis Evidence Level I (for adults); II-2 (for children)	Ceftriaxone	50–75 mg/kg/d (up to 2 g/dose) once a day	14 d (range: 10–28 d)	Risks associated with indwelling catheters, including infection and pseudolithiasis.
	Cefotaxime	150–200 mg/kg/d (up to 2 g/dose) divided every 8 h	14 d (range: 10–28 d)	Risks associated with indwelling catheters, including infection.

Continued

Table 17-3 *(cont)*

Condition and Level of Evidence	Drug[a]	Dosage	Duration	Comments
Cranial nerve palsy without clinical evidence of meningitis[c] Evidence Level II-3	Doxycycline[d] (patients ≥8 y) Amoxicillin (patients <8 y) Cefuroxime axetil (patients <8 y)	4 mg/kg/d (up to 100 mg/dose) divided 2 times/d 50 mg/kg/d (up to 500 mg/dose) divided 3 times/d 30 mg/kg/d (up to 500 mg/dose) divided 2 times/d	21 d (range: 14–21 d) 21 d (range: 14–21 d) 21 d (range: 14–21 d)	See comments in Erythema migrans row. Note there is not good evidence that treatment changes the outcome of facial palsy, but it prevents additional sequelae of infection.
Carditis Evidence Level III	Same oral agents as for erythema migrans; parenteral agents as for meningitis	Same dosages as for erythema migrans or meningitis if parenteral agent is used	14 d (range: 14–21 d)	Patients who are symptomatic should be hospitalized, monitored, and treated initially with a parenteral agent, such as ceftriaxone. Some patients with advanced heart block require a temporary pacemaker. Once advanced heart block resolves, treatment may be completed with an oral agent.
Arthritis[e] Evidence Level I (for doxycycline and amoxicillin); III (for cefuroxime)	Same oral agents as for erythema migrans	Same drugs and dosages as for erythema migrans or meningitis if parenteral agent is used	28 d	Nonsteroidal anti-inflammatory drugs are often helpful adjunctive treatment. For patients in whom arthritis persists or recurs, most experts recommend a second 28-d course of oral treatment; 14–21 d of parenteral treatment is an alternative (Evidence Level III). If clinical suspicion of concurrent neurologic disease, consider lumbar puncture and treatment parenterally as for meningitis but for 2–4 wk (Evidence Level III). In rare cases of persistent synovitis despite repeat treatment with antimicrobials, a rheumatologist should be consulted.

Abbreviations: CNS, central nervous system; GI, gastrointestinal.

[a] See text for alternative drugs if all preferred drugs are contraindicated.

[b] For multiple erythema migrans, some would treat for 21 d.

[c] See text about indications for lumbar puncture. If evidence of accompanying meningitis, treat as for meningitis.

[d] Doxycycline can be considered for children <8 y who are intolerant of alternative drugs. Likewise, alternative drugs can be considered if doxycycline is contraindicated.

[e] If uncertainty whether arthritis is acute bacterial infection or Lyme disease, parenterally administered cefuroxime is an appropriate drug to use for methicillin-susceptible *Staphylococcus aureus*, *Streptococcus pneumoniae*, *Streptococcus pyogenes*, and *Borrelia burgdorferi* while awaiting definitive diagnosis.

twice a day for 14–21 days), erythromycin (50 mg/kg/day, maximum: 500 mg/
dose, administered in divided doses 4 times a day for 14–21 days). First-
generation cephalosporins, such as cephalexin, are not effective treatment for
Lyme disease. Clinical trials in adults have demonstrated that doxycycline is
as effective as ceftriaxone for treating multiple erythema migrans (Evidence
Level I [in adults]; III [in children]).

Potential advantages of using doxycycline to treat Lyme disease include
excellent penetration into the central nervous system compared with alternative
oral agents and that it is effective in treating human granulocytic anaplasmosis,
an illness that may occur as a coinfection with Lyme disease. Doxycycline is
generally not recommended for children younger than 8 years because it may
cause staining of their permanent teeth or for women who are either pregnant
or lactating. A sun-induced dermatitis occurs in 15% to 30% of patients who
take doxycycline, so precautions should be taken to protect their skin from
the sun.

Early Disseminated Disease

Orally administered treatment is recommended for most patients with early
disseminated disease, including carditis except for those with severe carditis (eg,
complete heart block or those who are symptomatic from the carditis), who
should receive ceftriaxone or cefotaxime at least initially until the complete
block or symptoms resolve (Evidence Level III). A temporary cardiac pace-
maker may be necessary. Although there is some controversy, most experts
treat patients with cranial nerve palsies, except for those with concomitant signs
or symptoms of meningitis, with orally administered antimicrobials (doxycycline is preferred when possible). Treatment of patients with facial nerve palsy is
recommended to prevent other manifestations of Lyme disease. There is no
evidence that it affects outcome of the facial nerve palsy. Corticosteroids are not
indicated to treat patients with either facial nerve palsy or carditis caused by
Lyme disease. If the eye does not close completely, drops to lubricate it should
be administered several times a day.

A large clinical trial of European adults with Lyme meningitis found that
treatment for 14 days with doxycycline (200 mg a day) was as effective as
treatment with ceftriaxone (2 g intravenously [IV] once a day for 14 days)
(Evidence Level I). However, there are no data for US patients or children, so a
course of ceftriaxone is still recommended to treat children with Lyme meningitis, although oral treatment could be considered as an alternative treatment. It
is also important to monitor and manage elevated intracranial pressure in
patients in whom there is evidence that it persists despite antimicrobial
treatment.

Note that penicillin G (200,000–400,000 U/kg/day, maximum 18–24 million
U/day, in divided doses administered IV every 4 hours) is an alternative to
ceftriaxone or cefotaxime for treatment of Lyme disease when parenteral
therapy is indicated (Evidence Level I).

Late Disease

Lyme arthritis should be treated with orally administered doxycycline (amoxicillin for those <8 years) for 4 weeks unless these drugs are contraindicated. Cefuroxime is an alternative agent and particularly useful for empiric treatment while awaiting results of cultures if a patient presents with acute arthritis and methicillin-susceptible *Staphylococcus aureus, Streptococcus pneumoniae,* or *Streptococcus pyogenes* as part of the differential diagnosis in addition to Lyme disease. If Lyme arthritis recurs or persists 4 to 8 weeks after treatment is completed, a second course of oral treatment or, in some instances, 14 to 21 days of ceftriaxone administered IV is recommended (Evidence Level III). If the arthritis still does not resolve, consider either a persistent immune-mediated arthritis (which is relatively rare in children) that is not responsive to antimicrobials because the organism has invariably already been killed or alternative diagnoses; referral to a specialist is usually indicated. Nonsteroidal anti-inflammatory drugs may also be helpful for treating pain or inflammation associated with Lyme arthritis.

Post–Lyme Disease Syndrome and "Chronic Lyme Disease"

In some children who receive recommended treatment for well-documented Lyme disease, subjective symptoms, such as fatigue, arthralgia, or myalgia, may persist for weeks or even longer despite resolution of objective signs of disease. These have been termed *post–Lyme disease symptoms* if they persist for less than 6 months and *post–Lyme disease syndrome* if they persist longer and can cause functional disability. The cause and even relative frequency of this problem is unclear, because such nonspecific symptoms are relatively common in the general population without Lyme disease, especially among adolescents and adults. Some experts believe there is some degree of association between infection with Lyme disease and subsequent nonspecific symptoms, which are more common in patients with disseminated neurologic or late Lyme disease and those for whom treatment is delayed. Nevertheless, in most affected patients, these nonspecific symptoms resolve over time without additional antimicrobial treatment. There is no evidence that additional antimicrobial treatment is beneficial in persons with only nonspecific symptoms and no clinical signs of Lyme disease. Resistance of *B burgdorferi* to recommended first-line antimicrobials has not been reported.

Extensive publicity about "chronic Lyme disease," a condition without either a case definition or scientific evidence for its existence, may enhance patients' and parents' anxiety about the outcomes of treatment and contribute to both hypervigilance for and reporting of persistent nonspecific symptoms. Multiple studies in both children and adults have documented overdiagnosis and overtreatment of Lyme disease in patients who never had objective signs of Lyme disease but only nonspecific symptoms. A number of carefully conducted randomized clinical trials of prolonged antimicrobial treatment of adults with post–Lyme disease syndrome after treatment for Lyme disease have shown no benefit and substantial risks of adverse effects. Consequently, prolonged treatment with antimicrobials after conventional therapy of patients with persistent subjective symptoms is not recommended for patients whose objective signs of Lyme disease resolve or for those who never had objective evidence of Lyme disease (Evidence Level I [for adults]; III [for children]). Positive laboratory test results alone, especially those done at "Lyme specialty laboratories" that often perform diagnostic tests that are unconventional or use unconventional interpretations of conventional tests, are generally not considered reliable evidence of Lyme disease.

Management of Persons Bitten by an *Ixodes* Tick in Endemic Areas

The risk of Lyme disease after a bite by its vector tick, even in areas in which Lyme disease has the highest incidence, is only 2% to 3%. The tick must be infected (rates of infection of ticks vary from about 2%–50% depending on local area and stage of the tick) and must be attached for at least 36 to 48 hours before the risk of transmission becomes substantial. In fact, most persons develop Lyme disease from a bite by a nymphal stage tick that is unrecognized. In addition to the low risk of Lyme disease after a recognized bite, since identification of the species and duration of feeding requires expertise that may not be available, routine chemoprophylaxis for tick bites is not recommended (Evidence Level III). If there is certainty that the tick is either a nymphal or adult stage of *Ixodes* that is at least partially engorged, and the bite occurred in an area in which the risk that the tick is infected is at least 20% (which is generally true only in certain areas of New England and the eastern mid-Atlantic states as well as some parts of Wisconsin and Minnesota), a single dose of doxycycline (4 mg/kg, maximum: 200 mg), given with food to minimize nausea, may be offered to children 8 years and older to prevent Lyme disease (Evidence Level I). Other antimicrobials, such as amoxicillin or cefuroxime, should not be substituted for doxycycline for children younger than 8 years or those with a contraindication to doxycycline, because of different pharmacokinetics and lack of evidence of the effectiveness of single-dose prophylaxis with these agents (Evidence Level III). Follow-up tests for antibody against *B burgdorferi* in patients who had a tick bite but have no subsequent signs of Lyme disease are not indicated because the positive predictive value of such tests is poor. Routine testing of ticks for infection with *B burgdorferi* is also not indicated because there is no evidence that results of such tests are predictive of the risk of infection in the person who was bitten.

Long-term Monitoring

In general, long-term monitoring is unnecessary because treatment is usually highly effective. Moreover, follow-up depends on assessment of clinical signs and symptoms (persistent arthralgia or myalgia may be treated with nonsteroidal anti-inflammatory drugs). Patients with early localized disease should be instructed to return if any complications develop (eg, new neurologic findings, such as facial nerve palsy) or if the rash or associated symptoms do not resolve. Patients with early disseminated or late Lyme disease should be seen in follow-up to be certain the signs have resolved and no additional manifestations (eg, new neurologic signs) develop. Facial palsy due to Lyme disease generally resolves completely, but mild, sometimes clinically inapparent, weakness may persist in some patients who undergo careful neurologic testing. Uncommon cases of persistent synovitis that last longer than 3 months or are severe should be referred to a rheumatologist. Repeating antibody titers is rarely useful for monitoring Lyme disease. As with most infections, once antibodies against *B burgdorferi* develop, they (both IgM and IgG antibodies) may last for many years despite clinical cure. They are not a measure of activity of the disease. Furthermore, there is substantial variability in results of assays from batch to batch, so assessing whether antibody titers have changed over time as a means of assessing progression or cure of disease is generally unreliable.

Suggested Reading

Feder HM Jr, Johnson BJB, O'Connell S, et al. A critical appraisal of "chronic Lyme disease." *N Engl J Med*. 2007;357(14):1422–1430

Kalish RA, McHugh G, Granquist J, Shea B, Ruthazer R, Steere AC. Persistence of immunoglobulin M or immunoglobulin G antibody responses to *Borrelia burgdorferi* 10-20 years after active Lyme disease. *Clin Infect Dis*. 2001;33(6):780–785

Sanchez E, Vannier E, Wormser GP, Hu LT. Diagnosis, treatment, and prevention of Lyme disease, human granulocytic anaplasmosis, and babesiosis: A review. *JAMA*. 2016;315(16):1767–1777

Seltzer EG, Shapiro ED. Misdiagnosis of Lyme disease: when not to order serologic tests. *Pediatr Infect Dis J*. 1996;15(9):762–763.

Shapiro ED. Clinical practice. Lyme disease. *N Engl J Med*. 2014;370(18):1724–1731

Shapiro ED. Doxycycline for tick bites: not for everyone. *N Engl J Med*. 2001;345(2):133–134

Skogman BH, Glimåker K, Nordwall M, Vrethem M, Ödkvist L, Forsberg P. Long-term clinical outcome after Lyme neuroborreliosis in childhood. *Pediatrics*. 2012;130(2);262–269

Thompson A, Mannix R, Bachur R. Acute pediatric monoarticular arthritis: distinguishing Lyme arthritis from other etiologies. *Pediatrics*. 2009;123(3):959–965

Tory HO, Zurakowski D, Sundel RP. Outcomes of children treated for Lyme arthritis: results of a large pediatric cohort. *J Rheumatol*. 2010;37(5):1049–1055

Wormser GP, Dattwyler RJ, Shapiro ED, et al. The clinical assessment, treatment, and prevention of Lyme disease, human granulocytic anaplasmosis, and babesiosis: clinical practice guidelines by the Infectious Diseases Society of America. *Clin Infect Dis*. 2006;43(9):1089–1134

CHAPTER 18

Meningococcal Disease

Joshua Wolf, MBBS, and B. Keith English, MD

Key Points

- Invasive meningococcal disease is confirmed if *Neisseria meningitidis* is isolated from blood, cerebrospinal fluid, synovial fluid, pleural fluid, pericardial fluid, or skin scrapings from suspect skin lesions.

- Empiric therapy includes cefotaxime or ceftriaxone, but addition of empiric vancomycin should be considered because pneumococcal or staphylococcal infection can mimic meningococcal disease.

- Treatment of shock in meningococcal sepsis, and of increased intracranial pressure in those with severe meningitis, is essential.

- Close contacts of those with invasive meningococcal disease are at high risk for infection, so prophylaxis should be promptly provided to child care contacts and people who have been exposed to the patient's oral secretions, who slept in the same dwelling during the 7 days prior to onset of index case disease, or who were seated next to an infected individual during an airplane flight longer than 8 hours.

- Meningococcal vaccines are available that target serogroups A, C, Y, W-135, and B; recommendations support routine use in those 11 years and older and infants who are at high risk.

Overview

Meningococcal disease, caused by infection with *Neisseria meningitidis,* is a serious disease predominantly affecting children and adolescents. Infection usually presents as meningitis or bacteremia. Hallmarks of this disease are overwhelming sepsis associated with disseminated intravascular coagulation (DIC), multiorgan dysfunction, skin necrosis, and gangrene of the limbs. The course may be devastating, and disease progresses so rapidly that a previously well child is facing death within hours.

The disease occurs both sporadically and in epidemics. Modifiable risk factors for sporadic disease in adolescents include close or intimate contact with large numbers of people (eg, day care, military barracks, college dormitory, bar, or disco), close contact with a known case, smoking (active or passive), and deep tongue kissing with multiple partners. Other risk factors include genetic predisposition, parental smoking, complement deficiency, and recent upper respiratory tract infection.

Causes and Differential Diagnosis

Neisseria meningitidis (also called meningococcus) is a gram-negative bacterium most commonly appearing as diplococci (twin cocci joined together with a symmetric bean shape). The early symptoms and signs are often indistinguishable from those of very common benign febrile conditions, such because viral upper respiratory tract infection. Similarly, no specific clinical features definitively differentiate meningococcal disease from other causes of sepsis or meningitis, such as meningitis from *Streptococcus pneumoniae* or sepsis from *S pneumoniae*, group A *Streptococcus,* or *Staphylococcus aureus.* The presence of a rash, although suggestive, is not diagnostic of meningococcal disease because it can occur with many other infections, including systemic viral illnesses and tick-borne infections such as Rocky Mountain spotted fever and human monocytic ehrlichiosis. Purpura fulminans is highly suggestive of meningococcemia and rarely occurs in other bacterial infections.

Clinical Features

The main clinical presentations of invasive meningococcal disease are acute meningococcemia and meningitis. Acute meningococcemia may present as overt sepsis, or initially appear as undifferentiated fever sometimes called unsuspected meningococcal disease, and may not be associated with meningitis. Similarly, meningitis may occur without overwhelming sepsis. Other, less common, syndromes include chronic meningococcemia, pneumonia, conjunctivitis, and other focal infections. Once meningococcal bacteremia is established, it almost always progresses to serious illness without appropriate antibiotic treatment. There are rare reports of spontaneous resolution in which patients have recovered before blood culture results are reported as positive.

Sepsis

Coryza and sore throat are commonly seen in the early phase of meningococcal sepsis and are often the first symptoms to develop. These symptoms may falsely reassure medical staff that the patient has a viral respiratory tract illness. Progression to more specific or concerning symptoms usually occurs over a few hours. The clinical presentation may be further complicated if meningococcal disease is preceded by viral respiratory tract infection such as influenza.

General signs of sepsis such as cold hands and feet, leg pain, inability to walk, severe muscle pain, and abnormal skin color (such as pallor or mottled appearance) are frequently seen early in meningococcal disease and may be the first clues to seriousness of the illness. These signs and symptoms are reportedly less common in self-limiting viral infections, but cool peripheries and pallor occasionally occur in these benign conditions; there is the potential to create unnecessary alarm if these symptoms are overvalued. Other nonspecific signs and symptoms (eg, drowsiness, confusion, nausea, vomiting, and headache) are also more common in meningococcal disease than specific symptoms such as purpuric rash or meningism. Fever, tachycardia, and hypotension may also occur.

Rash occurs in around two-thirds of patients with meningococcal disease and is often visible at presentation. It classically appears petechial or purpuric, but can also be maculopapular. It often starts on the trunk or lower limbs. Careful examination may initially reveal petechiae only on conjunctivae or mucosal surfaces. Purpura fulminans, large coalescing regions of intradermal hemorrhage progressing to skin necrosis, is a very serious sign.

Meningitis

Patients with meningococcal meningitis may present with any of the features of sepsis, but these may also be absent. Common presenting symptoms include headache, fever, neck stiffness, lethargy, nausea, and vomiting. The classic "meningitis triad" of neck stiffness, photophobia, and altered conscious state is frequently incomplete. Only about 1 in 4 adults with meningococcal meningitis had the full triad in one study. Bulging fontanel can be present in young infants.

Acute neurologic complications of meningococcal meningitis are less common than in other bacterial causes but can include altered conscious state, coma, seizures, and cranial nerve palsies. Subdural effusion is usually sterile, but empyema occasionally occurs.

Other acute complications of meningococcal disease include DIC, the syndrome of inappropriate antidiuretic hormone, acute adrenal insufficiency due to adrenal hemorrhage, and myocarditis or pericarditis. Sepsis and DIC may paradoxically worsen with administration of antibiotics because of release of endotoxin. Distal limb ischemia is a serious complication of meningococcemia and may also progress despite appropriate maximal therapy. Patients with limb or skin ischemia may be left with significant areas of gangrene, leading to amputation or other serious orthopedic complications.

Rapid development of shock or development of purpura fulminans seems to be associated with mortality risk. Overall, the death rate of meningococcal disease is 10% in the modern era, and higher death rates are reported in adolescents. Death rate in patients with purpura fulminans is up to 50%, and most survivors have significant orthopedic complications. Paradoxically, presence of meningitis appears to reduce risk of mortality; children with meningitis have a somewhat lower mortality of around 8%.

Chronic Meningococcemia

Chronic meningococcemia is a rare presentation of meningococcal disease. Patients present with up to several weeks of fever and chills, joint pain, tenosynovitis, and painful rash. The rash is frequently intermittent and tends to correspond temporally with fever. Over several weeks, the disease can progress to focal infection such as meningitis, endocarditis, retinitis, or epididymitis. Focal infection appears rarely in children, and in this group some episodes resolve spontaneously. Because of the similar appearance, the disease may be mistaken for noninfectious vasculitides such as Henoch-Schönlein purpura, but meningococcal infection rapidly responds to antibiotic therapy.

Host immune factors play an important role in susceptibility to chronic meningococcemia. Risk factors include terminal complement pathway dysfunction, properdin deficiency, hypogammaglobulinemia, specific IgG subclass deficiency, and anatomic and functional asplenia. Pathogen factors such as lipopolysaccharide variations may also play a role in this modified presentation.

Arthritis and Serositis

Acute joint pain and swelling may be seen in conjunction with acute or chronic meningococcemia in about 10% of cases. It is occasionally caused by septic arthritis or hemarthrosis secondary to severe coagulopathy. Large joints are most commonly involved. Immune complex disease is often delayed, occurring after 5 days of illness, typically corresponding with clinical resolution of the acute illness, whereas infectious arthritis tends to present early in the course or is present at admission. Similarly, serositis can affect the pericardium, peritoneum, and pleural cavity. In contrast to arthritis, serositis is frequently caused by direct infection, although reactive sterile inflammation can also occur.

Pneumonia

Neisseria meningitidis is an uncommon but described cause of pneumonia. Studies of this are difficult to interpret in the absence of a control group because colonization is common in some groups and may coexist with an alternative cause for bacterial or viral pneumonia. Outbreaks can occur in closed communities, such as military camps, and are often caused by atypical serotypes not usually associated with sepsis or meningitis.

Conjunctivitis and Other Rare Presentations

Meningococcal conjunctivitis presents as purulent eye discharge with conjunctival injection, eyelid edema, or chemosis. Photophobia may be present, but most patients do not have fever or systemic symptoms at presentation. The syndrome is rare and clinically indistinguishable from other causes of bacterial conjunctivitis. Gram-negative diplococci are usually seen on Gram stain of a conjunctival swab. The differential diagnosis includes gonococcal disease and colonization with nonpathogenic *Neisseria* species. In one study, the time to development of systemic meningococcal disease was 41 hours on average (range: 3–96 hours); invasive disease was much more common (19 times) in patients who had received topical therapy alone for conjunctivitis than in those who had received systemic therapy. Other uncommon manifestations of meningococcal infection include endophthalmitis, neonatal sepsis, and cellulitis.

Evaluation

The clinical presentation of invasive meningococcal disease can be very difficult to differentiate from other causes of sepsis or meningitis in children, so patients are usually treated empirically until the organism is identified. In most cases of meningococcal sepsis, inflammatory markers are elevated and white blood cell counts are abnormal (ie, high or low).

Many patients with meningococcal disease have C-reactive protein (CRP) concentration greater than 100 mg/L, but the range of CRP values for meningococcal disease in children overlaps with those for viral illness and other bacterial infections. Paradoxically, CRP concentration appears to be lowest in patients at highest risk of septic shock or death from sepsis. High procalcitonin levels appear to predict poor clinical outcomes, but there is marked overlap between good and poor outcomes, and between meningococcal disease and benign febrile illnesses.

Culture of blood or cerebrospinal fluid (CSF) is the most common and definitive means for identification of the causative organism in cases of sepsis. Specimens for culture should be transported immediately for processing and incubation because the organism is fragile in cold or unfavorable conditions. Even with appropriate handling, up to 40% of blood cultures are sterile. The organism is rapidly killed by antibiotics, so blood culture results collected after antibiotics are almost always negative (>95%). Negative culture result, therefore, does not exclude the disease in a compatible clinical situation, especially after antibiotic therapy.

Cerebrospinal fluid should be collected as soon as the diagnosis is suspected if lumbar puncture is not contraindicated. Ideally, CSF is collected prior to administration of the first dose of antibiotic to maximize sensitivity of the test, but antibiotics should not be delayed if lumbar puncture is contraindicated. Cerebrospinal fluid abnormalities such as elevated protein concentration, depressed glucose concentration, and neutrophil-predominant pleocytosis may be present, but CSF parameters can be normal, especially early in the disease and in cases of sepsis without meningitis. Similar to blood culture, CSF is rapidly sterilized by antibiotic therapy. Most samples collected after any intravenous antibiotics are sterile, and 5 hours after antibiotic administration almost all are sterile. However, Gram stain of CSF may provide a clue to the diagnosis by showing gram-negative diplococci.

Where rash is prominent, Gram stain and culture of aspirated fluid, skin scrapings, or biopsies from lesions may yield the diagnosis. Meningococci can also be identified by culture of samples from other sites, including synovial fluid, conjunctival discharge, and sputum. Isolation of meningococci from throat or nasopharyngeal swab is difficult to interpret because they are a component of normal flora.

Molecular testing for meningococcal disease by polymerase chain reaction (PCR) of blood, CSF, or other specimens offers hope of improving the speed and sensitivity of diagnosis. Importantly, PCR is less affected than culture by prior antibiotic therapy since nonviable organisms can be detected. The performance of various PCR targets may differ, and false-negative results may occur because of mutations in target genes. A US Food and Drug Administration–approved multi-organism molecular test for diagnosis of meningitis or encephalitis is now available for CSF (FilmArray ME). The panel includes meningococcus, and may be useful especially in culture-negative or pretreated cases. Other such tests may become available in the near future.

Susceptibility testing is recommended by some experts for all meningococcal isolates as resistance to fluoroquinolones, penicillin, and even ceftriaxone has been reported. Resistance to penicillin and ceftriaxone is very rare in the United States but more common in some other countries. Knowledge of local epidemiology is important if meningococcal disease occurs in a returned traveler.

Investigation for Acute Complications

In addition to usual investigations undertaken for routine management of sepsis, such as clotting studies and arterial or venous pressure monitoring as indicated, there are a number of additional considerations in children with meningococcal disease.

Hyponatremia associated with syndrome of inappropriate antidiuretic hormone can occur in meningitis from any cause and requires careful management to prevent brain injury. Daily sodium and fluid balance monitoring can help prevent severe hyponatremia by guiding fluid management.

Waterhouse-Friderichsen syndrome describes adrenocortical dysfunction caused by bilateral adrenal gland hemorrhage and is an uncommon but important complication of meningococcal disease and other causes of sepsis. It should be considered in cases of persistent hypotension despite aggressive management, and may be diagnosed by serum cortisol and ACTH stimulation testing and imaging of the adrenal glands with computed tomography, magnetic resonance, or ultrasound while empiric treatment is initiated.

Routine head imaging is not recommended for patients with meningococcal sepsis or meningitis. Indications for brain imaging include localizing neurologic signs, coma, hydrocephalus, and persistent fever for more than 9 days or recurrent fever after initial defervescence.

Investigation for Predisposing Conditions

Complement deficiency or dysfunction is associated with markedly increased risk for meningococcal disease. Patients with these conditions often have milder disease and a lower chance of death but an elevated risk of recurrent meningococcal infection. The risk is highest in those with recurrent disease, older age at presentation (>10 years), or infection with an unusual serogroup. Where available, all patients with meningococcal disease should undergo CH50 assay for complement function. Positive results should prompt education, early empiric treatment for future potential episodes, meningococcal vaccination, and testing of relatives.

X-linked properdin deficiency is associated with increased severity of meningococcal disease, with a fatality rate of up to 75%. Patients, especially males, with severe disease should therefore undergo AP50 assay for properdin deficiency, with consideration of more sensitive and specific tests if the result is in the low-reference range. Abnormal results should again prompt education, early empiric treatment for future potential episodes, meningococcal vaccination, and testing of relatives. Patients with fatal disease should undergo testing for properdin deficiency because of implications for family members.

Investigations in Recurrent Meningococcal Disease

Most reports of recurrent meningococcal disease have identified classical complement pathway abnormalities, but alternative pathway abnormalities also occur. Alternative complement pathway testing by AP50 is appropriate in a patient with recurrent meningococcal disease who has normal CH50 determination.

Management

The first priority in management of bacterial sepsis is supportive care and treatment of shock. Management of the child with presumed bacterial sepsis must include empiric antimicrobial therapy that is active against meningococci and other potential pathogens. While the child with fever and purpura is likely to have meningococcemia, purpura fulminans has occasionally been associated with bacterial sepsis caused by other pathogens, including *Haemophilus influenzae*, group A *Streptococcus, S aureus,* and *S pneumoniae.* Thus, empiric therapy of severe bacterial sepsis (with or without purpura) should include cefotaxime or ceftriaxone plus vancomycin. Vancomycin may not be required in areas where penicillin-resistant pneumococci and methicillin-resistant *S aureus* are rare. Definitive therapy of bacterial sepsis is based on identification of the organism and susceptibility testing. However, susceptibility testing for meningococci is poorly standardized and the rate of resistance to penicillin or third-generation cephalosporins in the United States is extremely low. Thus, penicillin G, ampicillin, cefotaxime, or ceftriaxone may be used as definitive therapy. Cefotaxime or ceftriaxone is preferred for travelers from areas where penicillin resistance has been reported. Five to 7 days of therapy is generally adequate.

As for bacterial sepsis, the first priority for treatment of children with presumed bacterial meningitis is supportive care, correction of hemodynamic instability, and management of increased intracranial pressure in severe cases. Empiric antimicrobial therapy for children with definite or probable bacterial meningitis who are older than 1 month should include cefotaxime or ceftriaxone, plus vancomycin. The addition of vancomycin is necessary because pneumococcal sepsis and meningitis can mimic meningococcal infection, and until cultures allow for definitive therapy, vancomycin should be included in the empiric regimen.

Definitive therapy of meningococcal meningitis in the United States may be provided by either penicillin G, ampicillin, cefotaxime, or ceftriaxone. Five to 7 days of therapy is generally adequate. Persistent fever with appropriate therapy is rarely because of microbiologic failure and often caused by drug fever or the presence of sterile subdural effusion or inflammatory arthritis.

Unless cefotaxime or ceftriaxone is used to treat the primary disease, the patient should receive secondary prophylaxis as outlined below because penicillin does not eliminate meningococcal carriage.

Steroids, activated protein C (now withdrawn from the market), and other potential adjunctive therapies for patients with meningococcemia and other forms of bacterial sepsis have been studied more extensively in adults than children, but minimal evidence supports their use. Because of the lack of supportive evidence, especially in pediatric populations, adjuvant therapies are not currently recommended.

All cases of meningococcal disease should be reported to the appropriate local or state health department immediately, and to the Centers for Disease Control and Prevention within 14 days. Droplet isolation should be utilized until 24 hours of appropriate therapy has been provided.

Primary Prevention

Primary prevention of meningococcal disease is an important public health goal. Two quadrivalent meningococcal conjugate vaccines (MenACWY) are licensed in the USA, and are the preferred vaccines to prevent infections caused by serogroups A, C, Y, and W-135. Routine immunization with MenACWY is recommended for children 11 or 12 years of age with a booster dose at age 16 years. For those who receive the initial dose of MenACWY at 13 to 15 years, a booster dose should be given at 16 to 18 years. For those who have received a first dose of vaccine at 16 years or older, a booster dose is not currently recommended. For those 21 years or older, routine meningococcal vaccine is not currently recommended. A bivalent conjugate vaccine (MenCY-TT) is also available.

Infants at high risk of meningococcal disease include those who have persistent complement deficiency or functional or anatomic asplenia (including infants with congenital heart disease associated with asplenia and some with HIV infection), children who will travel to regions where meningococcal disease is hyperendemic or epidemic, or children who are at risk during a community outbreak caused by a vaccine serogroup strain. These infants should receive vaccination with an appropriate conjugate vaccine series (MenACWY-CRM, Hib-MCY-TT, or MenACWY-D depending on age, indication for vaccination, and risk of exposure to serogroups A and W-135).

Two vaccines against serogroup B meningococcus are available in the United States (MenB-FHbp and MenB-4C); the two vaccines are not interchangeable so the same vaccine should be used for all doses. Serogroup B vaccine may be considered for all patients aged 16 to 23 years and is recommended for all patients 10 years and older who are at high risk of meningococcal disease (as above) and during outbreaks of serogroup B meningococcal disease. Although these vaccines are not approved for use in younger children, data for safety and efficacy are available and the rate of serogroup B disease is highest in young infants. Therefore, vaccination of younger children at high risk may be recommended in the near future.

Secondary Prevention

Close contacts of people with invasive meningococcal disease are at risk of subsequent invasive meningococcal disease and should receive chemoprophylaxis. Close contacts include household contacts (and anyone who frequently slept in the same dwelling during the 7 days prior to illness onset), child care or preschool contacts at any time during the 7 days before illness onset, anyone with direct exposure to secretions of the index patient (including mouth-to-mouth resuscitation or unprotected contact during endotracheal intubation), and passengers seated directly next to the index patient during airline flights lasting more than 8 hours. Prophylaxis should only be given if the most recent contact was within the past 14 days.

Rifampin is the drug of choice for chemoprophylaxis for most children, including the index patient if the treatment of invasive meningococcal disease did not include ceftriaxone or cefotaxime (which also eradicates nasopharyngeal carriage). Ciprofloxacin is effective chemoprophylaxis for adult contacts but should not be used in regions where ciprofloxacin-resistant strains of meningococci have been detected (azithromycin is an alternative) (Table 18-1).

Long-term Implications

Although most children with meningococcal meningitis make a complete recovery, hearing loss, seizures, developmental delay, and other neuropsychological or behavioral sequelae can occur. The risk of major neurologic problems appears to be highest in children who had complicated/prolonged seizures or coma during their primary treatment course, and is lower in children with meningococcal versus pneumococcal meningitis. More subtle behavioral or academic difficulties may not become apparent until adolescence or even adulthood.

Caregivers and clinicians should be aware of the risks, and survivors of meningitis should have long-term developmental follow-up to identify opportunities for educational or psychologic intervention.

After a diagnosis of meningitis, hearing should be tested as soon as the patient is well enough, ideally before hospital discharge.

Table 18-1. Recommended Chemoprophylaxis Regimens for High-risk Contacts and People With Invasive Meningococcal Disease

Age of Infants, Children, and Adults	Dose	Duration	Efficacy, %	Cautions
Rifampin[a]				
<1 mo	5 mg/kg, orally, every 12 h	2 days		
≥1 mo	10 mg/kg (maximum 600 mg), orally, every 12 h	2 days	90–95	Can interfere with efficacy of oral contraceptives and some seizure and anticoagulant medications; can stain soft contact lenses
Ceftriaxone				
<15 y	125 mg, intramuscularly	Single dose	90–95	To decrease pain at injection site, dilute with 1% lidocaine
≥15 y	250 mg, intramuscularly	Single dose	90–95	To decrease pain at injection site, dilute with 1% lidocaine
Ciprofloxacin[a,b]				
≥1 mo	20 mg/kg (maximum 500 mg), orally	Single dose	90–95	Not recommended routinely for people younger than 18 years of age; use may be justified after assessment of risks and benefits for the individual patient
Azithromycin				
	10 mg/kg (maximum 500 mg)	Single dose	90	Not recommended routinely; equivalent to rifampin for eradication of *Neisseria meningitidis* from nasopharynx in one study

[a] Not recommended for use in pregnant women.

[b] Use only if fluoroquinolone-resistant strains of *N meningitidis* have not been identified in the community.

From American Academy of Pediatrics. Meningococcal infections. In: Kimberlin DW, Brady MT, Jackson MA, Long SS, eds. *Red Book: 2015 Report of the Committee on Infectious Diseases*. 30th ed. Elk Grove Village, IL: American Academy of Pediatrics; 2015: 552.

Suggested Reading

Christensen H, May M, Bowen L, Hickman M, Trotter CL. Meningococcal carriage by age: a systematic review and meta-analysis. *Lancet Infect Dis.* 2010;10(12):853–861

Crosswell JM, Nicholson WR, Lennon DR. Rapid sterilisation of cerebrospinal fluid in meningococcal meningitis: implications for treatment duration. *J Paediatr Child Health.* 2006;42(4):170–173

Haj-Hassan TA, Thompson MJ, Mayon-White RT, et al. Which early 'red flag' symptoms identify children with meningococcal disease in primary care? *Br J Gen Pract.* 2011;61(584):e97–e104

Hoek MR, Christensen H, Hellenbrand W, Stefanoff P, Howitz M, Stuart JM. Effectiveness of vaccinating household contacts in addition to chemoprophylaxis after a case of meningococcal disease: a systematic review. *Epidemiol Infect.* 2008;136(11): 1441–1447

Kanegaye JT, Soliemanzadeh P, Bradley JS. Lumbar puncture in pediatric bacterial meningitis: defining the time interval for recovery of cerebrospinal fluid pathogens after parenteral antibiotic pretreatment. *Pediatrics.* 2001;108(5):1169–1174

Thompson MJ, Ninis N, Perera R, et al. Clinical recognition of meningococcal disease in children and adolescents. *Lancet.* 2006;367(9508):397–403

Tully J, Viner RM, Coen PG, et al. Risk and protective factors for meningococcal disease in adolescents: matched cohort study. *BMJ.* 2006;332(7539):445–450

CHAPTER 19

Pertussis

Jennifer Vodzak, MD, and Sarah S. Long, MD

Key Points

- Pertussis is a highly contagious, vaccine-preventable respiratory tract infection associated with a classic clinical presentation in children and adolescents and a less typical syndrome in young infants.

- Classically, a catarrhal phase of illness is followed by a prolonged paroxysmal cough stage and then a recovery phase, with total disease course often lasting several months.

- Complications of pertussis are most commonly seen in younger infants and include a wide spectrum from conjunctival hemorrhage and rectal prolapse to apnea, secondary bacterial pneumonia, seizures, encephalopathy, pulmonary hypertension, and death.

- Diagnosis relies on recognition of the clinical disease, with confirmation by culture or polymerase chain reaction testing specific for *Bordetella pertussis*.

- Treatment with macrolide therapy may affect the course of disease if initiated before the paroxysmal phase and decreases contagiousness.

- Pregnant women should receive a dose of tetanus toxoid, reduced diphtheria toxoid, and acellular pertussis vaccine during each pregnancy, optimally between 27 and 36 weeks of gestation, to provide passive protection of the neonate. Additionally, a vaccine "cocoon" strategy is recommended and should target all members of the household and any caregivers or close contacts.

Overview

Pertussis is an acute respiratory illness, commonly known as whooping cough, that affects individuals of all ages. The clinical syndrome is caused by *Bordetella* species, most commonly *Bordetella pertussis* followed by *Bordetella parapertussis*. Infection is classically noted to have 3 distinct phases followed by prolonged, frequent paroxysmal cough. The clinical course varies in young infants, as well as in older children and adults with partial immunity, and in immunocompromised persons.

Causes and Differential Diagnosis

The most common cause of pertussis is infection with the bacterium *B pertussis,* an aerobic, fastidious, small gram-negative coccobacillus that infects only humans. It can be difficult to grow in the laboratory, usually requiring specialized growth media, such as Bordet-Gengou or Regan-Lowe agar. *Bordetella pertussis* produces a number of toxins and adhesins, including pertussis toxin and pertactin, which enhance its virulence and transmissibility. *Bordetella parapertussis* can also cause pertussis, but symptoms are generally less severe and the course is shorter overall.

The differential diagnosis for pertussis includes other infections and noninfectious etiologies that can cause cough (especially episodic) with a prolonged course or apnea in the young infant (Table 19-1). Occasionally, other *Bordetella* species, including *Bordetella bronchiseptica* and *Bordetella holmesii,* have been identified in patients (usually immunocompromised) with a pertussis-like syndrome. Clinicians should maintain high suspicion for pertussis to differentiate the cough syndrome from other causes, especially in infants with an obstructive airway event and other persons with a cough illness that is escalating after the first week of illness. Of note, identification of a virus in young infants may not exclude concomitant *B pertussis* infection. Studies have suggested that as many as one-third of hospitalized infants with pertussis may have coinfection with a respiratory virus, particularly respiratory syncytial virus.

Clinical Features

The clinical presentation of pertussis can vary by host factors, including age, immune status, vaccine status, and pertussis exposure history. Classic symptoms include paroxysmal coughing followed by forced inspiration that produces a whoop sound. Non-classic presentations occur in young infants and partially immune persons. Prolonged or more severe symptoms can occur in immunocompromised individuals. Because of the high contagiousness of *B pertussis* (ie, >95% infectivity for unimmunized persons in close contact) and significant morbidity and mortality for very young infants, early recognition and management of patients with pertussis is crucial.

Key clinical features in classic pertussis (usually in unimmunized toddlers and children) include an initial 1- to 2-week catarrhal phase of nonspecific symptoms, including rhinorrhea and mild cough. This is followed by the 2- to 6-week paroxysmal phase, notable for increasing intensity of paroxysmal coughing episodes with characteristic whoop and post-tussive vomiting, sometimes associated with cyanosis and apnea. The final convalescent phase is defined by improving cough episodes, with decreased intensity and frequency, but can last for weeks to months. During this final phase, cough may be exacerbated by acquisition of common viral upper respiratory tract infections. Generally, fever is uncommon and persons appear well between coughing episodes. Classic pertussis, or whooping cough, follows a predictable course in

Table 19-1. Etiologies and Differentiating Clinical Features of Episodic or Prolonged Cough Illnesses That Can Mimic Pertussis

Etiology	Potential Differentiating Features From Pertussis		
	Symptoms	Examination	Studies
Bacteria			
Mycoplasma pneumoniae	Fever, headache, fatigue, and myalgias	Rales and hypoxemia	Interstitial marking on chest radiograph Specific serology or PCR
Chlamydophila pneumoniae	Fever, fatigue, and myalgias	Rales and hypoxemia	Interstitial marking on chest radiograph Specific serology or PCR
Chlamydia trachomatis	Young infants only: staccato cough	Purulent conjunctivitis, tachypnea, hypoxemia, and rales	Interstitial marking on chest radiograph Positive culture or PCR
Tuberculosis	Constitutional symptoms and hemoptysis	Focal lung findings	Positive PPD tuberculin and chest radiograph Positive interferon-γ release assay
Viruses			
Adenovirus	Fever, sore throat, myalgias, and anorexia	Ill appearing and pharyngitis conjunctivitis	Positive viral culture or PCR
Respiratory syncytial virus	Fever	Wheezing and hypoxemia	Positive viral culture or PCR
Parainfluenza virus	Fever	Wheezing and hypoxemia	Positive viral culture or PCR
Rhinovirus	Fever	Wheezing	Positive viral culture or PCR
Influenza virus	Fever, fatigue, myalgias, and anorexia	Ill appearing and pharyngitis	Positive viral culture or PCR
Noninfectious			
Foreign body aspiration	Intermittent cough	Focal wheezing or rales	Imaging Bronchoscopy as indicated
Asthma or reactive airway disease	May be associated with allergic symptoms	Wheezing	Trial of asthma/allergy therapy

Abbreviations: PCR, polymerase chain reaction; PPD, purified protein derivative.

unimmunized toddlers and children and presents in 3 distinct clinical phases (Table 19-2). Symptoms and complications are less common in older children. Non-classic presentations occur in young infants and older children, adolescents, and adults. In young infants, early infection can be more difficult to

Table 19-2. Clinical Features of Pertussis by Age

Clinical Phase	Age: <3 mo (Unimmunized or 1 Dose)	Unimmunized Older Infants, Toddlers, and Children	Immunized Children, Adolescents, and Adults
	Unique Presentation	Classic Pertussis	Non-classic Symptoms
Catarrhal	• Shorter phase (1–5 d long). • May not be recognized clinically. • Fever is uncommon.	• Usually lasts 1–2 wk. • Rhinorrhea and mild cough. • Minimal constitutional symptoms. • Fever is uncommon.	• Can last 1–2 wk. • Nasal congestion and rhinorrhea. • Nonspecific symptoms may not be clinically recognized. • Fever is uncommon.

Paroxysmal	• May not have cough.
	• If cough present, usually occurs without whoop.
	• Common symptoms include apnea, gagging, choking or gasping, or an apparent life-threatening event.
	
	• Post-tussive vomiting.
		• Usually lasts 2–6 wk.
		• Cough is predominant symptom.
		• Starts as dry, intermittent cough.
		• Progresses to paroxysms.
		  o Uncontrollable cough burst associated with reddened face and anxious appearance
		  o Followed by forced inspiratory effort, making the classic whoop sound
		  o Occurs with minimal airway irritation or spontaneously
		
		• Post-tussive vomiting.
		• Upper body petechiae or conjunctival hemorrhages.
			• Usually lasts 2–6 wk.
			• Cough is predominant symptom.
			• Paroxysms may be heralded or associated with a feeling of suffocating or gasping for air.
			• Can be lack of classic paroxysms.
			  o Forceful coughing episodes not associated with a whoop
			  o Can be confused with other diagnoses
			   – Primary atypical pneumonia in adolescents
			   – Bronchitis or COPD exacerbation in adults
			• Post-tussive vomiting.
			• Upper body petechiae or conjunctival hemorrhages.

	• Feeding difficulty with gagging/cough episodes. • Fever or hypoxia should prompt evaluation for secondary bacterial pneumonia. • Highest risk for serious complications, including pulmonary hypertension (<4 wk of age), secondary bacterial pneumonia, respiratory failure, death.	• Anorexia and disrupted sleep. • Fever or hypoxia should prompt evaluation for secondary bacterial pneumonia. • Complications are less common, especially in older children.	• Mild anorexia. • Disrupted sleep due to coughing episodes. • Complications are uncommon.
Convalescent	• Cough may be more predominant. • Apnea events decrease. • Subsequent viral URTIs can exacerbate cough throughout first year of life.	• Cough gradually lessens over weeks to months (decreased severity and frequency). • Appetite/feeding and sleep improve. • Subsequent viral URTIs can exacerbate cough.	• Cough gradually lessens over weeks to months (decreased severity and frequency). • Appetite and sleep patterns improve. • Subsequent viral URTIs or pollutants can exacerbate cough.

Abbreviations: COPD, chronic obstructive pulmonary disease; URTI, upper respiratory tract infection.

identify. This age group has a high risk for severe disease and complications; thus, young infants (<2–3 months) often require hospitalization and careful monitoring for disease progression or complications over 24 to 48 hours. Babies younger than 6 months, and particularly those younger than 3 months, often have a shortened catarrhal phase; may present with gagging, gasping, or apnea as the chief symptom; and can have more complicated courses. Immunized older children, adolescents, and adults may have less severe symptoms, or the clinical course may not follow the 3 phases as clearly. Clinicians must maintain high suspicion for pertussis and test accordingly. In all age groups, postinfectious cough (usually episodic) can last for weeks to months after acute infection and can be exacerbated by subsequent viral upper respiratory tract infections; these episodes are *not* "relapses" of *B pertussis* infection.

Complications occur most often in babies younger than 6 months, with rates as high as 25%, and include apnea and secondary bacterial pneumonia most commonly. Of children hospitalized with pertussis, studies suggest that more than 75% are in this age group. Babies younger than 4 weeks infected with pertussis have the highest associated morbidity and mortality of any age. In adequately immunized infants (generally >6 months), pertussis infection can occur despite immunization, but complications are less common (Table 19-3).

Evaluation

Clinicians should consider pertussis in anyone with a prolonged cough illness that is worsening into the second week of symptoms, and in any infant with apnea, cyanosis, or apparent life-threatening events as the presenting concern. Diagnosis of pertussis is confirmed by testing respiratory secretions from a carefully collected deep nasopharyngeal sample, with highest yield when obtained during the catarrhal or early paroxysmal phase and prior to antibiotics. A number of diagnostic studies are available; culture remains the criterion standard, but polymerase chain reaction testing has become both more reliable and more available. Complete blood cell count with differential should be performed to evaluate for concerning features, including hyperleukocytosis (lymphocytosis), thrombocytosis, neutrophilia, or bandemia (related to secondary bacterial infection), because these may be signs of complications. Previously immunized persons with pertussis usually do not have the characteristic lymphocytosis and culture, or polymerase chain reaction is positive in 20% or fewer; diagnosis is made serologically (Table 19-4).

Radiologic evaluation may be helpful when the diagnosis is uncertain or if secondary bacterial pneumonia is suspected. Chest radiographic findings are generally normal in pertussis, but may show nonspecific peribronchial thickening or perihilar markings (eg, butterfly appearance), especially in infants.

Table 19-3. Complications Associated With Pertussis

Primary Disease/Acute Pertussis	
Apnea	• Infants <1 y (most common: <6 mo). • Infants <3 mo may require hospitalization/intubation. • Premature infants at increased risk for poor recovery from apneic episodes, possibly requiring mechanical ventilation.
Pulmonary hypertension with hyperleukocytosis (lymphocytosis), right-sided heart failure, and respiratory failure	• Uncommon complication. • Infants <4 wk at highest risk. • Evaluate for pulmonary hypertension in infants with impending respiratory failure or without clear signs and symptoms of pneumonia. • High mortality.
Secondary Bacterial Infections	
Pneumonia	• Can occur at any age (more common in infants and young children). • Common pathogens include *Streptococcus pneumoniae*, *Staphylococcus aureus*, and oropharyngeal flora. • Fever, hypoxia between paroxysms, or tachypnea should prompt evaluation for pneumonia.
Acute otitis media	• Can occur at any age, including older children
Central Nervous System Involvement	
Seizures	• Hypoxic brain injury secondary to prolonged apnea • May be secondary to hyponatremia
Encephalopathy	• Hypoxic brain injury secondary to prolonged apnea
Mechanical Issues (Increased Pressure During Paroxysms)	
Petechiae (usually upper body) and conjunctival hemorrhages	
Pneumothorax, pneumomediastinum, or subcutaneous emphysema	
Urinary incontinence or rectal prolapse	
Rib fractures (uncommon)	
Intracranial hemorrhage (uncommon)	

Management

Patients with cough illness compatible with pertussis should be placed in respiratory droplet isolation, and appropriate personal protective equipment, including surgical masks, should be worn by health care personnel. Evaluation should occur expeditiously to confirm pertussis, begin therapy, and limit exposures.

Management strategies should be considered for both the individual patient and the community because of the contagiousness of *B pertussis*. Patient management goals include antibiotic treatment; determining need for

Table 19-4. Laboratory Evaluation for Pertussis Infection

Laboratory Study	Features	Limitations
Diagnostic		
Culture	Remains criterion standard. High yield in unimmunized persons if collected properly.	Fastidious organism that is difficult to cultivate. Positive in <20% of immunized persons or in those who have received macrolides.
DFA	Quick turnaround time. Specific for *Bordetella pertussis*.	Only reliable in laboratories with highly experienced technologists.
PCR	Quick turnaround time. Specific for *B pertussis*. More sensitive than culture.	Highest yield in early disease. Requires appropriate technology. Can have false-positive results/contamination.
EIA for serologic tests	IgG-specific antibody to *B pertussis* components (especially pertussis toxin). Useful in unimmunized persons; ≥90 EU/mL highly suggestive of pertussis.	Cannot differentiate between disease and vaccine response. Poor standardization between laboratories.
Supportive		
CBC count with differential	Normal or high total WBC count due to absolute lymphocytosis (absolute lymphocyte count >10,000/mcL). Lymphocytic leukemoid reaction and thrombocytosis (>750,000/mcL) can occur in young infants and are risk factors for death.	Less common in partially immunized children, adolescents, or adults or if late in disease course.
Confounding		
Respiratory viral testing (viral culture, DFA, or PCR)	Concomitant viral infections can occur and may lead to more severe clinical course in some cases.	Positive respiratory viral testing does not exclude pertussis.
CBC count with differential	Neutrophilia or bandemia.	Abnormalities not associated with pertussis. May represent different diagnosis or secondary bacterial infection.

Abbreviations: CBC, complete blood cell; DFA, direct fluorescence assay; EIA, enzyme immunoassay; PCR, polymerase chain reaction; WBC, white blood cell.

assistance with recovery from paroxysms; monitoring for complications, especially in higher risk patients; optimizing nutrition and recovery; and educating caregivers about disease course. For the community, goals include decreasing transmission, providing appropriate postexposure prophylaxis (PEP), and limiting further exposures.

The highest benefit of antibiotic therapy is noted in infants presenting early in the disease course. For most patients presenting later, antibiotics are given generally to limit transmissibility rather than alter clinical course. Macrolides are standard treatment unless the patient has an underlying cardiac condition associated with long QT, with trimethoprim/sulfamethoxazole as alternative therapy in these patients and in infants older than 2 months (Table 19-5). In

Table 19-5. Antibiotics for Pertussis

Age Group	Antibiotic	Dose and Duration
<1 mo[a]	Azithromycin[b]	10 mg/kg once daily for 5 d
1–5 mo	Azithromycin[b] Clarithromycin Erythromycin *Alternative:* TMP/SMX[c,d]	10 mg/kg once daily for 5 d 15 mg/kg/d divided twice daily for 7 d 40–50 mg/kg/d divided 4 times daily for 14 d 8 mg (TMP component)/kg/d divided twice daily for 14 d
Infants ≥6 mo and children	Azithromycin[b] Clarithromycin Erythromycin *Alternative:* TMP/SMX[d]	10 mg/kg (maximum: 500 mg) once on day 1, then 5 mg/kg (maximum: 250 mg) once daily on days 2–5 15 mg/kg/d (maximum: 1,000 mg/d) divided twice daily for 7 d 40–50 mg/kg/d (maximum: 2,000 mg/d) divided 4 times daily for 14 d 8 mg (TMP component)/kg/d (maximum: 320 mg [TMP component]/d) divided twice daily for 14 d
Adults	Azithromycin[b] Clarithromycin Erythromycin *Alternative:* TMP/SMX[d]	500 mg once on day 1, then 250 mg once daily on days 2–5 500 mg orally twice daily for 7 d 500 mg orally 4 times daily for 14 d 160–800 mg (1 double-strength tablet) orally twice daily for 14 d

Abbreviation: TMP/SMX, trimethoprim/sulfamethoxazole.

[a] Idiopathic hypertrophic pyloric stenosis has been associated with macrolide use in infants, erythromycin much more so than azithromycin. Younger than 1 mo, erythromycin is not preferred because of increased risk of pyloric stenosis, and clarithromycin is not recommended. Azithromycin is the recommended antibiotic.

[b] Azithromycin may increase the risk of potentially fatal arrhythmias in certain persons with existing cardiac disease or arrhythmias.

[c] For infants <2 mo, TMP/SMX is contraindicated because of increased risk for displacing bilirubin and kernicterus. For infants ≥2 mo, TMP/SMX can be considered in patients with macrolide allergies or rare cases of proven macrolide resistance.

[d] TMP/SMX dosing is based on the TMP component.

patients with laboratory-confirmed or clinically suspected pertussis, antibiotics should be given to babies younger than 1 year within 6 weeks of cough onset and to anyone else within 3 weeks of cough onset.

The focus of care for infants and children with pertussis is to provide supportive care and appropriate monitoring. Generally, most babies younger than 3 months are hospitalized for at least 2 to 3 days to assess cough episodes and ability to recover unassisted and feed safely and to monitor for complications. Many infants 3 to 6 months of age are also hospitalized, depending on severity of symptoms and presence of concerning features. Factors that may decrease the clinician's threshold for hospitalization include lack of cough or whoop with paroxysms, poor recovery from cough episodes, witnessed apnea or cyanosis, poor feeding, and history of prematurity or chronic respiratory, cardiac, or neuromuscular disease. Environment and stimulation play key roles in management. Infants benefit from minimal disturbances and a quiet, calm environment to limit triggering the paroxysms. Oral feedings should be encouraged as tolerated and provided in smaller volumes to limit post-tussive vomiting. Finally, parental or caregiver education is very important to ensure understanding of disease course, especially after discharge.

Adjunctive medications are generally unhelpful for acute pertussis infection. Bronchodilator agents, such as albuterol, have not been shown to be beneficial and may irritate the denuded airway. Use of corticosteroids is not recommended; no prospective studies have been done to assess use in pertussis. Finally, cough suppressants are generally not recommended and may be detrimental if sedative effects occur in young infants.

Management of severe complications of pertussis requires skilled pediatric intensive care. Young infants are at higher risk for mechanical ventilation, prolonged apnea and bradycardia, secondary bacterial pneumonia, central nervous system involvement, pulmonary hypertension, and death.

Other Considerations

Isolation Measures and Limiting Exposures

Hospitalized patients with suspected or confirmed pertussis should be isolated according to hospital policy, following respiratory droplet precautions. Children should be excluded from day care and school until receipt of 5 days of effective therapy or for 21 days if not treated.

Postexposure Prophylaxis

Macrolide treatment is used for PEP in all household contacts and other close contacts (eg, child care providers), regardless of vaccine history or symptoms. In addition, the vaccine history should be reviewed and updated as appropriate. Local health departments should be consulted regarding antimicrobial PEP in community outbreaks, such as in schools or health care facilities.

Immunization

Pertussis vaccine is a critical component of personal protection and disease control. Pertussis-containing vaccine is included in universal primary pediatric immunization diphtheria and tetanus toxoids and acellular pertussis vaccine schedule at 2, 4, and 6 months and 4 to 6 years of age and booster tetanus toxoid, reduced diphtheria toxoid, and acellular pertussis (Tdap) vaccine dose at 11 to 12 years of age. All persons 11 years of age through elderly patients should receive a single dose of Tdap. All clinicians should have documentation of receipt of one dose of Tdap. Because morbidity and death rates are highest in young infants, a vaccine "cocoon" strategy is recommended and should target all members of the household and any caregivers or close contacts. Pregnant women should receive a dose of Tdap during each pregnancy, optimally between 27 and 36 weeks of gestation, to provide passive protection of the young infant. Because of short duration of protection following Tdap, re-immunization of individuals other than pregnant women is not cost effective or recommended.

Suggested Reading

Amirthalingam G. Strategies to control pertussis in infants. *Arch Dis Child.* 2013;98(7):552–555

Centers for Disease Control and Prevention. Pertussis epidemic—Washington, 2012. *MMWR Morb Mortal Wkly Rep.* 2012;61(28):517–522

Centers for Disease Control and Prevention. Updated recommendations for use of tetanus toxoid, reduced diphtheria toxoid and acellular pertussis vaccine (Tdap) in pregnant women and persons who have or anticipate having close contact with an infant aged <12 months—Advisory Committee on Immunization Practices (ACIP), 2011. *MMWR Morb Mortal Wkly Rep.* 2011;60(41):1424–1426

Centers for Disease Control and Prevention, American Academy of Pediatrics Committee on Infectious Diseases. Additional recommendations for use of tetanus toxoid, reduced-content diphtheria toxoid, and acellular pertussis vaccine (Tdap). *Pediatrics.* 2011;128(4):809–812

Liko J, Robison SG, Cieslak PR. Priming with whole-cell versus acellular pertussis vaccine. *N Engl J Med.* 2013;368(6):581–582

Wayne RA, Murray KT, Hall K, Arbogast PG, Stein CM. Azithromycin and the risk of cardiovascular death. *N Engl J Med.* 2012;366(20):1881–1890

Witt MA, Katz PH, Witt DJ. Unexpectedly limited durability of immunity following acellular pertussis vaccination in preadolescents in a North American outbreak. *Clin Infect Dis.* 2012;54(12):1730–1735

CHAPTER 20

Rat-Bite Fever

Laura M. Plencner, MD, and Mary Anne Jackson, MD

Key Points

- Symptoms of infection are often nonspecific, including fever, arthritis, arthralgias, and rash.

- Diagnosis can be difficult because of the need for specialized agar and incubation conditions for blood culture specimens. The anticoagulant in typical blood culture bottles may inhibit the growth of *Streptobacillus moniliformis*. Notify the laboratory if the diagnosis is suspected.

- Cases may resolve spontaneously within several weeks of infection, but if untreated, severe complications, including death, can occur.

- The treatment of choice is penicillin, although rarely, resistance to penicillin has been described.

Overview

Rat-bite fever is an uncommon zoonotic-transmitted illness and most commonly follows the bite or scratch of a rat. It is clear that a bite is unnecessary for disease transmission, and intimate contact of any kind may be a risk for infection.

Causes and Differential Diagnosis

Rat-bite fever is caused by *Streptobacillus moniliformis* or *Spirillum minus*. *Streptobacillus moniliformis* is the predominant pathogen in the United States, while *S minus* is more common in Asia. As few as 10% and as many as 100% of laboratory rats are colonized in the nasopharynx, and *S moniliformis* has also been found in rat urine.

Transmission to humans can occur via a scratch or bite of a rat but also by exposure to rat urine or feces, and cases are reported after intense intimate contact with oral secretions from colonized animals (children who kiss pet rats). Cases of rat-bite fever have also been described after contact with gerbils, squirrels, mice, or weasels.

Because the clinical symptoms of rat-bite fever are often nonspecific, the differential diagnosis is very broad (Box 20-1).

Box 20-1. Differential Diagnosis for Rat-Bite Fever

Bacterial Infections	Viral Infections	Other Infections	Noninfectious
GAS	EBV	Secondary syphilis	Juvenile idiopathic arthritis
Staphylococcal	Coxsackievirus		
Septic arthritis	Parvovirus		Drug reaction
Rocky Mountain spotted fever	Measles		Kawasaki disease
Ehrlichiosis			
Meningococcemia			
Disseminated gonococcal			
Leptospirosis			
Lyme disease			
Brucellosis			
Mycoplasma pneumoniae			
Chlamydophila pneumoniae			

Abbreviations: EBV, Epstein-Barr virus; GAS, group A *Streptococcus*.

Clinical Features

Characteristic clinical features of infection caused by *S moniliformis* ("streptobacillary fever" or rat-bite fever) are heralded by the development of fever and influenzalike symptoms, with vomiting, arthralgia, and myalgia 3 to 10 days after rat contact.

A distinctive rash may follow that includes macules, pustules, and vesicles on the upper and lower extremities; the palms and soles are often affected. Desquamation of the rash has also been described. This is followed by a nonsuppurative migratory polyarthritis in approximately 50% of affected patients. The knee is the most common joint affected by this infection, although any joint can be involved.

Spirillum minus is more likely to cause a local reaction at the site of the bite or scratch. After 7 to 21 days, the affected site becomes ulcerated and regional lymphangitis may be seen. A classic exanthem consisting of red or purple plaques is typical. In contrast to streptobacillary fever, arthritis is uncommon.

Complications of rat-bite fever include endocarditis; septic arthritis; local abscesses, including brain abscess; meningitis; pneumonia; persistent severe arthritis; severe diarrhea; and death. Untreated infection has a relapsing and remitting course for an average of 3 weeks. The mortality of rat-bite fever in untreated cases is approximately 10%.

Evaluation

Streptobacillus moniliformis is a nonencapsulated, nonmotile, pleomorphic, gram-negative rod, and *S minus* is a gram-negative spirochete.

While *S moniliformis* has been isolated in culture from blood, synovial fluid, and abscess fluid, it does not grow in typical sheep blood agar or MacConkey agar and specific agar and incubation conditions are required. If rat-bite fever is suspected, the clinician needs to alert the laboratory to the diagnosis and media enriched with blood, serum, or ascitic fluid will be used. The bacteria are quite slow growing, and growth may not be seen for 3 to 5 days. *Streptobacillus moniliformis* has also been identified by polymerase chain reaction testing, but testing is not routinely available in commercial laboratories.

Spirillum minus does not grow in standard culture, and diagnosis resides with identification by darkfield microscopy, using wet mounts of blood or exudates from lesions or lymph nodes.

Management

The treatment of choice for rat-bite fever is penicillin administered intravenously for 7 to 10 days. Administration of intravenous penicillin (250,000 U/kg/day divided every 4–6 hours; maximum dose of 24 million U/day) for 5 to 7 days with transition to oral penicillin (50 mg/kg/day divided every 8 hours; maximum dose of 3 g/day) for an additional 7 days may be considered in the patient who has rat-bite fever without endocarditis if a good response to therapy has been confirmed.

Rarely, resistance to penicillin has been reported; tetracycline, gentamicin, cefuroxime, and cefotaxime could be considered as second-line treatments, though the cephalosporins have not been well studied.

Alternative therapy for patients with a serious penicillin allergy include doxycycline if the child is at least 8 years of age (2 mg/kg/dose every 12 hours; maximum: 100 mg twice daily) or gentamicin (7.5 mg/kg/day divided every 8 hours).

In patients with endocarditis due to *S moniliformis,* therapy with high-dose intravenous penicillin (400,000 U/kg/day divided every 4–6 hours; maximum: 24 million U/day) for at least 4 weeks is recommended and the addition of gentamicin should be considered.

During hospitalization for *S moniliformis* infection, standard precautions are recommended.

Children with a known exposure to rat bite should be observed for symptoms, since the infection rate following a rat bite is approximately 10%. Some experts recommend postexposure prophylaxis with penicillin. People with frequent exposure to rats should wear gloves when handling rats and avoid hand to mouth contact to reduce the risk of infection.

Nontraditional pets, including rats, can put children at risk for zoonotic infections. Parents often look to pediatricians for guidance regarding safe pets and ways to reduce potential infection from a nontraditional pet. Children who are at the highest risk for zoonotic infection from a pet include children younger than 5 years and immunocompromised children, including children undergoing chemotherapy, children with HIV, and children who have received a solid organ transplant. Hand hygiene should be encouraged to help reduce the risk of zoonotic infection.

Suggested Reading

Albedawawi S, LeBlanc C, Shaw A, Slinger RW. A teenager with fever, rash, and arthritis. *CMAJ*. 2006;175(4):354

American Academy of Pediatrics. Rat-bite fever. In Kimberlin DW, Brady MT, Jackson MA, Long SS, eds. *Red Book: 2015 Report of the Committee on Infectious Diseases*. 30th ed. Elk Grove Village, IL: American Academy of Pediatrics; 2015

Andre JM, Freydiere AM, Benito Y, et al. Rat bite fever caused by *Streptobacillus moniliformis* in a child: human infection and rat carriage diagnosed by PCR. *J Clin Pathol*. 2005;58(11):1215–1216

Centers for Disease Control and Prevention. Fatal rat-bite fever–Florida and Washington, 2003. *MMWR Morb Mortal Wkly Rep*. 2005;53(51):1198–1202

Cunningham BB, Paller AS, Katz BZ. Rat bite fever in a pet lover. *J Am Acad Dermatol*. 1998;38(2 Part 2):330–332

Hockman D, Pence CD, Whittler RR, Smith LE. Septic arthritis of the hip secondary to rat bite fever: a case report. *Clin Orthop Relat Res*. 2000;(380):173–176

Khatchadourian K, Ovetchkine P, Minodier P, Lamarre V, Lebel MH, Tapiéro B. The rise of rats: a growing pediatric issue. *Paediatr Child Health*. 2010;15(3):131–134

CHAPTER 21

Staphylococcus aureus Infections

J. Chase McNeil, MD, and Sheldon L. Kaplan, MD

Key Points

- Staphylococci are the most common cause of skin and soft-tissue infections.

- Osteoarticular infection or pneumonia/empyema is most commonly noted in those with invasive staphylococcal infection.

- Drainage is generally sufficient to treat small skin abscesses, and oral antibiotics may be used for the well child in whom a larger abscess has been drained. All patients with staphylococcal skin or soft-tissue infection who are systemically ill should be hospitalized and treated with intravenous antibiotics and undergo appropriate drainage procedures.

- Magnetic resonance imaging is the modality of choice to confirm osteomyelitis because bone findings on plain radiographs are generally normal at presentation.

- Video-assisted thoracoscopic surgery or fibrinolytic infusion through the chest tube, depending on local standards, should be used in those with pleural empyema caused by *Staphylococcus aureus*.

- Culture and susceptibility data should be used to guide treatment of serious infections, and empiric treatment should factor in data derived from your local antibiogram.

Overview

Staphylococcus aureus is among the most common bacterial pathogens encountered in pediatric practice and is responsible for a wide spectrum of disease. Emergence of community-acquired methicillin-resistant *S aureus* (MRSA) among previously healthy children has led to an evolution in the severity and complications of these infections as well as their treatment. While there is potential for severe invasive disease, most infections in healthy children involve the skin and soft tissues.

Causes and Differential Diagnosis

Staphylococcus aureus are gram-positive, catalase-positive bacteria that classically appear like grape clusters on microscopic examination. Nasal or skin colonization occurs in 30% to 40% of otherwise healthy individuals, and the rates are higher in those with skin disorders.

Staphylococcus aureus is the principal pathogen in bacterial skin and soft-tissue infections (SSTIs) in children. For immunocompetent hosts the other primary organism of consideration in SSTI is group A *Streptococcus*. In immunocompromised hosts or those with a history of significant trauma, other organisms to consider include *Pseudomonas aeruginosa* and other gram-negative enteric organisms, *Vibrio* species, atypical mycobacteria, and fungi. *Pasteurella multocida* is seen with animal bites, and mixed aerobic and anaerobic organisms are common skin infections following human bites. For cellulitis in neonates, group B *Streptococcus* should be considered in the differential diagnosis.

The differential diagnosis of acute bone and joint infection is similar to that for acute limp. Cellulitis, fractures, sprain, and other trauma-related injuries must be considered, as well as the possibility of malignancy. Staphylococcal myositis and pyomyositis have emerged as common entities that can mimic bone and joint infection. The primary other infectious etiology to consider in these clinical situations is group A *Streptococcus*. The presence of trauma, a chronic presentation, or an immunocompromised host (including hemoglobinopathies) raises the possibility of other infectious etiologies including gram-negative organisms (including *Salmonella*), mycobacteria, and fungi. *Haemophilus influenzae* type b should be considered in unimmunized or under-immunized groups. In addition, in some countries, *Kingella kingae* is a very common cause of bone and joint infection in toddlers; less commonly, *Streptococcus pneumoniae* is seen.

The differential diagnosis of staphylococcal pneumonia is similar to that of other causes of pneumonia and includes bacterial and viral etiologies. The primary bacterial etiologies to consider include *S pneumoniae*, *H influenzae*, and *Mycoplasma pneumoniae*. In the setting of a recent influenza infection, in addition to *S pneumoniae* and *S aureus*, the other primary etiology to consider is group A *Streptococcus*.

Skin and Soft-Tissue Infections

Clinical Manifestations

Skin and soft-tissue infections most often present with localized erythema, tenderness, or swelling (Figure 21-1). Fever is variably present depending on the host and extent of disease. Presence of fluctuance and severe induration is highly suggestive of the existence of a drainable purulent collection.

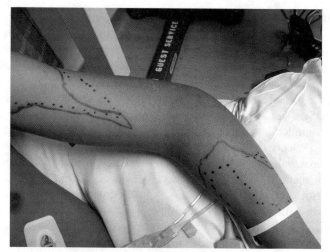

Figure 21-1. *Staphylococcus aureus* cellulitis.
The patient has areas of erythema encircled with a pen to follow
disease progression (solid versus dotted-lines).

Diagnosis

In most cases, a clinical diagnosis is made and the etiology is secured by
bacterial culture of wound exudates or surgical cultures. For immunocompetent children with minor SSTI or abscesses, the yield of blood cultures is low; in
general, blood cultures in SSTI should be reserved for those with severe disease
requiring drainage in the operating room, the immunocompromised, and those
who are systemically ill.

Management

Minor Skin Infections and Cellulitis

For minor skin infections, such as impetigo or mildly superinfected eczema
without systemic signs or symptoms of infection, the use of topical antimicrobials alone may be effective (Evidence Level III). Agents that may be used include
mupirocin, or retapamulin ointments. Cellulitis without an obvious focus that
can be drained can be adequately treated with oral antimicrobials on an
outpatient basis provided the patient is not systemically ill. Clindamycin,
trimethoprim/sulfamethoxazole (TMP/SMX), or doxycycline (for children
<8 years) is generally recommended if community-acquired MRSA is a
concern; cephalexin is commonly used for methicillin-susceptible isolates or if
community-acquired MRSA is not a common pathogen in the community
(Evidence Level II-2). The need to provide coverage for group A *Streptococcus*
for well-appearing children with non-purulent cellulitis is often a difficult
question in that a microbiologic etiology in such cases is usually undetermined,
and given the fact that TMP/SMX does not provide any group A *Streptococcus*
coverage. Drawing a line around the area of cellulitis with a marking pen may
help more objectively monitor clinical resolution or worsening.

Furuncles, Carbuncles, and Abscesses

For patients with purulent collections, the primary therapeutic intervention is performance of an incision and drainage of the infected focus (Figure 21-2). Thorough incision and drainage provides adequate treatment for small abscesses (<5 cm for children ≥9 years; <4 cm for children 12 months–8 years of age) even in the absence of systemic antibiotic therapy (Evidence Level I), although there was a trend for new lesions to develop less often in those with systemic antimicrobials in one study. Patients with larger abscesses are more likely to experience an increase in size of their lesion, re-accumulation of purulent material, and hospital admission when incision and drainage alone is used without effective antimicrobial therapy (Evidence Level II-2). Thus, for patients with an abscess greater than 5 cm for children 9 years or older, or greater than 4 cm for children 12 months to 8 years of age, incision and drainage and antibiotic therapy are recommended. For small abscesses, however, oral antibiotics in addition to incision and drainage should be considered for select clinical scenarios, including children with immunocompromising conditions, babies younger than 12 months, or children with an abscess on the face, hands, or perineum (Evidence Level III). Patients who are systemically ill should be admitted to the hospital, and parenteral antibiotics should be administered after performing a drainage procedure (Evidence Level III). Vancomycin or clindamycin intravenously (IV) is the recommended agent for hospitalized children with SSTI if community-acquired MRSA is a concern. Use of empiric clindamycin for suspected community-acquired MRSA is an option when the rate of clindamycin resistance for community *S aureus* isolates is less than 10% to 15% (Evidence Level III).

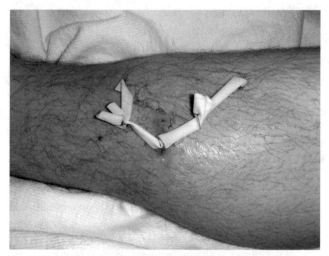

Figure 21-2. *Staphylococcus aureus* abscess of the lower extremity following drainage.
The patient underwent an incision and drainage procedure for a large soft tissue abscess with the placement of round rubber drains.

Recurrent Staphylococcal Skin Infections

Up to 20% of SSTIs are associated with recurrence or reinfection. Most children with recurrent skin infections are otherwise healthy; however, clinicians should be alert to potential warning signs of immunocompromising conditions that could increase the patient's risk for infections. If patients are exhibiting additional warning signs of immune dysfunction, such as failure to thrive, pneumonia, chronic diarrhea, other infections, or generalized lymphadenopathy, an immune evaluation should be considered.

Most experts recommend strict adherence to personal and family hygienic measures to minimize the recurrence of staphylococcal skin infections (Evidence Level III). These measures include regular bathing and avoiding reuse or sharing of personal items (eg, towels, razors, linens) that have direct contact with skin. Given that greater than 75% of children are colonized with *S aureus* at some point, much interest has developed in the use of a variety of agents to eradicate or decrease staphylococcal colonization and minimize recurrence of infection (Table 21-1); however, the specific dosing and duration of use of these agents are not fully understood. Hygienic measures alone are helpful in decreasing colonization in some cases; however, greater degrees of eradication were achieved in one study with the use of hygienic interventions plus intranasal mupirocin and either chlorhexidine or bleach baths (Evidence Level I). Furthermore, the intervention of hygienic measures, intranasal mupirocin, and chlorhexidine in combination for 5 days has been shown to result in reduced incidence of SSTI in the index patient and in family members when all

Table 21-1. Proposed Regimens for Preventing Recurrent Staphylococcal Skin and Soft-Tissue Infection

Intervention	Administration	Comments
Hygienic measures	Do not use soaps or lotions in jars; rather, pump or squeeze bottles. Refrain from sharing personal hygiene items that have been in contact with skin (eg, razors, towels, hairbrushes). Wash bed linens weekly in hot water and towels/washcloths after each use.	None.
Mupirocin	Applied intranasally 2–3 times daily.	The optimal duration of use is unclear.
Chlorhexidine gluconate	Solution used for bathing.	Used for up to 5 d in a row.
Diluted bleach baths	1 tsp (5 mL) of standard household bleach/gal of bathwater limiting time in tub to 15 min; repeat at twice-weekly intervals.	Optimal concentration, duration, and timing of bleach baths, as well as effectiveness, are unclear at this time. Do not use simultaneously with chlorhexidine products.

household occupants participated (Evidence Level I). Thus, a multipronged approach including use of high levels of personal hygiene, decolonization procedures, and involvement of the entire family should be considered in patients with recurrent *S aureus* SSTI.

Bone and Joint Infections

Clinical Manifestations

Hematogenous osteomyelitis most commonly affects the metaphysis of long bones such as the femur, tibia, fibula, and humerus. Osteomyelitis of the long bones frequently presents with fever, tenderness to palpation, swelling, and erythema of the overlying skin. Involvement of long bones of the lower extremity is frequently associated with inability to bear weight on the affected leg. Infection involving the pelvic bones frequently has a more insidious presentation and often a delay in diagnosis; ambulating children may develop a waddling or Trendelenburg gait.

Septic arthritis most frequently involves the hip, knee, or shoulder and is associated with similar concerns as above, although symptoms may localize to a specific joint. Joint redness, warmth, effusion, and restricted range of motion are the usual physical findings (Figure 21-3). Involvement of the hip joint is typically associated with flexion and external rotation of the hip. Concomitant septic arthritis and osteomyelitis are common in all age groups and typically involve contiguous sites.

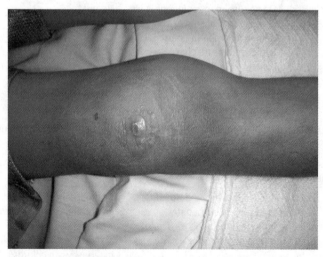

Figure 21-3. *Staphylococcus aureus* **septic arthritis.**
The photograph illustrates the erythema, swelling, and taut skin overlying the septic joint.

Diagnosis of Osteoarticular Infection

Figure 21-4 provides a diagnostic algorithm.

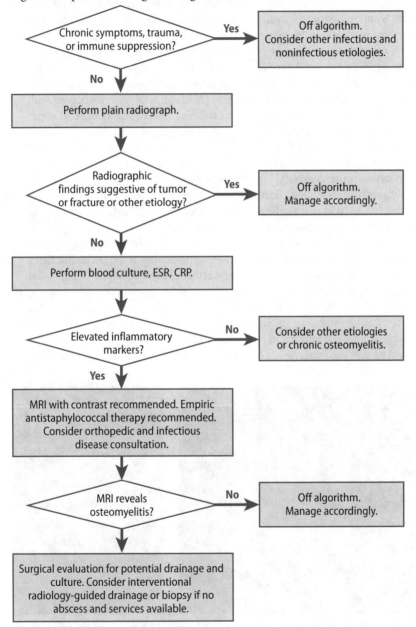

Figure 21-4. Proposed algorithm for the evaluation of suspected *Staphylococcus aureus* acute osteomyelitis.

Abbreviations: CRP, C-reactive protein; ESR, erythrocyte sedimentation rate; MRI, magnetic resonance imaging.

Note: Clinical algorithms are meant to assist with decision-making but are not a substitute for a thorough clinical evaluation and sound clinical judgement. If at any time a patient exhibits signs and symptoms of sepsis, antibiotics along with other supportive measures should be initiated immediately.

Sensitivity of C-reactive protein (CRP) for the diagnosis of acute osteomyelitis is approximately 98% (Evidence Level II-1), while sensitivity of white blood cell counts greater than 12,000/mcL is only 35%. Up to 52% of patients with *S aureus* osteomyelitis also have bacteremia; thus, blood culture is recommended in patients with suspected osteoarticular infection.

Conventional radiography has poor sensitivity for the diagnosis of acute osteomyelitis; however, most experts in the field continue to recommend its use to rule out other causes of bone pain (eg, tumor or fracture) (Evidence Level III). Use of magnetic resonance imaging (MRI) technology is associated with improved sensitivity and specificity for the diagnosis of staphylococcal bone and joint infections compared with nuclear imaging studies, and MRI is the preferred imaging modality for the diagnosis of staphylococcal osteoarticular infection (Figure 21-5, Evidence Level II-2). Sensitivity of MRI for the diagnosis of *S aureus* musculoskeletal infection was 98% compared to 53% for nuclear scintigraphy in one study. Furthermore, extraosseous sites of infection are identified on MRI in up to 68% of patients with *S aureus* osteomyelitis, which frequently leads to additional surgical interventions.

Ultrasound of the involved joint is highly sensitive for the diagnosis of staphylococcal septic arthritis, with a sensitivity approaching 100% (Evidence Level II-2). For patients with suspected septic arthritis, arthrocentesis and synovial fluid Gram stain and culture are recommended. Magnetic resonance imaging is useful for detection of complications outside the joint. The presence of bacteremia, a CRP greater than 100 mg/L, or longer than 2 days of fever after initiation of antimicrobial treatment in patients with *S aureus* septic joints is highly suggestive of the presence of contiguous osteomyelitis (Evidence Level II-2).

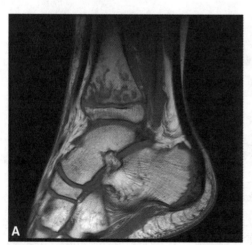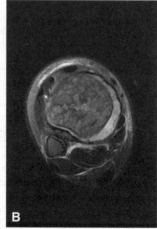

Figure 21-5. Magnetic resonance imaging of methicillin-resistant *Staphylococcus aureus* osteomyelitis of distal tibia.
Panel A, Sagittal T1 weighted images. Panel B, Axial T2 weighted images of the right tibia. This 12-year-old boy presented with a week of fever, lower extremity pain, and limp. He was found to have methicillin-resistant *Staphylococcus aureus* bacteremia and osteomyelitis with multiple subperiosteal and intraosseous abscesses.

Management of Osteoarticular Infection

The management of staphylococcal bone and joint infection relies heavily on cooperation among surgeons, generalists, and infectious diseases specialists. Surgical intervention is recommended for both diagnostic and therapeutic purposes. If surgical intervention is not necessary and blood cultures are negative after 24 to 48 hours, obtaining specimens via interventional radiology is recommended, if possible. Tissue or purulent fluid should be sent for Gram stain and culture to help identify the etiologic agent and refine antimicrobial therapy. Tissue biopsy with microscopic examination by a pathologist should also be considered if the diagnosis is in doubt. For areas of necrotic bone or large subperiosteal abscesses, surgical debridement is recommended also to expedite patient recovery. For septic joints, drainage and irrigation is essential to prevent long-term damage to the joint, especially in the hip and shoulder.

The need to delay antimicrobials until surgery can be performed to maximize culture yield is often a difficult decision to make. For patients who are clinically stable and for whom a prolonged (>24 hours) delay to surgery is unexpected, some experts would recommend delaying initiation of antimicrobials until cultures can be obtained (Evidence Level III). However, a recent study found that IV antibiotic therapy for less than 72 hours prior to obtaining cultures did not significantly affect culture results (Evidence Level II-3). For patients who are toxic appearing or if bacteremia is suspected, the initiation of antibiotics should not be delayed.

Empiric antimicrobial therapy should be directed against *S aureus* with coverage for other more uncommon agents as the scenario may dictate. Once culture and susceptibility data are available, therapy should be narrowed to the most specific agent possible. For patients with culture-negative osteomyelitis, targeting presumptive staphylococcal disease generally results in good outcomes (Evidence Level II-3).

For acute osteomyelitis, antimicrobial therapy should be continued for 4 to 6 weeks, based on data showing an increase in complications associated with treatment for 3 weeks or less (Evidence Level II-3). While traditionally a complete course of IV therapy was thought necessary, for most patients the evidence indicates that early transition to oral therapy in uncomplicated bone and joint infection leads to outcomes equivalent to those following complete IV courses of treatment (Evidence Level II-2). Septic joints in the absence of complications can be treated with 3 to 4 weeks of antibiotic therapy after drainage (Evidence Level III).

Long-term Monitoring and Complications

A combination of acute phase markers is often followed to evaluate for resolution of osteoarticular infection. These include white blood cell and platelet counts, erythrocyte sedimentation rate, and CRP (Evidence Level III). Many infectious diseases physicians obtain plain radiographs just before the completion of antibiotic therapy to evaluate for healing of the bone, which is one factor used to determine when to discontinue antibiotics and allow resumption of normal activities (Evidence Level III).

Staphylococcal osteomyelitis and septic arthritis are serious infections with potential for long-term sequelae. Among the most common complications of *S aureus* osteoarticular infections are the development of venous thromboses, which may be associated with septic pulmonary embolism. The development of pathologic fractures is also a concern and complicated up to 4.7% of *S aureus* osteomyelitis in one series. Fractures were associated with the presence of subperiosteal abscess, abscesses greater than 50% of the bone circumference, intramuscular abscesses, and the need for multiple surgical procedures (Evidence Level II-2). Growth abnormalities are common in patients who develop pathologic fractures. Long-term growth sequelae develop in up to 3% of cases of septic arthritis.

Staphylococcus aureus Pneumonia/Empyema

While traditionally thought to be an uncommon cause of pneumonia in healthy children, *S aureus,* especially MRSA, has emerged as a prominent cause of community-acquired pneumonia and pneumonia with empyema. The increase in number of cases of staphylococcal pneumonia may be associated with some unexplained characteristic of community-acquired MRSA isolates; these phenomena are currently under investigation. The coinfection of influenza and *S aureus* has been well described since the period following the 1918 Spanish influenza pandemic and has an increased mortality compared to either infection alone.

Clinical Manifestations

The symptoms of staphylococcal pneumonia are similar to those of other forms of bacterial pneumonia and include tachypnea, fever, vomiting, and cough with or without sputum production. Up to 62% of patients develop pneumonia with empyema with common presenting symptoms of chest pain, fever, and respiratory distress; most children are hypoxic (Evidence Level II-2). Over one-half of cases are associated with need for intensive care unit admission and more than 30% with the need for mechanical ventilation. Preceding respiratory viral illnesses or viral coinfection are detected in up 25% of cases.

Exacerbation of pulmonary disease associated with *S aureus* in the cystic fibrosis population represents a special case; it can take a protracted course and is often associated with a progressive decline in pulmonary function.

Diagnosis of Staphylococcal Pneumonia

The diagnosis of pneumonia is by and large based on clinical history, physical examination, and radiographic findings. Necrotizing pneumonia and pneumatoceles are commonly associated with staphylococcal pneumonia. Chest ultrasound can detect complex effusions (septated or loculated) in up to 75% of patients with staphylococcal pneumonia and effusion (Evidence Level II-2). Microbiologic diagnosis of pediatric pneumonia and empyema is often challenging. In studies of all causes of pediatric empyema, an etiologic agent is isolated from pleural fluid cultures in only one-third of cases. *Staphylococcus aureus* can be isolated in blood culture in about 20% of children with staphylococcal pneumonia.

Management of Staphylococcal Pneumonia

For patients with empyema, surgical intervention with either chest tube placement followed by the instillation of fibrinolytics or video-assisted thoracoscopic surgery is recommended. In studies of all causes of empyema, video-assisted thoracoscopic surgery in the first 48 hours of presentation was associated with a shortened hospital stay (Evidence Level II-3). Any fluid obtained by a surgical intervention should be sent for culture (Evidence Level II-2).

A number of studies have shown a predilection for MRSA to cause pulmonary disease (Evidence Level II-2). Thus, most experts recommend vancomycin for empiric treatment of suspected staphylococcal pneumonia (Evidence Level III). In areas of a low prevalence of clindamycin resistance, empiric treatment with clindamycin could be considered. Furthermore, some experts recommend clindamycin because it concentrates in pulmonary tissues in experimental models, and case series and cohort studies of MRSA pneumonia have shown good outcomes with this agent (Evidence Level II-2). Once culture and susceptibility data are known, transition can be made to an oral agent such as clindamycin or linezolid for MRSA isolates to complete treatment as an outpatient. The optimal duration of treatment for staphylococcal pneumonia is unclear, but treating for approximately 21 days is generally recommended (Evidence Level III).

Long-term Complications

Pulmonary sequelae developed in up to 6% of patients in one series, including recurrent pneumothoraces, chronic lung disease caused by either obstructive or restrictive pathology, or bronchiectasis (Evidence Level II-2). Some experts recommend repeating chest imaging near the end of therapy to assess for presence of pulmonary complications (Evidence Level III).

Toxin-Mediated Disease

Staphylococcal Scalded Skin Syndrome

Staphylococcal scalded skin syndrome is a toxin-mediated disease that causes tender scarlatiniform eruptions, with localized bullous impetigo, along with generalized exfoliation. The hallmark sign includes cleavage of the stratum granulosum of epidermis (Nikolsky sign). Staphylococcal scalded skin syndrome is caused by circulating exfoliative toxins A and B. Bacteremia is rare, but dehydration and superinfection can occur; therefore, fluid management should be monitored along with meticulous skin and wound care. Healing without scarring occurs.

Toxic Shock Syndrome

Staphylococcus aureus toxic shock syndrome (TSS) is caused by TSS toxin type 1 or other staphylococcal enterotoxins. The toxins act as superantigens, causing capillary leak that can cause hypotension and multiorgan failure. Characteristics include fever, generalized erythroderma, rapid-onset hypotension, and multisystem organ involvement that can produce profuse watery diarrhea,

---

Box 21-1. *Staphylococcus aureus* **Toxic Shock Syndrome Case Definition**

Clinical Features

- Fever: ≥38.9°C (102.0°F)
- Rash: diffuse, macular erythroderma
- Desquamation: 1–2 wk after onset (particularly palms, soles, fingers, and toes)
- Hypotension: systolic blood pressure ≤90 mm Hg for adults, lower than 5th percentile for children and adolescents <16 y; orthostatic drop in diastolic pressure of ≥15 mm Hg from lying to sitting; orthostatic syncope or orthostatic dizziness
- Multisystem organ involvement: ≥3 of the following:
  o Gastrointestinal: vomiting or diarrhea at onset of illness
  o Muscular: severe myalgia or a creatine kinase concentration greater than twice the upper limit of the reference range
  o Mucous membrane: vaginal, oropharyngeal, or conjunctival hyperemia
  o Renal: a serum urea nitrogen or serum creatinine concentration greater than twice the upper limit of the reference range or a urinary sediment with ≥3 white blood cells per high-power field in the absence of a urinary tract infection
  o Hepatic: total bilirubin, aspartate transaminase, or alanine transaminase concentrations greater than twice the upper limit of the reference range
  o Hematologic: platelet count ≤100,000/mm³
  o Central nervous system: disorientation or alterations in consciousness without focal neurologic signs when fever and hypotension are absent

Laboratory Criteria

- *Negative* results on the following tests if obtained:
  o Blood, throat, or cerebrospinal fluid cultures (Blood culture may be positive for *Staphylococcus aureus*.)
  o Serologic tests for Rocky Mountain spotted fever, leptospirosis, or measles

Case Classification

- *Probable:* a case that meets the laboratory criteria and in which 4 of 5 clinical features are present
- *Confirmed:* a case that meets laboratory criteria and in which all 5 of the clinical findings, including desquamation, unless the patient dies before desquamation occurs, are present

Adapted from Wharton M, Chorba TL, Vogt RL, Morse DL, Buehler JW. Case definitions for public health surveillance. *MMWR Recomm Rep.* 1990;39(RR-13):1–43.

vomiting, conjunctival injection, and severe myalgias. Evidence of soft-tissue infection with severe increasing pain is common but additionally can be associated with tampon use. Although there has been a decline in TSS associated with tampons, because the manufacturers have removed 3 of the 4 synthetic ingredients (polyester, carboxymethylcellulose, and polyacrylate rayon), prolonged use of highly absorbent tampons can enhance bacterial growth. Diagnosis is made with clinical and laboratory criteria (Box 21-1). Treatment includes bactericidal cell wall inhibitor with β-lactamase–resistant staphylococcal antimicrobial along with toxin inhibitor. If necrotizing fasciitis is present, surgical evaluation is critical.

Specific Antimicrobial Therapy

As a general rule, empiric therapy for bacterial infections should be guided by local epidemiology and antimicrobial susceptibility, particularly regarding empiric coverage for MRSA. Final therapy should be based on the results of culture and susceptibility testing. An overview of the antimicrobial management of *S aureus* infections is provided in Table 21-2.

Strong evidence from in vitro as well as clinical studies in adults confirms the superiority of nafcillin or cefazolin over vancomycin for the treatment of methicillin-susceptible *S aureus* (MSSA) infections; thus, an antistaphylococcal penicillin or first-generation cephalosporin is recommended for disease caused by MSSA (Evidence Level II-2). Furthermore, for severely ill patients with known or suspected gram-positive infection, combination empiric therapy with vancomycin in addition to an antistaphylococcal β-lactam antibiotic is recommended by many experts until the results of culture and susceptibility or rapid molecular tests for the genes encoding for methicillin resistance are known (Evidence Level III).

For treatment of life-threatening or serious infections caused by MRSA, the use of vancomycin in children is recommended. The utility of monitoring vancomycin trough levels to optimize efficacy is controversial. Data from adults suggest that better outcomes are achieved with trough concentrations of 15 to 20 mcg/mL; in two pediatric studies, the outcomes were no better but nephrotoxicity increased in patients with the higher vancomycin trough concentrations (Evidence Level II-3). An increase in vancomycin minimal inhibitory concentrations ("vancomycin creep") has not been noted in MRSA isolates from children as it has in isolates from adults; the clinical significance of this creep as it applies to pediatrics is unclear.

Studies of gram-positive bacteremia and nosocomial pneumonia in children have illustrated the non-inferiority of linezolid to vancomycin (Evidence Level I). While linezolid is tolerated well by most children, the cost and potential for rare but severe adverse effects (eg, peripheral neuropathy or visual disturbances with prolonged use) generally limit its use for MRSA infections in which other agents cannot be used.

Table 21-2. Commonly Used Systemic Antimicrobials With Activity Against *Staphylococcus aureus*

Antimicrobial Class	Most Common Agents	Bactericidal	Dosing	Adverse Effects	Comments
Glycopeptides	Vancomycin	Yes	Children >1 mo: 15 mg/kg/dose IV every 8 h (15 mg/kg/dose IV every 6 h is recommended if seriously ill or in the setting of CNS infection.) Maximum dose: 1.5 g/dose, 4 g/d	Redman syndrome, renal insufficiency, ototoxicity, bone marrow suppression	The value of monitoring vancomycin levels for therapeutic efficacy in children is controversial.
Anti-staphylococcal penicillins	Nafcillin, oxacillin	Yes	Nafcillin 150–200 mg/kg/d IV in divided doses every 4–6 h Maximum dose: 12 g/d Oxacillin: 150–200 mg/kg/d IV in divided doses every 4–6 h Maximum dose: 12 g/d	Neutropenia, rash, nephritis (rare), phlebitis, transaminitis	Transaminitis is more frequent with oxacillin, which may cause less phlebitis than nafcillin.
1st-generation cephalosporins	Cefazolin, cephalexin	Yes	Cefazolin (infants and children): 50–100 mg/kg/d IV divided every 8 h Maximum dose: 2 g/dose, 12 g/d Cephalexin (infants and children): 25–100 mg/kg/d orally divided every 6–8 h Maximum dose: 4 g/d	Neutropenia, nephritis (rare)	Option for patients allergic to penicillins but with non-immediate hypersensitivity reactions.
Oxazolidinones	Linezolid	No	<12 y: 10 mg/kg/dose IV/orally every 8 h Maximum dose: 1,200 mg/d >12 y: 10 mg/kg/dose every 12 h Maximum dose: 600 mg every 12 h	Neutropenia, lactic acidosis, neuropathy, optic neuritis, visual disturbances with prolonged use, hypertensive crises with tyramine-rich foods	High cost can be prohibitive. This agent may be beneficial when combined with other agents for pneumonia.

Class	Drug	FDA approved	Dosing	Adverse effects	Comments
Lincosamide	Clindamycin	No	Children: 10–13 mg/kg/dose IV/orally every 8 h Maximum dose: 1.8 g/d orally or 900 mg/dose, 2.7 g/d IV	Rash, minor transaminitis, loose stools	Liquid formulations often not palatable to young children. Excellent penetration into lung parenchyma. Minimal CSF penetration.
Sulfonamides	TMP/SMX	Yes	Children: 4–6 mg/kg/dose of TMP component orally every 12 h or 15–20 mg/kg/d of TMP component IV divided every 6–8 h Maximum dose: 1 double-strength tablet every 12 h	Neutropenia, rash, renal impairment	Primarily for treating skin and soft-tissue infections. Limited data for treatment of bone and joint infections. Questionable penetration of deeply infected foci.
Tetracyclines	Doxycycline, minocycline	No	Doxycycline (children >8 y): 2–4 mg/kg/d divided every 12–24 h Maximum dose: 100 mg/dose, 200 mg/d	Nausea/vomiting, rash, photosensitivity, dental staining in young children (<8 y)	Primarily for treatment of skin and soft-tissue infections.
Lipopeptides	Daptomycin	Yes	Adults SSTI: 4 mg/kg/dose IV daily Bacteremia: 6 mg/kg/dose IV daily	Rhabdomyolysis, eosinophilic pneumonia	Not approved for use in children; optimal dosing under investigation.
Anti-staphylococcal cephalosporins	Ceftaroline	Yes	≥6 mo: 12 mg/kg IV for subjects weighing ≤33 kg and 400 mg for subjects weighing >33 kg infused over 60 min every 8 h <6 mo: 8 mg/kg infused over 60 min every 8 h	Rash, diarrhea, neutropenia	Approved for children >2 mo.

Abbreviations: CNS, central nervous system; CSF, cerebrospinal fluid; IV, intravenously; SSTI, skin and soft-tissue infection; TMP/SMX, trimethoprim/sulfamethoxazole.

Clindamycin is the most commonly used antibiotic for the management of non-bacteremic community-acquired MRSA infections in children. Primarily retrospective studies have shown clindamycin therapy to be as effective as treatment with vancomycin and β-lactam antibiotics for MRSA and MSSA, respectively (Evidence Level II-3). Rising rates of resistance to clindamycin, particularly among MSSA, have limited its use in some centers.

Virtually all *S aureus* isolates demonstrate in vitro susceptibility to TMP/SMX, and older series have reported good results regarding treatment of SSTI (Evidence Level II-2). Conflicting results have been seen, however, in a number of retrospective series for the treatment of SSTI in the community-acquired MRSA era. One showed equivalent outcomes compared with clindamycin, while the other suggested greater rates of treatment failure; these discrepancies may reflect differences of completeness in incision and drainage procedures. In a large randomized double blinded study in children and adults, clindamycin and TMP/SMX were found equivalent for treatment of uncomplicated cellulitis and abscesses (Evidence Level I). Increase in the prevalence of clindamycin resistance among *S aureus* has led to an increased use of TMP/SMX by clinicians in some centers with excellent results, but clinicians should be aware of the adverse drug reactions associated with its use. Use of TMP/SMX is recommended by the Infectious Diseases Society of America for the treatment of staphylococcal SSTI. However, data on the use of TMP/SMX to treat invasive staphylococcal infections are very limited.

Antibiotics of the tetracycline class should generally be avoided in children younger than 8 years. Data from the pre–community-acquired MRSA era also suggest efficacy of these agents for skin infections in children (Evidence Level II-3). These agents in adults have been shown in more contemporary studies to be associated with good outcomes for treatment of SSTI (Evidence Level II-3); however, they do not seem as efficacious for osteoarticular infection. When these agents are used in older children and adolescents, patients must be counseled regarding potential photosensitivity related with this to class of antimicrobials.

Daptomycin is a lipopeptide antibiotic that is rapidly bactericidal against MRSA in vitro. Studies in adults have shown daptomycin to be non-inferior to vancomycin for treatment of *S aureus* bacteremia and SSTI (Evidence Level I). Daptomycin is approved in adults for treating MRSA SSTIs and bacteremia but not pulmonary infections. In vitro and animal studies have shown daptomycin to be inactivated by pulmonary surfactant, and animals with pneumonia treated with daptomycin had an increased death rate compared to comparator drugs. Daptomycin is undergoing investigation in children to determine the optimal dose and establish its safety in this age group.

Ceftaroline fosamil is a recently approved cephalosporin for use in adults with expanded activity against MRSA and vancomycin-resistant enterococci. In phase 3 studies in adults, ceftaroline was non-inferior to vancomycin plus aztreonam for SSTI and non-inferior to ceftriaxone for the treatment of community-acquired pneumonia (Evidence Level I). Furthermore, ceftaroline had a similar adverse effect profile to other cephalosporins and was found to be better tolerated than vancomycin in adults. Ceftaroline is approved by the US Food and Drug Administration for children older than 2 months for treatment of skin and soft-tissue infections. Studies are ongoing to determine the safety and appropriate dosing of this agent in children for other sites of infection.

Suggested Reading

Browne LP, Mason EO, Kaplan SL, Cassady CI, Krishnamurthy R, Guillerman RP. Optimal imaging strategy for community-acquired *Staphylococcus aureus* musculoskeletal infections in children. *Pediatr Radiol.* 2008;38(8):841–847

Carrillo-Marquez MA, Hulten KG, Hammerman W, Lamberth L, Mason EO, Kaplan SL. *Staphylococcus aureus* pneumonia in children in the era of community-acquired methicillin-resistance at Texas Children's Hospital. *Pediatr Infect Dis J.* 2011;30(7):545–550

Carrillo-Marquez MA, Hulten KG, Hammerman W, Mason EO, Kaplan SL. USA300 is the predominant genotype causing *Staphylococcus aureus* septic arthritis in children. *Pediatr Infect Dis J.* 2009;28(12):1076–1080

Cenizal MJ, Skiest D, Luber S, et al. Prospective randomized trial of empiric therapy with trimethoprim-sulfamethoxazole or doxycycline for outpatient skin and soft tissue infections in an area of high prevalence of methicillin-resistant *Staphylococcus aureus. Antimicrob Agents Chemother.* 2007;51(7):2628–2630

Duong M, Markwell S, Peter J, Barenkamp S. Randomized, controlled trial of antibiotics in the management of community-acquired skin abscesses in the pediatric patient. *Ann Emerg Med.* 2010;55(5):401–407

Fritz SA, Camins BC, Eisenstein KA, et al. Effectiveness of measures to eradicate *Staphylococcus aureus* carriage in patients with community-associated skin and soft-tissue infections: a randomized trial. *Infect Control Hosp Epidemiol.* 2011;32(9):872–880

Fritz SA, Hogan PG, Hayek G, et al. Household versus individual approaches to eradication of community-associated *Staphylococcus aureus* in children: a randomized trial. *Clin Infect Dis.* 2012;54(6):743–751

Goldman JL, Jackson MA, Herigon JC, et al. Trends in adverse drug reactions to trimethoprim-sulfamethoxazole. *Pediatrics.* 2013;131(1):e103-e108

Hahn A, Frenck RW Jr., Allen-Staat M, et al. Evaluation of Target attainment of vancomycin area under the curve in children with methicillin-resistant Staphylococcus aureus bacteremia. *Ther Drug Monit.* 2015:37:619-625

Hyun DY, Mason EO, Forbes A, Kaplan SL. Trimethoprim-sulfamethoxazole or clindamycin for treatment of community-acquired methicillin-resistant *Staphylococcus aureus* skin and soft tissue infections. *Pediatr Infect Dis J.* 2009;28(1):57–59

Kaplan SL, Forbes A, Hammerman WA, et al. Randomized trial of "bleach baths" plus routine hygienic measures vs. routine hygienic measures alone for prevention of recurrent infections. *Clin Infect Dis* 2014;58(5):679-682.

Lee MC, Rios AM, Aten MF, et al. Management and outcome of children with skin and soft tissue abscesses caused by community-acquired methicillin-resistant *Staphylococcus aureus. Pediatr Infect Dis J.* 2004;23(2):123–127

Liu C, Bayer A, Cosgrove SE, et al. Clinical practice guidelines by the Infectious Diseases Society of America for the treatment of methicillin-resistant *Staphylococcus aureus* infections in adults and children. *Clin Infect Dis.* 2011;52(3):e18–e55

Malone JR, Durica SR, Thompson DM, Bogie A, Naifeh M. Blood cultures in the evaluation of uncomplicated skin and soft tissue infections. *Pediatrics.* 2013; 132: 454-459.

McNeil JC, Forbes AR, Vallejo JG, et al. Role of operative or interventional radiology-guided cultures for osteomyelitis. *Pediatrics.* 2016;137(5)

McNeil JC, Kok EY, Forbes AR, et al. Healthcare-Associated Staphylococcus aureus Bacteremia in Children: Evidence for Reverse Vancomycin Creep and Impact of Vancomycin Trough Values on Outcome *Pediatr Infect Dis J.* 2016;35(3);263-268

Miller LG, Daum RS, Creech CB, et al. Clindamycin versus trimethoprim-sulfamethoxazole for uncomplicated skin infections. *N Engl J Med.* 2015;372(12);1093-1103

Williams DJ, Cooper WO, Kaltenbach LA, et al. Comparative effectiveness of antibiotic treatment strategies for pediatric skin and soft-tissue infections. *Pediatrics.* 2011;128(3):e479–e487

CHAPTER 22

Tetanus

Renuka Verma, MD; Krithiha Raghunathan, MD; and Anna Katrina Tinio, MD

Key Points

- Tetanus is a neurologic disease that follows wounds contaminated with *Clostridium tetani*, a ubiquitous environmental organism that elaborates an exotoxin, which blocks inhibitory impulses to motoneurons.

- Disease manifestations vary but generally feature severe generalized muscle spasms that lead to respiratory failure and dysautonomia that lasts for several weeks.

- The diagnosis should be made when classic features follow a tetanus-prone wound and other diagnoses have been excluded.

- Treatment should include metronidazole, wound debridement, tetanus immune globulin to neutralize toxin, and supportive care to manage muscle spasms and treat associated complications.

Overview

Clostridium tetani is still an important cause of death in the developing world due to poor sanitation and suboptimal access to appropriate medical care.

Causes and Differential Diagnosis

Clostridium tetani is a gram-positive obligate anaerobe bacilli, found in the soil as well as the intestines of various animals. Mature bacteria develop into spores that can remain alive in the extremes of environment and soil. Spores cannot be completely destroyed by boiling. Autoclaving is a satisfactory means for elimination of spores.

Clinical Features

A portal of entry for infection is generally noted. Tetanus-prone wounds may range from trivial scratches to contaminated lacerations, penetrating wounds, burns, or animal bites with necrosis, and can follow abortions or child birth in non-sterile conditions. Lower limb wounds, postpartum wounds, and open fractures are most frequently implicated in cases of confirmed tetanus.

The *classic triad of tetanus* consists of muscle spasm, rigidity, and dysautonomia. Early presentation includes neck stiffness, sore throat, and difficulty in opening the mouth. Spasm of the masseter muscle leads to trismus and then spreads out to facial muscles, resulting in risus sardonicus affecting the orbicularis muscle and, subsequently, dysphagia. Rigidity of the neck muscle gives rise to retraction of the head, and truncal muscle rigidity leads to opisthotonos; respiratory distress may arise from decreased chest wall compliance. Besides increased muscle tone, patients also have muscular spasms, which may be mistaken for seizures. These spasms occur spontaneously or as a result of tactile, visual, auditory, or even emotional stimulations. On occasion, spasms are very forceful and may lead to fracture or tendon avulsion. Symptoms continue to progress in spite of treatment, because the toxin in the neurons remains unaffected by neutralizing antibodies. Respiratory difficulty develops in moderate to severe tetanus because of rigidity and spasm of chest muscles and diaphragmatic dysfunction. Laryngeal and pharyngeal spasms may lead to acute life-threatening airway obstruction.

Dysautonomia. Increased sympathetic tone or overactivity is responsible for tachycardia and hypertension. This sympathetic activity and catecholamine excess results in death, even in patients with respiratory stability. Patients with tetanus in general often have a protracted course, which may further be complicated by lung or nosocomial infections. In severely ill patients, "autonomic storms" can be observed with hypertension and tachycardia, followed by bradycardia and hypotension owing to rapid changes in the vascular resistance. Copious salivation, increased bronchial secretions, and sweating may also be noted.

Presentations

There are 4 types of presentations: generalized, localized, cephalic, and neonatal.

Generalized tetanus is the most common and severe presentation, in which all body muscles are involved, starting from the head and neck and progressing to the rest of the body, with spread of spasm and rigidity. Patients may present with headache, pain, rigidity, and muscle spasms. Even minor stimuli, such as noise or touch, can initiate spasms. Medical procedures such as intravenous (IV) or intramuscular injections, catheterization, or suction can also trigger the painful muscle spasms, including laryngeal spasm, which can lead to respiratory failure. In the initial phase of illness, spasms are more obvious; in the second phase of illness, autonomic features become more prominent. Rigidity of the muscles is usually a late feature. The spasm and rigidity require paralysis for extended periods to decrease the pain.

Localized tetanus is seen with a smaller quantity of toxin after peripheral injuries, leading to spasm and rigidity in a small area of the body. It is associated with low mortality.

Cephalic tetanus is localized tetanus by the area of involvement, which affects cranial nerves. Patients may have facial nerve weakness or extraocular muscle involvement. Even though it is a localized disease, it can result in severe disease and higher mortality.

Neonatal tetanus starts with nonspecific symptoms, such as vomiting, poor feeding, and convulsions, which may be mistaken for sepsis or meningitis. Poor birthing conditions and umbilical cord care, or an umbilical cord cut without sterile scissors, are generally the cause of this condition. The incubation period (8 days) and onset of symptoms (1–3 days) for neonatal tetanus and the progression of disease are shorter than in non-neonatal tetanus (hours), possibly because of smaller axonal length, requiring less time for transport of the toxin. Neonatal tetanus can be easily prevented with maternal vaccination.

Several grading systems have been described; however, Ablett classification of severity is the most commonly used one (Table 22-1).

Diagnosis

The diagnosis of tetanus is by and large clinical, based principally on the classic features, history of injury, and a high index of suspicion. Tetanus should be suspected in patients in the absence of or with inadequate vaccination, even with vague muscle spasm and rigidity, and treatment should be initiated empirically while urinary toxicology studies are pending to rule out strychnine poisoning, hypocalcemic tetany, or a conversion disorder. Occasionally, dystonic reactions related to medication use post-injury can be confused with tetanus symptoms.

A positive wound culture for *C tetani* does not translate into tetanus infection automatically because not all strains include the toxin-producing plasmid; nor does a negative wound culture for *C tetani* exclude the diagnosis. The cerebrospinal fluid analysis is usually normal, and electromyographic findings are nondiagnostic as well.

Table 22-1. Ablett Classification of Severity

Grade	Clinical Features
I (mild)	Mild trismus, general spasticity, no respiratory embarrassment, no spasms, no dysphagia
II (moderate)	Moderate trismus, rigidity, short spasms, mild dysphagia, moderate respiratory involvement, respiratory rate >30 breaths/min
III (severe)	Severe trismus, generalized spasticity, prolonged spasms, respiratory rate >40 breaths/min, severe dysphagia, apneic spells, pulse >120 beats/min
IV (very severe)	Grade III plus severe autonomic disturbances involving the cardiovascular system

From Cook TM, Protheroe RT, Handel JM. Tetanus: a review of the literature. *British J Anaesthesia.* 2001;87(3):477–487:481, by permission of Oxford University Press.

Management
. . . .

Management of the tetanus requires a multipronged approach incorporating prevention of toxin production and absorption; treatment of spasms; stability of the cardiac and respiratory function; and antibiotic therapy. With the advent of mechanical ventilation and availability of benzodiazepines, survival from tetanus has improved significantly.

Treatment Objectives

Stop toxin production at the site of infection. Antibiotic therapy is administered to decrease the toxin production by eliminating growth of bacteria. Even though the role of antimicrobials is not well proven, use of metronidazole, penicillin, cephalosporins, or imipenem has been part of regular treatment of tetanus. Oral or IV metronidazole (30 mg/kg/day divided every 6 hours; maximum: 4 g/day) is effective in decreasing the number of vegetative forms of *C tetani* and the antimicrobial of choice. Therapy for 7 to 10 days is recommended. Metronidazole use is associated with better survival, a shorter hospital course, or lower death rate when compared with penicillin (Evidence Level II-1). There is some evidence that penicillin may amplify tetanospasmin activity, but it is considered an alternative to metronidazole.

Wound care. Local wound care and debridement is an essential part of tetanus care, especially if there is significant wound necrosis. Improved wound care and debridement also improves antibiotic penetration in the tissues. In patients with deep wounds, or cases following septic abortion, meticulous removal of dead tissue is essential. In rare cases, hysterectomy may be indicated on the basis of severity of the infection.

Neutralize circulating toxin. Intramuscular tetanus immune globulin (TIG) is recommended for the treatment of tetanus. Even though the optimal therapeutic dose for TIG is not well established, it is recommended that 3,000 to 6,000 U be given as a single dose. A smaller dose of 500 U is recommended by some as it appears to be as effective as higher doses and causes less discomfort. Part of the dose is recommended to be given locally around the wound, although efficacy has not been proven. It is also recommended that TIG be given before wound debridement, because manipulation of the necrotic tissue may release more toxin in the body. A meta-analysis has failed to prove the utility and efficacy of intrathecal dosing of TIG, and it is not licensed or formulated for intrathecal or IV use in the United States.

Intravenous immune globulin is not licensed to use for tetanus treatment by the US Food and Drug Administration; however, it can be given if TIG is unavailable.

Management of muscle spasms. There are no controlled trials on the treatment of muscular spasms in acute tetanus; however, it has been observed that decreasing stimulation of any kind helps in reducing spasms.

Benzodiazepines may aid in muscle relaxation and sedation and thereby reduce pain. A meta-analysis reveals that those treated with diazepam alone had a better chance of survival than those treated with combination sedatives (Evidence Level I). Midazolam has less cumulative effect and, therefore, is a preferred drug.

Anticonvulsants, such as phenobarbital or phenothiazines, can also be used for additive sedation and relaxation effects. Propofol may provide sedation, and rapid recovery is typical once the drug is stopped. Morphine is another useful sedative that does not produce cardiac effects. Heavy sedation is generally adequate to control muscle spasms, but in some cases, muscle relaxants, such as pancuronium or vecuronium, can also be used.

Among other agents that can control spasms, dantrolene and baclofen use has been reported in the literature in small case series (Evidence Level II). Baclofen appears to be an ideal drug because of its action on polysynaptic and monosynaptic tendons; however, because it does not cross the blood-brain barrier, it should be administered intrathecally.

Supportive therapy. Autonomic instability can be recognized in a well-sedated patient by erratic tachycardia and blood pressure, even in the absence of spasms or external stimulation. Alpha- and beta-adrenergic blocking agents are useful in controlling hypertensive responses; however, they fail to respond during hypotensive phase. Labetalol and propranolol have shown detrimental results, leading to heart failure and death in patients. Morphine can also be used to reduce sympathetic tone by decreasing vascular resistance along with its sedative effects.

Management of complications. Respiratory failure is a common cause of mortality; therefore, the patient should be cared for in an intensive care unit, and airway control and management is essential. Airway management can be achieved by mechanical ventilation, sedation, and muscle paralysis. Prolonged ventilation dependence may benefit from early tracheotomy for airway maintenance and minimal stimulation. Nutritional support and vigilance in diagnosis of secondary infection is necessary in such patients.

Prognosis

Prognosis in the patient with tetanus can be predicted on the basis of incubation period and onset of the disease. Shorter incubation and onset predicts high mortality. Dysautonomia, as well, correlates with high mortality. Extremes of the age and low birthweight are associated with higher mortality, possibly because of lack of or waning immunity.

Suggested Reading

American Academy of Pediatrics. Kimberlin DW, Brady MT, Jackson MA, Long SS, eds. *Red Book: 2015 Report of the Committee on Infectious Diseases.* 30th ed. Elk Grove Village, IL: American Academy of Pediatrics; 2015

Apte NM, Karnad DR. Short report: the spatula test; a simple bedside test to diagnosis tetanus. *Am J Trop Med Hyg.* 1995;53(4):386–387

Ataro P, Mushatt D, Ahsan S. Tetanus: a review. *South Med J.* 2011;104(8):613–617

Ogunrin OA. Tetanus—a review of current concepts in management. *Benin J Postgrad Med.* 2009;11(1):46–61

Okoromah CN, Lesi FE. Diazepam for treating tetanus. *Cochrane Database Syst Rev.* 2004;(1):CD003954

Rodrigo C, Samarakoon L, Fernando SD, Rajapakse S. A meta-analysis of magnesium for tetanus. *Anaesthesia.* 2012;67(12):1370–1374

Roper MH, Vandelaer JH, Gasse FL. Maternal and neonatal tetanus. *Lancet.* 2007;370(9603):1947–1959

Tiwari SP. Tetanus. In: *Manual for the Surveillance of Vaccine-Preventable Diseases.* Atlanta, GA: Centers for Disease Control and Prevention; 2008. http://www.cdc.gov/vaccines/pubs/surv-manual/index.html. Accessed March 28, 2016

CHAPTER 23

Tick-borne Rickettsial Diseases

Victoria A. Statler, MD, MSc, and Gary S. Marshall, MD

Key Points

- Tick-borne rickettsial diseases include Rocky Mountain spotted fever, spotted fever due to *Rickettsia parkeri* or *Rickettsia* species 364D, human monocytic ehrlichiosis, human granulocytic anaplasmosis, and ehrlichiosis due to *Ehrlichia ewingii*.

- Most cases occur between April and September, but cases have been reported during the winter months.

- Initiation of treatment should not be delayed pending the results of serologic tests, and treatment should not be stopped if such tests are negative during the acute illness.

- Treatment is doxycycline, regardless of age.

- Physicians should be aware of the clinical overlap with other serious infections, such as meningococcemia, as well as the possibility of coinfection with other tick-borne infections.

Overview

In the United States, the main tick-borne rickettsial diseases (TBRDs) are Rocky Mountain spotted fever (RMSF), spotted fever caused by *Rickettsia parkeri,* or *Rickettsia* species 364D, human monocytic ehrlichiosis (HME), human granulocytic anaplasmosis (HGA), and ehrlichiosis caused by *Ehrlichia ewingii.* Early recognition of TBRD and early, expectant initiation of doxycycline is crucial to decreasing morbidity and mortality. Tick-borne rickettsial diseases continue to cause severe illness and death in the United States because they are often mistaken for self-limited viral illnesses, in which case no therapy is given, or other bacterial infections, in which case antibiotics without activity against rickettsiae are given.

Causes and Differential Diagnosis

Rickettsiae are pleomorphic gram-negative coccobacilli. Hard-bodied ticks are both vectors and natural reservoirs for these organisms; small mammals and humans are incidental hosts.

Rocky Mountain Spotted Fever and Other Spotted Fever Group Rickettsioses

Rocky Mountain spotted fever is the most common rickettsial disease and the most fatal tick-borne illness in the United States. The causative agent is *Rickettsia rickettsii*. The most recognized tick vectors are the American dog tick (*Dermacentor variabilis*) in south central and eastern states and the Rocky Mountain wood tick (*Dermacentor andersoni*) in western states. Approximately 64% of all spotted fever group rickettsioses are reported from 5 states that make up what is known as the "tick belt": North Carolina, Tennessee, Missouri, Arkansas, and Oklahoma. However, TBRDs have been reported from all 48 contiguous states.

The brown dog tick (*Rhipicephalus sanguineus*) was first identified as a vector for RMSF in 2005 in Arizona, a state that previously reported very few cases. One-third of cases from Arizona are reported from October through December, indicating that the diagnosis of RMSF should be considered well into the cold weather months.

Other spotted fevers recognized in humans are caused by *R parkeri* and *Rickettsia* species 364D. *Rickettsia parkeri* is found in ticks in states along the Gulf of Mexico and southern and mid-Atlantic states bordering the Atlantic Ocean; the tick vector for *Rickettsia* species 364D is found in Northern California and along the Pacific Coast.

Ehrlichiosis

The causative agent of HME is *Ehrlichia chaffeensis,* which infects monocytes in humans and other mammals. The primary vector is the lone star tick, *Amblyomma americanum,* which is endemic in the lower Midwest and southeast and along the lower east coast states.

Human granulocytic anaplasmosis is caused by *Anaplasma phagocytophilum,* which infects granulocytes and reproduces intracellularly. The principal vectors are *Ixodes scapularis* (the black-legged or deer tick) in north central, mid-Atlantic, and New England states and *Ixodes pacificus* (the western black-legged tick) in northern California. The deer tick is also the primary vector for the causative agents of Lyme disease and babesiosis, and coinfections with these organisms have been reported (these are critical to detect because antimicrobial choice can be affected). *Ehrlichia ewingii* causes disease in immunocompromised patients.

There is substantial overlap in the clinical features of TBRDs, although some differentiating features are determined by distinct cellular tropisms of the respective organisms (Table 23-1). Early on, symptoms can be nonspecific, a factor that contributes to delayed recognition. The differential diagnosis of TBRDs is broad; important entities to consider are listed in Table 23-2. The most important thing to keep in mind is that meningococcemia and TBRDs may be indistinguishable shortly after onset of illness; therefore, clinicians should be convinced that meningococcemia is not a possibility before limiting empiric therapy to antibiotics that are active only against rickettsiae.

Table 23-1. Clinical and Laboratory Findings in Children With Rocky Mountain Spotted Fever and Human Monocytic Ehrlichiosis

	Rocky Mountain Spotted Fever, %[a] N = 92	Human Monocytic Ehrlichiosis, %[b] N = 32
Clinical		
Fever	98	100
Any rash	97	57
Nausea/vomiting	73	57
Headache	61	77
Myalgia	45	77
Abdominal pain	36	62
Diarrhea	34	36
Conjunctival injection	33	14
Altered mental status	33	36
Lymphadenopathy	29	50
Triad of fever, rash, and headache	58	54
Laboratory		
Leukopenia (<4,000/mcL)	9	57
Thrombocytopenia (<150,000/mcL)	59	93
Sodium <135 mEq/dL	52	54
AST >55 U/L	NR	92
ALT >55 U/L	NR	85

Abbreviations: ALT, alanine transaminase; AST, aspartate transaminase; NR, not reported (the percent of children with AST or ALT >55 U/L was not reported in the study, but the median AST value was 83 U/L and the median value for ALT was 55 U/L).

[a] Data from Buckingham et al.

[b] Data from Schutze et al.

Derived from Buckingham SC, Marshall GS, Schutze GE, et al; Tick-borne Infections in Children Study Group. Clinical and laboratory features, hospital course, and outcome of Rocky Mountain spotted fever in children. *J Pediatr.* 2007;150(2):180–187, and Schutze GE, Buckingham SC, Marshall GS, et al; Tick-borne Infections in Children Study (TICS) Group. Human monocytic ehrlichiosis in children. *Pediatr Infect Dis J.* 2007;26(6):475–479 (only confirmed findings included).

Table 23-2. Differential Diagnosis of Tick-borne Rickettsial Diseases in Children

Disease	Differentiating Features and Comments
Kawasaki disease	Conjunctivitis, changes in the oral mucosa, and irritability usually prominent. Generalized, polymorphous exanthem; can be accentuated in groin. ESR usually markedly elevated. *Treatment with immune globulin may be warranted.*
Meningococcal disease	Fever and rash occur with abrupt onset. Early rash may not have petechial component. May have leukocytosis or leukopenia, depending on severity of illness. *Lumbar puncture and early empiric treatment with ceftriaxone may be warranted.*
Enteroviral infection	Nonspecific febrile illness. Rash not always present. Children may be well appearing.
Staphylococcal toxin–mediated disease	Can have bilateral conjunctivitis and erythema of mucus membranes. Erythroderma (as opposed to rash). May have a minor source of infection, such as a boil or infected wound, or may be colonized, as occurs with tampon use. *Treatment with vancomycin, clindamycin, or both may be warranted.*
Scarlet fever	Sore throat usually prominent. Erythematous tonsils. Sandpaper-like rash. Children can be well appearing. *Treatment with a penicillin may be warranted.*
Stevens-Johnson syndrome	Significant involvement of mucus membranes. Medication or viral infection may be inciting factors.
Exanthema subitum (due to *human herpesvirus 6* infection)	Fever occurs and resolves before onset of rash. More common in children <2 y of age.
Erythema infectiosum (also called fifth disease; due to parvovirus)	Low-grade fever and mild constitutional symptoms. Lacy-appearing rash on trunk. Slapped-cheek appearance.
Epstein-Barr virus	Sore throat and lymphadenopathy usually prominent. May not have rash, but rash may be prompted by antibiotic use.

Abbreviation: ESR, erythrocyte sedimentation rate.

Clinical Features

Tick-borne rickettsial diseases regularly manifest as febrile illnesses of sudden onset. Associated symptoms may include headache, chills, myalgias, and malaise, and children may have nausea, anorexia, and abdominal pain. Physical examination may show conjunctival injection or periorbital edema; rash and hepatosplenomegaly are not uncommon. Findings suggesting meningoencephalitis, including altered mental status, focal neurologic deficits, cranial or peripheral nerve palsies, and sudden transient deafness, may be present.

A complete blood cell count and comprehensive metabolic panel can be useful when TBRDs are in the differential diagnosis (Figure 23-1). The white

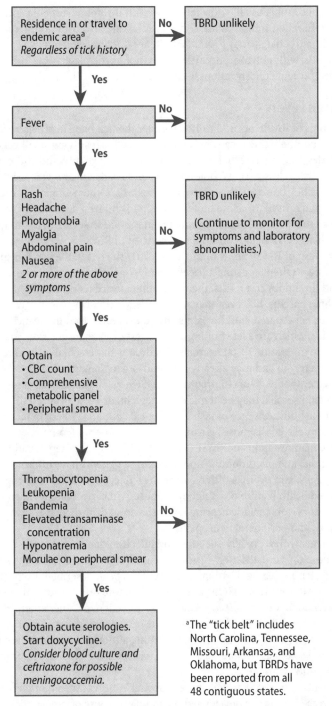

Figure 23-1. Suspecting and expectantly treating tick-borne rickettsial diseases.

Abbreviations: CBC, complete blood cell count; TBRD, tick-borne rickettsial disease.

blood cell count is usually normal or low, with thrombocytopenia and possibly anemia. Elevated transaminase concentrations are also common. Headache or mental status change may prompt a lumbar puncture, which may reveal aseptic meningitis, with polymorphonuclear or lymphocytic pleocytosis, moderately elevated protein concentrations, and negative bacterial cultures.

Spotted Fevers

Symptoms of RMSF occur 2 to 12 days after the tick bite. *Rickettsia rickettsii* infects endothelial cells, causing systemic vasculitis involving small vessels and capillaries, leading to rash, increased vascular permeability, and end-organ damage. The "classic triads" of fever, rash, and headache or fever, rash, and history of tick bite are not sensitive for diagnosis. Other symptoms such as nausea and refusal to eat are quite common in children. Likewise, vomiting and diarrhea may be seen, and abdominal pain may be so severe that it mimics appendicitis. Calf pain is anecdotally reported in RMSF.

The rash of RMSF appears 2 to 4 days after the onset of fever. It begins as blanching erythematous macules or maculopapules, classically appearing first around the ankles and wrists, then spreading inward (centripetally) to involve the trunk; parents, however, may not be able to articulate this progression. The face is usually spared, but the palms and soles are involved in most children. Petechiae, which are a late finding and suggest disease progression, may evolve into ecchymoses and distal necrosis. Children with petechial rashes are usually more severely ill and may already have end-organ damage.

Greater than 90% of children with RMSF develop some kind of rash, although in some it may be atypical, evanescent, or even localized to just one area of the body. Absence of rash does not rule out RMSF and, in fact, as a risk factor for delayed diagnosis, is associated with poorer outcome.

Late manifestations of RMSF include encephalopathy, hepatopathy, carditis, arrhythmia, and pneumonitis. About a third of patients have infiltrates on chest radiographs, and nearly a fifth have seizures. Encephalopathy can progress to coma and death if antibiotic therapy is not started early. Long-term complications in survivors include hearing loss, behavioral disturbance, learning disability, and peripheral neuropathy.

Patients with *R parkeri* infection and infection due to *Rickettsia* species 364D develop a crusted, non-pruritic, minimally tender eschar at the site of the tick bite; tender regional lymphadenopathy has been described. Eschars are not seen in RMSF, HME, or HGA and should therefore prompt consideration of *R parkeri* infection, *Rickettsia* species 364D infection, or other emerging spotted fever group rickettsioses. Some patients develop a maculopapular or vesiculopapular exanthem concentrated on the trunk, although involvement of the palms and soles has been reported. Other symptoms include fever, headache, myalgia, and arthralgia.

Patients with RMSF usually have a normal WBC count, although band forms are increased. They can develop hyponatremia (because of capillary leak) and hepatopathy, with elevated transaminase concentrations, hyperbilirubinemia, and prolonged prothrombin time. Anemia, thrombocytopenia, and elevated creatine kinase concentrations are also seen. Laboratory values in *R parkeri* infection include mild elevation of transaminases, thrombocytopenia, and leukopenia.

Ehrlichiosis

The clinical spectrum of ehrlichiosis ranges from subclinical or mild illness to life-threatening and fulminant disease. Common symptoms are shown in Table 23-1. Often, HME and RMSF are difficult to distinguish clinically; in fact, despite references to HME as "spotless" RMSF, up to 67% of children develop a rash. This occurs about 1 week after onset of fever and can be highly variable in appearance, usually involving the trunk but sparing the palms and soles. Less common symptoms include arthralgia, cough, conjunctivitis, pharyngitis, lymphadenopathy, hepatosplenomegaly, nausea, vomiting, diarrhea, abdominal pain, and jaundice. Peripheral and pulmonary edema are late findings. Severe manifestations of ehrlichiosis include acute respiratory distress syndrome, encephalopathy, meningitis, disseminated intravascular coagulation, spontaneous hemorrhage, and renal failure.

Descriptions of HGA in children are limited. In adults, HGA may be indistinguishable from HME. Rigors and chills can be prominent. Pharyngitis has been reported. Less than 10% of patients with HGA have a rash.

Leukopenia is more common in ehrlichiosis than in RMSF, and transaminase concentrations are more often elevated (>80% of patients). In fact, the combination of leukopenia and elevated transaminase concentrations in a febrile patient in the proper epidemiologic setting is highly suggestive of ehrlichiosis. Other laboratory abnormalities include elevated C-reactive protein concentrations or erythrocyte sedimentation rate and elevated lactate dehydrogenase concentrations. Wright stain of a peripheral blood smear obtained in the first week of illness may demonstrate morulae (clusters of bacteria) in the cytoplasm of monocytes (up to 20% of patients with HME) or neutrophils (20%–80% of patients with HGA). Morulae have many different shapes and sizes, and success in finding them depends directly on the experience of the microscopist. Absence of morulae on the peripheral blood smear does not exclude ehrlichiosis.

Evaluation
· · · · · · · · · ·

Up to 50% of patients do not give a history of tick bite—the site might have been obscure and the bite painless, particularly if the tick was small. In addition, because early symptoms are nonspecific and mimic those of common viral illnesses, clinicians must have a very high index of suspicion. Finally, no reliable tests can make a definitive diagnosis early on; therefore, treatment must be started to avoid a bad outcome.

Children with TBRD tend to see clinicians early in the course of illness. In fact, having a health care visit before hospital admission is correlated with *delayed* initiation of antirickettsial therapy, probably because of false reassurance that the illness is viral in nature. Figure 23-1 provides an algorithmic approach to recognition of TRBD.

Practically speaking, confirmation of rickettsial infection necessarily awaits convalescent serologic tests; acute-phase serologies are often negative (even specific IgM tests). Therefore, in most cases empiric treatment must be started before the diagnosis is definitively established, and treatment should not be stopped if acute-phase serologies are negative. Paired acute and convalescent (4 weeks after onset of symptoms) serologies, however, are worth performing—seroconversion is informative from epidemiology and public health standpoints and may provide some closure for the family. Both indirect immunofluorescence assays and enzyme-linked immunoassays are readily available to clinicians.

Nucleic acid detection by polymerase chain reaction (PCR) is available from the Centers for Disease Control and Prevention and state health and commercial centers. Polymerase chain reaction of whole blood is more useful to detect ehrlichia because the organisms replicate in circulating white blood cells. Polymerase chain reaction of whole blood for rickettsiae is less useful because these organisms infect endothelial cells.

Management

Doxycycline is the treatment of choice for all TBRDs in patients of any age. The dose is 2 mg/kg given twice daily (the intravenous and oral doses are equivalent), with a maximum of 100 mg/dose. Treatment is given for 7 to 14 days, or at least for 3 days after the patient becomes afebrile. Persistence of fever for more than 48 hours after initiation of doxycycline should prompt consideration of an alternative diagnosis.

Concern about staining of the permanent teeth by doxycycline used in young children who are being treated for TBRD is unwarranted. Chloramphenicol, which is no longer available in the United States, has been used for treatment of RMSF but has several potential adverse effects, including aplastic anemia. Because evidence for efficacy of chloramphenicol in ehrlichiosis is conflicting, doxycycline remains the best antimicrobial to treat both RMSF and ehrlichiosis.

Special consideration is given to treatment of HGA because of the possibility of coinfection with *Borrelia burgdorferi*, the causative agent of Lyme disease. Doxycycline is adequate therapy for Lyme disease but the treatment course is longer than for TBRD. Therefore, doxycycline should be given for 10 days in a patient with suspected HGA. Alternatively, amoxicillin or cefuroxime may be initiated after 5 to 7 days of doxycycline to complete a 14-day course of antibiotics. In regions where HGA is prevalent, clinicians must also be aware of possible coinfection with *Babesia microti,* which is not responsive to doxycycline.

Prevention and Reporting of Tick-borne Rickettsial Diseases

Tick-borne rickettsial diseases cannot be acquired without tick attachment. Insecticide skin sprays or lotions and treatment of clothing with tick or insect repellants like DEET aid in reducing the risk of tick attachment after exposure. Performing daily tick inspections of both humans and pets and promptly removing any attached ticks after outdoor activity is also important. Attached ticks should be removed by grasping the mouthparts close to the skin with forceps and gently pulling away from the skin with steady pressure.

All TBRDs are reportable in the United States. Clinicians who identify a potential case should notify the local or state health department, which will help in obtaining confirmatory testing.

Suggested Reading
· · · · · · · · · · · · · · · · · ·

American Academy of Pediatrics. *Ehrlichia* and *Anaplasma* infections (human ehrlichiosis and anaplasmosis). In: Kimberlin DW, Brady MT, Jackson MA, Long SS, eds. *Red Book: 2015 Report of the Committee on Infectious Diseases*. 30th ed. Elk Grove Village, IL, American Academy of Pediatrics; 2015:329–332

American Academy of Pediatrics. Rocky Mountain spotted fever. In: Kimberlin DW, Brady MT, Jackson MA, Long SS, eds. *Red Book: 2015 Report of the Committee on Infectious Diseases*. 30th ed. Elk Grove Village, IL, American Academy of Pediatrics; 2015:682–684

Buckingham SC, Marshall GS, Schutze GE, et al; Tick-borne Infections in Children Study Group. Clinical and laboratory features, hospital course, and outcome of Rocky Mountain spotted fever in children. *J Pediatr.* 2007;150(2):180–187

Biggs HM, Behravesh CB , Bradley KK et al. Diagnosis and management of tickborne rickettsial diseases: Rocky Mountain spotted fever, and other spotted fever group rickettsioses, ehrlichioses, and anaplasmosis—United States: a practical guide for healthcare and and public health professionals. *MMWR Recomm Rep.* 2016;65(RR-2):1–44

Schutze GE, Buckingham SC, Marshall GS, et al; Tick-borne Infectious in Children Study (TICS) Group. Human monocytic ehrlichiosis in children. *Pediatr Infect Dis J.* 2007;26(6):475–479

Tuberculosis and Nontuberculous Mycobacterial Infections

Andrea T. Cruz, MD, MPH, and Jeffrey R. Starke, MD

Key Points

- Tuberculosis (TB) remains one of the most prevalent infectious diseases in terms of morbidity and mortality; management varies by TB classification.

- The most common sites of TB disease are the lungs and peripheral lymph nodes, and the most dreaded site of disease is the central nervous system.

- The most common manifestation of nontuberculous mycobacteria (NTM) in an otherwise healthy child is lymphadenitis. *Mycobacterium avium* complex is the most common species. Surgical therapy is superior to medical therapy, and children generally recover without sequelae.

- Nontuberculous mycobacterial pulmonary disease is usually seen in patients with existing lung damage (eg, cystic fibrosis) or immunocompromised children. *Mycobacterium avium* complex and *Mycobacterium abscessus* are the most common species. Guidelines exist to facilitate the diagnosis of NTM pulmonary disease; even optimal medical therapy may not result in organism eradication, and long-term prognosis may be poor.

- Disseminated NTM disease is not seen in immunocompetent children. The most common species is *Mycobacterium avium* complex in children lacking central venous catheters; for the subgroup with central venous catheters, removal of the catheter is a necessary adjunct to parenteral therapy. Prognosis for children with disseminated NTM disease is poor, and outcome is tied to immune system recovery.

Tuberculosis

Overview

Tuberculosis (TB) remains among the 3 most prevalent infectious diseases (along with HIV and malaria) in terms of global morbidity and mortality.

Causes and Differential Diagnosis

Mycobacterium tuberculosis complex is a group of slow-growing, acid-fast bacilli (AFB) and includes *M tuberculosis, Mycobacterium bovis* (1%–2% of cases and transmitted by unpasteurized milk), and *Mycobacterium africanum* (rarely seen in the United States).

The relatively nonspecific signs and symptoms of childhood TB mean the clinician needs to have a high index of suspicion for TB and also that the differential diagnosis possibilities are broad. The differential diagnosis of pulmonary TB includes other causes of pulmonary parenchymal infiltrates (eg, community-acquired pneumonia, viral pneumonitis), other causes of intrathoracic lymphadenopathy (eg, fungal infections, mediastinal tumors), and other causes of pleural effusions (eg, complicated pneumonia, autoimmune processes, malignancy). The differential diagnosis of TB lymphadenopathy includes nontuberculous mycobacterial (NTM) infections, malignancy, cat-scratch disease (though TB nodes tend to be non-tender), and other causes of peripheral lymphadenopathy. The differential diagnosis of TB meningitis is somewhat limited, because the cerebrospinal fluid parameters and neuroimaging are characteristic. Other considerations include causes of subacute meningitis (ie, fungal, parasitic). However, because few cases of TB meningitis are seen annually in US children, the clinician's index of suspicion may be low and delays in diagnosis are quite common.

Clinical Manifestations

Children with TB exposure and infection are asymptomatic. The clinical manifestations of TB disease range from subtle to fulminant. In many countries in which active surveillance for TB is performed (eg, contact investigations to identify persons exposed to patients newly diagnosed as having TB disease), many children diagnosed as having disease have mild or no symptoms, but have radiographic findings defining TB disease. In contrast, most children with pulmonary TB in developing nations present only after they have been ill for weeks or even months.

The most common sites of TB disease are the lungs and peripheral lymph nodes, and the most dreaded site of disease is the central nervous system. Children with pulmonary TB may present with fever, failure to thrive, malaise, and cough. Examination often shows a lack of respiratory signs, and chest auscultation may be normal even in children with extensive disease. Children with TB lymphadenopathy have indolent, slowly growing non-tender cervical nodes, with or without overlying skin discoloration (please see Nontuberculous Mycobacterial Infections section). The symptoms of TB meningitis vary over the disease course. Early in the course, fever and constitutional symptoms predominate. As the child becomes more ill, signs of increased intracranial pressure, altered mental status, irritability, and cranial nerve palsies (especially cranial nerve VI) predominate.

Tuberculosis disease in children living with HIV is characterized by more rapid disease progression, increased risk of disease severity, and increased risk of extrapulmonary TB when compared with HIV-seronegative children. Additionally, diagnosis may be delayed because other opportunistic infections can mimic the clinical and radiographic findings of TB.

Evaluation

The American Academy of Pediatrics recommends that all children be screened for TB infection by using a questionnaire asking about risk factors. If a child's family answers yes to any of the screening questions, a tuberculin test should be placed or an interferon-γ release assay (IGRA) performed.

Children should be screened for TB risk factors at the annual well-child visit, because this may be their only encounter with their clinician. Box 24-1 shows how many millimeters of induration in response to a tuberculin skin test are considered positive and likely indicating TB infection, depending on a patient's risk factors (eg, epidemiologic and medical comorbidities). Measurement should occur between 48 and 72 hours after tuberculin test placement; any localized reaction within the first day should be discounted, because tuberculin skin tests measure delayed-type hypersensitivity. However, if induration or a blister occur later than 3 days after placement, the test result should be remeasured and this taken as the test result. The area of *erythema* should not be measured, only the indurated (or blistered) area. It is important to document the number of millimeters, as opposed to simply documenting "positive" or "negative," because the same measurement can be considered positive or negative on the basis of a child's risk factors and clinical presentation. The sliding scale for tuberculin skin test positivity reflects the desire to maximize tuberculin skin test sensitivity for patients at highest risk for either

Box 24-1. Tuberculin Skin Test Interpretation

≥5 mm induration is considered positive for
- Persons who had contact with known or suspected patients with contagious tuberculosis
- Persons with abnormal chest radiographic findings
- HIV-infected and other immunosuppressed patients

≥10 mm induration is considered positive for
- Babies and children <4 y
- Children in contact with adults at high risk
  - o Foreign-born persons from high-prevalence countries, or those who travel to high-prevalence countries
  - o Residents from nursing homes, and those who are imprisoned, institutionalized, or homeless
  - o Persons who inject drugs
  - o Persons with other medical risk factors
  - o Clinicians

≥15 mm induration is considered positive for persons with
- No risk factors

progression to disease or in patients who are less likely to mount an effective immunologic response. Even at 15 mm, most positive tuberculin skin test results will be false-positive in children who truly have no risk factors.

For immunocompetent children older than 4 years, an IGRA should be done in lieu of the tuberculin skin test. Interferon-γ release assays are blood tests evaluating the immune response to proteins more specific to *M tuberculosis* than proteins contained in the tuberculin skin test. One major advantage of IGRAs over the tuberculin skin test is enhanced specificity due to lack of cross-reaction between IGRAs and the BCG vaccine and between most NTM species; plus, it avoids the need for a repeat visit, which is necessary for the reading of a tuberculin test.

Figure 24-1 shows an algorithm for the incorporation of IGRAs into clinical practice. For high-risk patients, any test (tuberculin or IGRA) being positive counts and should prompt therapy.

Posteroanterior and lateral chest radiographs should be performed in all children suspected of having TB exposure, infection, or disease. For children in the first 2 categories, it is important to rule out disease prior to starting therapy. Inadvertently treating children with disease with monotherapy can rapidly select out for drug resistance. For children with disease, it is important to obtain a baseline radiograph, which can be followed at specified intervals or immediately if the child were to decompensate while on therapy. The lateral chest radiograph is particularly helpful to diagnose intrathoracic lymphadenopathy in the young child, in which a large thymus may obstruct visualization of the anterior mediastinum on the posteroanterior radiograph.

The most common radiographic findings in a child with intrathoracic TB include hilar or mediastinal lymphadenopathy, lobar infiltrates, atelectasis (caused by extrinsic bronchial compression by a lymph node resulting in distal obstruction), miliary disease, and pleural effusion. Of note, many young children with extrapulmonary disease (especially TB meningitis) have abnormal radiographic findings. Consequently, chest radiographs should be obtained even in children with suspected extrapulmonary disease.

Cavitary pulmonary lesions are uncommon before adolescence. While most infants and young children with pulmonary TB are not contagious, cavitary lesions in children of any age should result in immediate implementation of infection control precautions, including placement into a negative-pressure room, use of N95 respirators for clinicians, and N95 respirators or powered air-purifying respiratory and simple face masks for patients and families.

If a child has chest radiographic findings compatible with pulmonary TB, attempts should be made to obtain respiratory specimens for AFB stain and culture. For older patients, having children expectorate sputum may be feasible. In younger children, use of gastric aspiration or sputum induction (usually daily for 3 mornings) may be necessary. For well-appearing children beyond infancy who were identified through active surveillance (the person who has contagious TB is known) and have abnormal radiographic findings, respiratory specimens are often not obtained. Unfortunately, culture results are positive

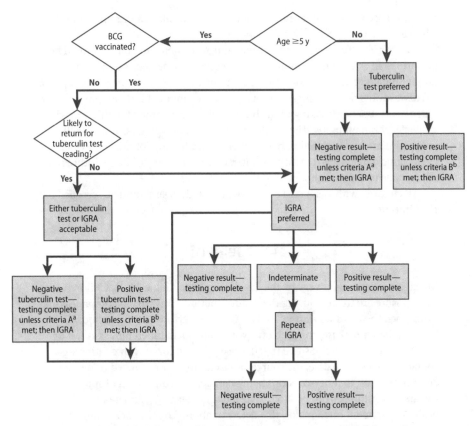

Figure 24-1. Algorithm for use of interferon-γ release assays in children who have risk factors from the screening questionnaire.

Abbreviation: IGRA, interferon-γ release assay.

ª Criteria A (one or both of the following criteria):

1. High clinical suspicion for tuberculosis
2. High risk for infection, progression, or poor outcome

ᵇ Criteria B (one or a combination of the following criteria):

1. Additional evidence needed to ensure adherence
2. Child healthy and at low risk
3. Nontuberculous mycobacteria suspected

from only 20% to 40% of children with TB; the diagnosis is often not microbiologically confirmed but instead based on the triad of epidemiologic risk factors for TB (especially recent exposure to a known case), immunologic evidence of TB infection (tuberculin skin test or IGRA), and compatible radiographic, clinical, or pathologic findings.

Evaluation of children with TB lymphadenopathy should include biopsy of the affected node, and material should be sent for AFB stain and culture, routine bacterial cultures, and histopathology. Ideally, the specimen should be obtained via fine-needle aspiration and not by incision and drainage of the node, because incision and drainage of nodes can result in a draining sinus tract (the same is true for NTM lymphadenopathy).

Lumbar puncture for routine studies and AFB stain and culture should be performed in any child in whom TB meningitis is suspected. Additionally, lumbar puncture should be considered for any infant about to begin therapy for TB disease outside the central nervous system. Computed tomography (CT) or magnetic resonance imaging of the brain should be obtained for children with suspected TB meningitis. The most common neuroimaging findings in TB meningitis are hydrocephalus, basilar meningitis, tuberculomas, and evidence of ischemic damage, particularly at watershed areas. Many of these findings are attributable to the vasculitis caused by *M tuberculosis*.

All children with suspected or confirmed TB disease should be screened for HIV infection.

Management

Management strategies vary by the TB classification (Table 24-1). Children with TB exposure are treated during the window period. This period comprises time from when the child was last in contact with the person with suspected TB (termed the *source case*) to when one would anticipate tuberculin skin test or IGRA result becoming positive (8–10 weeks). For children with continuing contact with a source case, the source case's cultures are evaluated frequently to determine when that person stops being contagious; conversion of sputum AFB smears and cultures from positive to negative are used to estimate this. The health department often makes this determination. After history, examination, and radiograph rule out disease, children younger than 5 years are started on monotherapy, usually isoniazid (INH), for prevention. If the second tuberculin skin test is less than 5 mm or the IGRA result is negative, the medication can be stopped. If the second tuberculin skin test is 5 mm or greater or the IGRA result is positive, the child is considered to have infection, and treatment is continued for a total of 9 months if INH is used (the 2 preceding months count toward therapy duration).

Children with latent TB infection should be treated to decrease the lifetime risk of progression to TB disease. The most data are available for 9 months of INH; this regimen, while highly effective, has the drawback of low adherence because of the duration of therapy. An alternative regimen is 4 to 6 months of rifampin (RIF). Four months of RIF is recommended for children exposed to persons whose *M tuberculosis* isolate is resistant to INH alone. This regimen may not be appropriate for children receiving antiepileptics, antiretrovirals, or other medications whose levels may be altered by RIF. A newer regimen of INH and rifapentine (a long-acting RIF derivative) given weekly for 12 doses was recently described. While there are not currently adequate data to support the use of this regimen in preadolescent children, the regimen is effective for children 12 years and older. Children being treated with either INH or RIF

Table 24-1. A Management Approach for Children With Tuberculosis Exposure, Infection, or Disease

Classification	Initial Treatment[a]	Duration of Therapy	Notes
Exposure, >4 y and immunocompetent	None	NA	Repeat tuberculin test or IGRA 2–3 mo after contact is broken.[b] If 2nd tuberculin test is ≥5 mm or the IGRA is positive, see Infection row.
Exposure, ≤4 y	1st-line: INH 2nd-line: RIF	2–3 mo[b] (Medication should be given via DOPT administered by the health department, if possible.)	Repeat tuberculin test 2–3 mo after contact is broken.[c] If 2nd tuberculin test is <5 mm, may stop medication. If 2nd tuberculin test is ≥5 mm, see Infection row.
Infection	INH	9 mo	Daily therapy via families or twice-weekly therapy via DOPT. 6 mo of INH is the international recommendation.
	RIF	4–6 mo[d]	Daily therapy via families or twice-weekly therapy via DOPT.
	INH + RIF	3 mo	Has been widely used in the United Kingdom with good results as daily therapy.
	INH + rifapentine	12 doses, administered once weekly via DOPT	For children ≥12 y.
Disease	Multidrug therapy, usually INH, RIF, PZA, EMB	6 mo for most pulmonary and extrapulmonary disease 9–12 mo for meningitis, disseminated disease, or cavitary lesions	Medications should be administered only via DOT to prevent nonadherence and selection of resistant bacteria. Adjunctive use of corticosteroids recommended in select circumstances (eg, meningitis, pericarditis). Expert consultation is recommended.

Abbreviations: DOPT, directly observed preventive therapy; DOT, directly observed therapy; EMB, ethambutol; IGRA, interferon-γ release assay; INH, isoniazid; NA, not applicable; PZA, pyrazinamide; RIF, rifampin.

[a] Number of medications and duration of therapy for children with confirmed or presumed drug-susceptible tuberculosis; the treatment of children with multidrug-resistant or extensively drug-resistant tuberculosis is beyond the scope of this chapter.

[b] Exposed infants are a very high-risk group, and tuberculin skin tests may be less reliable in this population. As such, tuberculin skin test results of siblings and other family members should be considered, and often children are kept on prophylaxis until they approach 6 mo and the tuberculin skin test becomes somewhat more reliable.

[c] Contact may be broken physically (eg, child has not seen the contagious adult since a certain date) or microbiologically (eg, on the basis of sputum smears and cultures, the person is deemed to no longer be contagious).

[d] Four months of rifampin is an accepted regimen for adults.

alone usually are seen 1 month after starting therapy and approximately every 2 months thereafter. Visits focus on adherence, barriers to medication administration, and tolerability; importance of latent TB infection therapy is stressed at each visit.

Isoniazid causes increased excretion in the urine of vitamin B_6 (pyridoxine). While clinical manifestations of this are rare in healthy children taking a normal American diet, supplementation should be given to babies (<1 year) who are exclusively breastfeeding, HIV-infected persons, adolescents, pregnant persons, children with diets lacking in milk or meat, and any child with nutritional deficiencies or risk of malabsorption. Pyridoxine will decrease the risk of peripheral neuropathy, but does not decrease the risk of hepatotoxicity. Most pediatric multivitamin formulations have adequate amounts (50–100 mg/day) of pyridoxine, and use of multivitamins in lieu of isolated vitamin B_6 supplementation may cost families less.

Children tolerate TB medications extremely well. Hepatotoxicity is rare, and routine measurement of serum liver enzyme levels is unnecessary unless the child has additional risk factors for liver abnormalities. Abdominal pain in the left upper quadrant occurring minutes after taking INH on an empty stomach is common and typically resolves within 60 minutes; it can be avoided by taking food with the medication. Right upper quadrant abdominal pain, generalized abdominal pain, icterus, or isolated vomiting may be signs of hepatotoxicity, and evaluation should be considered. Use of the INH suspension, which is sorbitol based, can result in an osmotic diarrhea or gastritis. For children receiving RIF, notifying the family of the orange urine discoloration (which can be mistaken for blood) will prevent frantic calls or emergency department visits. Adolescent girls receiving RIF need to be cautioned that it can render oral contraceptives ineffective and that alternative birth control strategies should be used.

Children with TB disease receive multidrug therapy, and this therapy should be administered via the health department as directly observed therapy. First-line therapy includes INH, RIF, pyrazinamide, and ethambutol (EMB). Isoniazid and RIF are the bactericidal agents, and children receive these drugs throughout therapy. Pyrazinamide is a drug used, in part, to shorten therapy to 6 months for intrathoracic TB. Ethambutol provides additional coverage in the event that a child has drug-resistant TB. Because EMB does not cross the blood-brain barrier efficiently, other drugs (ethionamide, aminoglycosides) are often substituted for EMB when children have TB meningitis. Drug resistance and multidrug resistance can be seen; therefore, local resistance rates should be evaluated until susceptibilities are available.

Children receiving TB medications often present to their primary care physicians with non–TB-related health issues that may arise while the child is taking TB medications. A brief overview of adverse effects and potential for drug interactions for anti-TB medications is shown in Table 24-2.

If there is concern for serious adverse effects (eg, jaundice or symptoms of hepatic dysfunction), children should immediately stop the medications and undergo a medical evaluation. The rates of hepatotoxicity are much lower in

Table 24-2. Potential Adverse Effects and Drug Interactions for Antituberculosis Medications

Medication	Adverse Effects	Drug Interactions	Notes
INH	Hepatotoxicity; peripheral neuropathy	Rare	Pyridoxine (a form of vitamin B_6) prevents peripheral neuropathy, but not hepatotoxicity. INH suspension causes osmotic diarrhea; convert to pills, which can be crushed and mixed with food, when infants are taking any pureed food.
RIF	Hepatotoxicity; idiosyncratic bone marrow suppression	Common	Important to warn parents and patients about orange discoloration to urine and (less commonly) other secretions.
PZA	Hepatotoxicity; increased serum uric acid; rash	Rare	While increased serum uric acid is seen in most children receiving PZA, joint concerns are rare.
EMB	Optic neuritis and red-green color discrimination difficulties	Rare	As children metabolize the drug more rapidly than adults, toxicity is very rare. EMB can be used even in the preverbal child in whom visual screening may be difficult.

Abbreviations: EMB, ethambutol; INH, isoniazid; PZA, pyrazinamide; RIF, rifampin.

children than adults, and routine monitoring of hepatic transaminase concentrations in the otherwise healthy child not receiving other hepatically metabolized medications is unnecessary. Clinicians should have a low threshold for measuring transaminase concentrations in a child receiving anti-TB medications who reports abdominal pain or vomiting. Timeliness and safety in the rare instance of true drug toxicity are facilitated when children are receiving medication via directly observed therapy or directly observed preventive therapy.

Long-term Monitoring and Implications

Most children with a diagnosis of TB disease do very well; the exception is children with TB meningitis. Children with intrathoracic TB often have improved but still abnormal radiographs at the end of therapy. With few exceptions, this does not affect their pulmonary function or change their duration of therapy, and their radiographs continue to improve in the first 1 to 2 years after therapy is stopped. The exception regarding duration of therapy would be the child who continues to have cavitary or extensive pulmonary parenchymal infiltrates after 6 months of therapy; extension of therapy to 9 months in these cases has been associated with lower relapse rates in adults.

One strategy for the timing of chest radiographs in children with intrathoracic TB disease is to obtain imaging before starting therapy, after 2 months (when 2 anti-TB medications are generally stopped, to be sure that there is not substantial radiographic worsening), and at the end of therapy, to establish a new radiographic baseline for the child. If a child's 2-month chest radiographic findings are normal, there is no need to repeat a chest radiograph at the end of therapy unless the child changes clinically. If the end-of-therapy chest radiographic findings remain abnormal, it would be reasonable to see the child again in 6 to 12 months to repeat the radiograph to see if its findings have normalized. If they have, the child needs no further evaluation and should be instructed that if she were to have a chest radiograph in the future showing anomalies, that would be a change from her post-TB treatment imaging.

Sequelae following TB disease are common in children with TB meningitis. Most of these children have motor or cognitive dysfunction. The extent of this dysfunction may not be evident until the child reaches school. All children with TB meningitis should have audiologic evaluation prior to hospital discharge and should be referred for additional developmental resources, such as Early Childhood Intervention.

Suggested Reading

American Thoracic Society, Centers for Disease Control and Prevention, Infectious Diseases Society of America. Targeted tuberculin testing and treatment of latent tuberculosis infection. *Am J Resp Crit Care Med.* 2000;161(4 Pt 2):S221–S247

American Thoracic Society, Centers for Disease Control and Prevention, Infectious Diseases Society of America. Treatment of tuberculosis. *MMWR Recomm Rep.* 2003;52(RR-11):1–77

Centers for Disease Control and Prevention. Trends in tuberculosis—United States, 2011. *MMWR Morb Mortal Wkly Rep.* 2012;61(11):181–185

Cruz AT, Starke JR. Pediatric tuberculosis. *Pediatr Rev.* 2010;31(1):13–25

Froehlich H, Ackerson LM, Morozumi PA; Pediatric Tuberculosis Study Group of Kaiser Permanente, Northern California. Targeted testing of children for tuberculosis: validation of a risk assessment questionnaire. *Pediatrics.* 2001;107(4):e54

Gie R. *Diagnostic Atlas of Intrathoracic Tuberculosis in Children: A Guide for Low-Income Countries.* International Union Against Tuberculosis and Lung Disease; 2003

Machingaze S, Wiysonge CS, Gonzalez-Angulo Y, et al. The utility of an interferon gamma release assay for diagnosis of latent tuberculosis infection and disease in children: a systematic review and meta-analysis. *Pediatr Infect Dis J.* 2011;30(8):694–700

Mazurek GH, Jereb J, Vernon A, LoBue P, Goldberg S, Castro K; IGRA Expert Committee, Centers for Disease Control and Prevention. Updated guidelines for using interferon gamma release assays to detect *Mycobacterium tuberculosis* infection—United States, 2010. *MMWR Recomm Rep.* 2010;59(RR-5):1–25

Nontuberculous Mycobacterial Infections
Overview

Nontuberculous mycobacterial organisms are mycobacterial species other than *M tuberculosis* complex and *Mycobacterium leprae*. Nontuberculous mycobacteria lack person-to-person transmission, but are environmentally ubiquitous. They can cause cutaneous disease at the site of skin trauma and cervical lymphadenopathy in otherwise healthy children. Nontuberculous mycobacterial species cause more invasive disease (ie, pulmonary, skeletal, bacteremia) in certain immunocompromised children. The rapidly growing species (including *Mycobacterium fortuitum, Mycobacterium abscessus,* and *Mycobacterium chelonae*) may grow within a week. Rapid growth may be the first laboratory indication that an acid-fast-positive organism is not *M tuberculosis*. Most other NTM species, including one of the most commonly isolated NTM species, *Mycobacterium avium* complex (MAC), take several weeks before growth is evident.

Just as children with HIV are more commonly affected by TB, certain comorbidities predispose to NTM disease. Interferon and interleukin receptor mutations increase risk for disseminated disease. Cystic fibrosis predisposes children to NTM pulmonary disease. Untreated, advanced HIV infection predisposes to disseminated NTM (primarily MAC) disease.

Causes and Differential Diagnosis

Mycobacterium fortuitum, M chelonae, and *M abscessus* represent species called "rapid growers," which grow sufficiently for diagnosis after just 3 to 7 days, in contrast to typical TB and other species of NTM, which take several weeks to grow.

The differential diagnosis of NTM lymphadenitis includes other bacterial causes of lymphadenitis (eg, streptococci, staphylococci, bartonellosis), viral infections (eg, Epstein-Barr virus, cytomegalovirus), *M tuberculosis,* and malignancy. One study compared children with TB and NTM lymphadenopathy, finding that children with NTM were younger (often preschool aged), born in countries with low TB prevalence, and had normal chest radiographic findings.

Pulmonary NTM occurs in already-diseased lungs. Consequently, the differential diagnosis is broad and includes *Stenotrophomonas* and *Pseudomonas aeruginosa* in cystic fibrosis patients. Nodular or reticulonodular lung disease may be confused with fungal pneumonitis or *Pneumocystis jiroveci*. For children with cystic fibrosis, a tree-in-bud or cavitary appearance on CT is suggestive of NTM infection. Plain radiographs may demonstrate worsening bronchiectasis, which can be caused by both progression of cystic fibrosis and other lung pathogens.

Cutaneous NTM disease can have a similar appearance to nocardiosis and sporotrichosis. In the immunocompromised patient, the disseminated nodular skin lesions seen with NTM can mimic cutaneous findings for disseminated cryptococcal disease, histoplasmosis, or aspergillosis. Disseminated NTM infection also mimics the symptomatology and radiographic manifestations of disseminated fungal disease.

Clinical Manifestations

The 2 most commonly encountered NTM scenarios in US children are the otherwise healthy preschool-aged child with NTM lymphadenitis and the cystic fibrosis patient with NTM pulmonary disease.

Nontuberculous mycobacterial lymphadenitis is the most common clinical manifestation of pediatric NTM disease. Children have slowly enlarging non-tender cervical nodes; lymphadenopathy is frequently unilateral. The nodes may become adherent to underlying soft tissues, the overlying skin, or both, which results in examination findings of fixed or apparently matted nodes. With time, the overlying skin often develops a violaceous discoloration.

Pulmonary NTM usually occurs in children with underlying lung pathology. Nontuberculous mycobacterial disease in patients with cystic fibrosis increases in frequency at adolescence, when routine bacterial lung flora often changes. Symptoms include worsening of existing pulmonary symptoms (cough, bronchodilator-refractory wheezing), deterioration of pulmonary function testing, or nonspecific constitutional symptoms (fatigue, weight loss). Fever is seen in some patients. The nonspecific nature of symptoms, occurring at a time when many adolescents with cystic fibrosis have other reasons for pulmonary decompensation, makes the diagnosis of NTM disease more challenging.

Patients can have NTM in their sputum as colonizing organisms, not causing pathologic changes in the lungs. Consequently, the American Thoracic Society (ATS) has identified clinical, radiographic, and microbiologic parameters to differentiate colonization from infection (Table 24-3). Radiographic changes may include worsening bronchiectasis, mucus plugging, and pulmonary nodules; however, these findings are nonspecific.

Skin and soft-tissue infections are seen most commonly with *Mycobacterium marinum*. The classic history is development of an indolent verrucous-appearing skin lesion, occasionally with adjacent tenosynovitis, after a child has had physical contact with a fish tank or waterborne animal. Superficial (folliculitis) and deeper soft-tissue infections (pyomyositis, osteomyelitis after penetrating injuries) have been described.

Disseminated disease has become much less common in the antiretroviral era. Bacteremia (including catheter-related bacteremia) and other disseminated forms (eg, meningitis, osteomyelitis) are now most common in solid organ and bone marrow transplant recipients and patients with specific immunologic

Table 24-3. American Thoracic Society Criteria for the Diagnosis of Nontuberculous Mycobacterial Pulmonary Disease (Both clinical and microbiologic categories must be fulfilled.)

Category	Criteria
Clinical	Pulmonary symptoms, chest radiographic findings (nodules or cavities), or CT findings (multiple nodules and multifocal bronchiectasis) *and*
	Exclusion of other diagnoses
Microbiologic	Positive cultures from >1 expectorated sputum samples *or*
	Positive culture from at least 1 bronchial wash/lavage *or*
	Transbronchial biopsy or other lung biopsy showing histopathologic features consistent with mycobacterial infection and that are culture positive for NTM *or*
	Transbronchial biopsy or other lung biopsy showing histopathologic features consistent with mycobacterial infection and sputum or bronchial wash/lavage specimen that is culture positive for NTM

Abbreviations: CT, computed tomography; NTM, nontuberculous mycobacteria.

deficits. Constitutional symptoms such as fever and weight loss predominate, and examination may demonstrate hepatosplenomegaly, diffuse nodular skin rash, and disseminated lymphadenopathy.

Evaluation

The optimal diagnostic technique and treatment for NTM cervical lymphadenitis is complete excision of the lymph node. In most cases, tissue should be sent for AFB stain, culture, and histopathology; in addition, routine aerobic and fungal cultures should be sent. Histopathology in NTM lymphadenitis is more likely to demonstrate microabscesses, positive AFB stain, and necrotizing granulomas, and less likely to demonstrate caseating granulomas than in TB lymphadenitis. Incision and drainage of lymph nodes with suspected NTM is not recommended, because this increases the risk of development of a chronically draining sinus tract.

Several NTM species can cause large areas of induration in response to the tuberculin skin test. One would expect the tuberculin skin test result to be positive and the IGRA result to be negative in most cases of NTM lymphadenitis, whereas positive tuberculin skin test and IGRA results would be more consistent with *M tuberculosis*.

The diagnosis of NTM pulmonary disease is much more difficult than the diagnosis of NTM infection in ordinarily sterile sites. Nontuberculous mycobacterial species can colonize healthy or diseased tissue, and they can also cause disease. To facilitate diagnosis, the ATS has developed criteria to differentiate colonization from NTM pulmonary disease (Table 24-3).

Table 24-4. Potential Adverse Effects and Drug Interactions for Medications Used to Treat Nontuberculous Mycobacteria Disease

Medication	Adverse Effects	Drug Interactions	Notes
Macrolides (azithromycin, clarithromycin)	GI distress; prolongation of QT interval	Rare	The only drug susceptibilities that correlate with in vivo results are for macrolides; they form the backbone of therapy for NTM disease.
RIF	Hepatotoxicity; idiosyncratic bone marrow suppression	Common	Important to warn parents and patients about orange discoloration to urine and (less commonly) secretions.
EMB	Optic neuritis and red-green color discrimination difficulties	Rare	As children metabolize the drug more rapidly than adults, toxicity is very rare. EMB can be used even in the preverbal child in whom visual screening may be difficult.
Aminoglycosides (amikacin, kanamycin, tobramycin)	Ototoxicity; nephrotoxicity	Rare	Toxicity is cumulative; serial evaluation of hearing and renal function is needed.
TMP/SMX	Rash; hypersensitivity reactions; idiosyncratic bone marrow suppression	Rare	IV formulation contains a substantial fluid volume.
Fluoroquinolones (ciprofloxacin, levofloxacin)	Prolongation of QT interval; tendon damage; exacerbated muscle weakness in myasthenia gravis patients	Rare	Particularly useful for *Mycobacterium fortuitum*.
Cephalosporins (cefoxitin)	Bone marrow suppression; interstitial nephritis	Rare	Adverse effects depend on cumulative dose.
Carbapenems (imipenem, meropenem)	Bone marrow suppression; interstitial nephritis; lower seizure threshold	Rare	Levels of antiepileptics may need to be increased.
Tetracyclines	Tooth discoloration in children <8 y	Rare	Risk of tooth discoloration and enamel hypoplasia in young children must be weighed against the potential benefit.

Abbreviations: EMB, ethambutol; GI, gastrointestinal; IV, intravenous; NTM, nontuberculous mycobacterial; RIF, rifampin; TMP/SMX, trimethoprim/sulfamethoxazole.

The most common radiographic findings include intrathoracic lymphadenopathy, tree-in-bud findings on CT, and cavitary lesions, the latter being more common in adolescent patients. For children with cystic fibrosis, comparison to prior CT scans is essential to assess for evolution of imaging findings. Expectorated cultures or sputum induction should be used to obtain specimens for AFB stain and culture. Throat swabs, as previously alluded to, have low culture yield.

Skin and soft-tissue disease caused by NTM often is identified by biopsy and culture; histopathology may demonstrate granulomas (less frequently seen with NTM than *M tuberculosis*), but no findings are pathognomonic. Granulomas are less common in immunocompromised children. Immunocompromised children with disseminated NTM infection often have positive mycobacterial blood cultures, and imaging may reveal pulmonary nodules.

Management

Given the adverse effect profiles of some of the medications used to treat pulmonary NTM, the duration of therapy, and that many antibiotics used to treat NTM are available only in a parenteral formulation, it is essential that clinicians are certain a child requires therapy (ie, that colonization is differentiated from disease). Table 24-4 describes some antibiotics used to treat NTM infections for children meeting ATS criteria (found in Table 24-3).

The treatment of choice for lymphadenopathy is complete excision of the lymph node. Surgery alone has been shown in several studies to be superior to medical therapy in terms of symptom duration and cosmesis. As with TB, combination multidrug therapy is used to decrease the risk of selecting for drug-resistant isolates. The most common regimen is a macrolide in combination with either RIF or EMB. Early studies used the first commercially available macrolide, clarithromycin. However, azithromycin seems as effective and offers the benefit of single daily dosing and a superior taste for the suspension formulation. Duration of therapy is 3 to 6 months.

Pulmonary NTM is primarily caused by MAC, *M abscessus,* and *Mycobacterium kansasii.* In vitro susceptibilities correlate with clinical response only for macrolides and MAC. Nonetheless, drug susceptibility testing is recommended for initial isolates and used to guide therapy. Table 24-5 shows ATS recommended regimens for the 2 most common NTM species isolated from the lungs of US patients.

Another common scenario is the one in which a child is being evaluated for both NTM and TB (either pulmonary or lymphadenopathy). One option is to start the child on a regimen of INH, RIF, EMB, and azithromycin. With this regimen, the child is receiving 3 drugs for TB and 3 for NTM. Of note, if the child ultimately is thought to have TB, the course of therapy would have to be extended to 9 months, because pyrazinamide was not included in the initial regimen.

Table 24-5. American Thoracic Society Treatment Regimens for Nontuberculous Mycobacterial Pulmonary Disease

Species	Disease Type	Initial Regimen	Continuation Regimen	Notes
MAC	Fibrocavitary or fibronodular	Macrolide, RIF, EMB daily (An aminoglycoside may be added for the first 8 wk for children with fibrocavitary disease.)	NA	Continue medications for 12 mo after smear conversion.
	Bronchiectatic	Macrolide, RIF, EMB thrice weekly	NA	
Mycobacterium abscessus	All	3 drugs to which there is documented susceptibility × 4–8 wk	2 drugs for 6–12 mo	Do not anticipate culture conversion[a]; follow patient clinically and radiographically.

Abbreviations: EMB, ethambutol; MAC, *Mycobacterium avium* complex; NA, not applicable; RIF, rifampin.

[a] Unlike for other nontuberculous mycobacterial species, culture conversion should not be the endpoint for therapy for *Mycobacterium abscessus* pulmonary disease, because this species is very persistent. Instead, efficacy of therapy is monitored by clinical (eg, improvement in pulmonary function tests (PFTs) and radiographic (eg, decreased pulmonary nodularity) improvement.

Nontuberculous mycobacterial skin and soft-tissue disease is usually caused by *M fortuitum*, *M marinum*, or *Mycobacterium ulcerans*. These species are often susceptible to oral agents. Combination therapy with 2 drugs to which the isolate has documented susceptibility is recommended. Therapy should be continued for approximately 4 months, but longer durations of therapy (minimum: 6 months) are recommended for NTM osteomyelitis. Surgical debridement may be a necessary adjuvant to medical therapy for children with deep-seated infections. Children with NTM skin/soft-tissue disease in association with disseminated disease should be treated as per the guidelines for disseminated NTM disease.

Disseminated NTM disease can occur in at least 2 scenarios. The first is the child with profound immunosuppression, and the second is the child with a central venous catheter who develops NTM bacteremia. In the first scenario, MAC is the most common organism, and therapy consists of a macrolide-based regimen with 2 other medications. After 1 to 2 months, 2 drugs (one of which should be a macrolide) can be used to complete the 6- to 12-month course of therapy. Treatment should continue for 6 to 12 months after blood culture conversion.

Long-term Monitoring and Implications

Immunocompetent children with NTM lymphadenitis can be monitored clinically for response to therapy. In the absence of therapy, complete symptom resolution was seen in two-thirds of children by 6 months and all children by 12 months in one study. However, draining sinus tracts and poor cosmetic outcomes are common in the absence of therapy.

Children with isolated NTM skin and soft-tissue disease do quite well with medical therapy alone. In instances of penetrating trauma and deep-seated infection, surgical debridement may be a useful adjuvant to medical therapy.

The outcome for children with other forms of NTM disease is not as good. In part, this is because of NTM's predilection for affecting already diseased tissues or people with weakened immune systems. Children with NTM pulmonary disease may never clear the organism from their lungs. This is particularly true for *M abscessus*. Instead of waiting for culture conversion, following symptoms, CT scans, and pulmonary function testing for response to therapy may be more realistic.

Children with disseminated NTM disease should be followed by blood cultures and anthropometric measurements. Prognosis is very poor for these patients, and survival is linked to immune system recovery. Primary prevention against disseminated MAC is recommended for children with low CD4$^+$ counts. Secondary prevention for children with a history of disseminated MAC is lifelong.

Suggested Reading

Blyth CC, Best EJ, Jones CA, et al. Nontuberculous mycobacterial infection in children: a prospective national study. *Pediatr Infect Dis J.* 2009;28(9):801–805

Carvalho AC, Codecasa L, Pinsi G, et al. Differential diagnosis of cervical mycobacterial lymphadenitis in children. *Pediatr Infect Dis J.* 2010;29(7):629–633

Detjen AK, Keil T, Roll S, et al. Interferon-gamma release assays improve the diagnosis of tuberculosis and nontuberculous mycobacterial disease in children in a country with a low incidence of tuberculosis. *Clin Infect Dis.* 2007;45(3):322–328

Griffith DE, Aksamit T, Brown-Elliott BA, et al. An official ATS/IDSA statement: diagnosis, treatment, and prevention of nontuberculous mycobacterial diseases. *Am J Respir Crit Care Med.* 2007;175(4):367–416

Kendall BA, Varley CD, Choi D, et al. Distinguishing tuberculosis from nontuberculous mycobacteria lung disease, Oregon, USA. *Emerg Infect Dis.* 2011;17(3):506–509

Mofenson LM, Brady MT, Danner SP, et al. Guidelines for the prevention and treatment of opportunistic infection among HIV-exposed and infected children: recommendations from the CDC, the National Institutes of Health, the HIV Medicine Association of the Infectious Diseases Society of America, the Pediatric Infectious Diseases Society, and the American Academy of Pediatrics. *MMWR Recomm Rep.* 2009;58 (RR-11):1–166

CHAPTER 25

Tularemia

Kari A. Simonsen, MD, and Jessica Snowden, MD

Key Points

- Tularemia is an acute febrile zoonosis with multiple possible clinical syndromes, depending on the route of infection (most commonly glandular and ulceroglandular).

- Suspect tularemia in patients with animal or tick exposure, presenting with non-healing skin lesions or lymphadenitis that is not responding to empiric β-lactam or macrolide antibiotics.

- If there is a clinical suspicion, start antibiotics empirically pending laboratory confirmation. Serologic confirmation is typically not possible until the second week of disease.

- Aminoglycosides (gentamicin or streptomycin) are currently the preferred treatment for all forms of tularemia. Alternatives include tetracyclines and fluoroquinolones in select cases.

- Hospital isolation of patients is not required because human-to-human transmission does not occur. However, laboratory personnel are at risk of exposure from culture specimens and should be notified of possible tularemia samples.

Overview

Tularemia is most often acquired through arthropodal bites, including multiple tick species and deer flies, in the United States. It can also be acquired by handling animal carcasses, especially rabbits and other hares; eating poorly cooked food contaminated with the bacteria; or drinking water that has been contaminated by infected animal carcasses. In the United States, most cases occur in the south central region during the months of June through October, and most infected patients have recreational or occupational risks that expose them to infected animals or arthropodal vectors and their habitats. Additionally, *Francisella tularensis,* the causative agent of tularemia, is capable of being transmitted as an agent of bioterrorism through aerosolization and is therefore classified by the Centers for Disease Control and Prevention as a Category A pathogen.

Causes and Differential Diagnosis

Francisella tularensis is a highly infectious gram-negative coccobacillus and can survive in multiple sources in nature, including water, wet soil, and animal carcasses, for several weeks.

The differential diagnosis of tularemia is broad and must be taken into clinical context, because the myriad features of tularemia may be associated with numerous other infectious etiologies. Clinical findings associated with the classic categories of tularemia may require consideration of a variety of conditions as noted in Table 25-1.

Clinical Features

Typically, the symptoms and physical examination findings of tularemia correlate with the route of inoculation. The incubation period averages 3 to 5 days, but the range is reported at 1 to 21 days. Initial nonspecific symptoms include abrupt onset of fever, chills, headache, fatigue, and anorexia. Additional systemic symptoms may include cough, myalgia, chest discomfort, sore throat, abdominal pain, nausea, and vomiting. Clinical presentation of tularemia can be variable and is divided into categories based on the most prominent physical findings: ulceroglandular, glandular, oculoglandular, oropharyngeal, pneumonic, or typhoidal (Table 25-2). Lymphadenopathy is the most commonly identified clinical feature, present in 96% of children with tularemia.

Evaluation

Diagnosis of tularemia requires a high clinical index of suspicion, accompanied by supportive laboratory findings, including serology or cultures. It can be cultured from the blood, spinal fluid, lymph node tissues, wound cultures, and other infected sites, but it can take up to 10 days for colonies to appear. Most suspected tularemia cases are confirmed using serologic testing analysis. A detectable antibody response to tularemia typically appears 10 to 14 days after the onset of symptoms. This can make acute diagnosis complicated because a patient may present in this sero-negative window. Acute and convalescent serology can be helpful in these cases, with a fourfold increase in titers considered positive. The most commonly used assays detect combined IgM and IgG specific to tularemia. Tube agglutination test result is considered positive with a single titer greater than 1:160 or a micro-agglutination titer greater than 1:128.

Table 25-1. Differential Diagnosis of Tularemia

Category of Tularemia	Condition
Glandular	• Staphylococcal and streptococcal (bacterial) adenitis • *Bartonella henselae* infections • Tuberculosis • Nontuberculous mycobacteria infections • *Toxoplasma gondii* infections • Rat-bite fever • Kawasaki disease • Mononucleosis • Plague
Ulceroglandular	• *Treponema pallidum* infections • Lymphogranuloma venereum • Sporotrichosis • Anthrax • HSV infections • Varicella-zoster virus
Oculoglandular	• HSV • Adenovirus infections • Mumps • *T pallidum* • *B henselae* • *Coccidioides immitis* diseases • Other bacterial conjunctivitis
Oropharyngeal	• Streptococcal pharyngitis • Adenovirus • HSV • Diphtheria
Pneumonic	• Tuberculosis • *Legionella* infections • *Mycoplasma* diseases • *Chlamydophila* infections • Psittacosis • Fungal infections • Rickettsial diseases
Typhoidal	• *Salmonella* species infections • Brucellosis • Legionnaires' disease • Q fever • Rickettsioses • Malaria • Disseminated fungal or mycobacterial infections • Other causes of bacterial sepsis or prolonged fever without localizing source

Abbreviation: HSV, herpes simplex virus.

Table 25-2. Physical Findings Associated With Tularemia

Category of Tularemia	Route of Infection	History/Physical Examination Findings
Ulceroglandular/glandular	Tick bite or handling infected animal tissue	• Most common in children • Painful maculopapular or vesicular lesion occurring at site of inoculation progressing to erythematous, slow-healing ulcer • Painful regional lymphadenopathy that may spontaneously drain • Most commonly head and neck lymphadenopathy in children due to tick bites on scalp
Oculoglandular	Direct inoculation of the conjunctiva with contaminated fingers (handling infected animals or insects) or via aerosols or splashes	• Painful, purulent conjunctivitis; lid edema; or chemosis • May have conjunctival ulcerations • May have regional lymphadenopathy
Oropharyngeal	Consumption of contaminated food or water	• Acute pharyngitis with or without tonsillitis or pharyngeal ulcerations • Regional lymphadenopathy • May also have gastrointestinal symptoms, which can lead to rapidly fulminant and fatal disease
Pneumonic	Due to inhalation of aerosols from farming, lawn mowing, or sheep shearing or within laboratory setting	• Patchy, bilateral infiltrates with associated pleural effusions • Hilar lymphadenopathy • Granulomas, similar to tuberculosis, possible • Nonproductive cough common • Rarely hemoptysis, shortness of breath, or pleuritic chest pain
Typhoidal	Can occur after dissemination of infection from any of the other forms of tularemia	• Significant fever, lymphadenopathy, chills, headache, nausea, vomiting, diarrhea, and evidence of endotoxemia • Critically ill with symptoms indistinguishable from other forms of sepsis

Routine laboratory evaluations, such as a complete blood cell count and inflammatory markers, are of limited utility in differentiating tularemia from other causes of lymphadenitis or fever. A complete blood cell count may be normal or demonstrate a slightly increased white blood cell count, and inflammatory markers may be only mildly elevated.

Management

The keys to successful treatment of tularemia are early clinical suspicion, diagnosis, and prompt initiation of appropriate antibiotics. The most favorable outcomes are observed in patients treated within 3 weeks of the onset of infection. Several in vitro studies and case series (Evidence Level II-2) support the role of streptomycin and gentamicin as first-line therapy. Because of the limited availability of streptomycin in the United States, gentamicin is usually the drug of choice. Patients are generally treated for 7 to 10 days with intravenous gentamicin, with longer courses for more severe illness. Tobramycin has not been shown to be effective in the treatment of tularemia.

In some cases, intravenous therapy may not be possible or there may be other contraindications to treatment with gentamicin or streptomycin. Alternative therapies include tetracyclines (doxycycline or tetracycline) or fluoroquinolones (ciprofloxacin or levofloxacin). Tetracycline has been shown to be effective in treating tularemia in the United States but is not considered first-line therapy because of the high relapse rate observed after discontinuing therapy; therefore, treatment with tetracycline should be continued at least 14 days (Evidence Level III). Several small case reports and case series in the United States have reported successful use of fluoroquinolones to treat tularemia (Evidence Level II-2), primarily in adults. Patients hospitalized with tularemia require only standard precautions because person-to-person transmission has not been reported. Laboratory personnel should be notified before any potential tularemia specimen is submitted for processing. Currently, no evidence supports antibiotic prophylaxis for tularemia after an insect bite or animal exposure.

Prognosis

With appropriate diagnosis and treatment, the death rate associated with tularemia infections is less than 1%. Elderly patients and those with other comorbidities, particularly immune dysfunction, are at higher risk for death, complications, or prolonged illness. Delays between the onset of symptoms and initiation of an effective antimicrobial treatment have been associated with a higher risk of lymph node suppuration and subsequent surgical drainage. Surgical drainage has been required in approximately 20% of reported pediatric cases of ulceroglandular or glandular tularemia. Relapse rates are highest in patients treated with a bacteriostatic antibiotic, such as tetracyclines. Tularemia-specific immunoglobulins can be detected for years after initial infection and are presumed to provide long-term protection, although this has not been completely evaluated.

Suggested Reading

Dennis DT, Inglesby TV, Henderson DA, et al. Tularemia as a biological weapon: medical and public health management. *JAMA*. 2001;285(21):2763–2773

Nigrovic LE, Wingerter SL. Tularemia. *Infect Dis Clin North Am*. 2008;22(3):489–504

Snowden J, Stovall S. Tularemia: retrospective review of 10 years' experience in Arkansas. *Clin Pediatr (Phila)*. 2010;50(1):64–68

Tärnvik A, Chu MC. New approaches to diagnosis and therapy of tularemia. *Ann N Y Acad Sci*. 2007;1105:378–404

Weber IB, Turabelidze G, Patrick S, Griffith KS, Kugeler KJ, Mead PS. Clinical recognition and management of tularemia in Missouri: a retrospective records review of 121 cases. *Clin Infect Dis*. 2012;55(1):1283–1290

PART

1

Infectious Diseases

CHAPTER 26

Cytomegalovirus

Amina Ahmed, MD

Key Points

- Cytomegalovirus (CMV) is commonly acquired asymptomatically in the immunocompetent host.

- Sensorineural hearing loss is associated with congenital CMV infection, with almost 50% of hearing loss developing after the newborn period. While it is the most common congenital infection, symptomatic disease occurs in only 10% of those infected.

- Lymphoproliferative disease associated with CMV is notable in immuno-compromised hosts, now most commonly in stem cell and solid organ transplant recipients.

Overview

Primary infection with cytomegalovirus (CMV) is common and usually asymptomatic but can cause a mononucleosis-type syndrome. Recurrent infection occurs with reactivation of a latent virus or reinfection with a different strain in an individual who is seropositive for CMV infection. Reactivation of viral infection is typically asymptomatic in the immunocompetent host, but it can result in horizontal or vertical transmission. Cytomegaloviral disease is most problematic in neonates infected congenitally and in the immunocompro-mised host.

Causes and Differential Diagnosis

Human CMV, as with other herpesviruses, establishes lifelong latency following primary infection. The virus is intermittently shed in body fluids, including urine, saliva, cervicovaginal secretions, and human milk, for months to years. Transmission of infection occurs by person-to-person contact, including sexual contact, with infectious virus in secretions. Vertical transmission from a mother to her neonate can occur through 1 of 3 routes: transplacental, resulting in congenital CMV infection; intrapartum, by exposure to infected cervical or vaginal secretions; or postnatally through breastfeeding.

The differential diagnosis of CMV mononucleosis includes mononucleosis-like syndromes caused by other viruses such as Epstein-Barr virus (EBV), adenovirus, hepatitis A, hepatitis B, or HIV. Most cases of infectious mononucleosis are caused by EBV, and CMV is responsible for most cases of heterophile-negative mononucleosis. Illness caused by CMV is typically milder than EBV-associated mononucleosis. Distinguishing features between the 2 infections are described in the Evaluation section. Serologic testing consistent with acute EBV confirms the disease. Toxoplasmosis can also cause a heterophile-negative mononucleosis-like illness. The syndrome is characterized predominantly by fever and lymphadenopathy. It rarely causes pharyngitis or abnormal elevation of transaminase concentrations and is unassociated with characteristic hematologic abnormalities. Adenoviral infections may manifest with symptoms that overlap those of mononucleosis, including pharyngitis with or without exudate. Often conjunctivitis and other upper respiratory tract symptoms predominate in adenoviral infection. Virus may be detected in throat or nasopharyngeal specimens by culture or molecular methods. Early viral hepatitis, including that caused by hepatitis A or B virus, may resemble CMV-related illness. The degree of hepatic involvement with hepatitis A or B virus quickly becomes more extensive than that seen with CMV, with transaminase values rapidly rising to above 1,000 IU/L. Primary HIV should be considered in any adolescent presenting with febrile illness resembling mononucleosis. Common findings include fever, sore throat, myalgia, and lymphadenopathy. Rash unassociated with antibiotic use is uncommon in mononucleosis caused by CMV but frequently observed in primary HIV infection within the first 48 to 72 hours after onset of fever. The diagnosis of HIV can be confirmed by serologic testing or polymerase chain reaction (PCR) testing.

Clinical Features

The clinical presentation of CMV infection depends on host factors.

Primary CMV infection in the immunocompetent child or adult typically results in minimal or no clinical disease. Adolescents and adults are more likely to exhibit symptoms of the mononucleosis syndrome, which is characterized by protracted fevers and malaise with limited localizing symptoms or signs. Severe or life-threatening disease occurs rarely with CMV infection in immunocompetent persons but may include pneumonitis, enterocolitis, myocarditis, pericarditis, and hemolytic anemia. Icteric or granulomatous hepatitis can occur. Cytomegaloviral meningoencephalitis has been reported and may occur as a complication of CMV mononucleosis or an isolated manifestation of primary CMV infection. The expected course of CMV mononucleosis in healthy hosts is recovery without sequelae. Typical duration of illness is 1 to 4 weeks, but symptoms may occasionally persist longer. Prolonged fatigue, as occasionally observed with EBV infection, is uncommon. With reactivation of infection or reinfection with new strains, individuals usually remain asymptomatic.

Among immunocompromised hosts, including those infected with HIV and solid organ and hematopoietic stem cell transplant recipients, primary or reactivation CMV infection can result in severe or life-threatening disease. Cytomegaloviral retinitis is by far the most common manifestation of CMV disease among HIV-infected individuals.

In those with AIDS, acquisition of CMV infection increases with age; thus, adults are more likely to be coinfected with HIV and CMV. Cytomegalovirus retinitis is typically unilateral at presentation but, in the absence of antiviral therapy or immune recovery, can progress to bilateral involvement. Patients present with blurred vision, decreased visual acuity, or visual field defects. Young children may exhibit strabismus as a result of visual compromise. Before the availability of combination antiretroviral therapy (cART), CMV retinitis was the leading cause of vision loss and blindness in this population. Additional clinical manifestations of CMV disease in AIDS include gastrointestinal diseases such as enterocolitis and esophagitis. Pneumonitis is less common than observed in other immunocompromised hosts. Central nervous system (CNS) disease attributable to CMV is uncommon but may present as encephalitis or polyradiculopathy.

Cytomegaloviral infection and disease classically present between 1 and 6 months after transplantation. Clinical manifestations range from asymptomatic viremia to a mononucleosis-like illness (CMV syndrome) to tissue invasive disease associated with significant morbidity and mortality. Cytomegaloviral syndrome is defined as clinical illness without evidence of end-organ involvement and is characterized by fever, malaise, leukopenia, thrombocytopenia, and transaminitis. End-organ disease is distinguished by detection of the virus from tissue from the involved organ.

The manifestations of disease in solid organ transplant (SOT) recipients vary by transplanted organ type but can include pneumonitis, hepatitis, enterocolitis, and encephalitis. Major indirect effects of CMV infection include both acute and chronic graft rejection, especially among renal and liver transplant recipients. Cytomegaloviral infection further depresses cell-mediated immunity, promoting opportunistic bacterial and fungal infections, development of EBV-associated posttransplant lymphoproliferative disease, and decreased patient survival.

In neonates, CMV is the most common cause of congenitally acquired infection. Although the infection is asymptomatic in most infected neonates, a substantial proportion of them develop permanent neurologic sequelae. Both primary and recurrent maternal infection during pregnancy can result in intrauterine transmission. The risk of transmission is substantially higher for mothers with primary infection (approximately 40%) versus mothers with recurrent infection (approximately 1%), but most cases of congenital CMV are a consequence of maternal CMV reactivation or reinfection. Infants born infected as a result of primary maternal infection are more likely to have symptomatic disease and, consequently, are at higher risk of neurologic sequelae associated with congenital CMV infection. Classic CMV disease is characterized by petechiae, hepatosplenomegaly, microcephaly, thrombocytopenia, jaundice, and intracranial (typically periventricular) calcifications. Clinical and laboratory findings for neonates with symptomatic congenital CMV infection are summarized in Table 26-1. Hepatosplenomegaly, although nonspecific to congenital CMV disease, is one of the more common manifestations of symptomatic infection. Petechiae and purpura are caused by thrombocytopenia, and may be present anywhere on the skin. Violaceous infiltrative papules or "blueberry muffin spots," more characteristic of congenital rubella syndrome, represent sites of extramedullary hematopoiesis. Approximately 5% to 30% of symptomatic infants have chorioretinitis. Other ocular abnormalities include microphthalmos, cataracts, and retinal necrosis and calcification. Microcephaly may be present at birth or progressive in the first year of life. Central nervous system involvement may also be exhibited by seizures, sensorineural hearing loss, and meningoencephalitis. Transient signs and symptoms such as hepatosplenomegaly, jaundice, and abnormal laboratory results gradually resolve over the course of the first several weeks of life. However, a significant proportion of both symptomatic and asymptomatic infants develop neurologic sequelae as a

Table 26-1. Clinical and Laboratory Findings in Neonates With Symptomatic Congenital CMV Infection

Finding	Percent With Abnormality
Clinical Findings	
Petechiae	76
Jaundice	67
Hepatosplenomegaly	60
Microcephaly	53
Intrauterine growth retardation	50
Chorioretinitis/optic atrophy	20
Purpura	13
Seizures	7
Laboratory Findings	
Elevated AST (>80 U/L)	83
Conjugated hyperbilirubinemia (direct bilirubin >4 mg/dL)	81
Thrombocytopenia (<100,000/mm³)	77
Elevated CSF protein (>120 mg/dL)	46

Abbreviations: AST, aspartate aminotransferase; CSF, cerebrospinal fluid.

From Ross SA, Boppana SB. Congenital cytomegalovirus infection: outcome and diagnosis. *Semin Pediatr Infect Dis.* 2004;16(1):44–49, with permission from Elsevier.

consequence of congenital infection, including cognitive deficits, cerebral palsy, visual impairment, and, most frequently, sensorineural hearing loss. It is estimated that 40% to 58% of symptomatic and 13.5% of asymptomatic infants develop permanent neurologic sequelae (Evidence Level II-2).

Perinatal and postnatal infections of the newborn occur through contact with CMV-infected maternal cervicovaginal secretions during delivery or through human milk ingestion after delivery. Transfusion-acquired CMV infection is now largely prevented by widespread use of CMV-negative and leukocyte-depleted blood products in neonatal intensive care units. Human milk plays a significant role in perinatal transmission, with up to 90% of seropositive lactating women shedding CMV in milk. Perinatal infection in term infants is most frequently asymptomatic. Premature infants, especially those with very low birthweight (<1,500 grams) are at risk for severe disease due to the lack of maternally transmitted CMV-specific antibodies. Infection becomes clinically apparent at 4 to 16 weeks of age. Infants may develop self-limited disease with hepatitis or pneumonitis. A sepsis-like syndrome has been described and is characterized by respiratory distress, poor perfusion, and hepatosplenomegaly. Laboratory abnormalities include neutropenia, thrombocytopenia, and transaminitis. Evidence suggests that, unlike congenital CMV infections, postnatal CMV infections are not associated with neurologic, audiologic, or ophthalmologic sequelae (Evidence Level II-2).

Evaluation

Infectious mononucleosis is most commonly caused by EBV, which is diagnosed by the presence of heterophile antibodies (monospot test) or EBV-specific serology. Cytomegalovirus is the most common cause of heterophile-negative mononucleosis-like illness.

Mononucleosis caused by CMV may be clinically indistinguishable from EBV-induced illness. Important distinctions between EBV- and CMV-associated mononucleosis are that CMV uncommonly causes exudative pharyngotonsillitis or cervical lymphadenopathy, findings that are hallmarks of symptomatic EBV infection. Splenomegaly, which occurs in up to 30% to 50% of individuals with EBV-associated mononucleosis, is less commonly observed in CMV infection. Exanthems associated with ampicillin treatment are commonly observed in children with both EBV- and CMV-associated mononucleosis.

As in EBV-associated mononucleosis, atypical lymphocytosis is noted consistently in CMV mononucleosis syndrome, with greater than 10% atypical lymphocytes detected on peripheral blood smear. Additional hematologic abnormalities such as anemia and thrombocytopenia that are typically observed in EBV-associated mononucleosis are uncommon with CMV. Mild to moderate elevations of hepatic transaminase concentrations are observed in more than 90% of patients with CMV infection, with peak concentrations typically not exceeding 300 to 400 IU/L.

In neonates, laboratory abnormalities include anemia in addition to thrombocytopenia, with platelet counts frequently less than 100×10^3/mcL. Hepatosplenomegaly may be accompanied by elevated transaminase concentrations and elevated direct and indirect bilirubin levels (see Table 26-1). Imaging of the brain with ultrasound, computed tomography, or magnetic resonance imaging techniques can demonstrate evidence of CNS involvement. The most common abnormality is periventricular calcifications, but ventriculomegaly, periventricular cysts, intracerebral calcifications, and cortical atrophy may also be noted (Figures 26-1, 26-2).

Serology provides indirect evidence of CMV infection by measuring antibodies at one or multiple time points in clinical illness and is the test of choice for the immunocompetent patient. The method most useful in determining whether a patient has ever had CMV infection is based on the presence or absence of CMV IgG. Cytomegaloviral-specific IgM antibodies are typically detectable within the first 2 weeks following onset of illness, whereas IgG antibodies are often undetectable until 2 to 3 weeks after onset of symptoms. Diagnosis of recent or acute infection may be made on the basis of detection of CMV IgM or fourfold rise in CMV-specific IgG in paired specimens obtained 2 to 4 weeks apart. However, IgM antibodies may be detectable for 4 to 6 months after primary infection and can often be positive with reactivation or reinfection. The accuracy of detection of CMV-specific IgM for the diagnosis of acute infection is limited by false-positive and false-negative results. IgG avidity assays are used to help distinguish acute CMV infection from more remote infection. These assays are based on the observation that IgG antibodies of low avidity are present during the first few months after onset of infection and take 16 to 20 weeks to mature to high levels. The presence of high avidity CMV IgG indicates long-standing infection.

The diagnosis of CMV infection has traditionally relied on isolation of the virus in cell culture. Cytomegalovirus can be isolated from multiple sites,

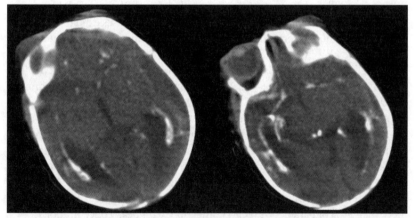

Figure 26-1. Intracranial calcifications in a neonate with congenital cytomegalovirus infection.

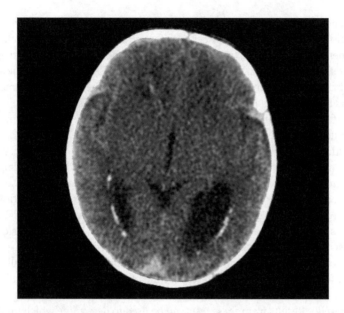

Figure 26-2. Periventricular calcifications in a neonate with congenital cytomegalovirus infection.

including blood, urine, oropharyngeal secretions, cerebrospinal fluid, bronchial washings, and tissue biopsy specimens. Although detection of CMV in culture indicates the presence of virus, it does not always confirm active infection because the virus may be shed intermittently in urine and saliva for months to years after acute infection. Results are based on observation of typical cytopathic effect in cells, which may take 2 to 3 weeks. The shell vial assay is a more rapid culture technique that has replaced conventional cell culture in many laboratories.

Antigenemia assays such as the pp65 assay have been used for more than a decade for quantification of CMV in blood specimens. The results correlate closely with viremia and are used to predict the severity of CMV infection and disease or monitor response to antiviral therapy in immunosuppressed populations such as transplant recipients. Use of the assay is limited in pediatrics, especially among those with leukopenia, because of the blood volume requirements.

Polymerase chain reaction is a widely available rapid and sensitive method of CMV detection based on amplification of nucleic acids. DNA can be extracted from whole blood, white blood cells, plasma, peripheral blood white blood cells, or any other tissue or fluid. Polymerase chain reaction tests for CMV may be qualitative or quantitative, although the latter are more widely used because of increased sensitivity and application.

Immunohistochemistry is used primarily for the detection CMV in tissue or body fluids. Detection of the virus in tissue confirms organ involvement.

Diagnosis of congenital CMV infection is proven by detection of the virus in body fluids in the first 2 to 3 weeks of life. Urine and saliva are the preferred specimens for testing, and, traditionally, CMV has been detected by conventional culture or shell vial assay culture. The role of PCR tests using urine and saliva has yet to be defined, but detection of viral genome in these specimens appears to be a promising alternative method for diagnosis (Evidence Level II-2). After 3 weeks of age, laboratory detection of virus does not confirm congenital CMV infection because it may represent natal or postnatal acquisition.

In immunocompromised hosts, serology and molecular diagnostics are used in conjunction to characterize risk for CMV disease and diagnose disease when suspected. Guidelines for evaluation of children for CMV are based on those published for adults. Diagnosis of CMV disease is typically made by isolation of the virus in culture or demonstration of CMV by PCR or by immunohisto-chemistry in the appropriate body fluids (eg, vitreous humor) or tissue.

In both SOT and hematopoietic stem cell transplantation (HSCT), all donors and recipients should be tested for the presence of CMV IgG antibody prior to transplantation (Evidence Levels I and II-2 for SOT and HSCT, respectively). Results from these tests can be used to determine which preventive strategy is most appropriate on the basis of risk stratification. After transplantation, antigenemia assays or PCR tests (typically quantitative or real-time PCR) are used to confirm infection or identify patients at risk for disease. The presence of viremia has been demonstrated to be a predictive factor for development of end-organ disease and is used for initiating preemptive therapy before overt disease is established. Serologic testing is rarely helpful after transplantation except to confirm seroconversion in a previously seronegative recipient. Urinary or salivary cultures are also unhelpful because isolation of virus may reflect shedding and may not correlate with disease. For suspected end-organ disease, diagnosis is confirmed by the demonstration of characteristic CMV histopathology or detection of virus by culture or molecular methods in tissue. In these patients, viremia has often been detected by PCR or antigenemia assay prior to or coincident with the development of symptoms and raises the suspicion for CMV disease.

Management

Treatment with antivirals is usually not indicated in the immunocompetent host with asymptomatic or mildly symptomatic CMV infection. Resolution of illness without sequelae is the expected outcome. Severe or life-threatening CMV disease in immunologically healthy hosts has been reported, and treatment of these patients should be considered (Evidence Level III). For immunocompromised hosts, treatment and prevention of disease is beneficial. For neonates with symptomatic CNS congenital CMV infection, treatment is beneficial in preservation of hearing.

There are 4 antivirals licensed for the treatment and prevention of CMV infection (Table 26-2): ganciclovir (GCV), valganciclovir (VGCV), cidofovir (CDV) and foscarnet (FOS). In addition, biologics such as immune globulin and CMV hyperimmune globulin may benefit select patients, and novel approaches such as adoptive immunotherapy are also being investigated.

Ganciclovir is currently approved for the treatment and long-term suppression of CMV retinitis in immunocompromised hosts and prevention of CMV disease in transplant recipients (Evidence Level I). However, it is widely used for the treatment of CMV infection and disease in the immunocompromised population (Evidence Level I). Both intravenous (IV) and oral formulations are available. An intraocular implant designed to deliver high concentrations of the drug into the vitreous of patients with CMV retinitis is also available. The most important adverse effect associated with GCV is bone marrow suppression. Dose-related neutropenia is the most consistent hematologic disturbance. It is reversible in most patients within a week of cessation of therapy.

Table 26-2. Antivirals for the Treatment of Cytomegaloviral Infection and Disease

Antiviral (Brand Name)	Drug Class/ Year of Approval	Approved Indication		Potential Adverse Effects
GCV (Cytovene)	Nucleoside analogue 1989	*Treatment*	CMV retinitis in immuno-compromised patients	Bone marrow suppression
		Prevention/ prophylaxis	CMV disease in transplant recipients	
VGCV (Valcyte)	Nucleoside analogue 2001 2003 2009	*Treatment*	CMV retinitis in patients with AIDS	Bone marrow suppression
		Prevention	CMV disease in high-risk kidney, heart, or kidney/ pancreas transplant recipients	
		Pediatric indication	Prevention of CMV disease in pediatric kidney and heart transplant patients aged 4 mo–16 y	
FOS (Foscavir)	Pyrophosphate analogue 1991	*Treatment*	CMV retinitis in patients with AIDS	Nephrotoxicity, electrolyte abnormalities
CDV (Vistide)	Acyclic nucleoside analogue 1996	*Treatment*	CMV retinitis in patients with AIDS	Nephrotoxicity

Abbreviations: CDV, cidofovir; CMV, cytomegalovirus; FOS, foscarnet; GCV, ganciclovir; VGCV, valganciclovir.

Adapted from Ahmed A. Antiviral treatment of cytomegalovirus infection. *Infect Disord Drug Targets.* 2011;11(5):475–503, with permission.

Valganciclovir is the oral prodrug of GCV, and its mechanism of action and safety profile is similar to that of GCV. With its significantly higher bioavailability and more convenient dosing schedule, oral VGCV has largely replaced oral GCV for the prevention of CMV infection and is commonly used in clinical practice in place of IV GCV. Valganciclovir is approved for the treatment of AIDS-related CMV retinitis. Valganciclovir is approved for the prevention of CMV infection and disease in high-risk kidney, kidney/pancreas, and heart transplant recipients. The notable exception is liver transplant recipients, in whom a significantly higher rate of disease occurred among those receiving VGCV compared with GCV. In practice, however, VGCV is the most commonly used antiviral for prophylaxis of all types of SOT recipients.

Cidofovir is highly active against CMV but, because of its potential for severe nephrotoxicity, remains a second-line treatment for CMV. Foscarnet is a pyrophosphate analog that is a noncompetitive inhibitor of viral DNA polymerase. It is indicated for the treatment of CMV retinitis in AIDS patients. The major adverse effects associated with FOS include nephrotoxicity and biochemical derangements, including hypocalcemia. Because of the unfavorable safety profiles, both drugs are reserved for second-line treatment of CMV infection or patients with failing treatment due to GCV-resistant strains.

There is currently no standard for treatment of congenital CMV infection. The Collaborative Antiviral Study Group demonstrated that 6 weeks of IV GCV treatment prevented best-ear hearing deterioration in children with congenital CMV disease involving the CNS, including microcephaly, intracranial calcification, abnormal CSF indices for age, chorioretinitis, and hearing deficits. Although treatment of neonates with symptomatic CMV infection appears to be beneficial (Evidence Level I), an expert panel cautions against GCV treatment of patients with milder disease than those included in the clinical trial (Evidence Level III). The decision to administer antiviral therapy to neonates with symptomatic congenital CMV disease thus remains at the discretion of the clinician. Ganciclovir is not recommended for the treatment of asymptomatic neonates with congenital CMV infection because of the significant risk of neutropenia and potential for carcinogenesis (Evidence Level III). More recent data suggest that treatment of neonates with 6 months of oral VGCV results in preserved normal hearing or improved hearing at 12 and 24 months of age more frequently than 6 weeks of VGCV; neurodevelopmental outcomes are also better in the longer treatment arm (Evidence Level III).

Children with congenital CMV infection should undergo regular evaluations for early detection and intervention. Cognitive deficits can be predicted by the presence of microcephaly or intracranial calcifications, both of which are associated with moderate to severe dysfunction. Infants with chorioretinitis should be monitored by ophthalmologic evaluations.

The treatment of CMV disease in patients with HIV has historically been directed toward CMV retinitis. Recommendations for the treatment and prevention of CMV disease in adolescents and adults with HIV have been published by the Centers for Disease Control and Prevention. Treatment is individualized on the basis of severity of disease and degree of immunosuppression. Oral VGCV, IV GCV followed by oral VGCV, FOS, and CDV are all effective treatments for CMV retinitis (Evidence Level I). Intravenous GCV or oral VGCV may be used along with intraocular GCV implants for sight-threatening disease. For patients not receiving cART, consideration should be given to initiating antiretroviral therapy. Although maintenance therapy with GCV was previously recommended indefinitely, in the era of cART, it may be discontinued once immune recovery is achieved (Evidence Level II-1).

There has been a significant decline in CMV-associated disease among SOT recipients. For the treatment of disease, IV GCV is recommended with oral VGCV as an option in nonsevere disease (Evidence Level I). For the treatment of CMV disease in children with severe or life-threatening disease, IV GCV is recommended (Evidence Level II-2). Valganciclovir may be used in nonsevere disease (Evidence Level III), but the dosing must be extrapolated for children.

Prevention of disease may be accomplished using either prophylaxis or preemptive treatment, but prophylaxis is generally recommended for pediatric patients, especially those at highest risk. Duration of prophylaxis varies by organ type, risk stratification, and institutional practice, but is typically 3 to 6 months. Once the threshold value is reached, treatment doses of IV GCV or VGCV should be started and continued until 1 or 2 negative test results are obtained (Evidence Level III). Testing while on treatment is usually conducted once or twice per week.

The treatment of end-organ disease caused by CMV in HSCT recipients is difficult, and morbidity and mortality remain significant. Intravenous GCV is usually used for induction for 2 to 3 weeks followed by maintenance therapy with either GCV or VGCV for a period of time based on clinical improvement and decline of viremia. Alternative agents such as CDV or FOS may be used to avoid the bone marrow suppression associated with GCV and VGCV. For pneumonitis, IV immune globulin or CMV hyperimmune globulin may be added for improved outcome (Evidence Level III).

Recommendations for the prevention of CMV disease among HSCT recipients have been provided by the American Society for Blood and Marrow Transplantation. As described for SOT, either the prophylaxis or preemptive therapy strategy may be used for all at-risk HSCT based on host factors and the laboratory support available. For prophylaxis, IV GCV is recommended from engraftment to 100 days after transplantation (Evidence Level I). Patients should be monitored for neutropenia and other evidence of bone marrow suppression. For preemptive therapy, once infection is identified by viremia or antigenemia, patients are treated with IV GCV twice daily for 1 to 2 weeks followed by maintenance therapy once daily until CMV is undetectable for several weeks (Evidence Level I). Although most data on the efficacy of these regimens are based on adult studies, the same strategies are generally extrapolated for use in children. Antiviral prophylaxis and preemptive therapy have both been effective in decreasing the incidence of CMV disease among HSCT recipients.

Suggested Reading

Ahmed A. Antiviral treatment of cytomegalovirus infection. *Infect Disord Drug Targets.* 2011;11(5):475–503

American Academy of Pediatrics. Cytomegalovirus infection. In: Kimberlin DW, Brady MT, Jackson MA, Long SS, eds. *Red Book: 2015 Report of the Committee of Infectious Diseases.* 30th ed. Elk Grove Village, IL; American Academy of Pediatrics; 2015: 317–322

American Academy of Pediatrics, Joint Committee on Infant Hearing. Year 2007 position statement: principles and guidelines for early hearing detection and intervention programs. *Pediatrics.* 2007;120(4):898–921

Elliott SP. Congenital cytomegalovirus infection: an overview. *Infect Disord Drug Targets.* 2011;11(5):432–436

Kotton CN, Kumar D, Caliendo AM, et al; Transplantation Society International CMV Consensus Group. International consensus guidelines on the management of cytomegalovirus in solid organ transplantation. *Transplantation.* 2010;89(7):779–795

Kotton CN. CMV: prevention, diagnosis and therapy. *Am J Transplant.* 2013;13(Suppl 3): 24–40

Luck S, Sharland M. Postnatal cytomegalovirus: innocent bystander or hidden problem? *Arch Dis Child Fetal Neonatal Ed.* 2009;94(1):F58–F64

Plosa EJ, Esbenshade JC, Fuller MP, Weitkamp JH. Cytomegalovirus infection. *Pediatr Rev.* 2012;33(4):156–163

Rafailidis PI, Mourtzoukou EG, Varbobitis IC, Falagas ME. Severe cytomegalovirus infection in apparently immunocompetent patients: a systemic review. *Virol J.* 2008;(5):47

Russell MY, Palmer A, Michaels MG. Cytomegalovirus infection in pediatric immunocompromised hosts. *Infect Disord Drug Targets.* 2011;11(5):437–448

CHAPTER 27

Encephalitis

Jo-Ann S. Harris, MD, and Robert R. Wittler, MD

Key Points

- The diagnostic evaluation for all patients should include a lumbar puncture and magnetic resonance image of the brain.
- Further diagnostic testing depends on epidemiologic factors, clinical presentation and course, and cerebrospinal fluid and magnetic resonance imaging results.
- Acyclovir should be started in all patients, pending results of diagnostic studies.

Overview

Encephalitis means inflammation of the brain parenchyma and in a strict sense is a pathologic diagnosis made if there is tissue confirmation, either at autopsy or on brain biopsy. Pragmatically, encephalitis is diagnosed in most patients on the basis of presence of an inflammatory process of the brain in association with clinical evidence of neurologic dysfunction. Surrogate markers of brain inflammation include inflammatory cells in the cerebrospinal fluid (CSF) or changes on brain imaging consistent with inflammation. The classic neurologic feature is altered level of consciousness.

Inflammation of the brain parenchyma can be associated with a meningeal reaction, spinal cord inflammation (ie, myelitis), or nerve root involvement (eg, radiculitis), in which case the terms *meningoencephalitis, encephalomyelitis, meningoencephalomyelitis, myeloradiculitis,* and *meningo-encephaloradiculitis* are used. *Limbic encephalitis* refers to encephalitis of the temporal lobes and often of other limbic structures. *Rhombencephalitis* refers to encephalitis affecting the hindbrain (ie, brainstem and cerebellum).

Causes and Differential Diagnosis

Viral infections are the most commonly identified causes of acute encephalitis (Box 27-1). However, even with extensive diagnostic testing, the etiology of encephalitis in most patients is undetermined. Bacteria, fungi, protozoa, and

Box 27-1. Causes of Acute Viral Encephalitis

Sporadic (not geographically restricted)
- Herpesvirus
  HSV, VZV, CMV, EBV, HHV-6
- Picornavirus
  Coxsackievirus; echovirus; enteroviruses D68, 70, and 71; parechovirus; poliovirus
- Paramyxovirus
  Measles, mumps
- Others
  Influenza, parvovirus, adenovirus, LCMV, rubella, HIV, chikungunya

Geographically Restricted (mostly arthropod-borne[a])
- The Americas
  West Nile virus, La Crosse encephalitis, St. Louis encephalitis, Powassan virus, Western and Eastern equine encephalitis, Venezuelan equine encephalitis, Colorado tick fever, dengue, rabies
- Europe/Middle East
  Tick-borne encephalitis, West Nile, rabies
- Africa
  West Nile, Rift Valley fever, Crimean-Congo hemorrhagic fever, dengue, rabies
- Asia
  Japanese encephalitis, West Nile, dengue, Murray Valley encephalitis, Nipah, rabies
- Australasia
  Murray Valley encephalitis, Japanese encephalitis

Abbreviations: CMV, cytomegalovirus; EBV, Epstein-Barr virus; HHV-6, *Human herpesvirus 6;* HSV, herpes simplex virus; LCMV, lymphocytic choriomeningitis; VZV, varicella-zoster virus.
[a] All viruses are arthropod-borne, except for rabies and Nipah virus.

helminths are also important causes of encephalitis or encephalitis-like syndromes (Box 27-2). It is important to try to differentiate between infectious encephalitis and postinfectious or postimmunization encephalitis or encephalomyelitis (ADEM, acute disseminated encephalomyelitis), which is thought to be mediated by an immunologic response to a preceding infection or immunization. Noninfectious diseases (eg, collagen vascular diseases, vasculitis, and paraneoplastic syndromes) can have similar clinical presentations to infectious causes of encephalitis (Box 27-2).

On the basis of the California Encephalitis Project, anti-*N*-methyl-D-aspartate receptor encephalitis was the leading cause (32 of 79 cases) with enteroviruses identified in 30 patients, *Human herpesvirus 1* in 7 patients, and varicella-zoster and West Nile viruses in 5 patients each.

Box 27-2. Nonviral Infectious and Noninfectious Causes of Acute Encephalitis or Diseases That Mimic Encephalitis

Bacteria
- Meningitis
- Brain abscess
- Tuberculosis
- *Borrelia burgdorferi*
- *Bartonella henselae*
- *Mycoplasma pneumoniae*
- Listeriosis
- Parameningeal infection
- Rickettsiae, ehrlichiosis, anaplasmosis
- *Coxiella burnetii*

Fungi
- Meningitis
- Brain abscess

Parasites
- Cerebral malaria
- Primary amoebic meningoencephalitis (*Naegleria fowleri*, *Acanthamoeba* species, *Balamuthia mandrillaris*)
- Toxoplasmosis
- Cysticercosis
- Helminths (*Baylisascaris procyonis*, *Angiostrongylus/Gnathostoma* species)

Postinfectious/Postimmunization
- ADEM
- Acute necrotizing encephalopathy

Autoimmune
- Anti-NMDAR encephalitis
- Basal ganglia encephalitis
- Systemic lupus erythematosus

Neoplasia
- Primary brain tumor or metastatic
- Paraneoplastic limbic encephalitis

Metabolic
- Hypoglycemia
- Hepatic or renal encephalopathy
- Toxic encephalopathy (alcohol, drugs)

Abbreviations: ADEM, acute disseminated encephalomyelitis; NMDAR, *N*-methyl-D-aspartate receptor.

The clinical features of acute encephalitis overlap with acute meningitis—patients with either syndrome may present with fever, headache, and altered mental status—and both diagnoses need to be considered. A decreased CSF glucose concentration suggests a bacterial, fungal, or protozoal etiology. Encephalitis also needs to be distinguished from encephalopathy (eg, secondary to metabolic disorders, hypoxia, ischemia, drugs, toxins, or systemic infection), which is defined by a disruption of brain function in the absence of direct inflammation of the brain parenchyma. The absence of fever, a more gradual onset of symptoms, and lack of pleocytosis or absence of focal changes on brain imaging can usually differentiate metabolic and toxic causes of encephalopathy from encephalitis.

Clinical Features

Pathogenicity of the etiologic agent, severity of involvement, anatomic localization of affected portions of the nervous system, and immune reaction of the host all act to determine the clinical findings. Thus, a wide range of clinical findings exist based on etiology and host response, and there is a wide range of severity of clinical manifestations even with the same etiologic agent. Diffuse neurologic involvement can present with behavioral or personality changes, decreased consciousness, and generalized seizures. Focal seizures, hemiparesis, movement disorders, ataxia (ie, rhombencephalitis), and cranial nerve defects (ie, rhombencephalitis) are evidence of localized involvement. Limbic encephalitis symptoms include memory loss, temporal lobe seizures, movement disorders, and affective or psychiatric findings. Limbic encephalitis in adults is often a paraneoplastic process with autoantibodies, but in children and adolescents, tumors are less frequent.

The initial manifestations of encephalitis often resemble an acute systemic illness with fever, headache, or irritability. As the illness progresses, neurologic symptoms and signs become more prominent. Table 27-1 lists epidemiologic risk factors, and Table 27-2 clinical findings associated with specific etiologies.

Diagnosis

Early identification of the etiology can have a major effect on both management and prognosis. In addition, identification of a specific etiologic agent, if possible, is important for potential prophylaxis, counseling of patients and families, and public health interventions. After initial stabilization of the cardiorespiratory status and control of any seizure activity, the evaluation should include a thorough history and physical examination, initial laboratory tests, lumbar puncture, neuroimaging, and electroencephalography.

The history and physical examinations can provide important epidemiologic clues in establishing the diagnosis. Often the patient is unable to answer questions because of age or altered consciousness, and the information must be obtained from parents, caregivers, or relatives. Prevalence of disease in the local community, ill contacts, travel history, social history, recreational activities (eg, freshwater swimming), toxin exposure, insect or animal contacts, vaccination history and timing, and history of recent infectious illness can help elucidate the cause. History of rash, cold sores, or stomatitis may also be helpful. The physical examination should include a careful neurologic examination including mental status, motor, sensory, cranial nerve, cerebellar, and reflex

Table 27-1. Possible Etiologies of Encephalitis Based on Epidemiology and Risk Factors

Risk Factor	Possible Etiology
Neonate	HSV, CMV, parechovirus, enterovirus, *Listeria monocytogenes*, toxoplasmosis, syphilis, rubella
Agammaglobulinemia	Enterovirus, *Mycoplasma pneumoniae*
Animal contact	
Bats	Rabies, Nipah virus
Cats	*Bartonella henselae*, toxoplasmosis, rabies, *Coxiella burnetii*
Raccoons	Rabies, *Baylisascaris procyonis*
Rodents	LCMV
Sheep and goats	*Coxiella burnetii*
Skunks	Rabies
Immunocompromised	VZV, CMV, HHV-6, *L monocytogenes*, *Mycobacterium tuberculosis*, toxoplasmosis, HIV
Ingestion items	
Raw or partially cooked meat	Toxoplasmosis
Unpasteurized milk	*L monocytogenes, C burnetii*
Insect contact	
Mosquitoes	West Nile virus, St. Louis encephalitis, La Crosse encephalitis, Eastern equine encephalitis, Western equine encephalitis, Venezuelan equine encephalitis, Japanese encephalitis, Murray Valley encephalitis, *Plasmodium falciparum*
Ticks	Tick-borne encephalitis, Powassan virus, *Rickettsia rickettsii, Ehrlichia chaffeensis, Anaplasma phagocytophilum, Borrelia burgdorferi*
Recent infection or vaccination	ADEM
Recreational activities	
Camping/hunting	All agents transmitted by mosquitoes and ticks
Spelunking	Rabies, *Histoplasma capsulatum*
Swimming/hot tubs	Enterovirus, *Naegleria fowleri, Acanthamoeba* species
Season	
Summer/fall	All agents transmitted by mosquitoes and ticks, enterovirus
Winter	Influenza
Soil contact	*Balamuthia mandrillaris*
Unvaccinated	VZV, influenza, measles, mumps, rubella, polio, Japanese encephalitis

Abbreviations: ADEM, acute disseminated encephalomyelitis; CMV, cytomegalovirus; HHV-6, *Human herpesvirus 6*; HSV, herpes simplex virus; LCMV, lymphocytic choriomeningitis virus; VZV, varicella-zoster virus.

Adapted from Tunkel AR, Glaser CA, Bloch KC, et al. The management of encephalitis: clinical practice guidelines by the Infectious Diseases Society of America. *Clin Infect Dis*. 2008;47(3):303–327, with permission from Oxford University Press.

Table 27-2. Possible Etiologies of Encephalitis Based on Clinical Findings

Clinical Presentation	Possible Etiology
General Findings	
Eosinophilia	Parasites
Hepatitis	*Coxiella burnetii,* EBV
Hypoglycemia, hyperammonemia, metabolic acidosis	Metabolic encephalopathy, toxic ingestion
Lymphadenopathy	EBV, CMV, *Bartonella henselae,* West Nile virus, toxoplasmosis, *Mycobacterium tuberculosis,* measles, rubella
Parotitis	Mumps
Rash	VZV, HHV-6, enterovirus, West Nile virus, *Rickettsia rickettsii, Mycoplasma pneumoniae, Borrelia burgdorferi, Ehrlichia chaffeensis, Anaplasma phagocytophilum*
Respiratory tract findings	Influenza, adenovirus, *M pneumoniae, M tuberculosis, Histoplasma capsulatum, C burnetii,* Venezuelan equine encephalitis, Nipah virus
Retinitis	CMV, *B henselae,* toxoplasmosis, West Nile virus, syphilis
Syndrome of inappropriate antidiuretic hormone	St. Louis encephalitis, HSV
Thrombocytopenia	Ehrlichiosis, rickettsiae
Neurologic Findings	
Cerebellar ataxia	VZV, EBV, mumps, St. Louis encephalitis, ADEM
Cranial nerve abnormalities	HSV, EBV, *Listeria monocytogenes, M tuberculosis, B burgdorferi, Balamuthia mandrillaris*
Intracranial calcifications	Congenital CMV, congenital toxoplasmosis
Movement disorders	Anti–*N*-methyl-ᴅ-aspartate receptor encephalitis, West Nile virus, Japanese encephalitis
Poliomyelitis-like flaccid paralysis	Enteroviruses (enterovirus 71, D68), West Nile virus, Japanese encephalitis, tick-borne encephalitis
Psychiatric symptoms	Anti–*N*-methyl-ᴅ-aspartate receptor encephalitis, rabies
Rhombencephalitis	HSV, West Nile virus, enterovirus 71, *L monocytogenes, M tuberculosis,* HHV-6, EBV
Space-occupying unifocal or multifocal ring-enhancing lesions on neuroimaging	Pyogenic abscess, fungal, *M tuberculosis, L monocytogenes,* neurocysticercosis, toxoplasmosis, amebic encephalitis
Multiple white matter lesions on neuroimaging	Acute disseminated meningoencephalitis

Abbreviations: ADEM, acute disseminated encephalomyelitis; CMV, cytomegalovirus; EBV, Epstein-Barr virus; HHV-6, *Human herpesvirus 6*; HSV, herpes simplex virus; VZV, varicella-zoster virus.

Adapted from Tunkel AR, Glaser CA, Bloch KC, et al. The management of encephalitis: clinical practice guidelines by the Infectious Diseases Society of America. *Clin Infect Dis.* 2008;47(3):303–327, with permission from Oxford University Press.

function. Other parts of the physical examination can suggest an etiologic agent, such as vesicular or maculopapular rash, lesions of hand-foot-and-mouth disease, and rash of Rocky Mountain spotted fever.

Laboratory and neuroimaging evaluations can also provide clues to the etiology and support the clinical diagnosis. Certain laboratory tests should be done on all patients with suspected encephalitis, but other tests are indicated only if there are consistent clinical or epidemiologic findings (eg, geographic location, season, exposure). Box 27-3 outlines the initial diagnostic evaluation for patients with encephalitis. Lumbar puncture should be performed in all patients unless contraindicated. This is usually done after neuroimaging to rule out mass lesion or shift in intracranial structures if indicated. Cerebrospinal fluid indices in patients with viral encephalitis can be similar to those in patients with viral meningitis and meningoencephalitis and overlap with bacterial meningitis. Characteristic CSF findings in viral encephalitis include pleocytosis (white blood cell [WBC] count ranges 0–500/mcL with a predominance of lymphocytes). Red blood cells are usually absent, and protein concentration is usually elevated. Glucose concentration is usually normal and greater than 50% of blood value. A decreased CSF glucose concentration suggests a bacterial, fungal, or protozoal etiology. In the California Encephalitis Project, patients with cases caused by viral and bacterial agents had a wide range of CSF WBC counts and protein concentrations, as did patients with cases caused by noninfectious etiologies. Patients with infectious encephalitis had significantly higher CSF WBC count compared to patients with noninfectious encephalitis (median CSF WBC count: 53.5 versus 9.5/mcL), but the difference in protein concentrations was not significant. It has been shown that 3% to 5% of patients with encephalitis have CSF findings that are completely normal.

Neuroimaging studies are useful in detection of early changes of encephalitis and can exclude other conditions with a clinical presentation similar to that of encephalitis, such as ADEM. Sedation for neuroimaging may be contraindicated, so consider contacting an anesthesiologist for general anesthetic if necessary. Some characteristic neuroimaging patterns are observed in patients with specific agents, such as herpes simplex virus (HSV) encephalitis, which can show significant edema and hemorrhage in the temporal lobes. Magnetic resonance imaging is the modality of choice because it is more sensitive and specific than computed tomography. Table 27.2 gives examples of clinical, laboratory, and neuroimaging clues to identifying the cause of encephalitis. Electroencephalogram (EEG) is a sensitive indicator of cerebral dysfunction and can be helpful in suggesting a specific agent, such as HSV. The EEG in HSV may show a temporal focus demonstrating periodic lateralizing epileptiform discharges. The EEG also has a role in identifying nonconvulsive seizure activity in patients with altered mental status.

Brain biopsy is rarely used today to establish the etiology of encephalitis. It is not routinely recommended. It may have a limited role and should be considered in cases of encephalitis of unknown etiology that deteriorate despite treatment with acyclovir. In some patients, definitive diagnosis can be

Box 27-3. Initial Diagnostic Evaluation for Patients With Encephalitis

General Studies
- CBC with differential analysis
- Renal function tests
- Serum hepatic enzyme
- Blood culture
- Coagulation studies
- Chest radiograph
- Ophthalmologic examination

Lumbar Puncture
- Opening pressure (when feasible)
- CSF WBC count with differential, protein, glucose, Gram stain, acid-fast stain
- Culture for bacteria
- PCR for HSV and other Herpesviridae (HHV-6, CMV, VZV)
- PCR for enterovirus
- PCR for parechovirus, influenza, West Nile virus, *Mycoplasma pneumoniae*, and other pathogens as indicated by history and epidemiology
- West Nile virus IgM and IgG, NMDAR antibody, specific arbovirus IgM and IgG (seasonal and geographic)
- Culture for fungus
- Culture for *Mycobacterium* (PCR is insensitive) if clinically indicated
- Cryptococcal antigen, *Histoplasma* antigen if clinically indicated
- *Toxoplasma gondii* PCR if clinically indicated
- CSF sample to hold for subsequent testing

Serum for Antibody
- Arbovirus (seasonal and geographic)
- EBV, CMV
- HIV
- *Bartonella henselae, M pneumoniae*
- Tick-borne pathogens based on season and geographic distribution
- Anti-NMDAR
- Acute serum to hold

Respiratory Secretions
- PCR or rapid test on respiratory tract specimen for enterovirus and influenza
- Viral culture on throat swab for HSV, enterovirus

Stool or Rectal Swab
- Viral culture of stool
- Enterovirus PCR

Urine
- Urinalysis
- Toxicology screening

Skin Lesions (if present)
- Biopsy for DFA and PCR for *Rickettsia rickettsii*
- Culture or PCR or DFA of skin lesions for HSV, VZV, and enterovirus

Neuroimaging
- Computed tomography
- Magnetic resonance imaging
- Electroencephalogram

Abbreviations: CBC, complete blood cell count; CMV, cytomegalovirus; CSF, cerebrospinal fluid; DFA, direct fluorescence assay; EBV, Epstein-Barr virus; HHV-6, *Human herpesvirus 6;* HSV, herpes simplex virus; NMDAR, *N*-methyl-D-aspartate receptor; PCR, polymerase chain reaction; VZV, varicella-zoster virus; WBC, white blood cell.

Adapted from Glaser C, Long SS. Encephalitis. In: Long SS, Pickering LK, Prober CG, eds. *Principles and Practice of Pediatric Infectious Diseases*. 4th ed. Philadelphia, PA: Elsevier Saunders; 2012:297–314, with permission.

established only by brain biopsy, but this has become uncommon with the routine use of magnetic resonance imaging and availability of diagnostic polymerase chain reaction and antibody assays.

Management

Encephalitis can be an acute life-threatening emergency that requires prompt intervention. Depending on how severely the patient is affected, intensive care may be required. Focus of the initial evaluation and management should be on treatable and common causes of encephalitis as well as supportive care. Box 27-4 lists the treatable or possibly treatable infectious and noninfectious causes of acute encephalitis-like syndromes.

Box 27-4. Selected Treatable or Possibly Treatable Infectious and Noninfectious Causes of Acute Encephalitis-like Syndromes

Infectious Causes

- **Viruses**
  - Herpesviridae
    - o HSV
    - o VZV
    - o CMV
    - o HHV-6
  - Influenza
  - HIV
  - Nipah
  - Rabies
- **Bacteria**
  - Meningitis
  - Brain abscess
  - *Listeria monocytogenes*
  - *Mycobacterium tuberculosis*
  - *Borrelia burgdorferi*
  - Bacterial toxins
  - *Rickettsia/Ehrlichia/Anaplasma* spp
  - *Mycoplasma pneumoniae*

- **Fungi**
  - Meningitis/brain abscess
- **Parasites**
  - *Toxoplasma gondii*
  - *Plasmodium* spp
  - Cysticercosis
  - Ameba
  - *Naegleria fowleri*
  - *Acanthamoeba* spp
  - *Balamuthia mandrillaris*

Noninfectious Causes

- **Parainfectious and autoimmune**
  - ADEM
  - Acute necrotizing encephalopathy
  - NMDAR encephalitis

- **Neoplasia**
- **Cerebrovascular**

Abbreviations: ADEM, acute disseminated encephalomyelitis; CMV, cytomegalovirus; HHV-6, *Human herpesvirus 6*; HSV, herpes simplex virus; NMDAR, *N*-methyl-D-aspartate receptor; spp, species; VZV, varicella-zoster virus.

Immediate management needs to focus on establishing hemodynamic stability, electrolyte and glucose normalization, and control of intracranial hypertension and seizures. Rapid assessment and management of increased intracranial pressure is critical to reduce cerebral edema, diminish cerebral anoxia, and minimize secondary brain injury. It is important to anticipate and be prepared for complications such as hyperthermia, inadequate respiratory exchange, fluid and electrolyte imbalance, aspiration and asphyxia, abrupt cardiac and respiratory arrest of central origin, cardiac decompensation, and gastrointestinal bleeding. Syndrome of disseminated intravascular coagulation can occur as well. Patients should be placed in appropriate infection control–based isolation precautions according to clinical and epidemiologic information. Consultation with neurology and infectious disease services may be helpful.

Empiric antimicrobial therapy should be started as early as possible. Appropriate treatment for bacterial meningitis, such as vancomycin and a third-generation cephalosporin, should be started if clinically indicated since the clinical presentation may overlap with encephalitis (Evidence Level III). If *Listeria* infection is suspected, the addition of ampicillin should be considered. Acyclovir should be initiated in all patients with suspected encephalitis as soon as possible pending the results of diagnostic studies because the earlier the treatment for HSV, the less likely that death or serious sequelae will result (Evidence Level III). In patients with clinical clues suggestive of rickettsial or ehrlichial infection, doxycycline should be added to empiric treatment regimens (Evidence Level III). Other empiric therapy may be indicated for other infectious causes of encephalitis suspected on the basis of clinical or epidemiologic information. An example would be to treat for influenza as indicated with oseltamivir (or appropriate antiviral based on influenza virus susceptibility data) during influenza season (Evidence Level III). A strategy for empiric therapy based on evaluation of CSF is shown in Figure 27-1.

Following the identification of a particular etiologic agent or noninfectious cause in a patient with encephalitis, appropriate antimicrobial therapy or other management should be initiated. Anti–*N*-methyl-D-aspartate receptor when identified is important, because it is a predominant cause of noninfectious encephalitis. Immunotherapy (corticosteroids, intravenous immune globulin, plasma exchange, or a combination of those) and removal of the tumor, if present, has been associated with improved outcome. In patients with ADEM, corticosteroids are recommended as initial therapy with intravenous immune globulin or plasma exchange used for patients who fail to respond adequately to corticosteroids. Suggested initial therapies for selected agents that cause encephalitis are presented in Table 27-3.

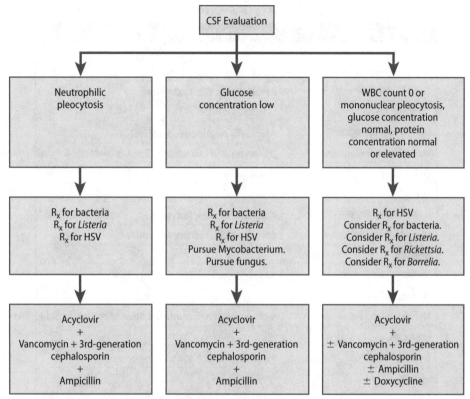

Figure 27-1. Strategy for empiric therapy based on cerebrospinal fluid evaluation.

Abbreviations: CSF, cerebrospinal fluid; HSV, herpes simplex virus; R_x, prescription; WBC, white blood cell.

Adapted from Long SS. Encephalitis diagnosis and management in the real world. In: Curtis N, Finn A, Pollard AJ, eds. *Advances in Experimental Medicine and Biology.* Vol 697. New York, NY: Springer; 2010:153–173, with permission.

Table 27-3. Suggested Initial Therapy for Selected Agents That Cause Encephalitis

Agent	Specific Therapy
Bacteria	
Borrelia burgdorferi	Ceftriaxone or cefotaxime
Coccidioides spp	Amphotericin B or fluconazole
Ehrlichia spp	Doxycycline
Listeria monocytogenes	Ampicillin + gentamicin; TMP/SMX
Mycoplasma pneumoniae	Doxycycline or macrolide or fluoroquinolone
Rickettsia spp	Doxycycline
Fungi	
Cryptococcus neoformans	Amphotericin B + flucytosine
Histoplasma capsulatum	Amphotericin B liposomal complex
Helminths	
Taenia solium (cysticercosis)	Albendazole + corticosteroids
Mycobacteria	
Mycobacterium tuberculosis	4-drug regimen (Consider addition of corticosteroid.)
Protozoa	
Toxoplasma gondii	Pyrimethamine + sulfadiazine or clindamycin
Viruses	
CMV	Ganciclovir or valganciclovir or foscarnet
Influenza A and B	Oseltamivir
HSV	Acyclovir
VZV	Acyclovir
HIV	cART

Abbreviations: cART, combination antiretroviral therapy; CMV, cytomegalovirus; EBV, Epstein-Barr virus; HSV, herpes simplex virus; spp, species; TMP/SMX, trimethoprim/sulfamethoxazole; VZV, varicella zoster virus.

Outcome and Long-term Monitoring

There are limited data on the long-term outcomes in children with encephalitis. Effects on the central nervous system may include intellectual, motor, psychiatric, epileptic, visual, or auditory sequelae. The short- and long-term outcomes depend in part on the etiologic agent, findings at the time of presentation, and age of the child. Rabies and *Naegleria fowleri,* for example, are known to have almost 100% mortality. Young infants usually have a worse prognosis than older children. Coma, convulsions, intensive care, or focal neurologic findings in the early phase of encephalitis are associated with worse outcomes. Herpes simplex virus encephalitis is the best studied and has a worse prognosis for survival and residual morbidity than enteroviruses. In a 12-year prospective study, children with HSV encephalitis had some form of neurologic debility in 63% of cases. For self-limited cases, it can take up to 1 year for complete recovery.

Long-term sequelae may not be identified in the acute phase of illness. Once the patient is discharged from the hospital, monitoring should continue for at least 1 year, including supportive care and rehabilitation, the extent of which depends on neurologic debility. Hearing evaluation should be performed at the time of discharge or soon after. Monitoring throughout childhood should include developmental assessments on a regular basis because these children are at risk for developmental or intellectual disability. Neuropsychological testing may be helpful as well, especially when developing an education plan for the child.

Suggested Reading

Bale JE. Virus and immune-mediated encephalitides: epidemiology, diagnosis, treatment, and prevention. *Pediatr Neurol.* 2015;53(1):3–12

Espositio S, Di Petro GM, Madini B, et al. A spectrum of inflammation and demyelination in acute disseminated encephalomyelitis (ADEM) in children. *Autoimmun Rev.* 2015;14(10):923–929

Gable MS, Sheriff H, Dalmau J, Tilley DH, Glaser CA. The frequency of autoimmune N-methyl-D-aspartate receptor encephalitis surpasses that of individual viral etiologies in young individuals enrolled in the California encephalitis project. *Clin Infect Dis.* 2012;54(7):899–904

Glaser CA, Honarmand S, Anderson LJ, et al. Beyond viruses: clinical profiles and etiologies associated with encephalitis. *Clin Infect Dis.* 2006;43(12):1565–1577

Long SS. Encephalitis diagnosis and management in the real world. In: Curtis N, Finn A, Pollard AJ, eds. *Advances in Experimental Medicine and Biology.* Vol 697. New York, NY: Springer; 2010:153–173

Ramanathan S, Mohammad SS, Brilot F, Dale RC. Autoimmune encephalitis: recent updates and emerging challenges. *J Clin Neurosci.* 2014;21(5):722–730

Thompson C, Kneen R, Riordan A, Kelly D, Pollard AJ. Encephalitis in children. *Arch Dis Child.* 2012;97(2):150–161

Tunkel AR, Glaser CA, Bloch KC, et al. The management of encephalitis: clinical practice guidelines by the Infectious Diseases Society of America. *Clin Infect Dis.* 2008;47(3):303–327

CHAPTER 28

Enteroviruses and Parechoviruses

José R. Romero, MD

Key Points

- Non-polio enteroviruses are common causes for nonspecific febrile illnesses in children and are implicated in common clinical syndromes (eg, coxsackievirus-associated hand-foot-and-mouth disease, summer aseptic meningitis).

- Life-threatening illness may follow infection in neonates, and the disease may mimic neonatal herpes simplex virus infection.

- Those with immunodeficiencies, both humeral and combined, may present with chronic central nervous system infection, a dermatomyositis-type illness, or disseminated infection.

- Polymerase chain reaction tests are helpful to confirm infection and may shorten duration of hospitalization for those with meningitis.

- Supportive care is generally recommended.

Overview

Non-polio enterovirus (EV) is a frequent pathogen in the pediatric population, and diverse clinical manifestations are notable, though some specific serotypes are associated with distinct clinical disease. Parechovirus (PeV) (typically presenting in late spring to summer) also appears to cause infection similar to EV (typically presenting in summer to early fall) during childhood. Most infections caused by members of the 2 genera occur in children younger than 5 years and, in particular, younger than 2.

Because of effective vaccination programs, poliovirus (PV) no longer circulates endogenously in the United States and most of the world.

Causes and Differential Diagnosis

Enteroviral and parechoviral infection in neonates may present similarly and mimic bacterial sepsis or infection caused by herpes simplex virus. In older children, the exanthema of hand-foot-and-mouth disease (coxsackievirus A16) may mimic chickenpox, herpes simplex virus, or eczema herpeticum. Other EV rashes are nonspecific, and drug hypersensitivity reaction and other viral exanthems should be included in the differential diagnosis. Included in the differential diagnosis of EV meningitis is Lyme disease, bacterial meningitis, and, rarely, drug-induced meningitis. In patients with myocarditis, other pathogens that may be considered in the differential diagnosis include adenovirus (most commonly types 2 and 5), cytomegalovirus, Epstein-Barr virus, hepatitis C virus, herpesvirus, HIV, influenza and parainfluenza viruses, measles, mumps (associated with endocardial fibroelastosis), *Human parvovirus B19,* rubella, and varicella. Other causes of cardiac dysfunction should be considered, including anatomic lesions (eg, aortic stenosis, anomalous coronary artery) and cardiomyopathies, including metabolic ones (eg, glycogen storage disease).

Clinical Features

Most EV and PeV infections are clinically silent.

Enteroviruses

Undifferentiated Febrile Illness

Febrile illness without an apparent focus of infection is a common symptomatic outcome of EV infection. The onset is abrupt with fever in association with any of the following findings alone or in combination: poor feeding, lethargy, irritability, vomiting, diarrhea, upper respiratory tract symptoms, or exanthems. Abdominal pain may be a concern in older children. Physical findings may be absent or minimal, consisting of mild pharyngeal and conjunctival injection, lymphadenopathy, and exanthems. The illness typically lasts less than 5 days.

Meningitis

The onset of EV meningitis is abrupt with fever in association with nonspecific symptoms such as vomiting, anorexia, rash, diarrhea, cough, sore throat, upper respiratory tract findings, and myalgias. In some, the fever may have a biphasic presentation. Nuchal rigidity is found in greater than 50% of children older than 2 years, but is uncommon in young infants. Headache is nearly universal in patients old enough to report it. Photophobia may be reported in older children. Neurologic abnormalities are seen in 10% or less of patients. These include febrile and nonfebrile seizures, syndrome of inappropriate antidiuretic hormone, coma, and increased intracranial pressure. Duration of the illness is usually less than 1 week in infants and children. However, in adolescents complete recovery may take up to 2.5 weeks.

Encephalitis

Enterovirus can cause nonfocal encephalitis. A prodrome of fever, myalgias, upper respiratory tract symptoms, vomiting, or diarrhea may precede the abrupt onset of central nervous system (CNS) symptoms. The latter may include headache, confusion, irritability, weakness, lethargy, and somnolence.

Progression to generalized seizures or coma may occur. In some children, focal seizures may develop that mimic those seen in herpes simplex encephalitis. Other reported focal neurologic findings include hemiplegia, hemichorea, and paresthesia. Physical findings are few and only sporadically observed and may include exanthems, meningeal signs, signs of increased intracranial pressure, apnea, truncal ataxia, cranial nerve abnormalities, and paralysis.

No individual EV serotype is associated with a unique encephalitic syndrome that sets it apart from the other serotypes with the exception of EV-A71. Infection with this serotype can result in a severe rhombencephalitis. The illness is characteristically biphasic, initially presenting with hand-foot-and-mouth disease or herpangina (both discussed below) followed by myoclonus, the principle CNS finding. Additional CNS findings include tremor, ataxia, cranial nerve involvement, and cardiopulmonary failure secondary to the development of neurogenic pulmonary edema. Morbidity and mortality of EV-A71 rhombencephalitis can be substantial. Rarely, other EV serotypes have been reported to cause rhombencephalitis.

Acute Flaccid Paralysis (Poliomyelitis)

Seventy-two percent of PV infections are subclinical in nature. Twenty-four percent of infections result in a nonspecific minor illness or abortive poliomyelitis characterized by fever, fatigue, headache, anorexia, myalgias, and sore throat, followed by complete recovery. Onset of major illness involving the CNS may be abrupt and follow flu-like minor illness. Meningitis, indistinguishable from that due to non-polio EV, also known as nonparalytic poliomyelitis, occurs with a frequency of 5%. A biphasic pattern of fever is seen in approximately one-third of children.

Less than 0.1% of PV infections under non-epidemic conditions and only 1% to 2% of infections during epidemics result in paralysis. Onset of paralysis is often preceded by severe myalgias, most commonly localized to the lower back and involved limbs. Hyperesthesias and paresthesias may be observed in the same muscle groups. Soreness and stiffness of the neck and back may be prominent. Development of weakness or paralysis is preceded by loss of superficial and tendon reflexes of the involved muscles. Paralysis appears 1 to 2 days after the onset of myalgias. It is typically asymmetric and flaccid and affects the proximal muscles. If the motor cortex is involved, the paralysis is spastic in nature. Single limb involvement commonly occurs. Respiratory failure can result from paralysis of muscles of the diaphragm. Progressive bulbar palsy can result from cranial nerve involvement, leading to difficulties in speech, swallowing, breathing, and eye and facial muscle movement. Involvement of the brainstem centers controlling respiration and vasomotor function can be potentially fatal.

Acute flaccid paralysis (AFP) may also occasionally be seen with infections caused by EV serotypes other than PV. Fever is usually absent at onset of the paralysis, and it tends to be milder. The upper extremities and face are more frequently affected.

Chronic Enteroviral Meningoencephalitis

In children with inherited or acquired humoral immunodeficiencies, EV can cause chronic CNS (or systemic) infection. This syndrome or variants have been described in patients with inherited mixed humoral and cellular immunodeficiencies, patients receiving chemotherapy or immunomodulatory therapy, or those undergoing bone marrow and solid organ transplantation. In children with X-linked agammaglobulinemia, the initial symptoms consist of persistent headache and lethargy. As the syndrome progresses, ataxia, loss of cognitive skills and memory, dementia, emotional lability, paresthesias, weakness, dysarthria, and seizures develop. In addition, non-neurologic manifestations may include a dermatomyositis-like syndrome, edema, exanthems, and hepatitis.

Other CNS syndromes that have been associated with EV are meningitis, encephalitis, febrile seizures, cerebellar ataxia, transverse myelitis, and Guillain-Barré syndrome. However, the association of some syndromes with EV infection causes difficulty in distinguishing the causality of a throat or stool isolate from coincidental shedding.

Myocarditis, Pericarditis, and Myopericarditis

Enterovirus is among the most frequent identifiable causes of viral myocarditis. History of a cold-like upper respiratory tract infection preceding the onset of cardiac signs and symptoms is frequently obtained. Patients often have fever if they present in the acute phase of infection. Cardiovascular symptoms can include palpitations, chest pain, and shortness of breath. Arrhythmias or sudden death may result from involvement of the cardiac conduction system. Patients with extensive cardiac involvement may have age-related signs and symptoms of congestive heart failure. In patients with pericarditis or myopericarditis, a pericardial friction rub may be auscultated.

While most patients recover uneventfully from clinically apparent myocarditis, many have residual electrocardiographic or echocardiographic abnormalities for months to years. Smaller percentages of patients develop congestive heart failure, chronic myocarditis, or dilated cardiomyopathy. Heart failure, chest pain, or arrhythmias may be the presenting signs in patients with dilated cardiomyopathy. Physical examination may reveal findings of mitral insufficiency, cardiomegaly, and congestive failure.

Exanthems and Hand-Foot-and-Mouth Disease

Enteroviral infections can result in a wide array of rashes. Any EV serotype is capable of causing several different types of rash, and no serotype is associated with a unique exanthem. Rashes are more frequently seen in individuals 15 years and younger and may occur with fever. Exanthems that have been described with EV infections include maculopapular, macular, papular, morbilliform, rubelliform, vesicular, urticarial, papulopustular, and scarlatiniform. A petechial rash similar to that seen with meningococcemia has also been reported.

Hand-foot-and-mouth disease has most frequently been associated with infection with coxsackievirus A16 in the United States and EV-A71 in countries of the Asia-Pacific rim. However, it may be seen with several other EV serotypes. During community outbreaks, children younger than 4 years are primarily affected. Onset is associated with a sore throat in the presence or absence of a low-grade fever. Constitutional symptoms such as anorexia or malaise may be present. Shortly after onset of the fever, an enanthem appears characterized by macules that rapidly become vesicles and, ultimately, ulcerate. Lesions are diffusely distributed over the oral structures, involving the buccal mucosa, palate, gums, tongue, uvula, pharynx, and lips. In most children, the presence of exanthem, consisting of small (3–5 mm in diameter) vesicles surrounded by a mildly erythematous halo, is noted on the dorsum of the fingers and the feet. Non-vesicular lesions may also be seen on the buttocks. The illness generally resolves in less than 1 week. In recent years, coxsackievirus A6 has been a significant cause of hand-foot-and-mouth disease in the United States, resulting in more severe disease with higher fever, more extensive rash, and papulo-bullous lesions.

Herpangina

Children 1 to 7 years of age have the highest incidence of herpangina. Onset of disease is typically abrupt with the presence of high fever in association with intense sore throat, dysphagia, and ptyalism. A vesicular enanthem, on an erythematous base, located on the anterior pillar of the fauces is typically observed. The soft palate, uvula, and, rarely, tonsils may also be involved. Over 2 to 3 days, the vesicles rupture and ulcerate. Associated findings include mild cervical lymphadenopathy, headache, myalgia, abdominal pain, and rarely parotitis or meningitis. The illness generally lasts 7 to 10 days.

Enterovirus may cause a number of upper and lower respiratory tract syndromes. Nucleic acid amplification tests (NAAT) have demonstrated that EV is etiologically linked to up to 15% of upper respiratory tract infections for which an etiology can be established and 18% of children hospitalized with lower respiratory tract infection.

Summer Cold

This syndrome consists of nasal congestion, rhinorrhea, and sneezing. Fever and sore throat are typically absent or, at worst, minimal in nature. Malaise and cough may occasionally be present. The illness lasts less than 1 week.

Pharyngitis, Tonsillitis, and Pharyngotonsillitis

These conditions have an abrupt onset consisting of fever in association with sore throat. On examination of the pharynx is erythema and inflammation of the throat, nasopharynx, tonsils, uvula, and soft palate. Petechia may be present. Cervical lymphadenitis is common. Recovery generally takes less than 1 week.

Pneumonia

Pneumonias caused by EV are clinically indistinguishable from those caused by other viral agents. A recent nationwide epidemic caused by EV-D68 resulted in several thousand cases of severe lower respiratory tract disease. Unlike bacterial pneumonias, the onset is gradual with coryza, anorexia, and a low-grade fever. Tachypnea, nonproductive cough, retractions, nasal flaring, and, in severe cases, cyanosis can be seen. If the child has associated bronchiolitis or bronchospasm, wheezing may be present.

Pleurodynia

Pleurodynia (variably known as Bornholm disease, epidemic myalgia, or devil's grip) is a misnomer for a muscular condition erroneously thought to be of pleuritic origin. In most patients, the onset of disease is abrupt, consisting of severe, paroxysmal pain that is referred to the lower ribs or sternum. In some, however, a prodrome lasting up to 10 days and consisting of headache, malaise, anorexia, and vague myalgia can occur. In patients old enough to characterize the pain, it may be described as stabbing, smothering, or catching. The pain is exacerbated by coughing, deep breathing, sneezing, or movement and may radiate to the shoulders, neck, or scapula. Deep breathing, coughing, sneezing, or movement accentuate the pain. During the paroxysms of pain, tachypnea, shallow breathing, and grunting respirations may be present. The pain may be so severe as to be associated with diaphoresis and pallor. Abdominal pain occurs in approximately half of cases and is more commonly seen in children. Associated symptoms may include anorexia, nausea, vomiting, headache, and cough. Physical findings may be sparse and include splinting of the chest and, occasionally, mild muscle tenderness on palpation. The average duration of the illness is less than 1 week.

Acute Hemorrhagic Conjunctivitis

Acute hemorrhagic conjunctivitis is very communicable, and secondary attack rates within households are high. The incubation period is 1 to 2 days. The onset is rapid with palpebral swelling, lacrimation, photophobia, blurring of vision, and severe ocular pain. Subconjunctival hemorrhages, the hallmark of the illness, vary in size from petechiae to large blotches. Preauricular lymphadenopathy and transient keratitis are common, but the latter seldom results in subepithelial opacities. Ocular mucopurulent discharge is occasionally present. The illness usually lasts 1 to 2 weeks with complete recovery generally being the rule. In some cases, a transient lumbar radiculomyelopathy and AFP-like illness may occur.

Neonatal Infections

Most PeV infections in neonates result in subclinical or benign febrile illness. If the latter occurs, the duration of illness is approximately 1 week. Nonspecific signs such as irritability, lethargy, anorexia, vomiting, and exanthems may be present.

Some neonates will develop severe disease following EV infection. The greatest risk for development of severe disease, as well as with significant morbidity and mortality, is when disease develops in the initial days to 2 weeks following birth.

In some, a biphasic presentation consisting of a mild, nonspecific illness precedes the development of severe disease. Nonspecific symptoms include fever, temperature instability, irritability, lethargy, hypotonia, poor feeding, vomiting, abdominal distention, apnea, retractions, grunting, and rashes. As the disease progresses, a multisystem organ syndrome develops with various combinations of hepatitis, meningoencephalitis, myocarditis, sepsis, coagulopathy, and pneumonia. Two major clinical presentations are recognized: encephalomyocarditis (severe myocarditis in association with heart failure and meningoencephalitis) and hepatitis-hemorrhage syndrome (severe hepatitis with hepatic failure and disseminated intravascular coagulopathy).

Neurologic involvement is manifested by lethargy, seizures, and focal neurologic findings. Signs of meningeal inflammation (eg, nuchal rigidity, bulging anterior fontanelle, Kernig and Brudzinski signs) may be absent. Neonates with myocarditis may have cardiomegaly, hepatomegaly, poor perfusion, cyanosis, signs and symptoms of congestive heart failure, metabolic acidosis, and arrhythmias. Hepatomegaly and jaundice are typical findings of severe hepatitis. If necrotizing hepatitis develops, evidence of disseminated intravascular coagulation is present. The sepsis-like clinical presentation is indistinguishable from those observed in severe bacterial infection. Additionally reported conditions include renal failure, intracranial hemorrhage, adrenal hemorrhage, necrotizing enterocolitis, and inappropriate secretion of antidiuretic hormone.

Parechovirus

Discussion of clinical syndromes associated with PeV will focus on those for which there have been well-characterized reports. A list of other possibly associated syndromes is provided (Box 28-1).

Box 28-1. Syndromes Possibly Associated With Parechoviral Infection

- Sudden infant death syndrome
- Reye syndrome
- Myocarditis
- Gastroenteritis
- Hand-foot-and-mouth disease
- Myositis
- Otitis
- Hemolytic uremic syndrome

Undifferentiated Febrile Illness

Fever and irritability are presenting concerns in nearly all infants. Rash (erythematous or maculopapular), rhinorrhea, cough, poor feeding, tachypnea, and tachycardia may occur. Some infants may have hypotension.

Meningitis

Clinically, infants with PeV meningitis present similarly to those with EV. Fever and irritability are present in nearly every patient. Exanthems are variably present. Vomiting, diarrhea, distention rhinorrhea, cough, tachypnea, apnea, and wheezing are seen in one-third to half of patients. Conspicuously absent in reports have been clinical findings indicative of increased intracranial pressure (eg, bulging fontanelle) or meningeal irritation (eg, nuchal rigidity, Kernig or Brudzinski signs).

Encephalitis

Human parechoviral encephalitis has been reported exclusively in neonates and young infants. Most cases have occurred in term neonates, with onset occurring in the first 2 weeks of life. In premature infants, the syndrome presents at 50 to 90 days of life. Seizures are present in most patients, and in one-third they are recurrent. Fever, irritability, apnea, and rash are seen in more than half of cases.

Acute Flaccid Paralysis

The onset of paralysis is acute. There is associated areflexia of the involved limb. Fever may be present. As with PV, the muscles of respiration may be involved and therefore paralysis can be life-threatening. Paraesthesia of the affected extremity and cranial nerve involvement may occur.

Neonatal Infections

Most EV infections in neonates result in subclinical or benign febrile illness. If the latter occurs, the duration of illness is approximately 1 week. Nonspecific signs such as irritability, lethargy, anorexia, vomiting, and exanthems may be present.

Hemorrhage-Hepatitis Syndrome

Although limited reports exist, this syndrome appears to be nearly identical to that described for EV.

Necrotizing Enterocolitis

Signs and symptoms of gastroenteritis, including bloody diarrhea, have been reported. Additional symptoms may include fever, apnea, tachypnea, respiratory distress, rhinorrhea, conjunctivitis, and rash.

Evaluation

Nucleic acid amplification tests (reverse transcription-polymerase chain reaction– and nucleic acid sequence based amplification–based) have supplanted viral culture for the detection of EV and PeV. Assays based on these methodologies have been shown to be significantly more sensitive than culture for the detection of these viral agents (Evidence Level I). This is particularly true for PeV and some of the EVs that have been shown to grow poorly or not at all in cell culture. Both methodologies have been adapted so that they may be used with multiple sample types (eg, cerebrospinal fluid [CSF], blood, tissue, pericardial fluid).

The evaluation of children with suspected EV or PeV undifferentiated febrile illness should focus on excluding bacterial infection, particularly in the neonate or young infant. Collection of blood, CSF, and urinary samples for bacterial (and viral, if appropriate) culture is paramount. No unique hematologic picture indicative of EV or PeV infection exists. Cytochemical analysis of the CSF may document evidence of viral meningitis.

In children with CNS syndromes consistent with either EV or PeV, cytochemical analysis of the CSF is essential in establishing the diagnosis. In EV meningitis, the CSF typically reveals a modest monocytic pleocytosis (100–1,000/mcL) with a normal or slightly depressed glucose concentration and a normal to slightly increased protein concentration. If lumbar puncture is preformed early in the course of illness, the CSF may demonstrate a polymorphonuclear cell predominance that shifts to a monocytic predominance if reexamined 24 to 48 hours later.

It is of note that most infants with PeV meningitis have no or minimal CSF abnormalities. If observed, the abnormalities are similar to those described for EV meningitis but less severe.

In cases of suspected EV and PeV meningitis, CSF should be submitted for EV and PeV genome detection using NAAT to establish the diagnosis. It is important to note that the current tests used to detect EV genome will not detect that of PeV. Serum may also be subjected to NAAT of the EV and PeV in these cases.

In cases of suspected EV and PeV encephalitis or AFP, CSF analysis should be performed as described above. However, CSF findings will be normal or show minimal abnormalities in most cases. This is particularly true in the case of PeV neonatal encephalitis in which CSF findings are normal. Enteroviral and PeV genome can be detected even when CSF cytochemical analysis is completely normal.

Neuroimaging may reveal abnormalities in greater than 50% of cases of EV encephalitis, but they are not unique enough to establish the etiology. In cases of EV-A71 rhombencephalitis, lesions of high signal intensity in the brainstem appear on T2-weighted images.

In all reported cases of neonatal PeV, encephalitic abnormalities have been detected using magnetic resonance imaging of the brain or cranial ultrasound. White matter changes consist of high intensity signals and punctate lesions. Cranial ultrasound demonstrates severe periventricular echogenicity.

All cases of suspected EV and PeV AFP should be reported to the health department. In addition to the evaluation listed above, stool should be collected for EV and PeV detection using cell culture and NAAT. In cases of AFP, spinal magnetic resonance imaging may show increased signal intensity in anterior horns of the spinal cord.

In patients with EV myocarditis, echocardiography may demonstrate decreased shorting fraction and poor ejection volume. Electrocardiographic findings vary and include low voltage QRS complexes, ST segment elevation, and T-wave inversions. Myocardial enzyme levels may be elevated in serum. Myocardial tissue for establishing a histologic diagnosis should be obtained by endomyocardial biopsy. The tissue should also be tested by NAAT for the presence of EV genome. In cases of pericarditis or myopericarditis, attempts to detect EV using NAAT should be performed on pericardial fluid.

Neonates with suspected EV or PeV CNS disease or any of the severe neonatal syndromes (sepsis, encephalomyocarditis, and hepatitis-hemorrhage syndromes) should have CSF and serum tested for the presence of viral genome using NAAT. Neonates or young infants with severe EV or PeV infections may have elevated levels of hepatic enzymes, hyperbilirubinemia, thrombo-cytopenia, and alterations of the prothrombin time and activated partial thromboplastin time.

The diagnosis of hand-foot-and-mouth disease, herpangina, pleurodynia, and hemorrhagic conjunctivitis is based primarily on clinical presentation of the child. No specific tests are generally required.

With the exception of the neonate, detection of an EV or PeV from a stool specimen (or throat swab) does not conclusively establish etiology of the syndrome being evaluated (Evidence Level III). In neonates younger than 3 weeks, detection of the EV or PeV in stool may correlate with the illness being evaluated because infection could have occurred only in the preceding 2 weeks. It is possible that an infant beyond a month of age or a child who had EV or PeV infection weeks earlier can present with an acute illness unrelated to them and have EV and PeV detected from the stool.

Management

The management of EV and PeV infections is symptomatic because no specific therapy is currently available. Physicians should focus on excluding bacterial and viral infections, particularly in the neonate or young infant. If appropriate, empiric therapy with antimicrobials that treat the most common age-appropriate bacterial and viral agents should be initiated until EV or PeV has been identified. Once an EV or PeV etiology has been confirmed, antimicrobials may be discontinued if the patient is doing well (Evidence Level I). If used appropriately, the results of NAAT will be available sooner than bacterial cultures and lead to a shorter length of hospitalization and use of antibiotics (Evidence Level I).

Antipyretics and analgesics may be given to control fever and muscular pain or headache. Intravenous fluids may be required to prevent dehydration in infants or young children unable to take or retain fluids. Immune globulin, given intravenously or intrathecally, has been used in neonates, infants, and immunocompromised individuals, such as children with agammaglobulinemia (Evidence Level III). However, its efficacy has not been established.

Supportive management of patients with myocarditis should include medical management of congestive heart failure and arrhythmias. Some children will benefit from the use of ventricular assist devices as a bridge to recovery during the acute phase of illness or as a bridge to cardiac transplantation (Evidence Level II-3). Reports of the use of intravenous immune globulin for treatment of EV myocarditis exist, but conclusive proof of its benefit is lacking (Evidence Level II-3). Similarly, reports of the use of immunosuppression (CD3, azathioprine, and prednisone) have documented improvement in myocardial function (Evidence Level II-3), but evidence is not conclusive. However, not all patients included in these reports were shown to have EV.

Parents should be instructed to wash their hands thoroughly to avoid household transmission (Evidence Level III). Infection control measures consist of contact precautions in addition to standard precautions (Evidence Level III) if the infant is in diapers or incontinent. These should remain in effect until the child leaves the hospital. Exclusion from day care is unwarranted.

Suggested Reading

Abzug MJ. Presentation, diagnosis, and management of enterovirus infections in neonates. *Paediatr Drugs.* 2004;6(1):1–10

Romero JR, Selvarangan R. The human parechoviruses: an overview. *Adv Pediatr.* 2011;58(1):65–85

Ruan F, Yang T, Ma H, et al. Risk factors for hand, foot, and mouth disease and herpangina and the preventive effect of hand-washing. *Pediatrics.* 2011;127(4):e898–e904

Stellrecht KA, Lamson DM, Romero JR. Enteroviruses and parechoviruses. In: Versalovic J, Carroll KC, Funke G, Jorgensen JH, Landry ML, Warnock DW, eds. *Manual of Clinical Microbiology.* 10th ed. Washington, DC: American Society for Microbiology Press; 2011:1387–1399

CHAPTER 29

Epstein-Barr Virus

Amina Ahmed, MD

Key Points

- Most children with primary Epstein-Barr virus (EBV) infection are asymptomatic.
- Classical infectious mononucleosis includes fever, exudative pharyngitis, and cervical lymphadenopathy.
- Atypical lymphocytosis is uniformly seen on peripheral smear review in patients with primary EBV infection.
- Heterophile antibody testing is unhelpful in making the diagnosis of EBV infection in the young child or during the first week of symptoms.
- Epstein-Barr virus antibody testing can confirm the diagnosis of primary EBV infection if IgM antibody to viral capsid antigen is found. If antibody to nuclear antigen is found, this is consistent with past infection and excludes primary EBV infection as the diagnosis.
- Polymerase chain reaction testing for EBV should be reserved for the immunocompromised host in whom a lymphoproliferative syndrome is suspected.
- Treatment is supportive, and corticosteroids should be reserved for those with impending airway obstruction.

Overview

Epstein-Barr virus (EBV) is a ubiquitous virus. While most infections are asymptomatic, the classic triad of fever, exudative pharyngitis, and cervical lymphadenopathy that is termed *infectious mononucleosis* is commonly seen and easily recognized by clinicians.

Causes and Differential Diagnosis

Epstein-Barr virus is a double-stranded DNA virus that is a member of the herpesvirus family. The age at acquisition of primary infection depends on geographic, cultural, and socioeconomic variables. Primary infection between

10 and 30 years of age tends to be associated with clinical symptoms, typically those of infectious mononucleosis.

The differential diagnosis for classic infectious mononucleosis includes cytomegalovirus, HIV, adenovirus, and toxoplasmosis (Table 29-1). Approximately 5% to 10% of cases of apparent infectious mononucleosis are from causes other than EBV. Cytomegalovirus (CMV) is responsible for most cases of heterophile-negative infectious mononucleosis. The syndrome caused by CMV is similar to but typically milder than EBV-associated infectious mononucleosis. Cervical lymphadenopathy is less prominent, and pharyngitis may be mild or absent. Cytomegalovirus disease exhibits a hematologic profile similar to that of EBV-associated infectious mononucleosis, with a high percentage of atypical lymphocytes. Subacute hepatitis is common in both CMV- and EBV-associated diseases. Serologic testing consistent with acute CMV infection in the absence of characteristic EBV serologic findings confirms the disease. Toxoplasmosis can also cause a heterophile-negative mononucleosis-like illness. It rarely causes pharyngitis or abnormal elevation of transaminase concentrations and is unassociated with characteristic hematologic abnormalities. Adenoviral infections may manifest with symptoms that overlap those of infectious mononucleosis, including pharyngitis with or without exudate. Virus may be detected in throat or nasopharyngeal specimens by culture or molecular methods such as polymerase chain reaction (PCR). Early viral hepatitis,

Table 29-1. Differential Diagnosis for Infectious Causes of Non- Epstein-Barr Virus-Associated Mononucleosis

Syndrome	Characteristics
Viral	
CMV	• Pharyngitis and lymphadenopathy less prominent • Positive for CMV antibodies in serum
Toxoplasmosis	• Exposure to cats • Positive for *Toxoplasma* antibodies in serum
HIV	• Sexually active • Positive for HIV, PCR, or antibody
HHV-6	• High fevers with subsequent rash on defervescence in younger children
Adenovirus	• Conjunctivitis, upper respiratory tract symptoms • Detection by viral culture or molecular test
Viral hepatitis	• More acutely elevated transaminase concentrations • Exposure history
Bacterial	
Streptococcal pharyngitis	• Absence of hepatosplenomegaly and atypical lymphocytes

Abbreviations: CMV, cytomegalovirus; HHV-6, *Human herpesvirus 6;* PCR, polymerase chain reaction.

Adapted from Marshall BC, Foxworth MK II. Epstein-Barr virus-associated infectious mononucleosis. *Contemp Pediatr.* 2012;29(10):52–64, with permission.

including that caused by hepatitis A virus and hepatitis B virus, may resemble EBV-related illness. However, neither hepatitis virus causes the pharyngitis or lymphadenopathy commonly observed with EBV infection. The degree of hepatic involvement with hepatitis A or B virus quickly becomes more extensive than that seen with EBV, with transaminase values rapidly rising to above 1,000 IU/L.

Primary HIV infection should be considered in any adolescent presenting with febrile illness resembling mononucleosis. Rash is less common in infectious mononucleosis caused by EBV but is frequently observed in primary HIV infection within the first 48 to 72 hours after onset of fever. False-positive heterophile antibody tests have been reported with HIV infection.

In addition to the infectious mononucleosis-like illnesses above, pharyngitis caused by *Streptococcus pyogenes* results in symptoms with considerable overlap to those of infectious mononucleosis. Both diseases are associated with fever, cervical lymphadenopathy, and pharyngitis with tonsillar exudates. However, streptococcal pharyngitis is usually unassociated with significant fatigue or splenomegaly on examination. Coinfection with both pathogens may occur, but with a pharyngeal carriage rate of approximately 25%, it is difficult to distinguish true infection with *S pyogenes* from colonization of bacteria when rapid streptococcal antigen testing or throat culture is positive. Failure of a patient to improve 2 to 3 days after initiating treatment of streptococcal pharyngitis should suggest the possibility of infectious mononucleosis.

If exudative pharyngitis is the primary finding, once *S pyogenes* disease is excluded, other viral etiologies including adenovirus and enterovirus and bacterial etiologies including *Neisseria gonorrhoeae* (in adolescents), *Arcanobacterium haemolyticum*, *Mycoplasma pneumoniae*, or *Fusobacterium necrophorum* (ie, Lemierre syndrome) may be considered.

Patients with infectious mononucleosis who empirically receive antibiotics (usually amoxicillin or other penicillins) may develop a generalized rash. In such cases, clinicians may consider the diagnosis of a tick-borne infection (Rocky Mountain spotted fever or ehrlichiosis) or leptospirosis.

In the patient with complications of EBV infection, differential diagnosis may vary depending on clinical manifestation. In those with central nervous system complications, viruses or other causes of aseptic meningitis or encephalitis may be considered (eg, herpes simplex viruses, enteroviruses, arboviruses, *Mycoplasma*). When primary EBV infection occurs with associated hematologic complications (eg, thrombocytopenia, agranulocytosis, hemolytic anemia, or hemophagocytic syndromes), leukemia or lymphoma should be excluded by appropriate evaluation.

Clinical Manifestations

Most primary EBV infections in immunocompetent individuals are asymptomatic or clinically inapparent.

Primary EBV infection in infants and young children is typically asymptomatic or mildly symptomatic. Nonspecific clinical symptoms include fever and upper respiratory tract findings such as rhinorrhea and pharyngitis. In a review of 113 children with documented EBV infection, mucopurulent nasal discharge and cough were present in 51% of the children younger than 4 years, compared with 15% in older children. The most frequent presenting signs and symptoms in children with infectious mononucleosis are fever, lymphadenopathy, and sore throat. Hepatomegaly is seen in 63% of children younger than 4 years, but only 30% of children and adolescents aged 4 to 16 years. Splenomegaly is also more common in younger children (51%) than older (15%).

The most widely recognized manifestation of symptomatic primary EBV infection is infectious mononucleosis, typically identified in adolescents and adults. The incubation period may be as long as 4 to 6 weeks. A prodrome of headache and malaise precedes characteristic features of the disease, which include fever, pharyngitis or sore throat, and lymphadenopathy. Fever may be as high as 39°C to 40°C (102.2°F–104°F) and can last up to 1 week, although in severe cases it may be prolonged. Tonsillopharyngitis develops during the first week of illness, with tonsils enlarged, reddened, and covered by exudates in 50% of patients. Pharyngitis caused by EBV may be indistinguishable from that caused by *S pyogenes*. Palatal petechiae may be noted in the first 2 weeks of illness, characteristically at the junction of the hard and soft palate. Eyelid edema, occasionally accompanied by facial puffiness, is a characteristic feature of primary EBV infection. The finding is described in as many as one-third of adult patients but occurs less frequently in children.

Lymphadenopathy is a hallmark of infectious mononucleosis and occurs in more than 90% of affected children and adults. Affected nodes are firm and tender. Symmetric involvement of cervical nodes is characteristic with posterior cervical nodes frequently more involved than the anterior chain. Mediastinal and hilar lymph node enlargement can infrequently lead to respiratory compromise. Generalized lymphadenopathy can also occur and involves occipital, axillary, epitrochlear, and inguinal chains.

An exanthem unassociated with antibiotic administration develops in up to 15% of affected cases. The rash typically occurs during the first few days of illness, is usually found on the trunk and arms, and can be erythematous, macular, papular, or morbilliform. Rarely, the rash is petechial or hemorrhagic, or it may resemble the exanthem of Gianotti-Crosti syndrome.

Splenomegaly occurs in approximately 50% of individuals with infectious mononucleosis and is more frequently noted in young children. Usually only the tip of the spleen is clinically palpable. Enlargement is noted between the second and third week of illness with resolution by the third or fourth week. Hepatomegaly may also be noted in up to 60% of young children with infectious mononucleosis but is less common in older age groups. Mild jaundice, caused by cholestasis or viral-induced hemolysis, affects fewer than 10% of patients, and may be accompanied by scleral icterus.

The 2 most common serious complications of infectious mononucleosis are airway obstruction and splenic rupture, which fortunately occur in less than 5% and 0.5% of infected patients, respectively. Obstruction of the upper airway occurs as a consequence of lymphoid hyperplasia and mucosal edema.

A commonly described complication of infectious mononucleosis is appearance of a morbilliform rash following administration of ampicillin and, less frequently, penicillin. The "ampicillin rash," as it is commonly known, occurs less frequently in children with infectious mononucleosis. The exanthem develops 5 to 10 days after initiation of ampicillin and resolves within a few days of discontinuation. Cutaneous lesions are characteristically maculopapular and pruritic, distributed mainly on the trunk and extremities but with potential to progress to a more extensive eruption. Development of the rash is not predictive of ampicillin allergy, and patients tolerate subsequent treatment with ampicillin without adverse effects.

Neurologic complications of primary EBV infection include Guillain-Barré syndrome, facial nerve palsy, meningoencephalitis, cerebellar ataxia, and optic neuritis. These syndromes may occur as the only manifestation of EBV infection or may be associated with typical infectious mononucleosis. Renal complications include interstitial nephritis and glomerulonephritis. Epstein-Barr virus has also been associated with pneumonia, myocarditis, pancreatitis, and genital ulceration. Infection-associated hemophagocytic syndrome is a secondary form of hemophagocytic lymphohistiocytosis, and the most common infectious trigger is primary EBV infection.

Complete recovery from infectious mononucleosis occurs uneventfully in most individuals, with symptoms gradually resolving over 2 to 4 weeks. Some patients experience prolonged signs and symptoms accompanied by fatigue and malaise for several weeks to as long as 6 months. No convincing evidence suggests that EBV infection or reactivation is responsible for chronic fatigue syndrome.

Less Common or Unusual Manifestations of Epstein-Barr Virus Infection

The most severe manifestations of EBV occur when the immune system fails to control primary or latent infection. Persons with compromised cellular immunity, such as those undergoing solid organ transplantation (SOT) or hematopoietic stem cell transplantation (HSCT), or those with congenital immunodeficiencies, such as the X-linked lymphoproliferative (XLP) syndrome, are at greatest risk for uncontrolled EBV-associated proliferations. With the potential for viral oncogenesis, an increased risk of malignancy is also associated with AIDS, organ transplantation, and congenital immunodeficiencies such as common variable immunodeficiency and Wiskott-Aldrich syndrome.

Posttransplant lymphoproliferative diseases (PTLDs) are lymphoid or plasmacytic proliferations that occur primarily in the setting of SOT or HSCT. Most PTLDs are B lymphocyte in origin and EBV associated. Susceptibility to PTLD is a consequence of immunosuppression caused by medications used to prevent graft rejection in SOT or conditioning regimens used for HSCT. Risk factors include intensity of immunosuppression and EBV serostatus. The risk in SOT is highest among EBV-negative recipients of EBV-positive donor organs. As a consequence, the frequency of lymphoproliferative disease appears to be higher in pediatric transplant recipients compared to adult recipients, who are more likely to be seropositive for EBV at transplantation. The clinical manifestations of disease are highly variable and can range from a nonspecific infectious mononucleosis-like illness with fever, sore throat, and lymphadenopathy to fatal illness characterized by lymphomas involving the gastrointestinal tract, central nervous system, or grafted organ.

X-linked lymphoproliferative syndrome is a rare congenital disorder associated with inability to produce a normal immune response to primary EBV infection. Individuals with XLP syndrome are at risk for fatal infectious mononucleosis and EBV-associated lymphomas. Early in infection, these individuals have features consistent with typical infectious mononucleosis, but they rapidly progress to fulminant disease. Causes of death include liver necrosis, acute hemorrhage, and meningoencephalitis, and widespread uncontrolled lymphoproliferation is found at autopsy. Approximately one-third of patients with XLP syndrome survive the initial EBV infection. Survivors develop dysgammaglobulinemia with increased susceptibility to bacterial infections and the development of malignancies. The only definitive therapy is stem cell transplantation.

The potential of EBV to induce malignancies has long been recognized. Neoplasms primarily associated with EBV include B-cell lymphomas and nasopharyngeal carcinoma. Additional malignancies associated with EBV include carcinoma of the salivary glands, thymomas, and T-lymphocyte lymphomas.

Evaluation

Hematologic complications are generally mild and occur in about 25% of cases. Leukopenia or leukocytosis may occur in the first week of illness, with greater than 50% of cells being lymphocytes. Atypical lymphocytes, most of which are activated T cells, may account for up 20% to 40% of the total white blood cells. In the absence of diagnostic serology, atypical lymphocytosis is the most reliable indicator of EBV-associated infectious mononucleosis. Mild thrombocytopenia is found in 25% to 50% of patients with infectious mononucleosis and is likely immune mediated. Severe thrombocytopenia ($<20 \times 10^9$/L) occurs rarely. Autoimmune hemolytic anemia occurs uncommonly, and aplastic anemia is rare. Mild transient neutropenia (2,000–3,000/mcL) occurs in more than 50% of cases, with a nadir in the third to fourth week of illness.

Although most patients with infectious mononucleosis do not have hepatomegaly on physical examination, asymptomatic mild to moderate elevations of serum glutamic pyruvate transaminase and serum glutamic oxaloacetic transaminase concentrations are seen in approximately 50% of uncomplicated cases.

The clinical diagnosis of infectious mononucleosis caused by EBV is based on the presence of typical symptoms in the absence of alternative explanations. In the immunocompetent host, diagnosis is further supported by serologic testing, either for the heterophile antibody or EBV-specific antibodies. Although detection of EBV DNA in plasma by PCR may be highly sensitive in this setting, the negative predictive value of the test is low. Thus, serology remains the criterion standard for diagnosis of infectious mononucleosis in immunocompetent persons. Among immunocompromised hosts, serology may not be interpretable in the setting of reactivated infection. Molecular methods such as PCR tests are commonly used in this population for diagnosis of disease as well as monitoring of response to treatment.

The heterophile antibody test, also known as the monospot, is the most rapid test available for the diagnosis of infectious mononucleosis. The tests detect antibodies in almost 90% of cases of EBV-associated infectious mononucleosis in older children and adults during the second week of illness. There are, however, several limitations. During the first week of illness, up to 25% of patients will not exhibit a positive heterophile response. More important, at least 40% of children younger than 4 years do not develop heterophile antibodies during primary infection. Because of its diminished sensitivity in this age group, the heterophile antibody test is not recommended for diagnostic testing of infectious mononucleosis in young children. Approximately 5% to 10% of cases of apparent infectious mononucleosis are not caused by EBV and will not have a heterophile antibody response. Finally, false-positive heterophile test results may occur in non-EBV infections such as CMV, adenovirus, hepatitis C, and malaria, as well as malignancies such as lymphoma and autoimmune diseases such as systemic lupus erythematosus.

Antibodies directed specifically against antigens of EBV confirm infection and are more useful for distinguishing between acute, recent, and past infection. Viral-specific serology is particularly helpful for diagnosis of EBV infection in children younger than 4 years with typical presentation of infectious mononucleosis, in patients with heterophile-negative infectious mononucleosis, or in those with prolonged or atypical disease. Antibodies to Epstein-Barr nuclear antigens (EBNA), early antigens, and viral capsid antigens (VCAs) are the most useful for diagnostic purposes. The presence of IgM antibodies to the VCA of EBV is transient, occurring within the first few weeks of infection and generally disappearing after 3 months. The presence of IgG antibody to the VCA of EBV occurs early in the disease, including during the acute phase, but then persists for life. Antibodies to early antigens are transiently detectable weeks to months after infection but may persist for months or intermittently for years. Antibodies to EBNA, a protein expressed during the latent phase, appear several weeks after infection, rise during convalescence, and subsequently persist at low but detectable titers for life.

Interpretation of serologic responses is outlined in Table 29-2. Acute primary EBV infection is characterized by the presence of IgM antibodies to VCA in the absence of antibodies to EBNA. Viral capsid antigen IgG antibodies may be present in acute infection, but usually in lower quantities than IgM. During convalescence (third week to third month after onset of illness), IgM antibodies to VCA decline as IgG antibodies rise, and recent infection is characterized by the presence of these antibodies with or without the presence of antibodies to EBNA. With the variability in appearance and persistence of early antigen antibodies, detection of antibody to early antigen by itself is insufficient to confirm or exclude a diagnosis of acute infectious mononucleosis. The presence of antibodies to EBNA denotes infection occurring at least 3 to 4 months previously, which may be any time during the life of the individual. In immunocompetent hosts, reactivation is not a clinically significant event, and its occurrence is difficult to confirm serologically in the absence of serial testing. In immunosuppressed or immunocompromised individuals, extremely elevated antibodies to VCA in the presence of antibodies to EBNA may be compatible with secondary or reactivated EBV infection.

Isolation of virus from body secretions or pathologic specimens by tissue culture is possible but labor intensive and not widely available. Because of latency of the virus and intermittent shedding in body fluids, detection of virus by tissue culture does not necessarily indicate acute infection.

If EBV-associated hemophagocytic syndrome is suspected, diagnostic criteria include cytopenia in at least 2 cell lines, hypertriglyceridemia or hypofibrinogenemia, and tissue demonstration of hemophagocytosis. Supporting evidence of disease includes elevated serum ferritin concentrations and

Table 29-2. Interpretation of Serum Epstein-Barr Virus (EBV) Serology Profiles

Infection	VCA IgG	VCA IgM	EA (D)	EBNA
No previous infection	−	−	−	−
Acute infection	+	+	±	−
Recent infection	+	±	±	±
Past infection	+	−	±	+

Abbreviations: EA (D), early antibody diffuse staining; EBNA, Epstein-Barr virus nuclear antigen; VCA IgG, immunoglobulin G antibody to viral capsid antigen; VCA IgM, immunoglobulin M antibody to viral caspid antigen.

From American Academy of Pediatrics. Epstein-Barr virus infections. In: Kimberlin DW, Brady MT, Jackson MA, Long SS, eds. *Red Book: 2015 Report of the Committee of Infectious Diseases*. 30th ed. Elk Grove Village, IL; American Academy of Pediatrics; 2015:336–340.

elevated levels of soluble interleukin-2 receptor CD25 (alpha chain of soluble IL-2 receptor) and low or absent natural killer cell activity.

Molecular diagnostic methods such as PCR are typically reserved for the diagnosis of EBV-associated diseases in immunocompromised patients because the serologic response to EBV antigens may be incomplete or uninterpretable. Polymerase chain reaction testing is not recommended for diagnosis of infectious mononucleosis in otherwise healthy children. Among solid organ and bone marrow transplant recipients, quantitative PCR for EBV DNA in peripheral blood is useful for the diagnosis of PTLD and for monitoring response to treatment. In end-organ disease, EBV can be identified in tissue by immunohistochemical methods. In transplant-associated lymphoproliferative disease, definitive diagnosis is made histologically with demonstration of the presence of EBV within the lesion by PCR or in situ hybridization.

Treatment

For most children and adults with infectious mononucleosis caused by EBV, no specific treatment is indicated. Most individuals recover uneventfully with resolution of symptoms within 1 to 2 weeks, but fatigue may persist in some for months.

Ampicillin or amoxicillin use in those with suspected coinfection with *S pyogenes* should be avoided and an alternative non–β-lactam antibiotic chosen. Acetaminophen or nonsteroidal anti-inflammatory drugs may be used for the treatment of fever, throat discomfort, or malaise.

While short-course corticosteroids can modestly ameliorate symptoms of sore throat, the beneficial effect is limited and use of steroids is not recommended for children with otherwise uncomplicated infectious mononucleosis (Evidence Level I). Prednisone or other corticosteroids may be used for those with impending airway obstruction and can be considered for those with massive splenomegaly, myocarditis, or hemolytic anemia.

A number of antivirals inhibit EBV replication in vitro, including acyclovir and ganciclovir, but these agents cannot eliminate the latent state of the virus. Available evidence does not support use of antivirals for the symptomatic treatment of infectious mononucleosis in immunocompetent hosts (Evidence Level I).

A meta-analysis substantiates these findings and reinforces the recommendation that acyclovir is not indicated for the treatment of infectious mononucleosis in immunocompetent hosts (Evidence Level I).

For pediatric patients with infectious mononucleosis who are involved in sports-related activities, an important management issue is the timing of resumption of athletic activities given the potential for splenic rupture. Bed rest is unnecessary, but athletes should refrain from contact sports during early or acute illness. Spontaneous or traumatic splenic rupture related to infectious mononucleosis is most likely in the 3 weeks after onset of illness, and most experts advise waiting at least 1 month after onset of illness and until splenomegaly has resolved before returning to athletics. According to the consensus statement of the American Medical Society for Sports Medicine, athletes should avoid all exercise for a minimum of the first 21 days after onset of illness (Evidence Level III), and some experts recommend avoidance of contact sports for 4 to 6 weeks. While resolution of splenomegaly may be documented by splenic palpation or radiographic evaluation, no guidelines recommend which method is preferable and the routine use of ultrasound is not indicated in most patients. Timing of return to sports should be individualized for each patient based on the onset of illness, degree of contact involved in athletic activity, and ability to establish resolution of splenomegaly.

For patients with EBV-associated hemophagocytic syndrome, treatment with etoposide, which decreases macrophage activity, and corticosteroids may be effective. Definitive therapy requires stem cell transplantation.

Reduction of immunosuppression is essential to the management of PTLD. Complementary interventions include rituximab, an anti-CD20 monoclonal antibody directed to B lymphocytes. The role of antivirals in the treatment of PTLD is unclear.

Suggested Reading

Candy B, Hotopf M. Steroids for symptom control in infectious mononucleosis. *Cochrane Database System Rev.* 2006;(3):CD004402

Gulley ML, Tang W. Using Epstein-Barr viral load assays to diagnose, monitor, and prevent posttransplant lymphoproliferative disorder. *Clin Microbiol Rev.* 2010;23(2): 350–366

Jenson HB. Epstein-Barr virus. *Pediatr Rev.* 2011;32(9):375–383

Marshall BC, Foxworth MK II. Epstein-Barr virus-associated infectious mononucleosis. *Contemp Pediatr.* 2012;29(10):52–64

Odumade OA, Hogquist KA, Balfour HH Jr. Progress and problems in understanding and managing primary Epstein-Barr virus infections. *Clin Microbiol Rev.* 2011;24(1):193–209

Putukian M, O'Connor FG, Stricker P, et al. Mononucleosis and athletic participation: an evidence-based subject review. *Clin J Sports Med.* 2008;18(4):309–315

CHAPTER 30

HIV

Diana L. Yu, PharmD; Marc Foca, MD; and Gordon E. Schutze, MD

Key Points

- Vertical HIV transmission is rare but still occurs in the United States.
- Human immunodeficiency virus infection rate is increasing in the adolescent population.
- Linkage to care with an HIV specialist and initiating antiretroviral therapy decreases HIV-associated morbidity and mortality and HIV transmission.
- Follow-up is essential to manage adverse effects of medications and evaluate adherence; treatment is a lifelong commitment.
- Treatment of the HIV-infected patient should be multidisciplinary; the primary care physician plays the key role of a medical home.

Overview

Human immunodeficiency virus infection in children is an uncommon infectious disease in the United States because of early identification of HIV infection in females of childbearing age and combination antiretroviral therapy (cART) that decreases the risk of vertical HIV transmission to less than 2%. On the other hand, HIV infections caused by high-risk practices are increasing in the adolescent population. It is important to recognize signs and symptoms of HIV infection in infants, young children, and adolescents because early initiation of cART can reduce morbidity and mortality associated with this infection. Care of an HIV-infected patient should occur in collaboration with a physician who has expertise in treating pediatric HIV patients to maximize outcomes.

Causes and Differential Diagnosis

Human immunodeficiency virus infection is caused by HIV, a retrovirus that infects immune cells that are $CD4^+$. There are 2 types of HIV: HIV-1 is the predominant type of HIV worldwide, whereas HIV-2 can be found in certain areas of the world (eg, West Africa). Although the methods of diagnosis are similar between HIV-1 and HIV-2, the management is different. Because HIV-2 is very uncommon in the United States, it will not be covered in this chapter.

Human immunodeficiency virus transmission occurs when a person contacts infected body fluids such as blood, semen, vaginal fluid, and human milk directly or non-intact skin or mucous membranes. Other body fluids, such as tears, saliva, and urine, have very low quantities of virus and are considered noninfectious. Human immunodeficiency virus infects CD4$^+$ cells, which include helper T lymphocytes, macrophages, monocytes, and dendritic cells, by integrating into the host DNA, using host mechanisms to replicate and build mature virions, which are released to infect other CD4$^+$ cells. As HIV replicates, the CD4$^+$ cell undergoes cell death, and if allowed to proliferate unchecked, both the innate and adaptive immunity are severely affected. Figure 30-1 illustrates the relationship between HIV plasma RNA and CD4$^+$ cell count over time in adolescent patients; although this figure cannot be extrapolated to infants or young children, the general correlation is similar. Morbidity and mortality from HIV are largely caused by secondary bacterial, fungal, or viral infections. Educating family and patients about HIV and how it affects the immune system is essential for prevention and medication adherence in those already infected.

Infants with perinatally acquired HIV infection who present with failure to thrive, lymphadenopathy, and recurrent sinopulmonary infection are generally evaluated for a variety of chronic diseases. The differential diagnoses in such patients would include other immunologic processes, such as severe combined

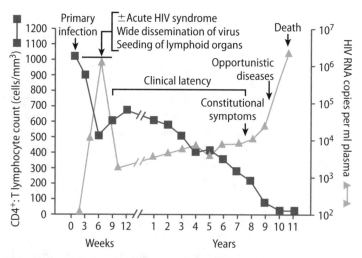

Figure 30-1. Relationship between HIV-1 RNA viral load and CD4$^+$ T-lymphocyte cell count over the course of untreated HIV-1 infection.

From Pantaleo G, Graziosi C, Fauci AS. The immunopathogenesis of human immunodeficiency virus infection. *N Engl J Med.* 1993;328(5):327–335, with permission.

immunodeficiency, common variable immunodeficiency, autoimmune and chronic benign neutropenia, failure to thrive, malabsorption syndromes, thyroid disease, chronic granulomatous disease, cystic fibrosis, and oncologic processes.

The differential diagnoses in older patients who present with acute HIV infection include Epstein-Barr virus, cytomegalovirus, influenza, syphilis, and streptococcal infection. During this time, the HIV plasma RNA is high and the patient may be especially infectious. The symptoms will wane after 1 to 2 weeks without any treatment, and patients may remain asymptomatic for many years. Patients may not report any illness because it is self-limiting and may be dismissed as a common cold.

Clinical Features

Untreated HIV-infected infants and young children may demonstrate significant morbidity and mortality within the first 5 years of life (ie, rapid progressors) or may not present with complications of infection until many years later (eg, ≥10 years; slow progressors). Often, children who have HIV infection present with failure to thrive or failure to reach early developmental milestones. Other symptoms that suggest infection include unexplained fevers, chronic lymphadenopathy, chronic diarrhea, parotid swelling, chronic oral candidiasis, recurrent otitis media or sinusitis, hepatomegaly, splenomegaly, recurrent pneumonias, or development of a chronic lung disease termed *lymphocytic interstitial pneumonia* (or LIP). The diagnosis of HIV is often not considered in infants and young children until an opportunistic infection (OI) or AIDS-defining illness occurs (eg, pneumocystis pneumonia [PJP], esophageal candidiasis, cytomegalovirus infection, disseminated *Mycobacterium avium* complex disease). Infants and children who present with these symptoms should undergo an immunologic and infectious workup that includes HIV testing.

Adolescent patients are most commonly infected through sexual contact or intravenous (IV) drug use and may present differently than infants and young children. Two to 6 weeks after initial infection with HIV, about one-half of patients experience signs and symptoms of acute primary infection. The symptoms are nonspecific and resemble infectious mononucleosis symptoms; patients may experience fever, lymphadenopathy, headache, pharyngitis, maculopapular rash on the trunk or face, or diarrhea, as well as myalgias or arthralgias. Patients with HIV diagnosed years after their acute infection may experience constitutional symptoms, such as fevers, unintentional weight loss, night sweats, and lymphadenopathy, as well as recurrent or serious bacterial infections. In the late stages of disease, patients may present with AIDS-defining illnesses, including those mentioned previously as well as disseminated histoplasmosis, cryptococcal meningitis, *Mycobacterium tuberculosis* infections, encephalitis caused by *Toxoplasma gondii,* and central nervous system effects (eg, encephalopathy or dementia).

Evaluation

Evaluation and Management of the HIV-Seropositive Mother

In the setting of mother-to-child-transmission of HIV, the maternal plasma RNA has the greatest effect on transmission. High-circulating viral load increases the risk of transmission; however, transmission has been observed to occur at any viral load. Mother-to-child-transmission typically occurs during the intrapartum period when the neonate is exposed to the mother's blood and vaginal secretions. Consequently, prolonged rupture of membranes and vaginal delivery in a female with a high HIV plasma RNA places the baby at risk of acquiring the infection. Other risk factors for HIV transmission are premature birth, chorioamnionitis, advanced HIV infection, and maternal substance use. Postnatal transmission is primarily caused by breastfeeding; therefore, in areas where formula is easily accessible, breastfeeding should be avoided (Evidence Level II). In addition, mothers should be instructed to not pre-masticate food for their infants and young children since transmission of HIV has been reported with this route of feeding as well (Evidence Level III).

The risk of mother-to-child transmission of HIV can be less than 2% if the mother is receiving cART and has optimal viral suppression (defined as undetectable circulating virus). Prior to the introduction of cART, the risk of transmission was as high as 20% to 30% in non-breastfed neonates. Although high-circulating maternal plasma HIV RNA has been associated with a higher risk of transmission, there is no plasma HIV RNA threshold in which transmission does not occur. Identifying females of childbearing age and managing HIV infection is key to decreasing the risk of transmitting HIV.

For adolescent girls and women who are known to be HIV seropositive and optimally treated with cART, continuation of current therapy is suggested. Efavirenz is known to be teratogenic in animals (Pregnancy Category D), which has traditionally led to clinicians recommending changes in cART if an adolescent girl or woman is found to be pregnant. The risk of neural tube defects is during the first 5 to 6 weeks of pregnancy; but, because pregnancy is rarely recognized prior to 4 to 6 weeks and the risk of neural tube defects appears lower than previously anticipated, the US Department of Health and Human Services (DHHS) recommends continuing efavirenz therapy during the first trimester (given optimal viral suppression) since changes in cART can lead to loss of viral control and other adverse effects and a fetal ultrasound can be performed at 18 to 20 weeks to assess for possible adverse effects (Evidence Level III). In the case of an expectant mother who has detectable levels of HIV RNA at any time during pregnancy, resistance testing should be performed. An HIV specialist should be consulted in anticipation of a change in cART. Additionally, adherence as well as other pregnancy-related issues (eg, vomiting) should be evaluated and addressed to optimize therapy.

Although initiation of cART is the mainstay for preventing mother-to-child transmission, females whose HIV is newly diagnosed and who are antiretroviral (ARV) naive may consider delaying antiretroviral therapy (ART) until after the first trimester or 12 weeks' gestation (Evidence Level III). This would depend on maternal $CD4^+$ cell count, HIV RNA levels, and maternal conditions, such as nausea and vomiting. The benefits of early initiation of cART should be weighed against the potential risk of fetal effects during the first trimester. Selection of initial cART during pregnancy should be done in conjunction with an HIV specialist.

Pregnant HIV-infected adolescent girls and women can be registered with the Antiretroviral Pregnancy Registry, which is highly encouraged by the DHHS. This is a voluntary cohort that collects data on ARV use during pregnancy and birth defects. It is international in nature, and data are reviewed every 6 months to update any associations with ARV use and birth defects. To date, benefits of ARV therapy for the mother and prophylaxis for the neonate far outweigh the potential risk of birth defects, of which few have been documented. The Antiretroviral Pregnancy Registry and its report can be found at www.apregistry.com.

The Pediatric AIDS Clinical Trials Group (or PACTG) 076 study showed that IV zidovudine (initial loading dose: 2 mg/kg IV over 1 hour, followed by continuous infusion of 1 mg/kg/hour until delivery) along with maternal antepartum and neonatal zidovudine decreased the risk of transmission by 66%. Thus, IV zidovudine should be considered for all mothers during the intrapartum period, especially in HIV-infected women with HIV plasma RNA of 400 or greater copies/mL or unknown HIV plasma RNA at time of delivery (Evidence Level I). For mothers who are virologically suppressed (HIV plasma RNA <400 copies/mL) near delivery, IV zidovudine is not necessary (Evidence Level II). A scheduled cesarean delivery should be considered when the HIV-infected mother is not virologically controlled (HIV plasma RNA >1,000 copies/mL), and IV zidovudine should be initiated 3 hours prior to the procedure (Evidence Level I). For mothers who are on zidovudine-containing cART and are initiated on IV zidovudine, oral zidovudine is not necessary and other oral ARV in the cART regimen should be continued as scheduled.

In the case of a mother with unknown HIV status who presents at the time of delivery, a rapid HIV antibody test should be performed (Evidence Level II). If the rapid test results are positive, IV zidovudine as well as combination neonatal prophylaxis (discussed in the following sections) should be initiated pending the confirmatory results (Evidence Level II). If the confirmatory results are negative, prophylaxis can be discontinued. If the confirmatory results are positive, neonatal prophylaxis should be continued and the mother should be connected to care for management of HIV infection (Evidence Level I). A summary of the strategies to reduce perinatal transmission is listed in Table 30-1.

Table 30-1. Intrapartum HIV Prophylaxis for Mother and Neonate

Clinical Situation	Recommended Peripartum Prophylaxis for the HIV-Infected Mother
HIV-positive mother, HIV RNA viral load ≥400 copies/mL or unknown near time of delivery	IV zidovudine at 2 mg/kg over 1 h, followed by 1 mg/kg/h until delivery (Evidence Level I)
HIV-positive mother, HIV RNA viral load >1,000 copies/mL near time of delivery	Scheduled cesarean delivery + IV zidovudine (Evidence Level I)
HIV-positive mother, HIV RNA viral load <400 copies/mL near time of delivery	IV zidovudine not required (Evidence Level II)
Unknown HIV status at time of delivery	Obtain rapid HIV antibody test. • If positive, start maternal (IV zidovudine) and neonatal (combination ARV) prophylaxis (Evidence Level II). • If confirmatory HIV test is positive, continue neonatal prophylaxis for 6 wk (Evidence Level I). • If confirmatory HIV test is negative, discontinue neonatal prophylaxis (Evidence Level III).
Clinical Situation	Recommended Prophylaxis Regimen for the HIV-Exposed Neonate
HIV-positive mother, on cART, virologically controlled	Zidovudine alone for 6 wk (Evidence Level I)
HIV-positive mother, *not* on cART prenatally	Zidovudine for 6 wk + 3 doses of nevirapine (Evidence Level I)
HIV-positive mother, on cART, *not* virologically controlled	Zidovudine for 6 wk + 3 doses of nevirapine or consult HIV specialist (Evidence Level III)
HIV-positive mother, on cART with known/suspected ARV resistance	Consult HIV specialist (Evidence Level III).

Abbreviations: ARV, antiretroviral; cART, combination antiretroviral therapy; IV, intravenous.

Adapted from HHS Panel on Treatment of HIV-Infected Pregnant Women and Prevention of Perinatal Transmission—A Working Group of the Office of AIDS Research Advisory Council (OARAC). *Recommendations for Use of Antiretroviral Drugs in Pregnant HIV-1-Infected Women for Maternal Health and Interventions to Reduce Perinatal HIV Transmission in the United States.* Washington, DC: US Department of Health and Human Services. http://aidsinfo.nih.gov/contentfiles/lvguidelines/perinatalgl.pdf. Accessed August 17, 2016.

Evaluation and Management of the HIV-Exposed Neonate

Neonates who are born to HIV-infected mothers should receive ARV prophylaxis for the first 6 weeks of life to decrease the risk of transmission and also undergo an assessment to exclude disease. A 4-week prophylaxis course can be considered for full-term neonates born to mothers on cART with full virologic suppression (Evidence Level II). A summary of the recommendations for ARV strategies to prevent perinatal transmission is listed in Table 30-1, and the dosing is listed in Table 30-2. If there is known perinatal exposure, HIV DNA polymerase chain reaction (PCR) testing should be performed at 2 to 3 weeks,

Table 30-2. Recommended Dosing of Antiretrovirals for Neonates

Antiretroviral	Gestational Age or Weight	Dosing
Zidovudine	≥35 wk	4 mg/kg/dose orally every 12 h for 6 wk
	30–34 wk	2 mg/kg/dose orally every 12 h for 2 wk; then increased to 3 mg/kg/dose orally every 12 h for 4 wk
	<30 wk	2 mg/kg/dose orally every 12 h for 4 wk; then increased to 3 mg/kg/dose orally every 12 h for 2 wk
Nevirapine	>2.0 kg	12 mg orally at birth, 48 h after 1st dose, and 96 h after 2nd dose
	1.5–2.0 kg	8 mg orally at birth, 48 h after 1st dose, and 96 h after 2nd dose

Adapted from HHS Panel on Treatment of HIV-Infected Pregnant Women and Prevention of Perinatal Transmission —A Working Group of the Office of AIDS Research Advisory Council (OARAC). *Recommendations for Use of Antiretroviral Drugs in Pregnant HIV-1-Infected Women for Maternal Health and Interventions to Reduce Perinatal HIV Transmission in the United States.* Washington, DC: US Department of Health and Human Services. https://aidsinfo.nih.gov/contentfiles/lvguidelines/perinatalgl.pdf. Accessed August 17, 2016.

1 to 2 months, and 4 to 6 months of age. Two positive virologic tests lead to definitive diagnosis of HIV infection. Human immunodeficiency virus type 1 infection can be presumptively excluded with negative virologic tests at 2 or more weeks and 4 or more weeks or negative virologic test at 8 or more weeks. Definitive exclusion of HIV-1 infection is defined as 2 negative virologic tests (at ≥1 month and ≥4 months) or negative antibody test at 12 to 18 months.

Evaluation of the Disease

If HIV infection is suspected in a neonate (without known or suspected HIV exposure at birth; if known or suspected at birth, please see Evaluation and Management of the HIV-Exposed Neonate section), infant, or young child, further investigation is warranted.

In babies and children younger than 18 months, methods that detect IgG antibodies, such as enzyme-linked immunosorbent assay, or rapid tests may provide the clinician the first clue about infection. If these antibody tests are negative, no further workup is required. If these tests are positive, further virologic testing will be necessary. A positive IgG based on test alone may represent true infection or passive maternal antibody detection, since these antibodies can be detected for as long as 18 months after birth. Virologic testing using molecular techniques (eg, a qualitative HIV DNA PCR or quantitative HIV RNA PCR) should be performed, and if the virologic test is positive, the infant or young child should be considered to be HIV infected. Human immunodeficiency type 1 culture and p24 antigen testing are no longer recommended for diagnosis of HIV infection in infants. After the age of 18 months, standard testing with enzyme-linked immunosorbent assay or rapid tests can be used to diagnose HIV infection.

Universal testing is recommended in patients who are 13 to 64 years of age during health care encounters unless the prevalence of HIV is low in the region (<0.1%) (Evidence Level III). Although the overall rate of new HIV diagnoses has remained stable, the rate of HIV-1 infection in persons aged 13 to 29 increased by 21% in 2009, and up to 20% of patients may be unaware of their diagnosis. Thus, the adolescent population is a very important group to test for HIV infection. Testing is highly recommended in patients who have risk factors for HIV infection, such as men who have sex with men (MSM), history of IV drug use, or history of sexually transmitted infections (Evidence Level II-3). The Centers for Disease Control and Prevention recommends that informed consent of HIV testing not be required, but the patient should be given the opportunity to opt out of testing. Most states require counseling and education prior to testing but may not require written consent; to review the HIV testing laws in your state, visit the National HIV/AIDS Clinicians' Consultation Center Web site (http://nccc.ucsf.edu/clinical-resources/hiv-aids-resources/state-hiv-testing-laws/). It is important to counsel and test persons at high risk for transmission; if test results are negative, it provides an opportunity for further safety education. If HIV testing is positive, coordinating the connection to care with HIV specialists is important, and consistent follow-up in the primary care setting provides the patient a complete health care network.

If a patient is diagnosed as having HIV infection, an evaluation should include a thorough history and physical examination. Baseline laboratory tests include HIV plasma RNA, $CD4^+$ cell count or percentage, complete blood cell count, serum chemistries, viral hepatitis panel, urinalysis, and liver function panel to monitor both HIV-1 infection and adverse effects from the medications (Evidence Level I). See Table 30-3 for additional suggested initial tests.

Antiretroviral resistance testing should be done prior to starting cART to help select the best regimen for treatment (6%–16% of ARV-naive adult patients are infected with drug-resistant virus); however, genotypic testing may not be successful if the HIV plasma RNA is less than 1,000 copies/mL (Evidence Level III). If considering abacavir as part of the cART regimen, major histocompatibility complex (or MHC) class I allele HLA-B*57:01 genetic screening should be performed prior to initiation to identify persons at risk for a hypersensitivity reaction; if the test is positive, abacavir should be avoided (Evidence Level I). If dapsone is needed for PJP prophylaxis because of sulfonamide allergy, the patient should undergo testing for glucose-6-phosphate dehydrogenase deficiency; if the patient is deficient, dapsone should be avoided and alternatives, such as atovaquone, can be used.

In adolescent and young adult patients with new diagnosis, a full workup to exclude concurrent sexually transmitted infections should be performed. Lastly, care of the HIV-infected patient should be patient centered and multidisciplinary; the patient and family should be evaluated for social, economic, substance use disorder, mental illness, comorbidity, and medical insurance concerns. If issues are identified, they should be managed accordingly because these factors can affect adherence to medications.

Table 30-3. Suggested Monitoring Schedule for HIV-Infected Patients

Parameter	Initial Visit	Prior to Antiretroviral Therapy	Antiretroviral Initiation[a]	First 1–2 mo[b]	Every 3–4 mo	Every 6–12 mo	Antiretroviral Modification
Clinical history and physical examination	X	X	X	X	X		X
Adherence evaluation	X		X	X	X		X
CD4+ cell count/percentage	X	Every 3–6 mo	X		X[c]		X
HIV plasma RNA	X	Every 3–6 mo	X	X	X[c]		X
CBC/differential[d]	X	Every 3–6 mo	X		X		X
Electrolytes[d]	X	Every 6–12 mo	X		X		X
Glucose[d]	X	Yearly	X		X		X
Serum urea nitrogen/creatinine[d]	X	Every 6–12 mo	X		X		X
AST/ALT/bilirubin[d]	X	Every 6–12 mo	X	X	X		X
Albumin/protein[d]	X	Every 6–12 mo	X			X	X
Lipid panel	X	Yearly	X			X	
Urinalysis	X		X			X	

Continued

Table 30-3 *(cont)*

Parameter	Initial Visit	Prior to Antiretroviral Therapy	Antiretroviral Initiation[a]	First 1–2 mo[b]	Every 3–4 mo	Every 6–12 mo	Antiretroviral Modification
Resistance test	X		X[e]				X
HLA-B*57:01 screening			X[f]				X[f]
Tropism test			X[g]				X[g]
Pregnancy test			X[h]				X[h]
Hepatitis B Screening[i]		X					

Abbreviations: ALT, alanine transaminase; AST, aspartate transaminase; CBC, complete blood cell count.

[a] If baseline laboratories were obtained within 30 to 45 days of initial visit, pre-initiation laboratories may not be necessary.

[b] When starting a new regimen, patients should be evaluated in person or by phone to screen for adverse effects and evaluate adherence; HIV RNA viral load may be obtained in the first few weeks of therapy to evaluate response.

[c] In clinically and virologically stable patients (HIV plasma RNA undetectable for >12 mo), clinicians can consider extending testing of HIV plasma RNA (to every 6 mo) and CD4$^+$ cell counts (to every 6–12 mo).

[d] Some chemistries may need to be more frequently monitored during the initial months of therapy, depending on the antiretroviral agent, or if abnormalities are observed.

[e] If resistance testing was obtained at the first visit, repeating resistance test prior to starting therapy is optional.

[f] HLA-B*57:01 screening should be performed if abacavir is being considered as part of antiretroviral therapy regimen; if positive, abacavir should be avoided.

[g] Tropism testing should be performed if CCR5 receptor antagonists (eg, maraviroc) are being considered as part of antiretroviral therapy regimen; if negative, CCR5 receptor antagonists should be avoided.

[h] Pregnancy testing should be performed in females of childbearing age if efavirenz is being considered as part of antiretroviral therapy regimen (Pregnancy Category D).

[i] If starting antiretroviral with hepatitis B activity (eg, lamivudine, emtricitabine, tenofovir) and if patient has not previously demonstrated immunity.

Adapted from DHHS Panel on Antiretroviral Guidelines for Adults and Adolescents—A Working Group of the Office of AIDS Research Advisory Council (OARAC). *Guidelines for the Use of Antiretroviral Agents in HIV-1-Infected Adults and Adolescents.* Washington, DC: US Department of Health and Human Services. http://aidsinfo.nih.gov/contentfiles/lvguidelines/adultandadolescentgl.pdf. Accessed August 18, 2016.

Management

. . . .

If a child has been diagnosed as having HIV infection, cART and supportive care are the keystones to management. Because there is no cure for HIV-1 infection, the primary goals of treatment are to reduce HIV-associated morbidity and mortality, maximize immunologic function, achieve durable suppression of viral replication, minimize ARV-associated toxicities, and reduce transmission of HIV. Care of an HIV-infected child should be provided with a team that includes a pediatric HIV specialist; however, the primary care physician plays the very important role of the medical home by providing continuity and coordinating care with other specialists as needed.

Antiretroviral therapy should be initiated in children and adolescents with the indications outlined in Table 30-4. Once treatment is started, poor adherence ($<95\%$ doses of medication) places the patient at risk for immunologic suppression and OIs. Moreover, in nonadherent patients, resistance mutations can accumulate and limit the number of ARVs available to treat HIV infection

Table 30-4. Clinical and Laboratory Indications for Initiating Antiretroviral Therapy in Pediatric and Adolescent Patients

Patient Age	When to Start Antiretroviral Therapy
<12 mo	Regardless of clinical symptoms, immune status, or HIV RNA viral load (Evidence Level II)
$1-<6$ y	• AIDS or significant HIV-related symptoms (Evidence Level I) • CD4$^+$ cell count <500 cells/mm^3 (Evidence Level I) • Moderate HIV-related symptoms (Evidence Level II) • CD4$^+$ cell count 500–999 cells/mm^3 (Evidence Level II) • Asymptomatic/mild symptoms, CD4$^+$ cell count ≥ 1000 cells/mm^3, and HIV plasma RNA ≥ 100K copies/mcL (Evidence Level II)

$6-<12$ y	• AIDS or significant HIV-related symptoms (Evidence Level I)
	• CD4$^+$ cell count ≤ 500 cells/mm^3
	  o <200 cells/mm^3 (Evidence Level I)
	  o 200–499 cells/mm^3 (Evidence Level II)
	• Moderate HIV-related symptoms (Evidence Level II)
	• Asymptomatic/mild symptoms, CD4$^+$ cell count ≥ 500 cell/mm^3 (Evidence Level II)

Adolescents	Regardless of clinical symptoms or immune status, including acute HIV infection (Evidence Level I)

Adapted from DHHS Panel on Antiretroviral Guidelines for Adults and Adolescents—A Working Group of the Office of AIDS Research Advisory Council (OARAC). *Guidelines for the Use of Antiretroviral Agents in HIV-1-Infected Adults and Adolescents.* Washington, DC: US Department of Health and Human Services. http://aidsinfo.nih.gov/contentfiles/lvguidelines/adultandadolescentgl.pdf. Accessed August 18, 2016; and HHS Panel on Antiretroviral Therapy and Medical Management of HIV-Infected Children—A Working Group of the Office of AIDS Research Advisory Council (OARAC). *Guidelines for the Use of Antiretroviral Agents in Pediatric HIV Infection.* Washington, DC: US Department of Health and Human Services. http://aidsinfo.nih.gov/contentfiles/lvguidelines/pediatricguidelines.pdf. Accessed August 18, 2016.

in the future. If factors associated with nonadherence are identified, clinicians may consider delaying therapy until adherence can be guaranteed, even if the patient qualifies for cART. On the other hand, if therapy can be started earlier, recent data have suggested early initiation of cART may decrease the risk of non–AIDS-related death. If a patient is strongly interested and able to demonstrate good adherence, he or she may be considered for early initiation.

Table 30-5 lists all available ARVs to treat HIV infection. Table 30-6 lists the ART regimens recommended as first-line therapy in children and adolescents by the DHHS Panel on Antiretroviral Therapy and Medical Management of HIV-Infected Children and Panel on Antiretrovirals Guidelines for Adults and Adolescents. In the rare situation when ART needs to be initiated emergently before the resistance panel is available, a protease inhibitor (PI)–based regimen should be used. Several alternative initial ART regimens are available in the HIV treatment guidelines.

In addition to discussing the importance of treatment and treatment adherence, it is important to discuss adverse effects of the medications. Adverse effects and long-term adverse effects of common ARVs and their management are listed in Table 30-7. Many patients and families who are not aware of the adverse effects and how to manage them may self-discontinue medications; supportive care, assurance, and education are critical in managing adverse effects. Additionally, some effects may not be visible to patients, and follow-up laboratory tests and physical examinations are necessary to monitor toxicities. In some cases, when the adverse effects are severe and affect quality of life, a change in the regimen may be necessary.

Nucleoside reverse transcriptase inhibitors (NRTIs) as a drug class have a warning for lactic acidosis and fatty liver; older NRTIs, such as zidovudine, stavudine, and didanosine, are at the highest risk of causing these symptoms. Patients should be educated to look for signs and symptoms of lactic acidosis, such as nausea, vomiting, abdominal pain, hyperventilation, muscular weakness, and lethargy. Other effects of mitochondrial toxicity associated with NRTIs include neuropathy, muscle pain, pancreatitis, and bone marrow suppression.

Non-nucleoside reverse transcriptase inhibitors (NNRTIs) are well-known to be associated with severe skin reactions and hepatotoxicity, especially nevirapine. Patients should be educated to follow up immediately if a rash is noted when starting an NNRTI; in some cases, discontinuation may be necessary. Additionally, hepatotoxicity is common so transaminases should be followed closely at the beginning of therapy. Efavirenz has central nervous system adverse effects, which rarely include psychiatric adverse effects, such as depression and suicidal ideation; additionally, it is a Pregnancy Category D medication and females of childbearing age should be educated to use contraception (preferably 2 forms).

One of the major adverse effects of PIs is gastrointestinal effects; most patients will experience diarrhea and nausea in the beginning of therapy.

Table 30-5. List of Antiretrovirals Available to Treat HIV Infection

Antiretroviral Class/Group	Generic Name (Trade Name)
NRTIs	Zidovudine (Retrovir) Lamivudine (Epivir) Emtricitabine (Emtriva) Abacavir (Ziagen) Tenofovir disoproxil fumarate (Viread) Didanosine (Videx or Videx EC) Stavudine (Zerit)
Combination NRTIs (fixed dose)	Zidovudine/lamivudine (Combivir) Abacavir/lamivudine (Epzicom) Abacavir/lamivudine/zidovudine (Trizivir) Tenofovir disoproxil fumarate/emtricitabine (Truvada) Tenofovir alafenamide/emtricitabine (Descovy)
NNRTIs	Nevirapine (Viramune) Efavirenz (Sustiva) Etravirine (Intelence) Rilpivirine (Edurant)
Combination NRTI/NNRTIs (fixed dose)	Tenofovir disoproxil fumarate/emtricitabine/efavirenz (Atripla) Tenofovir disoproxil fumarate/emtricitabine/rilpivirine (Complera) Tenofovir alafenamide/emtricitabine/rilpivirine (Odefsey)
PIs	Lopinavir/ritonavir (Kaletra) Atazanavir (Reyataz) Atazanavir/cobicistat (Evotaz) Darunavir (Prezista) Darunavir/cobicistat (Prezcobix) Fosamprenavir (Lexiva) Indinavir (Crixivan) Nelfinavir (Viracept) Ritonavir (Norvir) Saquinavir (Invirase) Tipranavir (Aptivus)
INSTI	Raltegravir (Isentress) Elvitegravir (Vitekta) Dolutegravir (Tivicay)
Combination NRTI/INSTI (fixed dose)	Abacavir/lamivudine/dolutegravir (Triumeq) Tenofovir disoproxil fumarate/emtricitabine/elvitegravir/cobicistat (Stribild) Tenofovir alafenamide/emtricitabine/elvitegravir/cobicistat (Genvoya)
Fusion inhibitor	Enfuvirtide (Fuzeon)
CCR5 receptor antagonist	Maraviroc (Selzentry)

Abbreviations: INSTI, integrase strand transferase inhibitor; NNRTI, non-nucleoside reverse transcriptase inhibitor; NRTI, nucleoside reverse transcriptase inhibitor; PI, protease inhibitor.

Table 30-6. US Department of Human and Health Services Recommended Initial Antiretroviral Therapy Regimens by Age (Evidence Level I)

Age	Recommended Regimen
14 d–<2 y	2 NRTIs + lopinavir/ritonavir
2–<3 y	2 NRTIs + lopinavir/ritonavir 2 NRTIs + raltegravir
3–<12 y	2 NRTIs + efavirenz 2 NRTIs + lopinavir/ritonavir 2 NRTIs + twice daily darunavir + ritonavir 2 NRTIs + atazanavir + ritonavir 2 NRTIs + raltegravir
Adolescents ≥12 y and not sexually mature	2 NRTIs + once daily darunavir + ritonavir 2 NRTIs + atazanavir + ritonavir 2 NRTIs + dolutegravir 2 NRTIs + elvitegravir + cobicistat
Adolescents ≥12 y and sexually mature	PI-based • Darunavir + ritonavir + emtricitabine/tenofovir disoproxil fumarate INSTI-based: • Dolutegravir/abacavir/lamivudine • Dolutegravir + emtricitabine/tenofovir disoproxil fumarate • Elvitegravir/cobicistat/tenofovir alafenamide/emtricitabine if ClCr >30 mL/min • Elvitegravir/cobicistat/tenofovir disoproxil fumarate/emtricitabine if ClCr >70 mL/min • Raltegravir + emtricitabine/tenofovir disoproxil fumarate
Preferred 2-NRTI Combination	
Birth–<3 mo	Zidovudine *plus* lamivudine or emtricitabine
3 mo–<12 y	Zidovudine *plus* lamivudine or emtricitabine Abacavir *plus* lamivudine or emtricitabine
Adolescents ≥12 y and not sexually mature	Abacavir *plus* lamivudine or emtricitabine Tenofovir alafenamide/emtricitabine
Adolescents ≥12 y and sexually mature	See above.

Abbreviations: ClCr, creatinine clearance; INSTI, integrase strand transferase inhibitor; NRTI, nucleoside reverse transcriptase inhibitor; PI, protease inhibitor.

Adapted from DHHS Panel on Antiretroviral Guidelines for Adults and Adolescents—A Working Group of the Office of AIDS Research Advisory Council (OARAC). *Guidelines for the Use of Antiretroviral Agents in HIV-1-Infected Adults and Adolescents*. Washington, DC: US Department of Health and Human Services. http://aidsinfo.nih.gov/contentfiles/lvguidelines/adultandadolescentgl.pdf. Accessed August 18, 2016; and HHS Panel on Antiretroviral Therapy and Medical Management of HIV-Infected Children—A Working Group of the Office of AIDS Research Advisory Council (OARAC). *Guidelines for the Use of Antiretroviral Agents in Pediatric HIV Infection*. Washington, DC: US Department of Health and Human Services. http://aidsinfo.nih.gov/contentfiles/lvguidelines/pediatricguidelines.pdf. Accessed August 18, 2016.

Table 30-7. Adverse Effects and Management for Common Antiretrovirals Used in the Treatment of HIV Infection in Children and Adolescents

Adverse Effect	Associated Antiretrovirals	Risk Factors	Prevention/Monitoring	Management
Bone marrow suppression	Zidovudine (macrocytic anemia, neutropenia, or both)	Premature birth Underlying hemoglobinopathy Poorly controlled HIV Concomitant marrow-toxic medications (trimethoprim/sulfamethoxazole, ribavirin, ganciclovir, and steroids)	CBC as part of routine care May consider monitoring CBC more frequently in neonates with risk factors and receiving zidovudine prophylaxis	Rarely needs intervention unless hemoglobin <7.0 g/dL, patient is symptomatic, or absolute neutrophil count <500/mm³. Discontinue other marrow-toxic medications; identify and treat underlying illnesses. Can consider changing zidovudine to another antiretroviral. Can consider trial of erythropoietin or granulocyte colony-stimulating factor. In neonates receiving prophylaxis, can consider discontinuation if ≥4 wk.
Rash	All NNRTIs PIs • Atazanavir • Darunavir • Fosamprenavir INSTI: raltegravir (uncommon) Elvitegravir (uncommon)	Sulfonamide allergy (to atazanavir, darunavir, or fosamprenavir)	Monitor for rash and assess severity.	Mild to moderate rash: Provide symptomatic treatment and medication can be continued (caution if rash is noted with nevirapine use). Severe rash: Discontinue ART and other possible agents and provide supportive therapy; when restarting therapy, avoid offending agent (especially if NNRTI).

Continued

Table 30-7 *(cont)*

Adverse Effect	Associated Antiretrovirals	Risk Factors	Prevention/Monitoring	Management
SJS/TEN	NRTI: case reports with zidovudine and didanosine	Adults/adolescents • Female sex • Race/ethnicity (African American, Hispanic, and Asian)	Nevirapine: 2-wk dose escalation. Counsel patients and families to report symptoms immediately.	Discontinue ART and other possible agents. Provide supportive therapy (hydration, wound care, or pain management). Do not reintroduce offending medication.
	NNRTI: nevirapine most common, but all NNRTIs			
	PIs: reported cases with atazanavir, darunavir, fosamprenavir, indinavir, lopinavir/ritonavir			
	INSTI: raltegravir (uncommon)			
Hypersensitivity reactions	NRTI: abacavir (Symptoms include fever/chills, rash, malaise, nausea, headache, myalgia/arthralgia, GI effects [diarrhea, vomiting, or abdominal pain], and respiratory symptoms.)	HLA-B*57:01 (more common in Caucasian than African American or Asian patients)	Avoid in patients who have positive screening for HLA-B*57:01. Screen for HLA-B*57:01 prior to starting abacavir. Counsel patients and families of signs and symptoms of hypersensitivity reaction and to report symptoms immediately.	Discontinue abacavir. Provide supportive therapy if needed. Do *not* rechallenge abacavir hypersensitivity reactions, because of risk of fatality.
	NNRTI: nevirapine (hypersensitivity syndrome of hepatic toxicity and rash) (Symptoms include fever, blisters, myalgia/arthralgia, conjunctivitis, lymphadenopathy, and facial edema.)	Adults/adolescents • Female sex • Males with pretreatment CD4$^+$ cell count >400/mm^3 and females with pretreatment CD4$^+$ cell count >250/mm^3 Children: Risk may be lower.	2-week lead-in period. Avoid use in males with pretreatment CD4$^+$ cell count >400/mm^3 and females with pretreatment CD4$^+$ cell count >250/mm^3. Counsel patients and families of signs and symptoms of hypersensitivity reaction and to report symptoms immediately.	Discontinue ART and other hepatotoxic medications. Provide supportive care as needed. Consider other causes of hepatitis. Avoid reintroducing nevirapine and other NNRTIs.

	INSTIs	Raltegravir: Seen when given with other medications known to be associated with hypersensitivity reactions Dolutegravir: <1% reported	Counsel patients and families of signs and symptoms of hypersensitivity reaction and to report symptoms immediately.	Discontinue ART. Provide supportive care as needed.
Cardiovascular effects	NRTIs • Abacavir • Didanosine (MI may be associated with use, but causal relationship unclear.)	Highest risk in patients with traditional cardiovascular disease risk factors	Counsel patients and families of signs and symptoms of cardiovascular issues and to report symptoms immediately.	Risk of MI has been primarily observational in the adult population; risk in the pediatric population is unknown.
	PIs: associated with MI and stroke in some studies PR prolongation: saquinavir + ritonavir or atazanavir + ritonavir or lopinavir/ritonavir	PR and QT prolongation Structural heart disease Cardiomyopathy Ischemic heart disease Concomitant PR- and QT-prolonging medications	Baseline electrocardiogram; consider monitoring throughout therapy. Evaluate for other QT-prolonging concomitant medications.	Risk of MI has been primarily observational in the adult population; risk in the pediatric population is unknown. Consider consultation with a cardiologist and possible ARV change. Consider discontinuation of other QT- or PR-prolonging medications.

Continued

Table 30-7 *(cont)*

Adverse Effect	Associated Antiretrovirals	Risk Factors	Prevention/Monitoring	Management
CNS effects	NNRTI: efavirenz (insomnia, abnormal dreams, impaired concentration, depression, psychosis, or suicidal ideation)	High efavirenz concentrations (>4 mcg/mL) Decreased metabolism of efavirenz (routine testing for CYP2B6 polymorphisms not currently recommended) History of psychiatric illnesses or use of psychotropic drugs	Administer on an empty stomach at bedtime to reduce effects. Monitor carefully in patients with history of psychiatric illness.	Assure patient that adverse effects are limited (typically 4 wk). Can consider obtaining trough concentration if symptoms persist.
	PI: lopinavir/ritonavir oral solution (contains ethanol and propylene glycol; has been associated with CNS depression, cardiotoxicity, and respiratory depression)	Neonates <42 wk' postmenstrual age or >14 d' postnatal age	Avoid use in neonates <42 wk' postmenstrual age or <14 d' postnatal age.	Discontinue medication; symptoms should resolve within 5 days.
	INSTI: raltegravir (headaches or insomnia)	History of insomnia	Evaluate for signs and symptoms of insomnia	Consider trial of discontinuation if insomnia is severe.
Peripheral neuropathy	NRTIs: stavudine, didanosine (aching, burning, or painful numbness bilaterally) (Stavudine can be associated with ascending neuromuscular weakness.)	Preexisting neuropathy Older age Poor nutrition Advanced HIV disease	Monitor for signs and symptoms of peripheral neuropathy.	Discontinue stavudine or didanosine. Neuropathy can be permanent and is difficult to treat; topical capsaicin may be effective.

			Prevention/Monitoring	Management
Diabetes mellitus or insulin resistance	Metabolic syndrome Lipodystrophy Obesity Family history of diabetes mellitus	NRTIs • Zidovudine • Didanosine • Stavudine PIs • Indinavir • Lopinavir/ritonavir (other PIs not studied) Less risk • Atazanavir • Fosamprenavir	Prevention: Lifestyle modification. Monitoring: Signs and symptoms of diabetes (polyuria, polydipsia, or polyphagia) or weight gain. Obtain random plasma glucose routinely with treatment; if random plasma glucose >140 mg/dL, obtain fasting plasma glucose.	Counsel on lifestyle modification. If random plasma glucose >200 mg/dL or fasting plasma glucose >126 mg/dL, patient meets diagnostic criteria for diabetes; refer to an endocrinologist for management. If fasting plasma glucose is 100–125 mg/dL, may be a sign of insulin resistance; refer to an endocrinologist for management.
Dyslipidemia	HIV infection Poor diet Obesity Lack of exercise Hypertension Metabolic syndrome Family history of dyslipidemia or cardiovascular disease	NRTIs: stavudine, zidovudine, didanosine (increase in triglycerides and LDL) NNRTI: efavirenz (increase in triglycerides, LDL, and HDL) PI: ritonavir-boosted regimens (increase in triglycerides, LDL, and HDL; lower incidence seen with atazanavir) INSTI: elvitegravir/cobicistat/tenofovir disoproxil fumarate/emtricitabine (increase in triglycerides, LDL, and HDL observed)	Prevention: low-fat diet and exercise, smoking cessation Monitoring • Adolescents—fasting lipid profile prior to initiating or changing ART. • Children—non-fasting screening lipid profile prior to initiating or changing ART; if abnormal, obtain fasting lipid profile.	Counsel patient on lifestyle modifications. Can consider changing ART that has less dyslipidemic effects. Pharmacologic management with fibrates or statins may be required; consider comanagement with a specialist.

Continued

Table 30-7 *(cont)*

Adverse Effect	Associated Antiretrovirals	Risk Factors	Prevention/Monitoring	Management
GI effects	NRTIs • Zidovudine (nausea or vomiting) • Didanosine, stavudine (pancreatitis)	Pancreatitis: concurrent use of didanosine and stavudine, concomitant use with other medications associated with pancreatitis, hypertriglyceridemia	Monitor for weight loss and adherence. Pancreatitis: Avoid in patients with history of pancreatitis.	Assure patient that nausea and vomiting will decrease over time. Antiemetics are not recommended for routine use but can be considered in severe cases. Pancreatitis: Discontinue offending agent and provide supportive care.
	All PIs (diarrhea, nausea, or vomiting [especially with nelfinavir and lopinavir/ritonavir]) INSTI: elvitegravir/cobicistat/tenofovir disoproxil fumarate/emtricitabine (nausea and diarrhea)	NA	Monitor for weight loss and dehydration. Can take with food to decrease nausea. Can rule out other infectious causes of diarrhea.	Assure patient that diarrhea will decrease over time. Can consider dietary modification, bulking agents, or antimotility agents if diarrhea is persistent.
Hepatotoxicity	NRTIs • Zidovudine, stavudine, didanosine (fatty liver) • Didanosine (non-cirrhotic portal hypertension with esophageal varices)	Concomitant didanosine and stavudine. Non-cirrhotic portal hypertension (with elevated transaminase and alkaline phosphatase concentrations and thrombocytopenia) associated with long-term didanosine has been observed in adults.	Avoid concomitant use of didanosine and stavudine (especially in pregnant women).	Rare cases of fatal lactic acidosis with hepatomegaly and fatty change have been reported; fatty liver generally appears with lactic acidosis. See Lactic Acidosis row for management.

All NNRTIs, but most common and severe with nevirapine	Nevirapine-associated hepatotoxicity Adolescents: males with pretreatment CD4+ cell count >400/mm³ and females with pretreatment CD4+ cell count >250/mm³	2-wk dose escalation. Avoid in adolescent boys with pretreatment CD4+ cell count >400/mm³ and females with pretreatment CD4+ cell count >250/mm³. Avoid in patients with baseline AST/AST >5–10 times ULN. Nevirapine is contraindicated in patients with Child-Pugh classification of B or C. Monitor AST and ALT as part of routine care; consider more frequent monitoring at beginning of therapy.	If symptomatic hepatitis is observed with nevirapine, nevirapine should be discontinued and not restarted; ART and other hepatotoxic medications should be discontinued.
All PIs (Fatalities associated with hepatotoxicity have been reported.) Atazanavir, indinavir (hyperbilirubinemia)	Coinfection with hepatitis B and C Concurrent hepatotoxic medications Elevated baseline AST and ALT concentrations Underlying liver disease Hyperbilirubinemia: none	Avoid in patients with baseline AST/AST >5–10 times ULN. Monitor AST and ALT as part of routine care. Monitor bilirubin periodically.	In asymptomatic patients with AST or ALT >5 times ULN, can consider discontinuation of ART or continue and monitor carefully. In patients with symptomatic hepatitis, discontinue ART and other potential hepatotoxic medications; avoid restarting offending agent. Look for other causes of hepatitis. Hyperbilirubinemia is primarily cosmetic. The offending agent does not have to be discontinued; may decrease over time.

Continued

Table 30-7 (cont)

Adverse Effect	Associated Antiretrovirals	Risk Factors	Prevention/Monitoring	Management
Lactic acidosis	All NRTIs, especially stavudine, didanosine, and zidovudine (mortality of up to 50% observed)	Adult/adolescent • Female sex • High BMI • Prolonged NRTI use • $CD4^+$ cell count $<350/mm^3$ • Pregnancy • African American ethnicity	Prevention: Avoid concomitant use of stavudine and didanosine. Monitoring: Routine serum lactate levels not recommended. Watch for signs and symptoms of lactic acidosis (fatigue, weakness, difficulty breathing, abdominal pain, nausea, vomiting); some patients may present with multiorgan failure.	Lactate level 19–45 mg/dL: Discontinue offending agent (stavudine, didanosine) and change to another agent. Lactate level >45 mg/dL: Discontinue ART and provide supportive therapy; when restarting therapy, select NRTI with less mitochondrial toxicity (abacavir, tenofovir, lamivudine) and monitor serum lactate monthly for at least 3 mo.
Nephrotoxicity/ nephrolithiasis	NRTI: tenofovir disoproxil fumarate (elevated serum creatinine levels or Fanconi syndrome)	Preexisting renal dysfunction Advanced HIV disease Concomitant didanosine or PI (especially lopinavir/ritonavir)	Monitor urinalysis; serum creatinine, phosphorous, and calcium.	If no other cause of nephrotoxicity is identified, consider changing tenofovir disoproxil fumarate to another NRTI.
	PIs • Indinavir, atazanavir (nephrolithiasis/ urolithiasis) • Indinavir (increased serum creatinine levels, hydronephrosis, or renal atrophy)	NA	Prevention: Adequate hydration decreases the risk of developing nephrolithiasis. Monitor urinalysis.	Provide adequate hydration and pain control. Consider changing therapy. If indinavir is associated with nephrotoxicity, change to alternative PI.

| Osteopenia/ osteoporosis | NRTI: tenofovir disoproxil fumarate

NNRTIs, PIs, and INSTI (lower bone marrow density observed in different combinations of cART) | Long duration of HIV infection
Low BMI
Lipodystrophy
Smoking
Steroid use
Medroxyprogesterone use
Nonblack race (Caucasian, Brazilian, Thai) | Tenofovir disoproxil fumarate should be avoided in children <12 y.
Prevention: Adequate calcium and vitamin D intake, weight-bearing exercise.
Monitoring: Assess nutritional intake, serum 25-hydroxyvitamin D levels, and dual energy x-ray absorptiometry scan every 6–12 mo in prepubertal children. | Ensure adequate intake of nutrition.
Correct vitamin D deficiency.
Weight-bearing exercise.
Reduce risk factors (smoking or steroid or medroxyprogesterone use).
Role of diphosphonates have not been established in children. |
| Lipodystrophy | NRTIs
• Stavudine
• Zidovudine
(facial/peripheral lipoatrophy)

Efavirenz, PIs, and raltegravir (central fat increase observed) | Obesity prior to cART

Obesity prior to cART | Monitor through patient report and physical examination.

Lifestyle modification.
Monitor BMI. | If possible, change stavudine or zidovudine to another NRTI.

Lifestyle modification |

Abbreviations: ALT, alanine transaminase; ART, antiretroviral therapy; ARV, antiretroviral; AST, aspartate transaminase; BMI, body mass index; cART, combination antiretroviral therapy; CBC, complete blood cell count; CNS, central nervous system; CYP2B6, cytochrome P450 2B6; GI, gastrointestinal; HDL, high-density lipoprotein; INSTI, integrase strand transferase inhibitor; LDL, low-density lipoprotein; MI, myocardial infarction; NA, not applicable; NNRTI, non-nucleoside reverse transcriptase inhibitor; NRTI, nucleoside reverse transcriptase inhibitor; PI, protease inhibitor; SJS/TEN, Stevens-Johnson syndrome/toxic epidermal necrolysis; ULN, upper limit of normal.

Adapted from DHHS Panel on Antiretroviral Guidelines for Adults and Adolescents—A Working Group of the Office of AIDS Research Advisory Council (OARAC). *Guidelines for the Use of Antiretroviral Agents in HIV-1-Infected Adults and Adolescents.* Washington, DC: US Department of Health and Human Services. http://aidsinfo.nih.gov/contentfiles/lvguidelines/adultandadolescentgl.pdf. Accessed August 18, 2016; and HHS Panel on Antiretroviral Therapy and Medical Management of HIV-Infected Children—A Working Group of the Office of AIDS Research Advisory Council (OARAC). *Guidelines for the Use of Antiretroviral Agents in Pediatric HIV Infection.* Washington, DC: US Department of Health and Human Services. http://aidsinfo.nih.gov/contentfiles/lvguidelines/pediatricguidelines.pdf. Accessed August 18, 2016.

Patients and family members should be assured that the adverse effect will resolve with time but may take up to 4 weeks before stooling patterns become normal. Hepatotoxicity and PR or QT prolongation are other adverse effects that have been noted with PIs; increased bleeding risk has been observed with PIs, so they should be avoided in patients with hemophilia. Metabolic issues, such as diabetes, dyslipidemia, and central obesity, are common with patients who are on PIs and should be monitored regularly; other ARVs, including NRTIs and efavirenz, can cause dyslipidemia or insulin resistance.

Integrase strand transferase inhibitors (INSTIs) are used as first-line therapy in children and adolescent patients and are generally well tolerated. Common adverse effects include nausea, headache, diarrhea, rash, and insomnia; serious adverse effects include hypersensitivity reactions. Raltegravir has been associated with myopathy and Stevens-Johnson syndrome. Elvitegravir should always be administered with a cytochrome P450 3A4 inhibitor (ie, cobicistat) for optimal pharmacokinetics and pharmacodynamics; additional adverse effects include dyslipidemia and serum creatinine elevation without affecting glomerular filtration (effect from cobicistat).

Lastly, drug-drug interactions should be evaluated. The NNRTIs can act as either an inducer or inhibitor of cytochrome P450 enzymes, and PIs and cobicistat are often strong inhibitors of cytochrome P450 enzymes. Additionally, adverse effects of ARVs can be compounded by other concomitant medications, such as antimicrobials for tuberculosis treatment, chemotherapy agents, and renal toxic medications (eg, prolonged nonsteroidal anti-inflammatory drugs, aminoglycosides). It is very important to review current medications, both prescription and over-the-counter, for possible drug-drug and drug-disease state interactions. Patients and families should be educated to contact clinicians if new medications are initiated.

The overall treatment goal of HIV is to prevent morbidity and mortality associated with OIs. It is important for the patient and family to understand that death associated with HIV is not from the virus itself, but rather the ultimate effect on the immune system, which puts the patient at risk for infections. As the $CD4^+$ cell count decreases, it is associated with acquisition of certain OIs or malignancies; however, AIDS-defining illnesses can occur at any $CD4^+$ cell count. Infants who have HIV infection are at high risk of death due to PJP; thus, it is recommended to initiate trimethoprim/sulfamethoxazole for prevention after completing the 6 weeks of zidovudine prophylaxis in HIV-exposed infants unless they are presumptively HIV negative with 2 negative HIV DNA PCRs obtained after 2 weeks of age. Indications and agents for primary prophylaxis to prevent OIs such as PJP, toxoplasmosis, and *M avium* complex disease are outlined in Table 30-8. The guidelines also provide recommendations for treatment and secondary prophylaxis for OIs.

In all patients, the immunization record should be reviewed and guidelines followed for HIV-infected patients. This ensures that the patient has been properly immunized and provides the opportunity for catch-up immunization if needed (Evidence Level III). Vaccines are effective tools in preventing

Table 30-8. Primary Prophylaxis for Opportunistic Infections in Children and Adolescents

Pathogen	Indication	First-line	Alternative
Pneumocystis jiroveci	Infants: aged 1–12 mo (including HIV-indeterminate) Children • Aged 1–<6 y: CD4$^+$ cell count <500/mm^3 or percentage <15% • ≥6 y: CD4$^+$ cell count <200/mm^3	Children: trimethoprim/sulfamethoxazole at 2.5–5/12.5–25 mg/kg orally twice per day (maximum: 320/1,600 mg/d) (Evidence Level I); alternative dosing for same daily dose: 3 consecutive or alternate days, 2 consecutive or alternate days, or 1 total daily dose	Children • Dapsone (children ≥1 mo) at 2 mg/kg orally daily (maximum: 100 mg) or 4 mg/kg once weekly (maximum: 200 mg) (Evidence Level I) • Atovaquone ○ 1–3 mo: 30-40 mg/kg orally daily ○ 4–24 mo: 45 mg/kg orally daily ○ ≥24 mo: 30-40 mg/kg orally daily (maximum: 1,500 mg) • Aerosolized pentamidine (children ≥5 y) at 300 mg nebulized every month (Evidence Level I)
	Adolescents: CD4$^+$ cell count <200/mm^3	Adolescents: trimethoprim/sulfamethoxazole, 1 double-strength tablet orally daily (Evidence Level I), or 1 single-strength tablet orally daily (Evidence Level I)	Adolescents • Trimethoprim/sulfamethoxazole, 1 double-strength tablet orally 3 times weekly (Evidence Level I) • Dapsone at 100 mg orally daily or 50 mg orally twice daily (Evidence Level I) • Dapsone at 50 mg orally daily + pyrimethamine at 50 mg orally weekly + leucovorin at 25 mg orally weekly (Evidence Level I) • Aerosolized pentamidine at 300 mg inhaled monthly (Evidence Level I) • Atovaquone at 1,500 mg orally daily (Evidence Level I) • Atovaquone at 1,500 mg orally daily + pyrimethamine at 25 mg orally daily + leucovorin at 10 mg orally daily (Evidence Level III)
MAC	Children • <1 y and CD4$^+$ cell count <750/mm^3 • 1–<2 y and CD4$^+$ cell count <500/ mm^3 • 2–<6 y and CD4$^+$ cell count <75/mm^3 • ≥6 y and CD4$^+$ cell count <50/mcL	Children • Clarithromycin at 7.5 mg/kg (maximum: 500 mg) orally twice daily (Evidence Level II) • Azithromycin at 20 mg/kg (maximum: 1,200 mg) orally once weekly (Evidence Level II)	Children • Azithromycin at 5 mg/kg (maximum: 250 mg) orally daily (Evidence Level II) • Rifabutin (children ≥6 y) at 300 mg orally daily (Evidence Level I) (Rule out active *Mycobacterium tuberculosis* disease prior to starting.)

Continued

Table 30-8 *(cont)*

Pathogen	Indication	First-line	Alternative
	Adolescents: CD4+ cell count <50/mcL	Adolescents • Azithromycin at 1,200 mg orally weekly (Evidence Level I) • Clarithromycin at 500 mg orally twice daily (Evidence Level I) • Azithromycin at 600 mg orally twice weekly (Evidence Level III)	Adolescents: rifabutin at 300 mg orally daily (Evidence Level I) (Rule out active *M tuberculosis* disease prior to starting.)

Toxoplasma gondii	Children
	• IgG antibody to *Toxoplasma* positive
	  • <6 y and CD4+ cell percentage <15%
	  • ≥6 y and CD4+ cell count <100/mm³
		Children: trimethoprim/sulfamethoxazole at 150/750 mg/m² orally once daily (maximum: 320/1,600 mg/d) (Evidence Level III); alternative dosing for same daily dose: once daily for 3 consecutive days, 2 divided doses daily, or 2 divided doses on 3 times weekly on alternate days	Children
			• Dapsone (children >1 mo) at 2 mg/kg or 15 mg/m² (maximum: 25 mg) orally daily + pyrimethamine at 1 mg/kg (maximum: 25 mg) orally daily + leucovorin at 5 mg orally every 3 d (Evidence Level I)
			• Atovaquone
			  ○ 1–3 mo: 30 mg/kg orally daily
			  ○ 4–24 mo: 45 mg/kg orally daily
			  ○ >24 mo: 30 mg/kg orally daily
			  ○ With or without pyrimethamine at 1 mg/kg or 15 mg/m² (maximum: 25 mg) orally daily + leucovorin at 5 mg orally every 3 d (Evidence Level III)

	Adolescents: IgG antibody to *Toxoplasma* positive and CD4+ cell count <100/mm³	Adolescents: trimethoprim/sulfamethoxazole, 1 double-strength tablet orally daily (Evidence Level II)	Adolescents • Trimethoprim/sulfamethoxazole, 1 double-strength tablet orally 3 times weekly (Evidence Level III) • Trimethoprim/sulfamethoxazole, 1 single-strength tablet orally daily (Evidence Level III) • Dapsone at 50 mg orally daily + pyrimethamine at 50 mg orally weekly + leucovorin at 25 mg orally weekly (Evidence Level I) • Dapsone at 200 mg orally weekly + pyrimethamine at 75 mg orally weekly + leucovorin at 25 mg orally weekly (Evidence Level I) • Atovaquone at 1,500 mg orally daily with or without pyrimethamine at 25 mg orally daily + leucovorin at 10 mg orally weekly (Evidence Level III)

Abbreviation: MAC, *Mycobacterium avium* complex.

Adapted from Panel on Opportunistic Infections in HIV-Infected Adults and Adolescents. *Guidelines for the Prevention and Treatment of Opportunistic Infections in HIV-Infected Adults and Adolescents: Recommendations from the Centers for Disease Control and Prevention, the National Institutes of Health, and the HIV Medicine Association of the Infectious Diseases Society of America.* Washington, DC: US Department of Health and Human Services. http://aidsinfo.nih.gov/contentfiles/lvguidelines/adult_oi.pdf. Accessed August 18, 2016; and Panel on Opportunistic Infections in HIV-Exposed and HIV-Infected Children. *Guidelines for the Prevention and Treatment of Opportunistic Infections in HIV-Exposed and HIV-Infected Children.* Washington, DC: US Department of Health and Human Services. http://aidsinfo.nih.gov/contentfiles/lvguidelines/oi_guidelines_pediatrics.pdf. Accessed August 18, 2016.

common bacterial and viral infections and should be used routinely in HIV-1–infected infants, children, and adolescents; thus, it is important to review the immunization status of the patient and ensure appropriate immunization status.

The vaccination schedule determined by the Advisory Committee on Immunization Practices should be followed to decrease morbidity and mortality from vaccine-preventable illnesses. Generally, inactivated vaccines are safe to use in immunocompromised patients; diphtheria and tetanus toxoids and acellular pertussis, hepatitis A and B, pneumococcal (conjugate and polysaccharide), meningococcal (conjugate and polysaccharide), influenza, *Haemophilus influenzae* type B conjugate, and poliovirus should be administered to all patients. Although the human papillomavirus (HPV) vaccine is not specifically recommended for patients with HIV infection, it can be administered according to schedule because it is an inactivated vaccine. Of note, HPV vaccine may not be fully effective in adolescent patients with a new diagnosis who have not received previous vaccination, since HPV is very common in persons who are sexually active. In the setting of live vaccines, there are some restrictions, especially in patients who are severely immunocompromised or have symptomatic HIV disease. Measles and varicella zoster virus infections can cause severe disease, and children with low-level immunosuppression should receive the measles-mumps-rubella vaccine and varicella vaccine on schedule; however, administration of live vaccines is contraindicated when the CD4$^+$ cell percentage is less than 15% in children younger than 5 years or count is less than 200/mm^3 in all other ages. Rotavirus vaccine can be considered in infants; although there are no safety or efficacy data in patients with compromised immune systems, in most infants HIV infection is not diagnosed by the first vaccination and the vaccine is substantially attenuated. Live influenza vaccines should be avoided in HIV-infected patients.

In HIV-1-infected patients, response to vaccines may be lower than that seen in healthy patients, since antibody response depends on CD4$^+$ T cell activation. Patients with advanced disease (CD4$^+$ cell percentage <15% or count <200/ mm^3) are more likely to have less response to vaccinations. Clinicians can consider obtaining serology to determine if patients achieved an adequate response; patients should be revaccinated as appropriate. The duration of immunogenicity for some vaccines is unknown in HIV-infected patients, and no data suggest revaccination will provide clinical benefit; clinicians can consider an additional revaccination 5 years after the first vaccination with the pneumococcal 23-valent polysaccharide vaccine, and booster doses of hepatitis B virus vaccine may be considered if immunogenicity wanes (Evidence Level III).

Long-term Monitoring

Currently, there is no cure for HIV. Treatment of HIV is a lifelong commitment, and although some long-term issues of HIV and ARVs are known, there may be others that have not been recognized. A good history and physical examination are needed at each patient visit to assess for OIs and adverse effects from ARVs. Additionally, evaluation of the patient's adherence should be done at each follow-up visit to encourage the patient's performance or identify barriers to adherence.

The HIV plasma RNA will also reflect the patient's adherence to cART; undetectable levels of virus suggest that the patient has been adherent. Virologic blips, which are defined as a detectable viral load after achieving viral suppression, are not uncommon but should be closely monitored. If the patient's HIV plasma RNA is persistently greater than 500 copies/mL, it may suggest either nonadherence to ART or virologic failure. Resistance testing should be performed if the HIV plasma RNA persists at greater than 1,000 copies/mL, and therapy should be changed if resistance is identified; alterations to cART regimen should be done in conjunction with an HIV specialist, and changes should never include just one drug (unless it is for an adverse effect of that drug). In these cases, discussion with the patient and family is necessary to identify barriers to adherence (eg, intolerance, polypharmacy, difficulty understanding regimen) as well as reinforce the importance of adherence to cART to prevent further development of HIV resistance. In some cases, patients may experience immunologic failure, which is defined as failure to improve $CD4^+$ cell percentage by greater than 5 percentage points in a child younger than 5 years with severe immunosuppression ($CD4^+$ cell percentage $<15\%$) or count greater than $50/mm^3$ in children 5 years or older with severe immunosuppression ($CD4^+$ cell count $<200/mm^3$). Unlike virologic failure, a change in the ART regimen may not improve immunologic failure; identifying other organic causes of immunosuppression, such as chronic steroid use, interferon use, zidovudine, or hematologic malignancies, and eliminating them is the best approach for managing immunologic failure.

Antiretrovirals have known long-term effects; some of these effects and their management are described in Table 30-7, and Table 30-3 provides a suggested general monitoring schedule for patients who are infected with HIV. Other specific monitoring should be completed according to the patient's history and cART regimen.

A long-term adverse effect from NRTIs is fat redistribution, especially lipoatrophy of the face and extremities. These effects have been mostly associated with the older NRTIs (eg, zidovudine, stavudine, didanosine), but effects of the newer NRTIs on lipoatrophy are still being determined. Protease inhibitors, efavirenz, and raltegravir containing cART have been associated with central fat disposition; however, the causal relationship has not been determined. While lipoatrophy may be associated with other effects, such as metabolic syndrome, it is primarily cosmetic; currently, there are no recommendations on interventions such as recombinant growth hormone, steroid use, autologous fat transplantation, or suction lipectomy in the pediatric population. Metabolic issues from cART have been well recognized; NRTIs, NNRTIs, and PIs are associated with dyslipidemia or insulin resistance. Lipid panel and serum glucose monitoring should be performed at least on a yearly basis. Hypertriglyceridemia, elevated low-density lipoprotein levels, and diabetes should be managed with a specialist; lifestyle changes and additional pharmacotherapy may be required.

Although cART has dramatically decreased morbidity and mortality, HIV-1-infected patients are at a high risk for other non-AIDS–related illnesses, such as cardiovascular disease, liver disease, cancer, and neurocognitive impairment. Recognizing symptoms and management of secondary disorders will improve quality of life; thus, a multidisciplinary approach and long-term follow-up for the HIV-1–infected child will provide the best care. Additionally, the care of the HIV-infected patient is constantly evolving; readers are highly encouraged to visit the AIDSinfo Web site (http://aidsinfo.nih.gov/) for the most recent recommendations.

Suggested Reading

Cummins NW, Badley AD. Mechanisms of HIV-associated lymphocyte apoptosis. *Cell Death Dis.* 2010;1:e99

DHHS Panel on Antiretroviral Guidelines for Adults and Adolescents—A Working Group of the Office of AIDS Research Advisory Council (OARAC). *Guidelines for the Use of Antiretroviral Agents in HIV-1-Infected Adults and Adolescents.* Washington, DC: US Department of Health and Human Services. http://aidsinfo.nih.gov/contentfiles/lvguidelines/adultandadolescentgl.pdf. Accessed August 18, 2016

Division of HIV/AIDS Prevention. Centers for Disease Control and Prevention. Surveillance overview. http://www.cdc.gov/hiv/statistics/surveillance/. Updated May 26, 2015. Accessed June 12, 2016

HHS Panel on Antiretroviral Therapy and Medical Management of HIV-Infected Children—A Working Group of the Office of AIDS Research Advisory Council (OARAC). *Guidelines for the Use of Antiretroviral Agents in Pediatric HIV Infection.* Washington, DC: US Department of Health and Human Services. http://aidsinfo.nih.gov/contentfiles/lvguidelines/pediatricguidelines.pdf. Accessed August 18, 2016

HHS Panel on Treatment of HIV-Infected Pregnant Women and Prevention of Perinatal Transmission—A Working Group of the Office of AIDS Research Advisory Council (OARAC). *Recommendations for Use of Antiretroviral Drugs in Pregnant HIV-1-Infected Women for Maternal Health and Interventions to Reduce Perinatal HIV Transmission in the United States.* Washington, DC: US Department of Health and Human Services. http://aidsinfo.nih.gov/contentfiles/lvguidelines/perinatalgl.pdf. Accessed August 17, 2016

Panel on Opportunistic Infections in HIV-Exposed and HIV-Infected Children. *Guidelines for the Prevention and Treatment of Opportunistic Infections in HIV-Exposed and HIV-Infected Children.* Washington, DC: US Department of Health and Human Services. http://aidsinfo.nih.gov/contentfiles/lvguidelines/oi_guidelines_pediatrics.pdf. Accessed August 18, 2016

Panel on Opportunistic Infections in HIV-Infected Adults and Adolescents. *Guidelines for the Prevention and Treatment of Opportunistic Infections in HIV-Infected Adults and Adolescents: Recommendations from the Centers for Disease Control and Prevention, the National Institutes of Health, and the HIV Medicine Association of the Infectious Diseases Society of America.* Washington, DC: US Department of Health and Human Services. http://aidsinfo.nih.gov/contentfiles/lvguidelines/adult_oi.pdf. Accessed August 18, 2016

Rubin LG, Levin MJ, Ljungman P, et al. 2013 IDSA Clinical Practice Guideline for Vaccination of the Immunocompromised Host. *Clin Infect Dis.* 2014;58:309-18

Samiuddin Z, Andrade RA. Care of the adult HIV-infected patient. In: Rakel RE, Rakel DP, eds. *Textbook of Family Medicine.* 8th ed. Saunders; 2011:248–260

Scarlatti G. Paediatric HIV infection. *Lancet.* 1996;348(9031):863–868

CHAPTER 31

Influenza

Roya Samuels, MD; Michelle Sewnarine, MD;
and Henry Bernstein, DO, MHCM

Key Points

- While epidemics inevitably occur each winter in the United States, the influenza virus is unpredictable in terms of both circulating strain and timing.

- Influenza vaccine is the mainstay for prevention of disease. Since 2010, it has included the influenza A (H1N1) pdm09 pandemic strain.

- Influenza vaccine effectiveness depends on the seasonal match of vaccine virus strains to circulating virus and the age and underlying conditions of the host.

- Diagnosis of influenza infection should be considered in children with acute onset of respiratory symptoms, regardless of whether or not there is a fever. Infected patients generally are highly febrile with sore throat and cough, lasting 3 to 7 days. Severe myalgia, headache, and rigors are commonly noted at onset.

- Diagnosis may be made on clinical grounds, with testing and early institution of treatment recommended for high-risk patients.

- Morbidity and mortality are greatest in the very young, the elderly, and those with cardiopulmonary, metabolic, neurologic, and immunocompromising conditions.

Overview

Influenza virus infection is a notable cause of upper respiratory tract illness in children, causing significant morbidity and mortality in this vulnerable population. Influenza viruses also have the potential for causing periodic global pandemics, as exemplified by the 2009 H1N1 outbreak.

Causes and Differential Diagnosis

Influenza viruses are orthomyxoviruses of 3 types (A, B, and C). They are single-stranded RNA viruses with 2 major surface proteins, which define the serotype of the virus: hemagglutinin and neuraminidase. Influenza virus types

A and B are the principal pathogens indicated in epidemic disease. Influenza virus type C is known to cause sporadic, mild influenza-like illness in children. Influenza type A subtypes currently include the H1N1 and H3N2 viruses. Influenza B viruses are not separated into subtypes, but are further divided into different lineages.

Annual winter epidemics of influenza A (H1N1 and H3N2) and B are predictable and generally associated with significant mortality in elderly and certain other high-risk populations. Annual *antigenic drift* in subtype relates to minor variation in the virus, and produces the seasonal changes in circulating virus. *Antigenic shift,* on the other hand, occurs only when influenza A virus is the fuel of pandemics. Since viral shedding in nasal secretions can persist for 7 to 10 days, and longer in young children and immunodeficient patients, the virus efficiently circulates, especially in close-knit populations. Specific antibodies to these various antigens, especially to hemagglutinin, are important determinants of immunity. Rates of communal immunity, in turn, influence incidence rates of the influenza virus.

Upper respiratory tract infections caused by other infectious pathogens share the same host of symptoms. These non-influenza etiologies include, but are not limited to, rhinovirus, adenovirus, respiratory syncytial virus, parainfluenza virus, human bocavirus, *Human metapneumovirus, Bordetella pertussis, Mycoplasma pneumoniae,* and *Chlamydophila pneumoniae.* Influenza generally presents with a greater severity of symptoms (eg, fever, chills, myalgia) than the more common upper respiratory tract infection (eg, nasal congestion, rhinorrhea).

Clinical Manifestations

The virus is commonly marked by a host of symptoms including acute onset of high fever, chills, rigors, malaise, headache, diffuse myalgia, and nonproductive cough. Subsequent signs and symptoms include nasal congestion, rhinitis, sore throat, and persistent cough. Less notable symptoms include abdominal pain, vomiting, diarrhea, nausea, and conjunctival injection.

Typical duration of the febrile illness is 2 to 4 days. Cough may persist for longer periods, and indication of small airway disturbance is often found weeks later. Although most children with influenza recover fully after 3 to 7 days, previously healthy children may demonstrate severe symptoms and complications.

Reported sequelae of the influenza virus include a variety of secondary illnesses. Complications may include acute otitis media, neurologic complications (eg, encephalopathy, seizures), myocarditis, pneumonia, bronchiolitis, sepsis, myositis, parotitis, and nephritis. Reye syndrome has been associated with influenza, and children with influenza or suspected influenza should not be given aspirin.

A post-influenza myositis may follow either influenza A or B, though more commonly the latter. Affected patients, usually school-aged boys, generally develop severe calf pain 3 to 4 days into their clinical illness and refuse to weight bear. Laboratory testing may reveal leukopenia and occasionally thrombocytopenia with blood creatine kinase elevated concentrations in the range of 1,000 to 5,000 U/L. Rhabdomyolysis leading to renal failure occurs rarely, and more commonly in girls.

Influenza is particularly severe in children with predisposing conditions such as hemoglobinopathies, diabetes mellitus, chronic renal disease, malignancy, cardiopulmonary disease, cardiomyopathy, and chronic lung disease, including bronchopulmonary dysplasia, asthma, cystic fibrosis, and neuromuscular diseases, which affect the accessory muscles of breathing.

Mortality secondary to the influenza virus has been reported in children with underlying chronic disease as well as previously healthy children. Invasive secondary infections with group A *Streptococcus, Staphylococcus aureus, Streptococcus pneumoniae,* or other bacterial pathogens may result in severe disease and death.

Evaluation

Most patients demonstrating clinical symptoms consistent with uncomplicated influenza disease, while residing in an area with known circulating cases of influenza, do not require influenza diagnostic testing for clinical management.

Other laboratory tests, such as a complete blood cell count, are also not necessarily indicated in confirming the diagnosis of influenza disease. A complete blood cell count or blood culture, however, may prove helpful in cases when bacterial superinfection or concomitant bacterial disease is suspected.

Chest radiograph is nonspecific. In patients with confirmed disease, it may demonstrate hyperaeration, peribronchial thickening, diffuse interstitial infiltrates, or bronchopneumonia in severe cases. Enlarged hilar lymph nodes and pleural effusion are rare in uncomplicated influenza. Radiologic studies may be obtained if there is a question of bacterial coinfection, which may affect clinical decision-making or need for expanding antimicrobial coverage.

A high index of suspicion for the diagnosis is influenced by the seasonality of influenza. Influenza testing should be performed in any of the following populations:

- Patients hospitalized with suspected influenza
- Patients for whom a diagnosis of influenza will warrant changes in clinical care (Box 31-1)
- Treatment of close contacts of patients who died of an unspecified acute illness in which influenza was suspected

Respiratory tract specimens should be collected shortly after illness onset, preferably within the first 72 hours of illness. Specimen collection after 5 days of illness onset may result in false-negative results because of a marked decrease in quantity of viral shedding over time.

Box 31-1. People at Higher Risk of Influenza Complications Recommended for Antiviral Treatment for Suspected or Confirmed Influenza

- Children <2 y
- Adults ≥65 y
- People with chronic pulmonary (including asthma), cardiovascular (except hypertension alone), renal, hepatic, hematologic (including sickle cell disease), or metabolic (including diabetes mellitus) disorders or neurologic and neurodevelopment conditions (including disorders of the brain, spinal cord, peripheral nerve, and muscle, such as cerebral palsy, epilepsy [seizure disorders], stroke, intellectual disability, moderate to severe developmental delay, muscular dystrophy, or spinal cord injury)
- People with immunosuppression, including that caused by medications or HIV infection
- Women who are pregnant or postpartum (within 2 wk after delivery)
- People <19 y who are receiving long-term aspirin therapy
- American Indian/Alaska Native people
- Residents of nursing homes and other chronic care facilities

Derived from American Academy of Pediatrics Committee on Infectious Diseases. Recommendations for prevention and control of influenza in children, 2016–2017. *Pediatrics.* 2016;138(4):e2016–e2527.

Optimal specimens in infants and young children include nasal aspirates and swabs. Nasopharyngeal aspirates and swabs are preferable in older children and adults. Oropharyngeal and sputum specimens result in a lower yield for influenza virus detection. In patients undergoing mechanical ventilation, upper and lower respiratory tract samples should be obtained. Lower respiratory tract samples include endotracheal aspirates and bronchoalveolar lavage.

Specimens of nasopharyngeal secretions obtained by swab, aspirate, or wash should be placed in appropriate transport media for culture. After inoculation into eggs or cell culture, influenza virus usually can be isolated within 2 to 6 days.

If antiviral therapy is to be prescribed, treatment should be started as soon after illness onset as possible and should not be delayed while waiting for a definitive influenza test result. Clinical benefit is greatest when treatment is initiated within 48 hours of onset of symptoms.

Influenza testing techniques are varied, and the particulars of a given clinical scenario will dictate which type of influenza test is the best option. Each method of testing has its own advantages and disadvantages, as described in Table 31-1.

It is imperative to use clinical judgment in deciding whether any patient with an influenza-like illness should be treated regardless of test results, especially because of the poor sensitivity of rapid influenza diagnostic testing. A false-positive screening result is most likely to occur in the context of low local disease prevalence. Confirmatory testing (viral culture or reverse transcriptase-polymerase chain reaction) should be considered in these instances to confirm accurate results.

Table 31-1. Comparison of Types of Influenza Diagnostic Tests

Influenza Diagnostic Test	Method	Availability	Typical Processing Time	Sensitivity, %	Distinguishing Subtype Strains of Influenza A	Cost
Rapid influenza diagnostic tests[a]	Antigen detection	Wide	<15 min	10–70	No	$
Rapid influenza molecular assays[b]	RNA detection	Wide	<20 min	86–100	No	$$$
Nucleic acid amplification tests (including RT-PCR)	RNA detection	Limited	1–8 h	86–100	Yes	$$$
Direct and indirect immunofluorescence assays	Antigen detection	Wide	1–4 h	70–100	No	$
Rapid cell culture (shell vials and cell mixtures)	Virus isolation	Limited	1–3 d	100	Yes	$$
Viral cell culture	Virus isolation	Limited	3–10 d	100	Yes	$$

Abbreviations: CLIA, Clinical Laboratory Improvement Act; RT-PCR, reverse transcriptase-polymerase chain reaction.

[a] Commercial rapid immunoassay diagnostic tests are CLIA-waived.

[b] Some rapid influenza molecular assays are CLIA-waived, depending on the specimen.

Adapted from Centers for Disease Control and Prevention. Guidance for clinicians on the use of rapid influenza diagnostic tests. http://www.cdc.gov/flu/professionals/diagnosis/clinician_guidance_ridt.htm. Updated May 26, 2016. Accessed August 25, 2016.

Management
. . . .

Regardless of influenza vaccination status and whether or not the onset of illness has been less than 48 hours, treatment should be offered or considered for specific patients, as described in Box 31-2.

Clinical judgment is an important factor in treatment decisions for pediatric patients presenting with influenza-like illness. Antiviral treatment should be started as soon as possible after illness onset and should not be delayed while waiting for a definitive influenza test result. Earlier treatment provides more optimal clinical responses, although treatment after 48 hours of symptoms in the child with moderate to severe disease or progressive disease may still provide some benefit. Treatment should be discontinued approximately 24 to 48 hours after symptoms resolve.

Children with severe influenza should be evaluated carefully for possible coinfection with bacterial pathogens (eg, *S aureus*) that might require antimicrobial therapy. Antipyretic agents for control of fever are of critical importance in young children, because fever and other symptoms of influenza could exacerbate underlying chronic conditions. Children and adolescents with influenza should not receive aspirin or any salicylate-containing products because of the potential risk of developing Reye syndrome.

In the United States, 2 classes of antivirals currently are available for treatment or prophylaxis of influenza: adamantanes (amantadine and rimantadine) and neuraminidase inhibitors (oseltamivir and zanamivir). Adamantanes should not be used to treat influenza. Circulating influenza A viruses continue to have extremely high levels of resistance to adamantanes, and influenza B viruses are intrinsically resistant to adamantanes. Since January 2006, neuraminidase inhibitors (eg, oseltamivir, zanamivir) have been the only recommended influenza antivirals because of this widespread resistance to the adamantanes and activity of neuraminidase inhibitors against influenza A and B viruses. A 5-day course of antiviral therapy has been studied and deemed an effective time course of treatment (Table 31-2). Peramivir, a third neuraminidase

Box 31-2. Summary of Antiviral Treatment for Clinical Influenza During the 2016–2017 Season

OFFER treatment as soon as possible to children...	CONSIDER treatment as soon as possible for...
• Hospitalized with presumed influenza • Hospitalized for severe, complicated, or progressive illness attributable to influenza • With presumed influenza (of any severity) and at high risk of complications	• Any healthy child with presumed influenza • Healthy children with presumed influenza who live at home with a sibling or household contact that is <6 mo or has a medical condition that predisposes to complications

Derived from American Academy of Pediatrics Committee on Infectious Diseases. Recommendations for prevention and control of influenza in children, 2016–2017. *Pediatrics*. 2016;138(4):e2016–e2527.

Table 31-2. Recommended Dosage and Schedule of Influenza Antivirals for Treatment and Chemoprophylaxis for the 2016–2017 Influenza Season: United States

Medication	Treatment (5 d)	Chemoprophylaxis (10 d)
Oseltamivir[a]		
Adults	75 mg twice daily	75 mg once daily
Children ≥12 mo		
Body weight		
≤15 kg	30 mg twice daily	30 mg once daily
16–23 kg	45 mg twice daily	45 mg once daily
24–40 kg	60 mg twice daily	60 mg once daily
≥41 kg	75 mg twice daily	75 mg once daily
Infants 9 mo–<12 mo[b]	3.5 mg/kg/dose twice daily	3.5 mg/kg/dose once daily
Term infants 0–<9 mo[b]	3 mg/kg/dose twice daily[c]	3 mg/kg/dose once daily for infants 3–<9 mo; not recommended for infants <3 mo, unless situation judged critical, because of limited safety and efficacy data in this age group
Zanamivir[d]		
Adults	10 mg (two 5-mg inhalations) twice daily	10 mg (two 5-mg inhalations) once daily
Children (≥7 y for treatment, ≥5 y for chemoprophylaxis)	10 mg (two 5-mg inhalations) twice daily	10 mg (two 5-mg inhalations) once daily

[a] Oseltamivir is administered orally without regard to meals, although administration with meals may improve gastrointestinal tolerability. Oseltamivir is available as Tamiflu in 30-, 45-, and 75-mg capsules and as a powder for oral suspension that is reconstituted to provide a final concentration of 6 mg/mL. For the 6-mg/mL suspension, a 30-mg dose is given with 5 mL of oral suspension; a 45-mg dose, 7.5 mL oral suspension; a 60-mg dose, 10 mL oral suspension; and a 75-mg dose, 12.5 mL oral suspension. If the commercially manufactured oral suspension is unavailable, a suspension can be compounded by retail pharmacies (final concentration: also 6 mg/mL), based on instructions that are present in the package label. In patients with renal insufficiency, the dose should be adjusted on the basis of creatinine clearance. For treatment of patients with creatinine clearance 10–30 mL/min: 75 mg once daily for 5 d. For chemoprophylaxis of patients with creatinine clearance 10–30 mL/min: 30 mg once daily for 10 d after exposure or 75 mg once every other day for 10 d after exposure (5 doses). See www.cdc.gov/flu/professionals/antivirals/antiviral-drug-resistance.htm.

[b] Approved by the US Food and Drug Administration down to 2 wk of age. Given its known safety profile, oseltamivir can be used to treat influenza in both term and preterm infants from birth.

[c] **Oseltamivir dosing for preterm infants.** The weight-based dosing recommendation for preterm infants is lower than for term infants. Preterm infants may have lower clearance of oseltamivir because of immature renal function, and doses recommended for term infants may lead to very high drug concentrations in this age group. Limited data from the National Institute of Allergy and Infectious Diseases Collaborative Antiviral Study Group provide the basis for dosing preterm infants using their postmenstrual age (gestational age + chronologic age): 1.0 mg/kg/dose orally twice daily for those <38 wk' postmenstrual age; 1.5 mg/kg/dose orally twice daily for those 38–<41 wk' postmenstrual age; 3.0 mg/kg/dose orally twice daily for those ≥41 wk' postmenstrual age.

[d] Zanamivir is administered by inhalation using a proprietary Diskhaler device distributed together with the medication. Zanamivir is a dry powder, not an aerosol, and should not be administered using nebulizers, ventilators, or other devices typically used for administering medications in aerosolized solutions. Zanamivir is not recommended for people with chronic respiratory diseases, such as asthma or chronic obstructive pulmonary disease, which increase the risk of bronchospasm.

Derived from Centers for Disease Control and Prevention. Antiviral agents for the treatment and chemoprophylaxis of influenza: recommendations of the Advisory Committee on Immunization Practices (ACIP). *MMWR Recomm Rep.* 2011;60(RR-1):1–24 and Kimberlin DW, Acosta EP, Prichard MN, et al; National Institute of Allergy and Infectious Diseases Collaborative Antiviral Study Group. Oseltamivir pharmacokinetics, dosing, and resistance among children aged <2 years with influenza. *J Infect Dis.* 2013;207(5):709–720.

inhibitor, was licensed on December 19, 2014, for use in adults 18 years and older and is being studied in children. Intravenous use of peramivir is approved for adults. Intravenous zanamivir is still being investigated, but can be used in consultation with infectious diseases specialists. It may also be obtained on a compassionate-use basis for seriously ill children, as currently supported by the US Food and Drug Administration through the manufacturer. Intravenous zanamivir is being studied in pediatric patients, but the manufacturer has not publicly released any information regarding plans to file for licensure in adults or children.

Options for treatment or chemoprophylaxis of influenza in the United States depend on influenza strain resistance patterns. Clinicians should remain aware of the predominant circulating strain and its susceptibility profile. Recommendations will depend on local activity and may change throughout the season (refer to www.cdc.gov/flu/weekly for weekly updates on antiviral resistance). Adverse effects of these antivirals are listed in Box 31-3.

The US Food and Drug Administration recently licensed oseltamivir down to 2 weeks of age. Given its known safety profile, oseltamivir can be used to treat influenza in both term and preterm infants from birth (see Table 31-2).

Oseltamivir is available in capsule and oral suspension formulations. The manufactured liquid formulation has a concentration of 6 mg/mL. If the commercially manufactured oral suspension is unavailable, the capsule may be opened and contents mixed with a sweetened liquid by retail pharmacies to a final concentration of 6 mg/mL.

Box 31-3. Adverse Effects of Antivirals

Adamantanes
- CNS adverse effects (more common with amantadine than rimantadine).
- Nervousness, anxiety, difficulty concentrating, lightheadedness.
- GI adverse effects.
- Nausea, loss of appetite.
- Delirium, hallucinations, agitation, and seizures are more common among persons with long-term illnesses.

Neuraminidase Inhibitors
- Oseltamivir
  - o GI adverse effects.
  - o Nausea, vomiting.
  - o Neuropsychiatric events.
  - o Rare cases of self-injury and delirium, mostly among pediatric patients, primarily in Japan.
  - o It is unknown what effect oseltamivir may have on behavior, but unusual patient behavior should be reported immediately to a clinician.
- Zanamivir
  - o Decreased respiratory function and bronchospasm, especially among those with asthma or other chronic lung disease.
  - o Diarrhea, nausea, sinusitis, nasal infections, bronchitis, cough, headache, and dizziness have occurred in <5% of persons who have received the drug.
  - o This drug is not typically recommended for anyone with underlying lung disease.

Abbreviations: CNS, central nervous system; GI, gastrointestinal.

Amantadine, oseltamivir, and zanamivir are licensed for chemoprophylaxis of influenza A. Chemoprophylaxis should not be considered a substitute for immunization. Although immunization is the preferred approach to prevention of infection, chemoprophylaxis for a 10-day course during an influenza outbreak, as defined by the Centers for Disease Control and Prevention (CDC), is recommended

- For children at high risk of complications from influenza for whom influenza vaccine is contraindicated
- For children at high risk during the 2 weeks after influenza immunization
- For family members or clinicians who are unimmunized and likely to have ongoing, close exposure to either of the following populations:
  o Unimmunized children at high risk
  o Unimmunized babies and toddlers who are younger than 24 months
- For control of influenza outbreaks for unimmunized staff and children in a closed institutional setting with children at high risk (eg, extended-care facilities)
- As a supplement to immunization among children at high risk, including children who are immunocompromised and may not respond to vaccine
- As postexposure prophylaxis for family members and close contacts of an infected person if those people are at high risk of complications from influenza
- For children at high risk and their family members and close contacts, as well as clinicians, when circulating strains of influenza virus in the community are not matched with seasonal influenza vaccine strains, on the basis of current data from the CDC and local health departments

Prevention

Seasonal influenza vaccination is the most effective method for the prevention of influenza and its associated morbidities. Routine annual influenza vaccination for all persons 6 months and older who do not have contraindications has been recommended by the Advisory Committee on Immunization Practices of the CDC and the American Academy of Pediatrics since 2010. It is recommended that the vaccine be provided by the end of October, if possible, prior to the expected annual influenza season; however, since the onset of influenza season is variable and unpredictable, immunization should be administered throughout the winter and even early spring. Providers may continue to offer vaccine until June 30 of each year, marking the end of the influenza season.

People with the following conditions are at increased risk of severe complications from influenza, and it is especially important they receive annual immunization:

- Asthma or other chronic pulmonary diseases, including cystic fibrosis
- Hemodynamically significant cardiac disease
- Immunosuppressive disorders or therapy

- HIV infection
- Sickle cell anemia and other hemoglobinopathies
- Diseases that require long-term aspirin therapy, including juvenile idiopathic arthritis or Kawasaki disease
- Chronic renal dysfunction
- Chronic metabolic disease, including diabetes mellitus
- Any condition that can compromise respiratory function or handling of secretions or can increase the risk of aspiration, such as neurodevelopmental disorders, spinal cord injuries, seizure disorders, or neuromuscular abnormalities

Inactivated influenza vaccines (IIVs) are available in both trivalent (IIV3) and quadrivalent (IIV4) forms. Note that the abbreviation IIV has replaced TIV (trivalent influenza vaccine) because IIVs now contain either 3 or 4 viral strains. Influenza quadrivalent vaccines include an additional influenza B virus.

Although most IIV vaccines are produced in eggs and contain measurable amounts of egg protein, recent data have shown that IIV administered in a single age-appropriate dose is well tolerated by recipients with a history of egg allergy of any severity. Recent literature has shown that egg allergy does not impart increased risk of anaphylactic reaction to vaccination with IIV. The Joint Task Force on Practice Parameters, representing the American Academy of Allergy, Asthma & Immunology and the American College of Allergy, Asthma & Immunology, states that special precautions regarding medical setting and waiting periods after administration of IIV to egg-allergic recipients beyond those recommended for any vaccine are no longer warranted. The recommended waiting period for influenza vaccine, as for any vaccine, is 15 minutes after vaccination for all recipients to decrease the risk of injury should the patient faint. Standard vaccination practice should include the ability to respond to acute hypersensitivity reactions.

Two trivalent influenza vaccines manufactured using new technologies that do not utilize eggs are now available for people 18 years or older during the 2016–2017 season: cell culture-based IIV3 (or ccIIV3) and recombinant influenza vaccine (or RIV3). It is anticipated that ccIIV4 will be available for people 4 years and older during the 2016–2017 season.

Most years, 1 or more strains are altered in the vaccine. Even when composition of the influenza vaccine does not change from the previous season, antibody titers in children may be reduced by as much as 50% within 12 months after vaccination, highlighting the value of annual receipt of vaccine.

Annual influenza vaccine is also indicated for household members and caregivers of children at high risk for disease morbidity, healthy children younger than 5 years, and babies younger than 6 months. Cocooning, or immunization of people who are in close contact with children with high-risk conditions or any child younger than 5 years, is an important means of protection for these children.

Inactivated influenza vaccines do not contain live virus and are available for both intramuscular (IM) and intradermal (ID) use in both trivalent and quadrivalent formulations. Intramuscular formulations of IIV4 are available from several manufacturers. Different formulations have different age indications, but there are brands licensed for use in children as young as 6 months of age. An ID formulation of IIV4 is licensed for use in people 18 through 64 years of age, and is available only as IIV4. Intradermal vaccine administration involves a microinjection with a shorter needle than needles used for IM administration. There is no preference for IM or ID immunization in people 18 years or older. Therefore, pediatricians may choose to use either the IM or ID product in their late adolescent and young adult patients, as well as for any adults they may be vaccinating (ie, as part of a cocooning strategy). Prior recommendations for immunization determined by age and risk factors were replaced with the promotion of universal immunization based on elevated morbidity and mortality rates from influenza in the unimmunized population. Inactivated influenza vaccine may be administered concurrently with other live and inactivated vaccines.

The current American Academy of Pediatrics and CDC interim recommendation regarding quadrivalent live attenuated influenza vaccine (LAIV4) is that it not be used in any setting during the 2016–2017 influenza season. Observational data from the US Flu Vaccine Effectiveness Network demonstrated poor effectiveness of LAIV4 for several consecutive influenza seasons; therefore, IIV is considered the best preventive measure against influenza. During the 2013–2016 influenza seasons, children who received LAIV4 were found to have greater than 2.5 times the risk of developing influenza compared to those who received IIV vaccination.

Antivirals may serve as an adjunct to vaccination when used for chemoprophylaxis after an exposure to influenza virus.

Influenza vaccines are not licensed for administration to babies younger than 6 months. Two doses of vaccine (0.25 mL for 6–36 months of age; 0.5 mL for 3–8 years of age) at least 1 month apart are recommended for primary immunization of children younger than 9 years. Children 9 years and older should receive one dose of vaccine each year. Evidence from several studies demonstrates that children 6 months through 8 years of age require 2 doses of influenza vaccine during their first season of vaccination to optimize immune response.

Recommendations for influenza vaccination in children 6 months through 8 years of age are as follows:
- Children need 2 doses if they have received fewer than 2 doses of any trivalent or quadrivalent influenza vaccine (IIV or LAIV) prior to July 1, 2016. The interval between the two doses should be at least 4 weeks. If receiving the seasonal influenza vaccine for the first time, the child should receive a second dose this season at least 4 weeks after the first dose.
- Children require only 1 dose if they have previously received 2 or more total doses of any trivalent or quadrivalent influenza vaccine (IIV or LAIV) prior to July 1, 2016. The 2 previous doses need not have been received during the same influenza season or consecutive influenza seasons. Despite recent evidence for poor effectiveness of LAIV4, receipt of LAIV4 in the

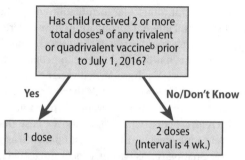

Figure 31-1. Number of 2016–2017 seasonal influenza vaccine doses for children 6 months through 8 years of age.
[a] The 2 doses need not have been received during the same season or consecutive seasons.
[b] Receipt of LAIV4 in the past is still expected to have primed a child's immune system, despite recent evidence for poor effectiveness. There currently are no data that suggest otherwise.
Derived from American Academy of Pediatrics Committee on Infectious Diseases. Recommendations for prevention and control of influenza in children, 2016–2017. *Pediatrics*. 2016; in press.

past is still expected to have primed a child's immune system. There currently are no data that suggest otherwise. Therefore, children who received 2 or more doses of LAIV4 prior to July 1, 2016 may receive only 1 dose of IIV for the 2016–2017 season (see Figure 31-1).

Prevention of influenza following immunization with IIV in healthy children older than 2 years is approximately 50%. Limited data suggest that IIV efficacy is lower in children 6 through 23 months of age than in children older than 23 months. Several years ago, there was a presumed association of febrile seizures with influenza vaccine noted in children vaccinated with Afluria in the southern hemisphere. During the 2 influenza seasons spanning 2010–2012, there were increased reports of febrile seizures in the United States in young children who received IIV3 and the 13-valent pneumococcal conjugate vaccine (or PCV13) concomitantly. Overall, the benefits of timely vaccination with same-day administration of IIV and pneumococcal conjugate vaccine or diphtheria and tetanus toxoids and acellular pertussis (or DTaP) vaccine outweigh the risk of febrile seizures, which rarely have any long-term sequelae, with simultaneous administration, and the Advisory Committee on Immunization Practices and American Academy of Pediatrics recommendations have not changed. Further research is needed to determine what relationship, if any, exists between IIV in toddlers and febrile seizures.

Suggested Reading

American Academy of Pediatrics Committee on Infectious Diseases. Recommendations for prevention and control of influenza in children, 2016–2017. *Pediatrics.* 2016;138(4):e2016–e2527

Centers for Disease Control and Prevention. Prevention and control of seasonal influenza with vaccines: recommendations of the Advisory Committee on Immunization Practices, United States, 2016–17 influenza season. *MMWR Recomm Rep.* 2016;65(5):1–54

Centers for Disease Control and Prevention. Influenza (flu): guidance for clinicians on the use of rapid influenza diagnostic tests. CDC Web site. http://www.cdc.gov/flu/professionals/diagnosis/clinician_guidance_ridt.htm. Accessed April 1, 2016

Centers for Disease Control and Prevention. Vaccine Information Statements (VIS): inactivated influenza VIS. CDC Web site. http://www.cdc.gov/vaccines/hcp/vis/vis-statements/flu.html. Accessed April 1, 2016

Lessin HR, Edwards KM; American Academy of Pediatrics Committee on Practice and Ambulatory Medicine, Committee on Infectious Diseases. Immunizing parents and other close family contacts in the pediatric office setting. *Pediatrics.* 2012;129(1):e247–e253

US Food and Drug Administration. Influenza virus vaccine for the 2015–2016 season. FDA Web site. http://www.fda.gov/biologicsbloodvaccines/guidancecomplianceregulatoryinformation/post-marketactivities/lotreleases/ucm454877.htm. Accessed April 1, 2016

CHAPTER 32

Measles, Mumps, Rubella

J. Michael Klatte, MD, and Barbara Pahud, MD, MPH

Key Points

- Measles and rubella have effectively been eradicated in the United States, but cases imported from outside of the United States sporadically occur and occasionally cause outbreaks. Mumps outbreaks also occur infrequently within the United States.

- Pediatricians should be able to identify the classic manifestations of these diseases and know that diagnosis in the susceptible host can generally be established by detection of IgM antibody early in the course of disease.

- Effective antiviral therapy does not exist for these diseases, and supportive care is the mainstay for treatment. In addition, all children with measles should be treated with vitamin A (once daily for 2 days, then a third dose in 2–4 weeks for any child who is determined to be vitamin A deficient).

- Congenital rubella syndrome may follow maternal rubella, and an increased risk for disease is noted in women born outside the United States.

- Appropriate isolation precautions should be used for hospitalized patients with measles (airborne for 4 days after rash), mumps (droplet for 5 days after parotid swelling), and rubella (droplet for 7 days after rash), with extended period of contact isolation for those with congenital rubella syndrome.

Overview

Measles, mumps, and rubella are viral illnesses that continue to cause global outbreaks of disease. Prompt disease identification is especially important in an outbreak setting to prevent spread of disease.

Causes and Differential Diagnosis

Measles

During the prodromal stage of a measles infection, the clinical presentation is typically indistinguishable from numerous viral upper respiratory tract illnesses that present with fever, nasal congestion, and rhinorrhea. Even when conjunctivitis and photophobia appear, the differential diagnosis remains large, including respiratory viruses, such as adenovirus or Epstein-Barr virus (EBV), and bacterial causes like *Streptococcus pneumoniae*. Characteristic pattern of fever and evolution of rash generally suggests the diagnosis of measles to the experienced clinician, but other viral diagnoses such as *Human parvovirus B19* (B19V), *Human herpesvirus 6*, rubella, influenza, and enteroviral infections are often considered. *Streptococcus pyogenes*- or *Staphylococcus aureus*-associated scarlet fever; noninfectious entities such as Kawasaki disease, drug eruption, and serum sickness–like reaction; and rheumatologic diseases like juvenile arthritis may also possess a number of clinical findings similar to measles.

Mumps

The differential diagnosis of mumps is classically one that encompasses the differential diagnosis of acute parotitis. When combined with prodromal stage symptoms, including headache, myalgias, decreased appetite, and malaise, the differential diagnosis of mumps should lead one to consider alternative viral diagnoses such as influenza or parainfluenza virus, EBV, cytomegalovirus, enteroviral, *Human herpesvirus 6*, lymphocytic choriomeningitis virus, and HIV infections. Assessment for bacterial sources of acute parotid swelling or sialadenitis, particularly *S aureus*, should be performed, especially if purulent discharge is able to be expressed from the salivary glands. Noninfectious causes of parotid swelling to consider include rheumatologic conditions, such as sarcoidosis and Sjögren syndrome, as well as salivary tract calculi.

Rubella

The differential diagnosis for rubella includes other viral infections such as measles, parainfluenza virus, B19V, EBV, adenovirus, enterovirus, and bacterial infections, such as scarlet fever. *Mycoplasma pneumoniae* infections may be considered in school-aged children, and the rash may be confused with noninfectious entities such as contact dermatitis.

Clinical Features
. . . .

Measles

Measles is an acute viral illness classically characterized by a prodrome consisting of fever, cough, coryza, and conjunctivitis followed by a maculopapular rash with cephalocaudal distribution.

A 2- to 4-day fever prodrome occurs after which the patient develops the characteristic triad of cough, coryza, and non-purulent conjunctivitis. Fevers, which may be as high as 40.6°C (105.1°F), are noted during the prodrome along with upper respiratory tract symptoms and a mucosal enanthem known as Koplik spots, which may be seen at the end of the prodrome before rash develops. Koplik spots are bluish white specks classically noted on the lower buccal mucosa adjacent to the Stensen duct and opposite the lower molars; however, they may also occur on the labial as well as palatal mucosae. The enanthem, which rest on an erythematous base, may develop a gray discoloration and ulcerated appearance as the infection progresses. Disappearance of Koplik spots coincides with initial spread of the exanthem.

The rash of measles, which develops between 12 and 14 days after initial exposure, is initially discrete, maculopapular, and erythematous and first appears on the scalp and behind the ears, with progressive sequential spread to the face, neck, trunk, and extremities, including hands and feet. Once progression is complete, the rash begins to coalesce over 3 to 4 days, in a pattern similar to appearance of the original rash, and lasts in total approximately 6 days. In the absence of complications, fevers abate at approximately the same time as rash coalescence begins. As the rash resolves in the same pattern as it appeared, a brownish copper-colored skin discoloration appears that does not blanch with pressure. Other symptoms that may present during the exanthem include pharyngitis, anorexia, abdominal pain, diarrhea, and lymphadenopathy.

If fever persists beyond day 10 of illness, measles-associated complications should be considered. Measles complications are more common in children with nutritional deficiencies or who are immunocompromised, and are responsible for the high mortality associated with measles. Transient immunosuppression caused by measles may lead to secondary infections or reactivation of latent infections. The most common complication is acute otitis media, but life-threatening complications, especially in developing countries, include pneumonia, diarrhea, and encephalitis. Other less common but well-described complications include thrombocytopenia, hepatitis, toxic shock syndrome, keratitis, pericarditis, myocarditis, and mastoiditis. Hemorrhagic measles, a severe presentation characterized by hemorrhage from skin and mucosa that may result in death, has been reported mostly during widespread epidemics.

Modified measles infection refers to development of an attenuated clinical presentation, which occurs as a result of the patient possessing partial immunity to measles. This type of infection has been observed in those who have been previously vaccinated (including children who have received both 1 and 2 doses of measles vaccine), those who have previously been infected with measles, susceptible children exposed to measles infection who have been administered intravenous immune globulin, and infants who have residual immunity due to transplacental passage of maternal antibodies. The clinical features of measles remain the same in these patients with some notable exceptions. The incubation period may be longer, prodromal period is shorter, and Koplik spots may be absent. Though the exanthem follows a pattern of spread similar to classic infection, the rash is of shorter duration, is more discrete, and does not coalesce. Fever, when present, is shorter in duration and does not typically reach the maximum temperatures associated with classic measles.

The clinical presentation and progression of measles infection in the immunocompromised child differ from those of an otherwise healthy host.

Children with cell-mediated immune defects, including those with HIV, organ or hematopoietic stem cell transplant recipients on high-dose immunosuppressive therapy, or children with malignancies, are at highest risk for severe morbidity and mortality from measles infection. Clinical findings vary according to the degree of immunosuppression, and the severity is likely a result of impaired cell-mediated immunity. Immunocompromised children with measles often have an incubation period similar to classic measles but have a protracted course. Following a prodromal stage, the rash may be delayed or absent. Development of respiratory distress or hypoxia that coincides with the exanthem should raise concern for giant cell pneumonia, often rapidly fatal in this pediatric subpopulation. Patients who survive remain at risk for development of measles inclusion body encephalitis, a type of encephalitis, specific to the immunosuppressed patient, that develops between 5 weeks and 12 months after initial measles infection. The condition is characterized by development of focal seizures, with progressive deterioration in neurologic function and mental status. Duration from onset of initial symptoms until death ranges from 1 week to 2 months. As with giant cell pneumonia, intranuclear inclusion bodies are found on histopathologic examination of brain tissue specimens.

Subacute sclerosing panencephalitis (SSPE) is a slowly progressive and debilitating complication observed in those previously infected with wild-type measles. Children 2 years and younger and HIV-infected children who contract measles are at elevated risk for future development of SSPE. The average interval between measles infection and SSPE onset is 7 years, with death occurring in 95% of individuals within 1 to 3 years. Disease progression is categorized into 4 stages, on the basis of clinical signs and symptoms. Subacute sclerosing panencephalitis stage 1 signs and symptoms include personality changes and progressive intellectual deterioration. Those in stage 2 exhibit seizures, myoclonic jerks, and progressive dementia. Stage 3 is defined by rigidity and a progressive degree of unresponsiveness, while patients in stage 4 are often comatose or in a persistent vegetative state. The incidence of SSPE has declined sharply since implementation of measles vaccination.

Mumps

In children with mumps, a prodromal stage of 1 to 2 days is common and is marked by fever between 38.9°C and 39.4°C (102°F–103°F), headache, diffuse myalgias, decreased appetite, and malaise. Upper respiratory tract symptoms, such as congestion and rhinorrhea, are also common during this stage. Up to a third of infections are asymptomatic, and up to half manifest only with nonspecific symptoms.

Symptomatic patients present with parotid gland swelling, preceded by localized tenderness over the parotid and adjacent areas (otalgia). Many patients begin with unilateral swelling, but after a discrete time period, up to 75% will have involvement of the opposite parotid gland. Other glands, including the submaxillary and sublingual glands, may be involved as well. Swelling is marked by the distinct presence of edema, but not erythema, over the affected glands. The edematous areas are typically tender to palpation, and normal movements of the jaw are often limited because of pain. In contrast to the skin overlying the parotid, the Stensen duct appears inflamed, enlarged, and erythematous during the period of acute parotid swelling, with gradual resolution. Swelling of affected glands reaches its peak intensity over a period of 3 days, with a gradual recession in size thereafter. Complete normalization of gland size occurs approximately 10 days after swelling onset.

Lymphocytic choriomeningitis is the second most common manifestation of clinical mumps infection after parotitis. The degree of central nervous system involvement varies widely, and in part depends upon age at infection. In subjects with mumps meningitis in the pre-vaccine era, pleocytosis was commonly found, though only 5% to 10% exhibited overt clinical signs of meningitis. Meningitis was reported before, during, or after parotitis. Nuchal rigidity and severe headache were more often observed in older children and adolescents than younger children with mumps, likely because of better recognition in these age groups. Other neurologic complications of mumps include encephalitis, deafness, and various demyelinating disorders. Death secondary to mumps is rare but usually related to mumps-associated encephalitis. Mumps-associated encephalitis was the most frequent case of viral encephalitis in the 1960s but has virtually disappeared since vaccine introduction.

Epididymo-orchitis and oophoritis occur in about 15% and 7% of postpubertal adolescents infected with mumps, respectively. Findings are most often unilateral, but may be bilateral in 20% to 40% of cases. Time to onset and resolution of symptoms, including fever and testicular pain, plus scrotal swelling and erythema, generally coincides with development and regression of parotid swelling. Infertility even following bilateral orchitis is infrequent.

Pancreatitis is relatively rare, and occurs in 3% to 4% of those patients with clinically evident mumps infection. Pancreatitis may present concurrently with parotid swelling, but it might also precede onset of parotid swelling. Clinically significant glomerulonephritis secondary to mumps infection is a rare finding presenting within the first 5 to 14 days after onset of symptoms. Acute or subacute sensorineural hearing impairment was reported in less than 5% of clinically evident cases of mumps, though it may occur following subclinical infection. High-frequency hearing impairment from mumps infection is often transient, and bilateral in nature. Finally, mumps-associated arthropathy is infrequent but more common in males.

It is unclear if vaccination truly modifies clinical presentation. Current literature suggests that vaccinated cases present with lower complications, and when they do occur, severe complications are reported in adults more than children. The clinical presentation, symptoms, and course of mumps in immunocompromised children has not been well studied. In the transplantation population, reports of fatal meningoencephalitis and severe nephritis resulting in permanent renal failure have been reported after bone marrow transplantation and renal transplantation, respectively.

Rubella

Infected children are often asymptomatic during the 7 days following exposure and may not exhibit any prodromal symptoms besides mild rhinorrhea and nasal congestion. Adolescents, however, are more likely to have prodromal symptoms such as low-grade fevers, conjunctival injection, pharyngitis, headache, and diffuse myalgias. Petechial lesions on the palate may occasionally be observed.

Lymphadenopathy, a commonly observed finding in rubella infection, arises most often during the second week after exposure; however, it may develop as early as 4 days after exposure, and can precede rash onset by 1 week or more. Lymphadenopathy caused by rubella is characterized by its posterior auricular, suboccipital, and posterior cervical locations, though generalized lymphadenopathy may be observed. The total duration of lymphadenopathy averages approximately 7 days, but has been observed up to 14 days after rash onset.

The exanthem of rubella appears within 3 weeks after exposure. Up to 40% of symptomatic rubella infections may present without a rash, though the total number of those with rubella who do not develop rash is difficult to assess, given the large number of those with subclinical infection. The characteristic rash has been described as mild, discrete, and erythematous, with a maculopapular appearance. The rash first appears on the face and neck, with subsequent spread to the trunk and finally extremities, in a centrifugal spread similar to measles. Unlike measles, however, the duration of exanthem presence is brief, with most lasting an average of 3 days from onset until complete resolution. In adolescents, the rash may be pruritic, further differentiating it from the exanthem of measles. The rash may coalesce, but skin does not develop the copper discoloration of a characteristic resolving measles exanthem.

Transient polyarthritis and arthralgias may occur, though these findings are more common in adolescent girls and adults. Joint symptoms develop 1 to 7 days after exanthem eruption, and often persist for 1 to 2 weeks.

Acute rubella encephalitis is an uncommon feature of rubella infection, and is estimated to occur in approximately 1 in 6,000 cases. Encephalitis symptoms commonly commence between 2 and 4 days following exanthem appearance, though in some instances they may not occur until 1 week or more after rash development. Greater than 80% of those with rubella encephalitis recover without sequelae, though severe, protracted courses have been reported.

Congenital Rubella Syndrome

Congenital rubella syndrome (CRS) is the result of fetal rubella infection in utero. In general, timing of maternal infection acquisition correlates with severity of infection, with the greatest number of abnormalities observed in children whose mothers acquired rubella during the first or second trimester of pregnancy. Typical clinical manifestations of CRS include growth retardation, blueberry muffin lesions (characteristic dermal sites of erythropoiesis), cataracts, congenital glaucoma, congenital heart disease, pigmented retinitis, hepatosplenomegaly, and radiolucent bone disease. Neonates may have meningoencephalitis and interstitial pneumonitis. Late-onset findings reported in children born with CRS include behavioral disorders, mental retardation, continued growth retardation, and endocrine deficiencies, such as diabetes mellitus and thyroid dysfunction.

Evaluation

Measles

In the unimmunized susceptible host, a positive enzyme immunoassay (EIA) from serum demonstrating the presence of IgM antibody is diagnostic and may persist for 30 days after infection. The presence of IgM antibody may be transient in those who have had 1 or 2 doses of measles-containing vaccine. False-negative results are common within the first 72 hours after rash onset; thus, testing should be repeated if the clinical suspicion remains high.

IgG antibody levels begin to appear between 5 and 10 days after rash onset. Comparison of IgG antibody titers in paired acute and convalescent sera, obtained approximately 2 weeks apart, can be used to diagnose acute measles infection. A fourfold rise in antibody titer is confirmatory.

In an outbreak setting, a positive IgM or IgG antibody cannot be used to confirm wild-type measles infection in a person who was recently vaccinated (6–45 days prior to rash onset). In this subpopulation, differentiation between IgM produced by wild-type virus versus vaccine virus is not possible, unless viral genotyping performed on an isolate from culture or reverse transcriptase-polymerase chain reaction (RT-PCR) can be obtained. IgG antibody levels are boosted following reexposure, though confirmation requires a second level to be drawn 14 to 30 days after the initial IgG titer. In outbreak settings, RT-PCR testing or culture should be obtained if serology is inconclusive.

Measles virus is difficult to cultivate but can be isolated in viral culture of nasopharyngeal, urinary, or throat swabs, in addition to blood specimens. It is the preferred method of diagnosis in an immunocompromised host in whom serology is unreliable. Specimens obtained within 72 hours after rash onset are most likely to yield positive growth on culture, with a progressive decline in virus isolation between 4 and 10 days after rash onset. Given the significant variability in isolation (depending on when the specimen is obtained), technical difficulty with measles virus isolation in culture, and necessity of sending specimens out for confirmation, viral culture is not the initial preferred method for diagnosis.

Nucleic acid amplification testing by RT-PCR testing on blood, urinary, nasopharyngeal, or throat swab specimens can also be used for diagnosis and is available through state public health laboratories or the Centers for Disease Control and Prevention Measles Laboratory. Genotyping may be useful in determining epidemiology and differentiating infection caused by wild-type virus versus a vaccine virus strain. As with viral culture, results of RT-PCR are very sensitive to the timing of collection and handling of specimen; thus, a negative result does not necessarily rule out disease. Diagnostic criteria for measles are found in Box 32-1.

Box 32-1. Diagnostic Criteria for Measles

Suspected: Any febrile illness that is accompanied by rash and does not meet the criteria for probable or confirmed measles or any other illness.

Probable: In the absence of a more likely diagnosis, an illness characterized by all of the following findings:
- Generalized rash lasting ≥3 d
- Temperature of 38.3°C (≥101°F)
- Cough, coryza, or conjunctivitis
- No epidemiologic linkage to a confirmed case of measles
- Noncontributory or no serologic or virologic testing

Confirmed: Confirmed cases should be reported to the CDC via the NNDSS.
- Laboratory confirmation[a] by any of the following findings:
  o Positive serologic test for measles IgM antibody
  o Significant rise in measles antibody level by any standard serologic test
  o Isolation of measles virus from a clinical specimen
  o Detection of measles virus-specific nucleic acid by PCR

or

- An illness characterized by all of the following findings:
  o Generalized rash lasting ≥3 d
  o Temperature of 38.3°C (≥101°F)
  o Cough, coryza, or conjunctivitis
  o Epidemiologic linkage to a confirmed case of measles

Abbreviations: CDC, Centers for Disease Control and Prevention; NNDSS, National Notifiable Diseases Surveillance System; PCR, polymerase chain reaction.

[a] A laboratory-confirmed case does not have to have generalized rash lasting ≥3 d, temperature of 38.3°C (≥101°F), or cough, coryza, or conjunctivitis.

Mumps

A number of different laboratory methods are useful for diagnosis of mumps in the nonimmune host. Guidance should be sought from the Centers for Disease Control and Prevention regarding specimen collection through their Web site or the state health department. Testing for IgM antibody to mumps by EIA is preferred over fluorescence immunoassay, and antibody can be detected within 5 days after the onset of clinical symptoms. Levels peak at approximately 7 days, and can remain elevated for weeks to months after symptom onset.

A diagnosis of mumps infection may also be made by documentation of seroconversion by EIA or obtaining both acute and convalescent paired sera demonstrating a fourfold rise in IgG titers. In addition, mumps virus is readily detected in oral secretions, cerebrospinal fluid (CSF), and other body fluids. Swabbing of the buccal mucosa/Stensen duct often yields the highest concentration of virus. Reverse transcriptase-polymerase chain reaction testing for mumps from buccal mucosa swabs, throat swabs, or saliva has gained favor because of the test's high sensitivity and specificity and rapid turnaround time when compared with detection by viral culture. In the susceptible host, mumps virus may be isolated from buccal mucosa between 10 and 14 days after the onset of symptoms. Obtaining a buccal swab for RT-PCR testing or viral culture is most likely to generate a true positive result when obtained within 72 hours after symptom onset.

In the vaccine era, parotitis is far more likely to be caused by other viral agents than mumps. In addition, there are inherent difficulties in making the diagnosis of mumps in an immunized individual. Therefore, consultation with an infectious diseases specialist may be helpful before undertaking a diagnostic evaluation in such cases.

Reverse transcriptase-polymerase chain reaction testing (and to a lesser extent viral culture) appears to be the best diagnostic modality for those with partial or preexisting immunity to mumps and in the immunocompromised host. Specimens from parotid secretions or CSF obtained for RT-PCR testing should be obtained in the first 72 hours of symptom onset, during the greatest period of viral replication. Unlike in the nonimmune host, however, obtaining this specimen may be critical in the diagnosis given the obstacles faced with serologic diagnosis and theoretical risk of decreased shedding duration and quantity.

In the patient with meningitis in whom mumps is suspected, the CSF profile resembles that of enteroviral infection; however, hypoglycorrhachia is a characteristic feature in mumps meningitis, with CSF glucose values in the 10- to 20-mg/dL range.

Rubella

In the susceptible host, laboratory methods to diagnose rubella are similar to those used for measles and mumps. Rubella-specific IgM antibody typically appears in the blood between 4 and 30 days after onset of symptoms, but adequate production may not occur until after 72 to 96 hours following onset of symptoms. Thus, repeat rubella IgM testing should be performed 5 days after onset of rash in patients in whom suspicion is high for rubella infection. False-positive results are often seen with rubella-specific IgM antibody testing. This is due in part to testing cross-reactivity with other viral antibodies, including B19V IgM and the heterophile antibody of EBV. Other noninfectious sources such as elevated rheumatoid factor may also be responsible for false-positive rubella IgM test results.

Recent rubella infection may also be determined by measuring the rise in rubella-specific IgG levels in paired acute and convalescent sera. In the susceptible host, rubella IgG is typically present within 8 days after symptom onset.

Rubella can be isolated from nasal swabs and throat swabs, as well as CSF in cases of rubella encephalitis. Unlike mumps, rubella virus can also be isolated from blood specimens. A sharp decline in the concentration of detectable virus in the blood often coincides with rash onset. Virus can be isolated from oropharyngeal secretions during the period beginning with prodromal symptom onset, up to and including 14 days after exanthem appearance. Oropharyngeal specimens obtained within the first 4 days after rash onset typically yield the highest concentration of virus. Reverse transcriptase-polymerase chain reaction testing for rubella virus (sensitivity averaging 80%–90% and specificity of near 100%) is preferred for diagnosis in the immunocompromised host. Diagnostic criteria for rubella are found in Box 32-2.

Box 32-2. Diagnostic Criteria for Rubella

Suspected: Any generalized rash illness of acute onset that does not meet the criteria for probable or confirmed rubella or any other illness.

Probable: In the absence of a more likely diagnosis, an illness characterized by all of the following findings:
- Acute onset of generalized maculopapular rash
- Temperature >37.2°C (99.0°F), if measured
- Arthralgia, arthritis, lymphadenopathy, or conjunctivitis
- Lack of epidemiologic linkage to a laboratory-confirmed case of rubella
- Noncontributory or no serologic or virologic testing

Confirmed: A patient with or without symptoms who has laboratory evidence of rubella infection confirmed by 1 or more of the following laboratory test results:
- Isolation of rubella virus
- Detection of rubella virus–specific nucleic acid by PCR
- Significant rise between acute- and convalescent-phase titers in serum rubella IgG antibody level by any standard serologic test
- Positive serologic test for rubella IgM antibody

or

An illness characterized by all of the following findings:
- Acute onset of generalized maculopapular rash
- Temperature >37.2°C (99.0°F)
- Arthralgia, arthritis, lymphadenopathy, or conjunctivitis
- Epidemiologic linkage to a laboratory-confirmed case of rubella

Abbreviation: PCR, polymerase chain reaction.

Congenital Rubella Syndrome

The diagnosis of CRS involves a thorough assessment of potential clinical and laboratory findings in addition to laboratory testing. Either cell culture or RT-PCR may be used to confirm the diagnosis of CRS. Samples with the highest diagnostic yield include throat swabs, nasal swabs, and urinary specimens. Other specimens from which rubella virus can be isolated include CSF, blood, and surgically obtained lens aspirates in those with congenital cataracts. Virus can be shed from the cornea for over a year in those with CRS.

Serologic testing in neonates or infants with CRS often reveals rubella-specific IgM presence at birth. Rubella-specific IgM antibody may persist until

12 months after birth in patients with CRS, though levels often gradually decline prior to this time. Differentiation between maternally acquired antibodies and rubella-specific IgM produced by the infant as a result of congenital infection, however, is often extremely difficult. In these circumstances, repeat IgM along with IgG levels should be obtained between 6 and 8 months. In infants whose initial and repeat rubella-specific IgM titers are positive, CRS is extremely probable. Case definitions for CRS are found in Box 32-3.

Box 32-3. Case Definitions Approved by the Council of State and Territorial Epidemiologists for Congenital Rubella Syndrome

Suspected: A neonate or an infant who does not meet the criteria for a probable or confirmed case but has 1 or more of the following clinical findings:
- Cataracts or congenital glaucoma
- Congenital heart disease (most commonly patent ductus arteriosus or peripheral pulmonary artery stenosis)
- Hearing impairment
- Pigmentary retinopathy
- Purpura
- Hepatosplenomegaly
- Jaundice
- Microcephaly
- Developmental delay
- Meningoencephalitis
- Radiolucent bone disease

Probable[a]: An infant who does not have laboratory confirmation of rubella infection but has at least 2 of the following findings without a more plausible etiology:
- Cataracts or congenital glaucoma[a]
- Congenital heart disease (most commonly patent ductus arteriosus or peripheral pulmonary artery stenosis)
- Hearing impairment
- Pigmentary retinopathy

or

An infant who does not have laboratory confirmation of rubella infection but has at least 1 or more of the following findings without a more plausible etiology:
- Cataracts or congenital glaucoma[a]
- Congenital heart disease (most commonly patent ductus arteriosus or peripheral pulmonary artery stenosis)
- Hearing impairment
- Pigmentary retinopathy

and

One or more of the following findings:
- Purpura
- Hepatosplenomegaly
- Jaundice
- Microcephaly
- Developmental delay
- Meningoencephalitis
- Radiolucent bone disease

Continued

Box 32-3 *(cont)*

Confirmed: An infant with at least 1 symptom (listed on the previous page) that is clinically consistent with CRS and laboratory evidence of congenital rubella infection as demonstrated by any of the following results:
- Isolation of rubella virus
- Detection of rubella-specific IgM antibody
- Infant rubella antibody level that persists at a higher level and for a longer period than expected from passive transfer of maternal antibody (ie, rubella titer that does not drop at the expected rate of a twofold dilution per month)
- A specimen that is PCR positive for rubella virus

Infection only: An infant without any clinical symptoms or signs of rubella but with laboratory evidence of infection as demonstrated by any of the following results:
- Isolation of rubella virus
- Detection of rubella-specific IgM antibody
- Infant rubella antibody level that persists at a higher level and for a longer period than expected from passive transfer of maternal antibody (ie, rubella titer that does not drop at the expected rate of a twofold dilution per month)
- A specimen that is PCR positive for rubella virus

Abbreviations: CRS, congenital rubella syndrome; PCR, polymerase chain reaction.

a In probable cases, either or both of the eye-related findings (cataracts and congenital glaucoma) count as a single complication. In cases classified as infection only, if any compatible signs or symptoms (eg, hearing loss) are identified later, the case is reclassified as confirmed.

Management

Measles

Measles decreases serum concentrations of vitamin A, accentuating the problem in previously deficient children. For this reason, vitamin A administration once daily for 2 days is universally recommended in children with measles, particularly those who may be deficient. Recommended dosing is as follows: 50,000 IU/day for infants younger than 6 months, 100,000 IU/day for infants 6 to 11 months of age, and 200,000 IU/day in children 12 months or older (Evidence Level I). A third dose should be given in 2 to 4 weeks for any child who is determined to be vitamin A deficient. Vitamin A decreases overall mortality in infected children younger than 2 years and reduces pneumonia-specific mortality and morbidity caused by croup. Ribavirin is not approved for use in the United States but has been used in patients with measles who are severely immunocompromised (Evidence Level III).

Airborne precautions should be utilized for hospitalized children with measles and continued for 4 days following the onset of rash and the entire duration of illness in the immunocompromised host.

Immunization with measles-mumps-rubella (MMR) vaccine is the cornerstone of care for children exposed to measles and who are not appropriately immunized with 2 doses of MMR vaccine. If administered within 72 hours of exposure, MMR vaccination may modify the course of infection, should infection develop. In outbreak settings, children between the ages of 6 and 11 months may be candidates for MMR vaccination, though doses administered prior to 12 months of age should not be counted toward completion of the 2-dose vaccine series. Immune globulin may also be indicated for babies younger than 1 year and the immunocompromised host. Exposed unvaccinated children should be quarantined (excluded from school/day care or any other public areas) until 21 days after onset of rash of the last case of measles or until vaccinated. Administration of 1 MMR dose is sufficient to prevent quarantine, and a second dose should be given to those who are eligible. Given the inherent difficulty with imposing quarantine measures in schools, quarantine is not routinely recommended in the event of a measles outbreak. Exceptions to this might include outbreaks in schools attended by large numbers of students who refuse vaccination.

The dosing regimen for intramuscular immune globulin (IMIG) for measles postexposure prophylaxis is as follows: 0.5 mL/kg intramuscularly in the child younger than 12 months and all otherwise healthy exposed children who do not have evidence of preexisting immunity (maximum dose: 15 mL). Dosing for the severely immunosuppressed child, including HIV-1–infected children with severe immunosuppression, is 400 mg/kg intravenous immune globulin (IMIG is no longer recommended for this population). All other eligible HIV-infected children may receive 0.5 mL/kg IMIG (maximum dose: 15 mL).

Mumps

As with measles, no proven effective antiviral therapy exists for mumps, and treatment consists of supportive measures and rest. Hospitalization may be necessary for pain and hydration support. Steroids should not be used for treatment of mumps orchitis, because they can decrease testosterone concentrations, leading to a greater chance of testicular atrophy and sterility. Interferon-α2B has been studied as a possible intervention for testicular atrophy and sterility prevention in postpubertal boys with mumps orchitis, but further studies are needed in this area (Evidence Level III). Intravenous immune globulin may be indicated in treatment of autoimmune-based sequelae of mumps infection, such as thrombocytopenic purpura (Evidence Level III).

Droplet isolation for patients hospitalized with mumps should continue for 5 days following parotitis onset. Infected children should be isolated and excluded from school, child care, and other community settings for a minimum of 5 days after onset of parotitis to prevent transmission and for outbreak control.

In the event of a mumps outbreak, children who have previously received 1 or 2 doses of MMR vaccine may return to school, ensuring completion of vaccination series for those needing the second dose. Children who have not received any dose of MMR should be excluded but may be readmitted immediately following vaccination. Children who cannot receive mumps vaccine should be excluded from school for a minimum of 26 days after the onset of parotitis in the last infected person. A third dose of vaccine has been considered in certain outbreak settings and is currently being investigated.

Rubella

No antiviral therapy exists for the treatment of rubella. Care should therefore be directed toward management of rubella complications. In those who develop arthritis secondary to rubella infection, rest and nonsteroidal anti-inflammatory drugs alone are indicated. Those who develop refractory thrombocytopenia with severe bleeding may also be candidates for intravenous immune globulin administration, though thrombocytopenia is typically self-limited.

In neonates and infants with CRS, management of the numerous potential sequelae of infection, including respiratory, cardiac, and neurologic complications, should be in the same manner as with rubella-negative infants. Prompt recognition of ophthalmologic abnormalities is advised, because corneal clouding may indicate the presence of glaucoma and subsequent need for operative intervention. Determination of retinopathy or cataract presence should also be made, though most ophthalmologists choose to defer surgical management for these conditions until the child is at least 12 months of age.

Children with CRS may shed virus for at least 12 months, and contact precautions should be continued indefinitely for the hospitalized child and used for each subsequent hospitalization. Isolation can be discontinued if after 3 months of age the child has 2 negative viral cultures taken a month apart. Children with CRS should be considered for exclusion from child care facilities until they are no longer considered infectious, and all their contacts, especially women of childbearing age, should be tested for immunity to rubella and vaccinated if not immune.

For hospitalized children with postnatally acquired rubella infection, droplet isolation precautions should be maintained for 7 days following rash onset. Quarantine is essential for limiting outbreaks. Children with postnatally acquired rubella infection should be excluded from school, child care, and other community settings for 7 days after rash onset. In a school outbreak setting, children who do not have evidence of immunity should be excluded until immunized. Those who refuse vaccination should be excluded until 21 days after onset of rash in the last infected person.

Immunization of the eligible child exposed to rubella has not been shown to prevent or modify the course of rubella infection; however, controlled trials regarding this assumption are lacking. On the basis of outbreak studies performed during the 1970s and 1980s, vaccination of eligible children and adults may curb the spread of outbreaks in a more rapid fashion than if no immunizations were administered. Eligible children who have not received 2 doses of MMR vaccine should be immunized per current Advisory Committee on Immunization Practices recommendations, regardless of exposure, because immunization will provide protection in the event of a future exposure to rubella.

Suggested Reading

American Academy of Pediatrics. Measles; mumps; rubella. In: Kimberlin DW, Brady MT, Jackson MA, Long SS, eds. *Red Book: 2015 Report of the Committee of Infectious Diseases.* 30th ed. Elk Grove Village, IL; American Academy of Pediatrics; 2015: 540–542

Centers for Disease Control and Prevention. *Manual for the Surveillance of Vaccine-Preventable Diseases.* Atlanta, GA: Centers for Disease Control and Prevention; 2012. http://www.cdc.gov/vaccines/pubs/surv-manual/index.html. Accessed March 31, 2016

Hamborsky J, Kroger A, Wolfe S, eds. *Epidemiology and Prevention of Vaccine-Preventable Diseases.* 13th ed. Washington, DC; Public Health Foundation; 2015

Plotkin SA, Orenstein WA, Offit PA, eds. *Vaccines.* 6th ed. Philadelphia, PA: Saunders; 2012

CHAPTER 33

Parvovirus

James Christopher Day, MD

Key Points

- Infection caused by *Human parvovirus B19* is associated with 2 classic exanthems: erythema infectiosum (common; school-aged children) and papular petechial glove and stocking syndrome (uncommon but distinctive; young adults).

- Arthropathy is uncommon in children, reported most often in adult women, and usually features a symmetric polyarthropathy involving knees and hands.

- Severe anemia may be seen in those with hematologic conditions (eg, sickle cell anemia, other hemoglobinopathies, hereditary spherocytosis) and immunodeficiencies, particularly in solid organ transplant recipients, HIV-infected patients, and those receiving immunosuppressive therapies.

- Pregnancy-associated parvoviral infection may cause fetal death when acquired early in pregnancy and is a cause of fetal hydrops.

- Treatment is unnecessary in the otherwise healthy child with erythema infectiosum or papular petechial glove and stocking syndrome.

Overview

Human parvovirus B19 (B19V) is the cause of erythema infectiosum (ie, fifth disease), and a prominent cause of several other clinical syndromes, including aplastic crisis in sickle cell disease, pure red cell aplasia in immunocompromised hosts, polyarthropathy, fetal hydrops, and fetal demise. Red blood cell precursors are the cells most commonly infected by parvovirus, which leads to the decreased red blood cell (RBC) production seen in several of these clinical syndromes.

Causes and Differential Diagnosis

The differential diagnosis for parvovirus disease depends on the clinical syndrome. Other viral exanthems may resemble erythema infectiosum. A variety of hematologic and rheumatologic diseases may be considered in settings where RBC precursor cell lines are affected. A wide range of diagnoses should be considered in the setting of fetal hydrops, including Rh isoimmunization, metabolic/genetic syndromes, cardiovascular diseases, and lymphatic/vascular tumors, as well as thoracic, extrathoracic, or urinary tract defects.

Clinical Features

Most commonly, parvoviral infections result in no or minimal symptoms. In the minority of affected patients, several syndromes can be seen.

Erythema infectiosum, or fifth disease, presents as a distinctive rash on the face with moderately erythematous cheeks and circumoral pallor often described as "slapped cheeks." Over the next 1 to 4 days, the rash migrates to the trunk and limbs where it is pink, macular, and frequently reticular in pattern. The rash may reappear or intensify in response to sunlight or heat for weeks to months after the initial illness. There is often a prodrome 1 to 2 weeks before occurrence of the slapped-cheek rash that may include fever, malaise, myalgia, acute rhinitis, and headache. The incubation period ranges from 4 to as long as 21 days.

An additional distinctive skin manifestation of B19V is papular petechial glove and stocking syndrome. Almost exclusively occurring in young adults, it presents with painful, pruritic, symmetric papular and petechial lesions of the hands and feet. Oral manifestations may be noted and include petechiae, pharyngeal erythema, swollen lips, and painful oral ulcers. Symptoms abate over several days. Recognition of this entity can eliminate extensive additional testing, which may be considered in the setting of petechial rash.

In illnesses with a high rate of RBC turnover, such as sickle cell disease, other hemoglobinopathies, and hemolytic anemias, parvoviral infection of RBC precursors can result in an aplastic crisis. The subsequent anemia frequently requires blood transfusion. This anemia resolves after the infection has been cleared and RBC production resumes. The only infectious agent known to cause aplastic crisis is B19V, and in sickle cell patients it appears to be the cause of at least 80% of such crises.

Pure red cell or persistent anemia can occur with ongoing infection with the virus, which can occur in a number of immunodeficient states, including during cancer chemotherapy or while on immunosuppression following organ transplantation. This syndrome has also been seen in HIV.

Clinically significant arthropathy characteristically occurs in middle-aged women infected with B19V and is not as common in children, though it does occur. In children, the arthropathy, when it does occur, typically involves the knees and ankles. It may be symmetric or asymmetric. It typically resolves within 3 weeks. Older adolescents and adults most often have symmetric arthropathy involving the proximal interphalangeal and metacarpophalangeal joints. It usually self-resolves over a few weeks.

While most B19V infections during pregnancy do not harm the fetus, there is a risk of fetal loss because of the infection, particularly during the period with the highest risk of transplacental infection with the virus, from the ninth to 20th week of gestation. Fetal loss is generally linked to fetal hydrops. *Human parvovirus B19* causes a severe anemia and likely myocarditis, leading to congestive heart failure in the fetus. *Human parvovirus B19* is estimated to cause 10% to 20% of all cases of nonimmune hydrops and carries a 5% to 9% risk of fetal loss per infection when transplacental infection occurs. The risk of transplacental infection for a mother with a B19V infection during pregnancy is around 30%. If fetal loss does not occur, the risk of long-term sequelae is low. Risk factors for infection with B19V during pregnancy are generally not considered modifiable; the most significant risk factor is exposure to children in the household. Risks for individuals who work with children (eg, elementary school teachers or day care workers) have not been shown to be higher than for pregnant women in other occupations. Both the Centers for Disease Control and Prevention and American College of Obstetricians and Gynecologists have recommended against routinely excluding pregnant women from the workplace, even during endemic outbreaks of parvovirus. Pregnant women are encouraged to discuss their individual risk with their physician.

Evaluation

Most parvoviral infections, generally including erythema infectiosum, are mild and do not require laboratory evaluation. Laboratory diagnosis of more serious parvoviral syndromes depends on the clinical context. Viral culture of this pathogen is difficult and not clinically useful. IgG to parvovirus is not a useful indicator of current infection, because a high proportion of individuals have a past history of infection and these IgG antibodies will persist for life; however, it does indicate past infection. Specific IgM to parvovirus is often detectable in the serum of affected individuals soon after the onset of clinically apparent illness (eg, by the third day of aplastic crisis) and remains detectable for 2 to 3 months. *Human parvovirus B19* IgM can form complexes with viral particles during periods of high viremia, leading to a false-negative test result. Immunocompromised individuals may also have negative titers because of an inability to make antibodies. When IgM testing is negative but parvovirus continues to be suspected, polymerase chain reaction testing will be necessary to make a diagnosis. *Human parvovirus B19* polymerase chain reaction can detect viral DNA in the presence of acute infection, but viral DNA may also remain detectable in serum for months and in tissues, including bone marrow, for years after initial infection. Determination of the viral load may be helpful in an immunocompromised host who presents with aplastic crisis.

Management

No specific therapy is indicated for erythema infectiosum. By the time of the appearance of the rash, viremia has typically resolved.

In mothers known to have acquired B19V infection during pregnancy, monitoring for hydrops is done by prenatal ultrasound that includes Doppler ultrasonography of blood flow in the middle cerebral artery. The likelihood of fetal demise from complications of B19V (eg, anemia, hydrops) can be reduced from 50% to 18% by intrauterine RBC transfusion.

Reduction in immunosuppression and administration of intravenous immune globulin should be considered in patients with B19V aplastic crisis in the setting of solid organ transplantation or in HIV infection.

Suggested Reading

Florea AV, Ionescu DN, Melham MF. Parvovirus B19 infection in the immunocompromised host. *Arch Pathol Lab Med.* 2007;131(5):799–804

Heegard ED, Brown KE. *Human parvovirus B19. Clin Microbiol Rev.* 2002;15(3):485–505

Snyder M, Wallace R. Clinical inquiry: what should you tell pregnant women about exposure to parvovirus? *J Fam Pract.* 2011;60(12):765–766

Tolfvenstam T, Broliden K. Parvovirus B19 infection. *Semin Fetal Neonatal Med.* 2009;14(4):218–221

Young NS, Brown KE. Parvovirus B19. *N Engl J Med.* 2004;350(6):586–597

CHAPTER 34

Rabies

Sergio E. Recuenco, MD, MPH, DrPH

Key Points

- Encephalitis caused by rabies virus is invariably fatal and should be distinguished from other causes of encephalitis. Intensive care treatment and sedation is the mainstay for care, and use of the Milwaukee Protocol may be considered.

- The diagnosis should be suspected in cases of a rapidly progressive encephalitis or when encephalitis follows a high-risk bite encounter or exposure to a bat in sleeping infants or an incapacitated adult.

- To diagnose rabies, saliva, serum, cerebrospinal fluid, and nuchal skin biopsy material should be tested. Testing should include rabies virus polymerase chain reaction and culture for rabies virus, detection of rabies virus antigen by direct fluorescent assay, and measurement of IgG and IgM antibodies to rabies virus. Involvement of public health officials and an infectious diseases specialist is necessary.

- In the patient with an animal bite, postexposure prophylaxis is effective and should be considered urgently.

- In the setting of a dog, cat, or ferret bite, observation of the animal can be undertaken. If the animal remains well during observation for 10 days following the bite, rabies has been excluded.

- In those exposed to a bat or other high-risk wildlife bite, if available, the animal should be immediately euthanized and tested for rabies.

Overview

Rabies is a fatal disease, with rare opportunity for therapeutic interventions after clinical onset. Extremely rare recoveries in young individuals are documented, potentially as a result of a low-dose exposure to the virus or an early and robust immunologic response by the patient. Timely intervention with rabies postexposure prophylaxis (PEP) after a rabies exposure is sufficient to halt virus migration and progression to clinical onset.

Causes and Differential Diagnosis

A history of exposure to potentially rabid animals is essential to associate clinical encephalitis with rabies, but sometimes exposure history is missing and difficult to rule out in young children and impaired teenagers that may not be able to report accurately an animal exposure. All mammals are susceptible to contract rabies and able to transmit the virus during the infectious period when virus is present in saliva.

Bites from carnivores such as dogs, raccoons, or foxes, and most animals of similar size, can be easily identified, with notable exceptions among certain species of bats. Rodent bites (eg, mouse, rat, squirrel, guinea pig) have a very low risk for transmission and in natural and domestic settings are not considered a rabies exposure unless an aggressive unprovoked attack from the rodent is described.

Transmission has been documented from organ transplantation (eg, cornea, lung, liver, heart, kidneys) with an incubation period of less than 1 week to 18 months. Transmission is possible through inhalation of aerosolized rabies virus, which can occur in the laboratory and caves with very high density bat populations; however, air transmission of rabies should not be considered in normal outdoor and domestic settings. Human-to-human transmission by contact with saliva of a rabid individual is possible but of low concern with standard biosafety practices and infection control practices.

The contact of tissues or fluids containing viable rabies virus (eg, saliva of a rabid animal, brain tissue) with any opening of the skin or mucosae allowing access to nervous tissue is considered a rabies exposure. A contact of saliva from a rabid animal with intact skin is not a rabies exposure. Contact with blood, urine, stool, or milk from rabid animals or humans is not considered a rabies exposure. The incubation period after an exposure is 45 days in average, varying from less than a week to 6 months; exceptional incubation periods of up to 8 years have been documented.

Rabies prodromal symptoms tend to be nonspecific and can be easily confounded with other diseases. Rabies diagnosis is difficult, and the differential diagnosis will include not only other causes of acute encephalitis but also substance use and mental disorders (Table 34-1). Rabies outbreaks in children living in highly endemic areas can be confounded with pneumonia or influenza when a cluster of children presents with respiratory symptoms, ptyalism, and encephalitis.

Table 34-1. Rabies Differential Diagnosis

Etiology	Differential Diagnosis	Relevant Signs/Symptoms	Laboratory/Clinical Evidence
Viral Infection	HSV infection	Does not show the relapsing/remitting pattern of mental lucidity seen in rabies.	Bloody CSF (inconstant). HSV is detected in CSF by PCR with >95% sensitivity.
	Enterovirus meningoencephalitis	Fall seasons may overlap. Profound dysautonomia, as in rabies, with cardiomyopathy.	Enteroviruses are detected in CSF by PCR with >95% sensitivity.
	West Nile virus encephalitis	History of a mosquito bite. Generally, shows more parkinsonian findings or body rigidity than rabies.	West Nile virus–specific IgM in CSF is diagnostic.
	Other arbovirus encephalitides	History of a mosquito bite. Generally, shows more parkinsonian findings or body rigidity than rabies.	Serum anti-arbovirus antibodies are present.
	Japanese encephalitis	Parkinsonian symptoms are common. Patients develop hyperreflexia.	Presence of Japanese encephalitis virus RNA in tissue, blood, or CSF is diagnostic. Japanese encephalitis virus antibodies may be detected in CSF or serum.
	Zika fever	History of a mosquito bite. Alteration of mental status, progression to coma. Guillain-Barré syndrome.	RT-PCR and antibody testing in serum, CSF, or urine positive for Zika virus.

Continued

Table 34-1 *(cont)*

Etiology	Differential Diagnosis	Relevant Signs/Symptoms	Laboratory/Clinical Evidence
Bacterial/Rickettsial Infection	Rocky Mountain spotted fever and rickettsial encephalitis	Tick exposure is common with Rocky Mountain spotted fever. Petechial rashes and eschars are present.	WBC count usually low. Rocky Mountain spotted fever and other rickettsial serologic testing is diagnostic using acute and convalescent sera.
	Tetanus	Aerophobia, hydrophobia, and mental state changes are absent. The main sign is trismus (which results in a grimace described as *risus sardonicus*, or sardonic smile) associated with muscle rigidity, spasms, respiratory embarrassment, dysphagia, or dysautonomia.	Detection of tetanospasmin in plasma or clostridial culture from wound swab. CSF findings are normal.
	Bartonella encephalopathy	Associated with refractory seizures and regional lymphadenitis.	*Bartonella* serologic testing is diagnostic.
Noninfectious Causes	Guillain-Barré syndrome	Acute flaccid paralysis is similar to paralysis seen in rabies, especially paralytic rabies. Sphincter involvement is rare. There is no fever.	CSF shows elevated protein concentration with a normal cell count (albuminocytologic dissociation). Nerve conduction studies show slowing of nerve conduction velocities.
	Limbic encephalitis	Aerophobia and hydrophobia are absent, but other clinical features are very similar to rabies. Seizures are common with NMDA antibodies.	Serum antibodies to NMDA are positive.
	Acute disseminated encephalomyelitis	Aerophobia and hydrophobia are absent, but other clinical features are very similar to rabies.	Brain MRI shows white matter lesions.

Psychiatric Disorders/Substance Use Disorder	Alcohol withdrawal delirium	History of chronic alcohol use and either reduction or cessation of drinking before presentation. Prodromal illness is absent. Fever is rare.	The diagnosis is clinical.
	Cocaine overdose	History of cocaine use.	Cocaine may be detected in urine, blood, or gastric contents. The half-life in blood is short.
	Amphetamine overdose	History of amphetamine use disorder.	Urine is positive for amphetamines.
	Acute psychosis	Main symptoms are hallucinations, delusions, and thought disorder, possibly accompanied by agitation. The prodromal and physical manifestations of rabies are absent. Other clinical features depend on the cause.	No differentiating tests.

Abbreviations: CSF, cerebrospinal fluid; HSV, herpes simplex virus; NMDA, N-methyl-D-aspartate class of glutamate receptor; MRI, magnetic resonance imaging; PCR, polymerase chain reaction; RT-PCR, reverse transcription-polymerase chain reaction; WBC, white blood cell.

Clinical Features

Rabies onset often includes changes of behavior, hallucinations, sore throat, vomiting, headache, pain in limbs, and paresthesias. Fever may not be apparent at hospital admission but can be detected during the 24 to 48 hours following admission. Hydrophobia and ptyalism are important signs of rabies but not always identified because of fast progression of the patient to coma and death.

Animal exposure history or recent travel to rabies-endemic areas can trigger consideration of rabies in the differential. Rapid progression from conscience impairment to coma and general status deterioration is characteristic to rabies. Two main clinical presentations of rabies have been described: the encephalitic (furious) form, in which agitation and aggressiveness can be observed, and the paralytic form, in which ascending weakness can be observed, also affecting the control of sphincters. Changes in mental status are not observed in the paralytic form.

Evaluation

Rabies Exposure

Each potential rabies exposure needs case-by-case evaluation. Risk assessment for the exposure should consider probability of the animal involved in the exposure to be rabid (local epidemiology, animal species, health status, provoked or unprovoked attack), nature of the exposure (eg, bite, scratch, touch), and evidence of percutaneous injury. Wildlife considered high-risk in the United States includes raccoons, foxes, coyotes, bobcats, and skunks, and bite incidents in such instances are readily apparent. However, most human cases of rabies in the last decade in the United States have been confirmed to be bat related, and cases have occurred in which disease has been transmitted in absence of a bite history.

All animal bites should receive prompt wound care, including washing the wound with running water and soap for no less than 10 minutes. Tetanus immunization status should be verified and prophylactic antibiotics should be given for cat bites, crush or penetrating wounds, extensive bites, and those on the face, hands, feet, or genitals. Important information that should be collected regarding circumstances of the bite include species of the animal, general appearance and behavior of the animal, whether the encounter was provoked by the presence of a human, and severity and location of bites. If a rabies exposure is confirmed, immediate rabies PEP is indicated.

Because bat exposures are considered high-risk, PEP is recommended even in absence of a bite history in cases in which a bat is found in the room with a sleeping child or incapacitated adolescent or adult. In such cases, it is imperative that the bat be caught and tested for rabies and not released or destroyed. Specific instructions for capturing a bat are available at the Centers for Disease Control and Prevention Web site (www.cdc.gov/rabies/bats/contact/capture.html).

Postexposure prophylaxis includes a total of 4 rabies vaccine doses (cell culture-derived rabies vaccine) of 1 mL given intramuscularly on days 0, 3, 7, and 14 in the arm or deltoid area and should always include administration of rabies immune globulin at a dose of 20 IU/kg, infiltrating the wound with a maximum of 50% of the total dose and injecting the rest intramuscularly on day 0 or up to day 7. Rabies vaccine and rabies immune globulin should not be injected in the same arm.

In the United States, only 2 rabies vaccines are licensed for intramuscular use, the purified chick embryo cell vaccine and human diploid cell vaccine. Both can be interchanged in case allergies or adverse effects are observed, avoiding interruption of PEP. Rabies vaccine cultured on Vero cells is available in other countries. Purified chick embryo cell, human diploid cell, and Vero cell vaccines are recommended by the World Health Organization, for intramuscular and intradermal use.

When the animal involved in the exposure is available, euthanasia and rabies testing of the brain by a public health laboratory will determine whether the animal is rabid. In the case of dogs, cats, and ferrets, an observation period

Table 34-2. Rabies Postexposure Prophylaxis Guide—United States (Advisory Committee on Immunization Practices)

Animal Type	Evaluation and Disposition of Animal	Postexposure Prophylaxis Recommendations
Dogs, cats, and ferrets	Healthy and available for 10 d of observation.	Persons should not begin PEP unless animal develops clinical signs of rabies.[a]
	Rabid or suspected rabid.	Immediate PEP.
	Unknown (eg, escaped).	Consult public health officials.
Skunks, raccoons, foxes, and most other carnivores; bats[b]	Regarded as rabid unless animal proven negative by laboratory tests.[c]	Consider immediate PEP.
Livestock, small rodents, lagomorphs (rabbits and hares), large rodents (woodchucks and beavers), and other mammals	Consider individually.	Consult public health officials. Bites of squirrels, hamsters, guinea pigs, gerbils, chipmunks, rats, mice, other small rodents, rabbits, and hares almost never require PEP.

Abbreviation: PEP, postexposure prophylaxis.

[a] During the 10-d observation period, begin PEP at the first sign of rabies in a dog, cat, or ferret that has bitten someone. If the animal exhibits clinical signs of rabies, it should be euthanized immediately and tested.

[b] Postexposure prophylaxis should be initiated as soon as possible following exposure to such wildlife unless the animal is available for testing and public health authorities are facilitating expeditious laboratory testing or it is already known that brain material from the animal has tested negative. Discontinue vaccine if appropriate laboratory diagnostic test (ie, the direct fluorescent assay) is negative.

[c] The animal should be euthanized and tested as soon as possible. Holding for observation is not recommended.

Adapted from Manning SE, Rupprecht CE, Fishbein D, et al. Human rabies prevention—United States, 2008: recommendations of the Advisory Committee on Immunization Practices. *MMWR Recomm Rep.* 2008;57(RR-3):1–28.

of 10 days can be used, independent of the vaccine status of the animal. If the animal is still healthy at the end of the observation period, it is not rabid and rabies prophylaxis can be discontinued. Initiation of PEP could be delayed during the 10-day observation period or while the rabies laboratory is confirming diagnosis, unless the bite occurred on the head, neck, or hand; the bites are severe and profound; or the patient is a small child. For those situations, PEP should start without delay and can be stopped later if rabies is ruled out. If the patient has clinical symptoms suspicious of rabies, PEP is not indicated.

Patients receiving steroids in high doses, immunosuppressive medication (as feasible), or antimalarials should discontinue those treatments during administration of PEP. Immunocompromised patients must receive an additional fifth dose of rabies vaccine on day 28, and provide serum for rabies antibody testing 14 days later to confirm an immunologic response. If an inadequate antibody response is determined (rapid fluorescent focus inhibition test value ≥1:5 or ≥0.5 IU per Advisory Committee on Immunization Practices and World Health Organization), the case must be reevaluated in consultation with local public health authorities.

For situations potentially at high risk for rabies exposures, because of occupational risk or travel to endemic areas, a pre-PEP schedule is available using one 1 mL dose of the rabies vaccine intramuscularly on days 0, 7, and 21 or 28.

Suspected Rabies

Animal exposures should be further evaluated in any patient presenting symptoms of acute encephalitis. When the exposure is not apparent or suspected, rapid deterioration of the patient's condition is justification to reconsider rabies in the differential. Standard laboratory examination of body fluids such as serum, cerebrospinal fluid (CSF), and urine will be indicative of viral encephalitis but may not be specific for rabies. Magnetic resonance images and radiographs will show nonspecific signs of encephalitis, and typically findings are unremarkable at hospital admission. For this reason, rabies is often diagnosed using a rule-out approach. Testing available for other diseases in the differential diagnosis (eg, herpes simplex virus, West Nile virus, Lyme disease, limbic encephalitis) is completed according to medical evaluation during early stages of hospitalization, and negative results for any of those etiologies will increase the priority for a rabies diagnosis. To diagnose rabies antemortem, 4 samples are required: saliva, serum, CSF, and nuchal skin biopsy. All samples should be collected on the same day, or paired samples can be taken over successive days. Positive results in the serum of an unvaccinated individual or positive results in any of the other samples will confirm rabies. To rule out a diagnosis for rabies, all 4 samples from the patient must test negative. For encephalitic patients dying before an etiology is established, rabies post-mortem tests are available, requiring an autopsy to obtain samples from central nervous system tissues: brain stem, cerebellum, and parts of the brain.

Management

Patients exhibiting clinical rabies must be treated in an intensive care unit using standard precautions. Clinicians should know that the patient's saliva, CSF, and brain tissue is considered infectious. Clinicians who incur a bite from the patient or have an open wound or mucous membrane that has become contaminated with the patient's saliva, CSF, or brain tissue should receive PEP.

Salivary polymerase chain reaction and culture if positive confirm the diagnosis and that the patient is infectious. Serial determination can be made if the patient survives looking for reversion to negative results.

Most patients will not live longer than 2 weeks, even under optimal intensive care unit conditions. Management of the disease is based on palliative care and use of sedatives. No therapeutic options are available other than experimental therapeutics such as the Milwaukee protocol (www.mcw.edu/rabies).

Known clinical complications of rabies are respiratory failure, poikilothermy refractory to antipyretics, lactic acidosis, cardiac arrhythmias, hypotension that responds to administration of tetrahydrobiopterin, aspiration due to ptyalism, ileus beginning at day 5 to 7 after clinical onset, diabetes insipidus, cerebral edema, hyponatremia, urinary retention, and myocarditis. Vasospasm can be expected approximately at days 5 and 12 of hospitalization and can be managed using calcium channel blocking agents. Some experts who advocate the Milwaukee protocol suggest avoidance of barbiturates, propofol, and topiramate and suggest that vasopressor use may lead to vasoconstriction in those with tetrahydrobiopterin deficiency.

Case reports of spontaneous rabies recovery and abortive rabies deserve further study to understand factors that may lead to recovery. Early suspicion and diagnostic testing, with provision of supportive care and careful monitoring, increases the opportunities for survivorship in pediatric rabies cases.

Suggested Reading

Brown CM, Conti L, Ettestad P, Leslie MJ, Sorhage FE, Sun B. Compendium of animal rabies prevention and control, 2011. *J Am Vet Med Assoc.* 2011;239(5):609–617

Centers for Disease Control and Prevention. Investigation of rabies infections in organ donor and transplant recipients—Alabama, Arkansas, Oklahoma, and Texas, 2004. *MMWR Morb Mortal Wkly Rep.* 2004;53(26):586–589

Centers for Disease Control and Prevention. Rabies. http://www.cdc.gov/rabies. CDC Web site. Updated January 26, 2016. Accessed March 28, 2016

Manning SE, Rupprecht, CE Fishbein, et al. Human rabies prevention—United States, 2008: recommendations of the Advisory Committee on Immunization Practices. *MMWR Recomm Rep.* 2008;57(RR-3):1–28

Petersen BW, Rupprecht CE. Human rabies epidemiology and diagnosis. In: Tkachev S, ed. *Non-Flavivirus Encephalitis.* InTech; 2011

Recuenco S.E., Willoughby R, and Robertson K. Rabies-Online monograph. Epocrates BMJ. 2010. www.online.epocrates.com/noFrame/showPage.do?method=diseases& MonographId=903&ActiveSectionId=35. Accessed February 10, 2016

Rupprecht CE, Briggs D, Brown CM, et al. Use of a reduced (4-dose) vaccine schedule for postexposure prophylaxis to prevent human rabies: recommendations of the Advisory Committee on Immunization Practices. *MMWR Recomm Rep.* 2010;59(RR-2):1–9

CHAPTER 35

Respiratory Viruses

Christelle M. Ilboudo, MD, and Janet A. Englund, MD

Key Points

- Respiratory viruses in children may cause upper and lower respiratory tract infections.

- Most respiratory viruses have seasonal epidemics, which are usually in the fall through spring in temperate climates.

- Most children who are healthy and immunocompetent require only supportive care.

- Antimicrobials should not be used for children with viral upper respiratory tract infections.

- Diagnostic measures, especially newer rapid methods of molecular detection, such as polymerase chain reaction, may be useful in the diagnosis of moderate to severe disease in hospitalized patients, helping avoid the unnecessary use of antimicrobials and potentially initiating specific antiviral therapy for influenza.

- Prevention involves good hand hygiene and standard precautions in social and health care settings for most viruses, as well as immunization against influenza viruses.

Overview

Viral respiratory tract infections are the most common cause of illness in all age groups (Table 35-1). Both upper respiratory tract infections (URTIs), occurring above the epiglottis, and lower respiratory tract infections (LRTIs), occurring below the epiglottis, may result from viral infections. Most viral causes of respiratory tract infections have a seasonality pattern, and many have typical clinical characteristics associated with disease. Most viral respiratory tract infections do not warrant extensive evaluation and require only supportive care in immunocompetent hosts. In preterm infants, young infants, and immuno-compromised patients, respiratory viruses can cause a more severe or pro-longed illness or lead to complications. Respiratory viral coinfections are common, and the contribution of multiple viruses to clinical disease is under study. This chapter discusses the most common viral causes of respiratory tract

Table 35-1. Summary of the Most Common Respiratory Viruses

Clinical Diseases	Viruses	Age Group	Treatment
Common cold	Rhinovirus and HCoV	All	Supportive care, nasal irrigation, or vapor rub
Croup	PIV-1 and -2, RSV, and HCoV	All	Corticosteroids or nebulized epinephrine
Laryngitis and bronchitis	PIV-1, -2, and -3; RSV; rhinovirus; adenovirus; and HMPV	Adolescents and adults	Supportive care but no antibiotics for initial presentation (Consider in symptoms >1 wk or worse.)
Bronchiolitis	RSV, HMPV, and PIV-3	<24 mo	Supportive care; oxygen (CPAP with heliox); epinephrine + oral dexamethasone; or ribavirin for immunocompromised hosts
Pneumonia	RSV, HMPV, PIV-3, adenovirus, and rhinovirus	All	Supportive care for healthy school-aged children

Abbreviations: CPAP, continuous positive airway pressure; HCoV, human coronavirus; HMPV, *Human metapneumovirus;* PIV, parainfluenza virus; RSV, respiratory syncytial virus.

infections, including respiratory syncytial virus (RSV), parainfluenza virus (PIV), *Human metapneumovirus* (HMPV), rhinovirus, human coronavirus (HCoV), adenovirus, and human bocavirus (HBoV).

Causes and Differential Diagnosis

Most respiratory viruses typically cause upper respiratory tract symptoms associated with the common cold with annual epidemics starting in the fall and ending in the spring in temperate climates. Other viruses, such as PIV, rhinovirus, or HBoV, are endemic and cause disease year-round.

Rhinovirus is the worldwide leading cause of the common cold. Annual epidemics generally start in August or September and end in April or May in temperate climates but may occur year-round. The average incidence of the common cold in preschool-aged children is 5 to 7 per year, but 10% to 15% will have at least 12 infections per year, with children in day care settings being most commonly affected. There are 3 species of rhinovirus with well over 100 serotypes, and they are transmitted through small-particle aerosols (coughing followed by inhalation), large-particle aerosols (saliva expelled during sneezing), and direct contact (self-inoculation after contact with an infected object or person). Direct contact with secretions is the most effective mode of transmission. For infection to occur, the virus has to make direct contact with the nasal mucosa or conjunctiva. Rhinovirus is the most common virus detected in children with respiratory illness and frequently exacerbates asthma.

Human coronavirus is associated with the common cold (second to rhinovirus) and occasionally with acute otitis media and asthma exacerbation. Four types of coronavirus have been identified in humans: HCoV-229E, -OC43, -NL63 and -HKU1. Human coronavirus NL63 is more frequently associated with laryngotracheobronchitis (croup) and pneumonia in infants and immunocompromised hosts compared with the other types. SARS- and MERS-associated coronaviruses are thought to originate in animals and spread to humans as an incidental host; these viruses cause more severe symptoms than the other coronaviruses and tend to affect adults more than children. Modes of transmission have not been well defined.

Parainfluenza virus is the major cause of laryngotracheobronchitis. It also causes half of the cases of laryngitis and may be associated with as many as a third of the cases of LRTIs. There are 4 PIV types. Type 3 is endemic, causing year-round disease with a peak in the fall through spring, and is associated with bronchiolitis that affects mostly young children between 6 months and 3 years of age. Types 1 and 2 occur mostly in older children and have an epidemic peak every other year in the fall in temperate climates; PIV-1 is most commonly associated with croup. Type 4 has not been as well characterized yet but commonly presents as URTI. Transmission occurs via contamination of hands with secretions containing the virus followed by autoinoculation. Predisposing factors to severe disease with PIV include malnutrition, overcrowding, vitamin A deficiency, lack of breastfeeding, and environmental smoke and toxin exposure.

Human metapneumovirus is an important cause of respiratory disease worldwide and can cause both URTIs and LRTIs. First identified in 2001, 2 subgroups (A and B) have been identified. In temperate climates, HMPV causes disease in the winter and early spring, frequently overlapping with RSV and influenza season. Children presenting with HMPV have similar clinical characteristics to those with RSV. Primary infections occur in 90% to 100% of children by age 5 to 10 years. Children between 6 and 12 months of age are at greatest risk for hospitalizations and LRTI.

Respiratory syncytial virus is the most important respiratory virus in young children, and the leading cause of severe LRTI requiring hospitalization in children younger than 1 year. Severe disease is noted particularly in babies younger than 6 months, those with cyanotic heart or underlying pulmonary disease, and premature infants. Other risk factors for severe disease include underlying neurologic disabilities and immunodeficiencies. Respiratory syncytial virus disease occurs in annual epidemics during the winter and spring in temperate climates. Transmission is through direct or close contact to large-particle droplets or fomites from infected individuals.

Adenovirus is associated with both URTIs and LRTIs, keratoconjunctivitis, pharyngoconjunctival fever, and gastrointestinal tract disease. Disseminated disease may occur in the very young or in immunocompromised hosts. Outbreaks may occur in crowded situations, and institutional epidemics have followed (eg, through the use of contaminated ophthalmic instruments). Transmission of respiratory disease occurs through inhalation of aerosolized droplets, direct person-to-person contact, and contact with fomites.

Human bocavirus was recently discovered in secretions of symptomatic young children. This virus is mainly detected in young children, and symptoms may be more pronounced the first time a child has the virus detected. It has been associated with fever, URTIs, and LRTIs, but has not always been linked to disease when found in respiratory secretions and has not been linked to disease in immunocompromised or high-risk hosts. More commonly, HBoV is found in the presence of other pathogens, such as rhinovirus, adenovirus, and RSV, as well as bacterial pathogens, like *Streptococcus* species and *Mycoplasma pneumoniae.*

Depending on the clinical presentation, a variety of other viral, bacterial, or noninfectious (eg, foreign body, airway anatomic anomaly) should be considered. For children with common cold symptoms, differentiation between rhinovirus and the other viruses described is often difficult. Influenza viral infection should be considered in children with rhinorrhea, sore throat, and cough, usually with higher fever and more systemic symptoms (eg, malaise, myalgia) than with other respiratory viruses. It is important to consider influenza particularly during the influenza season, as antiviral treatment may be warranted early in the course and bacterial pneumonia may follow after several days. Kawasaki disease may be considered in the differential of children with adenoviral infection who present with fever, conjunctivitis, and rash. The differential diagnosis of croup caused by PIV includes bacterial tracheitis, foreign body, and airway anomaly (ie, hemangiomas, laryngeal papillomas). Asthma exacerbation may occur related to viral respiratory tract infection; rhinovirus, RSV, and HMPV are common pathogens associated with these exacerbations.

Clinical Features

Rhinovirus and HCoV; the Common Cold

Symptoms commonly include nasal congestion, nasal discharge (rhinorrhea), cough, sore throat, or scratchy throat. Objective findings include a low-grade fever in children during the first 2 to 3 days of illness, an enlargement of the cervical lymph nodes, and erythema of the nasal mucosa and oropharynx. Typical illness lasts 5 to 7 days, but can be as long as 12 to 14 days in children; viral shedding can persist long after symptoms have resolved. In preterm infants and children with underlying medical conditions, such as chronic pulmonary or neurologic disease, these viruses can cause severe disease.

Parainfluenza Virus, HCoV, and HMPV; Croup

The clinical manifestations of croup include fever, hoarseness, barking cough, laryngeal obstruction, and inspiratory stridor. Most patients will also have a low-grade fever. Disease can last 3 to 5 days in mild cases or progress rapidly and become fatal in certain instances.

Parainfluenza Virus, RSV, Rhinovirus, Adenovirus, and HMPV; Laryngitis and Bronchitis

These are primarily diseases of adolescents and adults. The clinical features of laryngitis are a change in pitch of the voice with hoarseness. Bronchitis is characterized by symptoms of URTIs lasting a few days and followed by a second phase of persistent cough, sputum production, or wheezing that can last 1 to 3 weeks.

Respiratory Syncytial Virus, HMPV, and PIV; Bronchiolitis

Bronchiolitis is a disease of babies and children younger than 2 years. It usually presents with 1 to 3 days of preceding URTI symptoms (nasal congestion, rhinorrhea, and cough) followed by fever, cough, and mild respiratory distress (increased respiratory rate and mild retractions). Respiratory syncytial virus is the most common virus associated with bronchiolitis. On examination, affected children have tachypnea, intercostal and subcostal retractions, expiratory wheezing, and a chest with hyperexpansion. They may have rales and a prolonged expiratory phase. Other findings include conjunctivitis, pharyngitis, and acute otitis media. It can lead to respiratory failure with hypoxemia or progressive hypercapnia. The highest morbidity is in healthy babies younger than 2 months, premature infants, and infants with chronic lung or congenital heart disease. The typical course of illness in an otherwise healthy child is 2 to 5 days, but the infection can last up to 3 weeks in severely affected children.

Respiratory Syncytial Virus, PIV, Adenovirus, Rhinovirus, and HMPV; Pneumonia

Signs and symptoms of viral pneumonia can be subtle. The patient is usually 1 to 3 years of age and has a gradual onset with upper respiratory tract symptoms initially followed by irritability, respiratory congestion, cough, post-tussive vomiting, and fever. Patients are not toxic appearing, although they can be hypoxemic. Neonates and young infants can present with difficulty feeding and fussiness. On lung examination, they can have rales, decreased breath sounds, egophony, bronchophony, tactile fremitus, and dullness to percussion. Wheezing is more likely in the setting of viral pneumonia.

Evaluation

Evaluation starts with determining acuity of the illness. Most children older than 2 years presenting with URTI do not require hospitalization. Children younger than 2, especially those younger than 6 months, are at the greatest risk for severe disease, and further evaluation may be warranted.

Initial evaluation includes history of illness, pertinent medical history, exposure history, and clinical signs and symptoms. Children presenting with upper respiratory tract symptoms generally do not require further evaluation unless symptoms persist or worsen.

Rapid detection of RSV by enzyme immunoassay (EIA) is sensitive and specific in younger children. Recent molecular development using nucleic acid amplification provides for the rapid detection of respiratory viruses, using nasopharyngeal specimen. New rapid multiplex polymerase chain reaction tests have been developed for the rapid detection of multiple respiratory viruses. These tests have been shown to be superior to conventional diagnostic methods in detecting a broad range of respiratory viral agents in children and identifying children who are infected with more than one virus. Older methods of detection consist of cell culture and direct fluorescent assay (DFA), methods that are less sensitive but still a reliable indicator of disease.

Management

Management of viral respiratory tract infections depends on severity of illness and immune status of the patient. Most immunocompetent children recover from their illness with minimal supportive care.

The Common Cold

There are no effective treatments for the common cold. Over-the-counter medications, including antihistamines, antitussives, expectorants, and decongestants, though readily available, have not proven beneficial in children. Cold and cough over-the-counter medications are among the top 10 substances leading to death in children younger than 5 years and therefore not recommended. Echinacea, a common herbal therapy for treatment of the common cold, is also not effective in children. Products that may improve symptoms in children include nasal irrigation, vapor rub, and zinc sulfate (Evidence Level I). Limited data support the use of herbal remedies, including *Pelargonium sidoides* (ie, geranium) extract and buckwheat honey, for treatment of cough. Hand hygiene is the most effective preventive measure.

Croup

Humidified air and mist are used for the treatment of croup; however, no randomized control trials have shown their benefit over room air (Evidence

Level I). Corticosteroids are routinely indicated for the treatment of croup. Dexamethasone and budesonide have been proven effective in relieving the symptoms of croup as early as 6 hours after treatment in randomized control trials (Evidence Level I). Nebulized epinephrine is associated with clinically and statistically significant reduction in symptoms of croup in moderate to severe cases 30 minutes after treatment (Evidence Level I). No evidence favors racemic epinephrine, racemic L-epinephrine, and nebulized epinephrine delivered by intermittent positive pressure breathing over simple nebulized epinephrine.

Laryngitis and Bronchitis

Antibiotic treatment for acute laryngitis or bronchitis is not beneficial (Evidence Level I). Inhaled bronchodilators and mucolytic agents are also discouraged. Supportive care is the mainstay of treatment.

Bronchiolitis

Most children with bronchiolitis can be treated at home with supportive care. Hypoxia, apnea, respiratory distress, and feeding difficulties are indications for admission and further interventions. Supportive care includes assisted feeding, minimal handling, gentle nasal suctioning, and oxygen administration. The use of mist inhalation via a vaporizer or tent has not been proven beneficial over room air. Oxygen administration is beneficial in respiratory distress and hypoxia. The use of continuous positive airway pressure (CPAP) either alone or with heliox showed no conclusive evidence that CPAP reduced the need for intubation or that its use with heliox was effective, because of poor methodology in the studies. However, these studies showed that the use of CPAP led to a decrease in PCO_2. Continuous positive airway pressure use can clinically reduce the need for mechanical ventilation (Evidence Level I). Heliox therapy in severe bronchiolitis reduces respiratory distress in the first hour of treatment but has no effect on the need for intubation or mechanical ventilation or on the length of stay (Evidence Level I). Bronchodilators in the form of β_2-agonists, anticholinergic agents (ipratropium bromide), and adrenergic agents (epinephrine) have shown short-term modest improvement in symptomatology (Evidence Level I). Epinephrine showed the greatest benefit, reducing the risk of admission within the first 24 hours when compared to placebo. None of the bronchodilators have an effect on length of hospital stay. Corticosteroids, whether inhaled or systemic, do not reduce the duration of hospitalization or severity of symptoms (Evidence Level I). The combination of nebulized epinephrine and oral dexamethasone has been shown to reduce the rate of hospitalization by 9% when compared to either treatment alone or placebo, but results are based on a single study (Evidence Level I). Ribavirin, a synthetic guanosine nucleoside analogue, inhibits RSV replication. Randomized control trials show conflicting results in its efficacy. It is not generally recommended for the treatment of RSV bronchiolitis in immunocompetent patients. It may be more effective in severely immunocompromised patients, including those with bone marrow or solid organ transplants. Prevention strategies for bronchiolitis include minimizing passive smoking exposure and limiting nosocomial transmission. Monthly administration of monoclonal anti-F antibody (palivizumab) through RSV season reduces the risk of hospitalization in infants with bronchopulmonary dysplasia, congenital heart disease, and prematurity.

Pneumonia

Antibiotics are not useful in healthy school-aged children with symptoms consistent with viral pneumonia, and they may lead to the development of antibiotic resistance.

Long-term Monitoring and Implications

Rhinovirus and adenovirus produce long-lasting immunity after infection; however, given the numerous serotypes, infections frequently recur. Bronchiolitis in infancy is associated with an increased risk of asthma in later childhood that wanes towards adolescence.

Suggested Reading

Bont L, Aalderen WM, Kimpen JL. Long-term consequences of respiratory syncytial virus (RSV) bronchiolitis. *Paediatr Respir Rev.* 2000;1(3):221–227

Gharabaghi F, Hawan A, Drews SJ, Richardson SE. Evaluation of multiple commercial molecular and conventional diagnostic assays for the detection of respiratory viruses in children. *Clin Microbiol Infect.* 2011;17(12):1900–1906

Henrickson KJ. Parainfluenza viruses. *Clin Microbiol Rev.* 2003;16(2):242–264

Jacobs SE, Lamson DM, St George K, Walsh TJ. Human rhinoviruses. *Clin Microbiol Rev.* 2013;26(1):135–162

Jartti T, Jartti L, Ruuskanen O, Söderlund-Venermo M. New respiratory viral infections. *Curr Opin Pulm Med.* 2012;18(3):271–278

Kroll JL, Weinberg A. *Human metapneumovirus. Semin Respir Crit Care Med.* 2011;32(4):447–453

Long SS, Prober CG, Pickering LK, eds. *Principles and Practice of Pediatric Infectious Diseases.* 4th ed. Philadelphia, PA: Saunders; 2012

Lynch JP III, Fishbein M, Echavarria M. Adenovirus. *Semin Respir Crit Care Med.* 2011;32(4):494–511

Nagakumar P, Doull I. Current therapy for bronchiolitis. *Arch Dis Child.* 2012;97(9): 827–830

CHAPTER 36

Rotavirus

Penelope H. Dennehy, MD

Key Points

- Studies of children with rotaviral infection have shown a spectrum of disease, ranging from asymptomatic shedding to severe dehydration, seizures, and even death. Typical symptoms are nonspecific and include vomiting, non-bloody diarrhea, and fever.

- Enzyme-linked immunosorbent assays and latex agglutination tests are the most widely used methods for detection of rotaviruses.

- The mainstay of supportive therapy is assessment of volume status and administration of oral rehydration salts. Refeeding an age-appropriate diet can begin once fluid deficits are corrected.

- Preventive measures for rotavirus gastroenteritis in children, other than vaccination, rely on hand hygiene and cleaning of potentially contaminated surfaces.

- Two rotavirus vaccines are licensed for use in infants in the United States and safe and effective in preventing moderate to severe rotaviral disease in children. These vaccines have reduced the burden of rotaviral disease in the United States.

Overview

In the United States, viruses are the most common pathogens causing acute gastroenteritis in children of all age groups. Prior to the introduction of rotavirus vaccine in 2006, rotaviruses were the most frequently observed pathogens in acute gastroenteritis, but these infections have decreased significantly since vaccination was universally recommended.

Causes

Rotaviruses were among the first viral agents to be identified as important causes of viral gastroenteritis.

Human rotaviruses are part of a large family of viruses causing neonatal diarrhea in a variety of domestic animals and birds. Group A rotaviruses are the most important cause of severe acute gastroenteritis in infants and young children worldwide.

Clinical Features

The incubation period for rotavirus diarrhea is short, usually less than 48 hours.

The clinical manifestations of infection vary and depend on whether it is the first infection or reinfection. Rotavirus predominantly infects children, but infection also occurs in adults. Immunosuppressed hosts, including children, appear to develop a more severe and protracted infection.

Studies of children with rotaviral infection have shown a spectrum of disease, ranging from asymptomatic shedding to severe dehydration, seizures, and even death. Typical symptoms are nonspecific and include vomiting, non-bloody diarrhea, and fever. Rotavirus gastroenteritis usually begins with acute onset of fever and vomiting followed 24 to 48 hours later by watery diarrhea. On average there are up to 10 to 20 bowel movements per day. Symptoms generally persist for 3 to 8 days, although protracted episodes have been noted on occasion. Fever is usually low-grade and occurs in up to half of all infected children. Some children may have high fevers. Rotaviral infection with fever may trigger seizures in children with a propensity for febrile seizures. Vomiting is non-bilious and occurs in 80% to 90% of infected children. Vomiting is usually brief, lasting 24 hours or less in most children. Dehydration and electrolyte disturbances are the major sequelae of rotaviral infection and occur most often in the youngest children. Respiratory symptoms may be seen in 30% to 50% of children with rotavirus gastroenteritis. However, ill children are frequently simultaneously infected with both respiratory and gastrointestinal viruses, making interpretation of these findings more difficult.

Although infection can occur at any age, rotavirus most commonly causes clinically significant disease in young infants and children. Dehydrating rotavirus gastroenteritis primarily occurs among infants and children aged 3 to 24 months. Babies younger than 3 months have relatively low rates of rotaviral infection, probably because of passive maternal antibody, and possibly breastfeeding.

Most children are infected with rotavirus more than once. First infections are more likely to result in severe gastroenteritis than subsequent infections. Protective immunity develops after rotaviral infection and is strongest against moderate to severe disease. Subsequent infections are usually milder or may even be asymptomatic. Adults usually have asymptomatic or mild disease because of immunity from previous exposure.

Most mothers have rotavirus antibody from previous infection that is passed transplacentally, protecting the neonate. As a result, most infected neonates will have asymptomatic or mild disease. An exception is the preterm infant, who is at greater risk of severe illness than the term infant because of the lack of transplacental maternal antibodies. Exposure of neonates (asymptomatically) to rotavirus is associated with a reduced likelihood of their developing severe rotavirus diarrhea later in infancy.

Severe and prolonged rotavirus gastroenteritis has been reported in children with immunodeficiency, particularly those with T-cell immunodeficiencies or severe combined immunodeficiency (SCID), and after bone marrow transplantation. In these cases, rotavirus may be associated with severe disease and may be fatal, and extraintestinal replication has been reported. Rotaviral infection of children after solid organ transplantation is usually self-limited but more severe than in healthy children. Rotavirus does not seem to be a common cause of severe or persistent diarrhea in individuals with HIV infection.

Rotavirus gastroenteritis has occurred in association with multiple other clinical syndromes, which may be etiologically associated with rotavirus. These clinical syndromes include gastrointestinal or central nervous system complications.

The gastrointestinal syndromes that may be associated with rotavirus include necrotizing enterocolitis, intussusception, biliary atresia, and prolonged diarrhea. Necrotizing enterocolitis has been associated with nosocomial rotaviral infections in neonates. Intussusception was reported in association with rotavirus gastroenteritis shortly after recognition of this virus. However, subsequent studies have never established a definitive etiologic link with natural rotaviral infection. Biliary atresia has also been reported in association with rotaviral infection. Although most children recover from rotavirus gastroenteritis completely, some children continue to have protracted diarrhea. Carbohydrate or lactase intolerance may persist after resolution of diarrhea. Epidemiologic studies have suggested that rotaviral infection does not increase the risk for subsequent persistent diarrhea in childhood.

Rotavirus gastroenteritis may be associated with central nervous system complications, particularly seizures and encephalopathy. Rotavirus has been detected by polymerase chain reaction in cerebrospinal fluid in some cases. However, it is unclear whether detection of rotavirus represents actual replication in the central nervous system, contamination at the time of lumbar puncture, or carriage of rotavirus RNA in cerebrospinal fluid lymphocytes.

Evaluation

Laboratory studies in symptomatic children are generally unremarkable. Dehydration with elevations in the serum urea nitrogen and hyperchloremic metabolic acidosis is a common finding. Hypocalcemia has also been reported. Peripheral blood white blood cell counts are usually normal in uncomplicated cases. Mild elevations in the serum aspartate transaminase concentration have been reported during acute illness without other evidence of hepatic injury, and these elevations may reflect damage to intestinal epithelial cells.

Diarrheal stools are described as watery or yellow without mucus or blood. Minimal to moderate numbers of stool white blood cells are seen in approximately one-third of samples.

Direct immune-based assays of stool and polymerase chain reaction techniques have been most frequently employed to make the diagnosis of a rotaviral infection. Because of ease of their performance, enzyme immunoassays and latex agglutination assays are the most widely used methods for detection of rotavirus antigen in stool in clinical settings. Choice of assay generally depends on the format and ease of use for a particular clinical laboratory.

Management

No antiviral is currently available to treat rotaviral infection. Orally administered human immune globulin, administered as an investigational therapy in immunocompromised patients with prolonged infection, has decreased viral shedding and shortened the duration of diarrhea.

The current mainstay of treatment of acute rotavirus gastroenteritis consists of oral rehydration therapy (ORT) and early introduction of feedings. Adequate fluid and electrolyte replacement and maintenance are the key to managing rotavirus gastroenteritis. Oral rehydration therapy is the preferred method unless the child has intractable vomiting, which would require intravenous (IV) rehydration (Evidence Level I). Hydration status in children can be assessed on the basis of easily observed signs and symptoms. Children who are not thirsty and have moist mucous membranes, wet diapers, and tears are not dehydrated and do not require oral rehydration salts (ORS). In the absence of dehydration, ORS should be used to replace ongoing stool losses only in severe cases in which the patient has already required rehydration and still has ongoing diarrhea.

Children who are mildly or moderately dehydrated should receive 50 to 100 mL/kg of ORS over 4 hours and should be reevaluated often for changes in hydration status. Children who are vomiting generally tolerate ORS. Oral rehydration salts are contraindicated in the child who is obtunded or at risk for aspiration. When ORT is complete, regular feeding should be resumed.

Hypotension is a late manifestation of shock in children. Mental status, heart rate, and perfusion are better indicators of severe dehydration and incipient shock. After initial treatment with IV fluids, these children can be given ORT.

Early refeeding is recommended in managing acute rotavirus gastroenteritis because oral feedings help facilitate mucosal repair following rotaviral infection (Evidence Level I). Introducing a regular diet within a few hours of rehydration or continuing the diet during diarrhea without dehydration has been shown to shorten duration of the disease. Early refeeding has not been associated with increased morbidity, such as electrolyte disturbances or a need for IV fluids.

Although ORS treat dehydration, they are not effective in shortening the duration of rotavirus-induced diarrhea. A growing body of literature is establishing the effectiveness of selected probiotics as an adjunct to rehydration therapy. In developed countries, *Lactobacillus* GG given in a daily dose of 10 billion colony-forming U/day has proven efficacy in rotavirus gastroenteritis to reduce the duration of diarrhea, risk of protracted diarrhea, and duration of hospitalization (Evidence Level I). The duration of diarrhea may be reduced as much as 1 to 2 days with the use of probiotics.

Nitazoxanide is a thiazolide antimicrobial with activity against anaerobic bacteria, protozoa, and viruses. Three randomized double-blind clinical trials have demonstrated effectiveness of nitazoxanide in treating rotavirus gastroenteritis in young children with significant reductions in time to resolution of symptoms. More data on nitazoxanide are needed before it can be considered for routine use (Evidence Level III).

Antidiarrheals are generally not recommended for treatment of rotavirus gastroenteritis. Over-the-counter medicines such as loperamide and bismuth subsalicylate can help relieve gastroenteritis symptoms in adults but are not recommended for children (Evidence Level I).

Antiemetics should not be routinely used in the treatment of children with acute rotavirus gastroenteritis (Evidence Level I). Although ondansetron use may decrease vomiting during the first hours after presentation, the need for IV fluids in the emergency department, and hospitalization rates in those patients who require IV fluids, its use may increase diarrheal episodes. In addition, most studies of ondansetron in children with acute gastroenteritis have been performed only on mildly dehydrated children. Of greatest concern is that the use of ondansetron may increase risk of developing prolongation of the QT interval (see www.fda.gov/Safety/MedWatch/SafetyInformation/SafetyAlertsforHuman-MedicalProducts/ucm272041.htm). Patients at risk for adverse effects include those with underlying heart conditions, such as congenital long QT syndrome; those who are predisposed to low levels of potassium and magnesium in the blood; and those taking other medications that lead to QT prolongation.

Prevention

The single most important procedure to minimize transmission of rotavirus is frequent hand-hygiene measures. Rotavirus can rapidly contaminate environmental surfaces because of the large number of viruses shed in an infected child's stool. Rotavirus is very stable and may remain viable in the environment for weeks or months if not disinfected. Hands may be contaminated from environmental surfaces, further facilitating spread of infection. Skin disinfectants such as chlorhexidine are ineffective against rotavirus. Studies have shown that hand washing with soap and water removes only 75% of virus from the hands. Agents containing alcohol are the most effective against rotavirus. To control the spread of rotavirus, hands should be cleaned of visible stool with soap and water and then an alcohol-containing hand rub should be used. Since general disinfectants such as bleach are ineffective against rotavirus, potentially contaminated surfaces, such as changing tables, should be cleaned of all visible stool and then disinfected with 95% ethanol or other alcohol-containing disinfectant. Although hand hygiene and cleaning of potentially contaminated surfaces are important control measures, vaccination is the only measure likely to have a significant effect on the incidence of severe dehydrating rotaviral disease.

In general, breastfeeding is associated with milder rotaviral disease and should be encouraged.

Two oral rotavirus vaccines, a monovalent attenuated human rotavirus vaccine (RV1, Rotarix, GlaxoSmithKline Biologicals, Rixensart, Belgium) and a pentavalent bovine–human reassortant vaccine (RV5, RotaTeq, Merck and Company), are available and recommended for routine immunization of all infants in the United States by the Centers for Disease Control and Prevention, American Academy of Pediatrics, and American Academy of Family Physicians. The licensed rotavirus vaccines have undergone large trials of safety and efficacy. In prelicensure studies, the rates of serious adverse effects and intussusception were the same among vaccine and placebo recipients.

Unlike efficacy studies conducted in a carefully controlled setting, studies on vaccine effectiveness compare the risks of disease outcomes in vaccinated or unvaccinated populations in a real-life setting. A complete series of RV5 showed effectiveness ranging from 78% to 100% in preventing severe rotaviral disease (hospitalizations or emergency department visits) and 96% in preventing outpatient visits.

In the United States, rotavirus vaccination significantly reduced the burden of rotavirus-related hospitalizations, ranging from 60% to 93% depending on vaccine coverage, age group, and rotavirus season studied. Reductions in all-cause gastroenteritis or diarrhea-related hospitalizations, emergency visits, and outpatient/physician office visits were also seen.

Current rotavirus vaccines were not associated with intussusception in large prelicensure trials. Although an increased risk of intussusception from rotavirus vaccine has not been documented in the United States, data currently available cannot exclude a risk as low as that detected in other locations. The benefits of rotavirus immunization include prevention of hospitalization for severe rotaviral disease in the United States and death in other parts of the world. Currently, benefits of these vaccines, which are known, far outweigh the rare potential risks.

Following are recommendations for use of rotavirus vaccines:
- Infants in the United States should routinely be immunized. Three doses of RV5 administered orally at 2, 4, and 6 months of age or 2 doses of RV1 administered orally at 2 and 4 months of age (Evidence Level I).

- Initiate the first dose of rotavirus vaccine from 6 through 14 weeks, 6 days, of age (the maximum age for the first dose is 14 weeks, 6 days).
  o Immunization should not be initiated for infants older than 15 weeks (Evidence Level III).
  o The minimum interval between doses of rotavirus vaccine is 4 weeks (RV5, Evidence Level I; RV1, Evidence Level III).
  o All doses of rotavirus vaccine should be complete by 8 months, 0 days, of age (RV5, Evidence Level I; RV1, Evidence Level III).
- Regarding interchangeability of products: Complete with the same product whenever possible.
  o Do not defer immunization if the product used for previous doses is unavailable or unknown; continue or complete the series with the product available (Evidence Level III).
  o If any dose in the series was RV5 or the product is unknown for any dose in the series, give a total of 3 doses of rotavirus vaccine (Evidence Level III).
- Concurrent administration of rotavirus vaccine with other appropriate-for-age childhood vaccines is recommended (Evidence Level I).
- The vaccine should not be deferred in infants with transient, mild illness with or without low-grade fever (Evidence Level III).
- Preterm infants may be immunized assuming the infant is at least 6 weeks of postnatal age and clinically stable.
  o Use the same schedule and with the same precautions as recommended for term infants (Evidence Level I).
  o The first dose of vaccine may be given at the time of discharge or after the infant has been discharged from the nursery (Evidence Level III).
- Infants living in households with immunocompromised people can and should be immunized. Infants living in households with pregnant women should also be immunized.
- Do not administer rotavirus vaccine to infants who have a history of a severe hypersensitivity reaction (eg, anaphylaxis) after a previous dose of rotavirus vaccine or to a vaccine component.
  o Do not administer RV1 to infants with a severe (eg, anaphylactic) latex allergy because the rubber oral applicator contained in the RV1 contains latex (Evidence Level III).
  o The RV5 dosing tube is latex-free.
- Absolute contraindications to both rotavirus vaccines include SCID and prior history of intussusception (Evidence Level III).
  o Severe diarrhea and prolonged shedding of vaccine virus are reported in infants who were administered live, oral rotavirus vaccines and later identified as having SCID.

- Precautions for administration of rotavirus vaccine include other immuno-deficiencies (SCID is a contraindication); moderate to severe illness, including gastroenteritis; preexisting chronic intestinal tract disease; and spina bifida or bladder extrophy (Evidence Level III).
- Rotavirus vaccine may be administered at any time before, concurrent with, or after administration of any blood product, including antibody-containing blood products (Evidence Level III).
- Breastfeeding infants should be immunized according to the same schedule as non-breastfed infants (Evidence Level I).
- Do not repeat the dose if an infant regurgitates, spits out, or vomits during or after vaccine administration (Evidence Level III).
- Use standard precautions for hospitalized infants who have been recently immunized with rotavirus vaccine (Evidence Level III).
- In infants who have had rotavirus gastroenteritis, it is still recommended that one initiate or complete the schedule following the standard age and interval recommendations (Evidence Level III).

Suggested Reading

American Academy of Pediatrics Committee on Infectious Diseases. Prevention of rotavirus disease: updated guidelines for use of rotavirus vaccine. *Pediatrics.* 2009;123(5):1412–1420

Cortese MM, Parashar UD; Centers for Disease Control and Prevention. Prevention of rotavirus gastroenteritis among infants and children. Recommendations of the Advisory Committee on Immunization Practices (ACIP). *MMWR Recomm Rep.* 2009;58(RR-2):1–25

Dennehy PH. Effects of vaccine on rotavirus disease in the pediatric population. *Curr Opin Pediatr.* 2012;24(1):78–84

Dennehy PH. Rotavirus infection: an update on management and prevention. *Adv Pediatr.* 2012;59(1):48–74

Guarino A, Albano F, Ashkenazi S, et al. European Society for Paediatric Gastroenterology, Hepatology, and Nutrition/European Society for Paediatric Infectious Diseases evidence-based guidelines for the management of acute gastroenteritis in children in Europe. *J Pediatr Gastroenterol Nutr.* 2008;46(Suppl 2):S81–S122

King CK, Glass R, Bresee JS, Duggan C. Managing acute gastroenteritis among children: oral rehydration, maintenance, and nutritional therapy. *MMWR Recomm Rep.* 2003;52(RR-16):1–16

CHAPTER 37

Varicella-Zoster Virus

Anne A. Gershon, MD

Key Points

- A pruritic vesicular rash characterizes classic varicella; severe complications are most common in the very young, adolescent-adults, and immunocompromised patients.

- Reactivation of varicella (ie, shingles) is characterized by a dermatomal-grouped painful or pruritic vesicular rash, although on occasion rash can be absent.

- Rarely, fetal embryopathy may follow maternal varicella that occurs during the first or second trimester.

- Direct fluorescence assay, culture, or polymerase chain reaction testing (most sensitive) of skin lesions or saliva can be used for laboratory diagnosis; genotyping can discriminate between wild-type and vaccine virus.

- Acyclovir, valacyclovir, or famciclovir are the drugs of choice and recommended for those with high-risk conditions, including immunocompromised hosts or patients with chronic cutaneous or pulmonary disease; those receiving aspirin; and those older than 12 years. Foscarnet is used for those with acyclovir-resistant infection.

- The US vaccination program has been highly successful in reducing the morbidity and mortality of varicella in the United States.

Overview

Varicella, the primary infection with varicella-zoster virus (VZV), is most often a mild to moderate pruritic, febrile rash illness in otherwise healthy children, but may be severe or even fatal in immunocompromised patients. Varicella also tends to be more serious with increased frequency of complications in infants and adults. A rare congenital varicella syndrome consisting in part of central nervous system (CNS) damage with limb hypoplasia, cutaneous scarring, and eye abnormalities occurs in offspring of approximately 2% of pregnant women with varicella in the first or second trimester.

Varicella-zoster virus causes latent infection in the following nerve ganglia: dorsal root, cranial nerve, and autonomic, including enteric. Reactivation may therefore produce signs/symptoms in skin (mainly seen on trunk and face), the gastrointestinal tract, and the CNS. Gastrointestinal and CNS reactivations particularly may occur without skin lesions.

Causes and Differential Diagnosis

The causative agent of varicella and herpes zoster (ie, shingles) is VZV (ie, *Human herpesvirus 3*). The differential diagnosis includes a variety of infectious and noninfectious agents that result in a papulovesicular exanthema. These include, most commonly, enteroviruses such as coxsackieviruses implicated in hand-foot-and-mouth disease and herpes simplex virus infections. Scabies, particularly in infants, may result in vesicular lesions, and rickettsial pox may produce a papulovesicular eruption days after an eschar is noted at the site of the bite of a house mouse mite. Insect bites, drug reactions, and contact dermatitis represent noninfectious entities that may produce clinical confusion with chickenpox.

Clinical Manifestations

The clinical manifestations and potential complications of varicella and herpes zoster are found in Table 37-1 and Table 37-2.

Table 37-1. Clinical Manifestations of Varicella and Herpes Zoster

Patient	Manifestations
Varicella	
Healthy host	250–500 pruritic vesicles concentrated on head and trunk, with extremities relatively spared; fever; itching; anorexia; malaise (All last approximately 5 d and are often more severe in adults than children.)
	Differential diagnosis: disseminated HSV infection, impetigo, insect bites, drug rash, contact dermatitis, enteroviral infection, rickettsial pox
Immunocompromised	Often >500 vesicles, which may be hemorrhagic; fever >40°C (104°F); high incidence of complications (Fatalities are possible unless antiviral therapy is given.)
Herpes Zoster	
Healthy host	Unilateral band-like patch of somewhat confluent vesicles, rash pruritic or painful. (Both last approximately 1–2 wk. Rash on face, including around eye, if trigeminal involvement.)
	Neurologic and gastrointestinal forms also exist (see text).
	Differential diagnosis: recurrent HSV infection.
Immunocompromised	Rash more extensive and may be hemorrhagic or generalize beyond dermatomal area to bilateral sites, fever, pain

Abbreviation: HSV, herpes simplex virus.

Table 37-2. Complications of Varicella and Herpes Zoster

Patient	Manifestations
Varicella	
Healthy host	Bacterial skin infection, especially from group A *Streptococcus;* bacterial pneumonia (uncommonly); viral pneumonia (very rarely); CNS complications (cerebellar ataxia, encephalitis, stroke [rarely]); glomerulonephritis; arthritis; hepatitis (rarely)
Immunocompromised (including children on >2 mg/kg/d of prednisone)	Extensive skin rash with hemorrhage; primary viral pneumonia; bacterial pneumonia; encephalitis; hepatitis
Herpes Zoster	
Healthy host	Meningitis (uncommonly); PHN with often severe and persistent neuropathogenic pain, seen especially in elderly patients; GI ulcers; pseudo-obstruction
Immunocompromised	PHN, encephalitis, vasculitis/vasculopathy (including stroke, cerebral hemorrhage)

Abbreviations: CNS, central nervous system; GI, gastrointestinal; PHN, postherpetic neuralgia.

Evaluation

The single best laboratory test for rapid diagnosis of VZV infection is by identification of viral DNA by polymerase chain reaction (PCR). This may be performed on skin swabs or biopsies, vesicular fluid, cerebrospinal fluid if there are CNS symptoms, and saliva specimens or buccal swabs. Details of PCR and other tests such as direct fluorescence assay and culture are listed in Table 37-3. Varicella-zoster virus DNA may be typed by using PCR and restriction enzyme technology to differentiate between vaccine (ie, Oka) and wild-type viruses. This testing is useful for evaluating patients with herpes zoster months to years following vaccination. It is performed free of charge by 2 sources, the Centers for Disease Control and Prevention (CDC) (404/639-0066) and a joint safety project of Merck and Columbia University (800/672-6372).

Antibodies to VZV are usually measured using commercial enzyme-linked immunosorbent assays. However, these assays lack sensitivity to identify persons who have vaccine-induced immunity and may also yield false-positive values (Evidence Level III). High values, however, may indicate either recent active disease or vaccine-induced immunity. Patients who develop herpes zoster usually have detectable VZV antibodies before developing the illness.

Table 37-3. Laboratory Diagnosis of Varicella-Zoster Virus

Test	Specimen	Time to Results	Comments
PCR	Vesicular fluid, skin swab, CSF, biopsy, scab	2–3 d	Sensitive, commercially and academically available; can use to distinguish HSV from VZV and Oka from wild-type VZV (Evidence Level I)
DFA	Swab from base of vesicle (must include epithelial cells)	Several hours	Availability limited (Evidence Level III)
Viral culture	Vesicular fluid, biopsy	3–7 d	Insensitive since VZV is labile, limited availability, very rare to isolate VZV from CSF (Evidence Level III)
Serology	Acute and convalescent serum specimens	2–3 weeks to obtain convalescent sera (Ideally, paired sera should be tested simultaneously)	IgG tests: lack sensitivity to identify vaccinees who are immune; IgG and IgM tests: may yield false-positive results (Evidence Level III)

Abbreviations: CSF, cerebrospinal fluid; DFA, direct fluorescence assay; HSV, herpes simplex virus; PCR, polymerase chain reaction; VZV, varicella-zoster virus.

Management and Prevention

Children with clinical varicella should not be given salicylates because this predisposes to development of Reye syndrome (Evidence Level I). Chronic salicylate therapy should be suspended for approximately 3 weeks if children receiving it are closely exposed to VZV (Evidence Level III).

Useful antivirals are available to treat VZV infections (Table 37-4). At times treatment is potentially lifesaving; other times the aim is to provide faster healing and decrease the time of acute pain. There is no evidence that antiviral therapy decreases the incidence of postherpetic neuralgia. Varicella-zoster virus infections may be treated with acyclovir (ACV), valacyclovir, or famciclovir. The latter 2 drugs are given only orally, and are usually reserved for patients older than 2 years; they result in higher blood levels than oral ACV. Acyclovir is available for oral and intravenous administration, which is used for sicker patients. The earlier in the course of infection that ACV is administered, the more effective the medication. At some point (ie, about a week after onset), antivirals against VZV may be of little utility. Acyclovir may be particularly lifesaving for immunocompromised patients who develop the primary VZV infection, varicella. Oral ACV in persons who are immunocompetent provides less dramatic effects against varicella. Oral ACV is usually reserved for otherwise healthy patients who are at risk to develop moderate to severe varicella that is not thought to be life-threatening. These might include unvaccinated individuals who have chronic cutaneous or pulmonary illnesses, those receiving long-term aspirin therapy or short or low doses of steroids, or those who are

Table 37-4. Dosages of Antivirals for Varicella-Zoster Virus Infections

Drug	Indication	Age	Recommended Dosage
ACV, orally	Varicella or herpes zoster in immunocompetent host	Up to 12 y	80 mg/kg/d in 4 divided doses for 5 d; maximum dose: 3,200 mg/d (Evidence Level I)
ACV, IV (hospitalized patients)	Varicella or herpes zoster in immunocompetent or immunocompromised host	Any	30 mg/kg/d in 3 divided doses for 5–10 d (Evidence Level I)
Valacyclovir,[a] orally	Varicella or herpes zoster in immunocompetent or immunocompromised host	≥12 y	20 mg/kg 3 times/d for 5 d; >12 y: 1 g 3 times/d for 5–7 d (Evidence Level I)
Famciclovir,[b] orally	Herpes zoster in immunocompetent or immunocompromised host	≥12 y	500 mg 3 times/d for 7 d (Evidence Level I)
FOS	VZV infection, ACV resistant; usually in immunocompromised host	Adult dose	40 mg/kg 3 times/d for up to 3 wk (Evidence Level III)

Abbreviations: ACV, acyclovir; FOS, foscarnet; IV, intravenously; VZV, varicella-zoster virus.

Note: On the basis of limited clinical experience, chemoprophylaxis with ACV at described doses beginning 7–10 d after exposure for 1 wk may be used in exposed immunocompromised patients if passive immunization is unavailable. Valacyclovir may be used as an alternative at a dose of 20 mg/kg/dose 3 times/d (Evidence Level III).

[a] *Red Book* 2015 recommends valacyclovir for children >2 y for VZV.

[b] *Red Book* 2015 does not recommend famciclovir for children.

being successfully treated for HIV infection. Secondary household varicella patients may be treated since they are at risk to develop more extensive infections. It is more compelling to treat adults with varicella than otherwise healthy children with this disease. It is rare for a vaccinated individual who develops break-through varicella to require antiviral therapy. Most adults with herpes zoster should receive antiviral therapy to hasten healing; antiviral therapy for children with herpes zoster should be given if the child is judged to be particularly uncomfortable or to have an extensive skin rash.

Because pregnant women are at increased risk from severe varicella, they should be given ACV. If the infection is severe, they should receive IV ACV. Children with varicella being treated for cancer should receive either oral or IV ACV; if oral therapy is used, close observation for signs of hepatitis, pneumonia, or encephalopathy is mandatory. If these are suspected, IV treatment should be promptly given.

Isolation of Hospitalized Patients

In the vaccine era, with approximately 90% of children being immunized, patients with VZV infections are infrequent and hospitalizations are unusual. Nevertheless, at times nosocomial exposures still occur, particularly from herpes zoster cases. Varicella-zoster virus spreads mainly from skin lesions by the aerosol route, although viral respiratory tract spread may also occur.

Standard, airborne, and contact precautions are recommended for patients with VZV infections. Isolation should be maintained until all lesions have crusted, usually about 5 days for varicella and longer for patients with herpes zoster, especially if they are immunocompromised. Immunized patients with mild varicella are potentially contagious, especially if they have more than 50 skin lesions.

Nonimmune individuals who have been exposed to VZV should remain isolated between days 8 and 21 after exposure; if passive immunization was given, they should remain isolated for 28 days after exposure. Similarly, neonates whose mothers have active varicella should also be isolated.

Recommendations for Hospital Exposures

Because of the possibility of spread of VZV in hospitals where there may be unimmunized children or immunocompromised patients, conservative approaches towards spread should be taken (Box 37-1).

Box 37-1. Recommendations for Varicella-Zoster Virus in the Hospital Setting

- Identify clinicians, patients, and visitors who may be susceptible to varicella.
- Vaccinate those without contraindications.
- Passive immunization should be given to individuals who need it.
- Exposed patients who lack immunity should be discharged as soon as possible.
- Exposed patients who cannot be discharged should be isolated.
- Exposed clinicians who have had 2 doses of vaccine should be observed for development of rash and fever and placed on sick leave if thought to have developed break-through varicella. Individuals who have received only 1 dose should be given a second dose and treated similarly to those who received 2 doses.

Control Measures in Child Care and School

Children may return to child care or school following varicella after all lesions have crusted. Those without vesicles may return 24 hours after no new maculopapular lesions have developed.

Immunization

Passive immunization should be given to individuals at high risk to develop severe varicella. In the United States in the post-vaccine era, the need for passive immunization has declined significantly. Therefore, varicella-zoster immune globulin is no longer being produced in the United States; its substitute, VariZIG, can be obtained by calling FFF Enterprises in Canada, 800/843-7477 (open 24 hours) under an investigational new drug protocol. VariZIG is given intramuscularly; the dose is 62.5 U for children weighing 2 kg or less, 125 U for children weighing 2.1 kg to 10 kg, 250 U for children weighing 10.1 kg to 20 kg, 375 U for children weighing 20.1 kg to 30 kg, 500 U for children weighing 30.1 kg to 40 kg, and 625 U for all people weighing more than 40 kg.

Varicella is extremely contagious; herpes zoster is approximately half as infectious as varicella. Passive immunization should be given for the following types of exposure to VZV: household, face-to-face indoor play for approximately 5 to 60 minutes, hospitalized in same 2- to 4-person bedroom or adjacent beds in large ward, face-to-face contact with any person deemed contagious, neonate whose mother developed varicella (*not* herpes zoster) 5 days before or 2 days after delivery (Evidence Level III).

Candidates for passive immunization include varicella-susceptible patients from the following groups: immunocompromised children, pregnant women, neonates whose mothers have varicella, hospitalized preterm infant (of ≥28 wk' gestation) if the mother did not have varicella or vaccine, and babies younger than 28 weeks regardless of the mother's varicella immune status (Evidence Level III).

Intravenous immune globulin can also be used for passive immunization, at a dose of 400 mg/kg/dose. While originally recommended only if less than 5 days had elapsed since the exposure, the CDC has recently extended the interval to 10 days postexposure (Evidence Level III).

Active immunization with live attenuated varicella vaccine is the mainstay for control of chickenpox today. The vaccine is available in 2 formulations: monovalent and quadrivalent, which is combined with measles-mumps-rubella (MMR) vaccines. Infants are usually immunized at 1 year of age with monovalent varicella vaccine and MMR vaccine, simultaneously but at different subcutaneous injection sites (Evidence Level III). The second dose is preferably given as MMR vaccine, if available, usually at about 4 years of age (Evidence Level II-2). Measles-mumps-rubella vaccine is licensed only for children aged 1 to 12 years. After that age, monovalent varicella vaccine must be used. The shortest acceptable interval between doses of varicella vaccine, however, is 1 month. Vaccine efficacy after 1 dose is approximately 85%, which increases to 98% after the second dose. Break-through varicella in vaccinees is almost always mild (Evidence Level II-2).

The incidence of varicella and its complications has fallen dramatically in the past 15 years (Evidence Level II-3). Deaths from varicella in the United States have become rare, with an 88% decrease in deaths because of varicella with vaccine coverage.

Prior to implementation of the 2-dose schedule, there were frequent varicella outbreaks at child care facilities and schools. Since 2008 or so, these outbreaks appear to have stopped.

Vaccinated children develop specific antibodies to VZV that appear to be long-lasting, but these antibodies are difficult to demonstrate using commercially available enzyme-linked immunosorbent assays, which are insensitive and may yield false-positive results. The fluorescent antibody to membrane antigen test is sensitive and accurate but not generally available (Evidence Level III). Therefore, the best indication of immunity to varicella is either medical documentation of disease or proof of immunization with 2 doses of vaccine. Patients with herpes zoster can be presumed to be immune to varicella. There is little evidence of waning immunity after 1 dose (Evidence Level II-2); studies examining persistence of immunity after 2 doses are not yet available. Protection of unvaccinated children who are exposed to varicella is usually achieved by postexposure immunization. Ideally, this should be done within 1 to 2 days after exposure, but can be performed at any time after an exposure. Vaccinees who do not develop varicella after an exposure should receive a second vaccine dose at least 1 month after the first.

The presence of serum antibodies to VZV usually indicates immunity to varicella. It is common, however, for individuals who develop herpes zoster to be seropositive for VZV since it is the cell-mediated immune response that is impaired in these persons.

Although it is uncommon, it appears that administration of ACV does not interfere with development of the immune response to VZV in individuals who have recently been vaccinated against varicella. Despite this observation, however, exposure of recent vaccinees to ACV is usually to be avoided.

Varicella vaccine has proven to be extremely safe (Evidence Level III). Worldwide some 100 million children and adults have been immunized. The most commonly observed adverse effect is development of a mild vesicular rash (that may include the injection site) in about 5% of vaccinees, about 1 month after immunization. Transmission of Oka VZV to others from these skin lesions is exceptionally rare. There have been 18 published reports of proven serious adverse effects due to Oka VZV, such as widespread rash, hepatitis, pneumonia, and herpes zoster with meningitis, in the world literature in recently vaccinated children and adolescents. These patients have had known, suspected, or occult immunodeficiency diseases, and roughly 90% survived these complications by administration of antiviral therapy. The clinical courses of these children underscore the importance of avoiding varicella immunization of immunocompromised individuals. The aim should be to protect immunocompromised children from varicella by herd immunity, which has been observed in highly immunized populations. One exception to the warning not to immunize the immunocompromised are children with HIV infection. These children may be given monovalent varicella vaccine as long as they have greater than 15% circulating CD4 cells and no defining symptoms of AIDS (Evidence Level III). Usually such children will be receiving antiretroviral therapy that includes protease inhibitors. Vaccinating these children against varicella is highly protective against herpes zoster as well.

Other very rare complications, overwhelmingly attributed to Oka VZV by temporal association only, include anaphylaxis, ataxia, death, Guillain-Barré syndrome, encephalitis, erythema multiforme, meningitis, neuropathy, Stevens-Johnson syndrome, stroke, secondary bacterial infection, seizures, and thrombocytopenia. In some instances, the illness was actually shown to be caused by wild-type VZV and not the vaccine (Oka) strain. It is clear that complications related to varicella vaccination are infinitely fewer than those from natural disease.

Other contraindications to administration of live attenuated varicella vaccine, in addition to immunosuppression, include pregnancy, salicylates (as mentioned in the package insert), and allergy to vaccine components such as gelatin and neomycin (Evidence Level III).

Herpes zoster has been reported in some 100 or so vaccinees. Interestingly, about one-half of the cases in which genotyping has been carried out to identify the virus as vaccine type or wild type have been found to be caused by wild-type VZV. It is hypothesized that these children had subclinical infection with wild-type VZV either before or after vaccination. Studies from the CDC indicate that the incidence of herpes zoster is between 4 and 10 times lower after vaccination than natural infection in healthy children. In immunocompromised vaccinees (studied mostly in the 1980s), the incidence of herpes zoster was about 6 times lower in vaccinees compared to patients who had the wild-type infection. The incidence of herpes zoster in middle-aged adults who were vaccinated as young adults is also exceptionally low. All of these studies indicate that herpes zoster is less frequent after vaccination than natural infection, yet another advantage of vaccination against varicella.

While there have been discussions about whether the decrease in circulation of wild-type VZV will lead to an increase in the incidence of herpes zoster in young and middle-aged adults who were not immunized, this seems unlikely. It has been noted that the incidence of herpes zoster has been increasing in the American population for the past 50 years; undoubtedly, this phenomenon is multifactorial. Potential reasons include the aging of the population, increased numbers of ambulatory immunocompromised patients, increased ascertainment of herpes zoster, and increasing stress in the population. While studies have suggested that exposure to children (some of whom have varicella) protects against herpes zoster, others, studying isolated populations, have shown that such exposure is not required for protection. In addition, it is becoming clear that individuals may experience subclinical reactivation of VZV periodically, which boosts their immunity to VZV. Fear of increased herpes zoster in the population should not impede use of varicella vaccine.

Suggested Reading

Breuer J, Grose C, Norberg P, Tipples G, Schmid DS. A proposal for a common nomenclature for viral clades that form the species varicella-zoster virus: summary of VZV Nomenclature Meeting 2008, Barts and the London School of Medicine and Dentistry, 24-25 July 2008. *J Gen Virol*. 2010;91(Pt 4):821–828

Gershon AA, Arvin AM, Levin MJ, Seward JF, Schmid DS. Varicella vaccine in the United States. A decade of prevention and the way forward. *J Infect Dis*. 2008;197(Suppl 2):S39–S40

Hardy I, Gershon A, Steinberg SP, LaRussa P; Varicella Vaccine Collaborative Study Group. The incidence of zoster after immunization with live attenuated varicella vaccine. A study in children with leukemia. *New Engl J Med*. 1991;325(22):1545–1550

Marin M, Güris D, Chaves SS, Schmid S, Seward JF; Centers for Disease Control and Prevention. Prevention of varicella: recommendations of the Advisory Committee on Immunization Practices (ACIP). *MMWR Recomm Rep*. 2007;56(RR-4):1–40

Marin M, Zhang JX, Seward JF. Near elimination of varicella deaths in the United States following implementation of the childhood vaccination program. *Pediatrics.* 2011;128(2):214–220

Shapiro ED, Vazquez M, Esposito D, et al. Effectiveness of 2 doses of varicella vaccine in children. *J Infect Dis.* 2011;203(3):312–315

Wineman S, Chun C, Schmid S, et al. Incidence and clinical characteristics of herpes zoster among children the varicella vaccine era, 2005-2009. *J Infect Dis.* 2013;208(11):1859–1868

PART

1

Infectious Diseases

Section 4

Fungal Infections

CHAPTER 38

Aspergillosis

Andreas H. Groll, MD; Charalampos Antachopoulos, MD;
Emmanuel Roilides, MD, PhD; and Thomas J. Walsh, MD, PhD

Key Points

- Filamentous fungi of the genus *Aspergillus* may cause a broad spectrum of conditions in children, including transient asymptomatic colonization, pulmonary hypersensitivity reactions, saprophytic colonization of pathologic airway structures, and life-threatening tissue invasive infection.

- The most common site of invasive aspergillosis is the lung, with dissemination particularly to the central nervous system occurring in approximately 30% of cases.

- Cornerstones for successful management of invasive aspergillosis include the prompt initiation of appropriate antifungal therapy, reversal of the patient's underlying deficiency in host defenses if feasible, and, in select circumstances, surgical interventions.

- Options for first-line antifungal treatment of invasive aspergillosis in patients 2 years or older includes voriconazole and liposomal amphotericin B; for children younger than 2 years, liposomal amphotericin B is the only first-line option with an existing pediatric dosage.

- Primary chemoprophylaxis of invasive aspergillosis may be indicated in high-risk populations with incidence rates of close to 10% or higher. These may include patients with acute leukemia, patients with bone marrow failure syndromes, and those following allogeneic hematopoietic stem cell transplantation, particularly when immunosuppression is augmented for graft-versus-host disease.

Overview

Filamentous fungi of the genus *Aspergillus* may cause a broad spectrum of conditions in children, including transient asymptomatic colonization, pulmonary hypersensitivity reactions, saprophytic colonization of pathologic airway structures, and life-threatening tissue invasive infections predominantly of the lung with or without dissemination in patients with congenital or acquired deficiencies in host defenses.

Causes and Differential Diagnosis

Most cases of human disease are caused by *Aspergillus fumigatus,* followed by *Aspergillus flavus* and, less commonly, *Aspergillus nidulans, Aspergillus niger,* and *Aspergillus terreus.* The usual portal of entry is the respiratory tract through inhalation of *Aspergillus* conidia; further potential sites of entry include the gastrointestinal tract and macerated surfaces of the skin.

The differential diagnosis for aspergillosis depends on the site of involvement and host immune status. A wide variety of bacterial and other fungal pathogens are generally considered. For target organs such as the lung, drug-induced injury also is a consideration.

Clinical Features

Hypersensitivity Reactions

Hypersensitivity reactions caused by *Aspergillus* species include allergic bronchopulmonary aspergillosis, extrinsic asthma, and hypersensitivity pneumonitis. Allergic bronchopulmonary aspergillosis in children is associated with chronic lung diseases such as asthma and cystic fibrosis. Symptoms include shortness of breath, cough, production of brownish sputum, and weight loss. Conventional chest radiographs show central bronchiectasis and a tubular branching pattern of mucoid impaction producing a "finger-in-glove" appearance. Without treatment, allergic bronchopulmonary aspergillosis may become chronic and lead to respiratory insufficiency.

Saprophytic Aspergillosis

Aspergilloma and other forms of saprophytic aspergillosis consist of macroscopically visible fungal mycelia in preformed anatomic structures (fungus balls) such as pulmonary cavities, bronchiectasis, and the paranasal sinuses without deep invasion of adjacent tissue. The characteristic radiographic appearance of an aspergilloma is that of a pulmonary nodule within a lung cavity with or without air crescent. Apart from intermittent cough, affected patients may be asymptomatic. However, patients may have constitutional symptoms or hemoptysis that may on occasion be life-threatening. Related entities described in adult patients with chronic destructive lung conditions include chronic pulmonary aspergillosis (multiple cavities with or without fungus balls), chronic fibrosing pulmonary aspergillosis (marked and extensive pulmonary fibrosis), and chronic necrotizing pulmonary aspergillosis (slow invasion of adjacent lung tissue without dissemination).

Invasive Aspergillosis

Invasive pulmonary aspergillosis is by far the most frequent entity, with disseminated disease predominantly in the central nervous system (CNS) found in approximately 30% of cases. Clinical manifestations of fever, cough, and dyspnea, although nonspecific and not obligatory, represent the main symptoms. Pleuritic chest pain and potentially life-threatening hemoptysis may occur with the angioinvasive form in granulocytopenic patients, particularly during the time of granulocyte recovery. Tracheobronchial forms of invasive aspergillosis may also occur and have been reported predominantly in patients with uncontrolled HIV infection and following lung transplantation at the site of the bronchial anastomosis. Central nervous system aspergillosis should be considered in immunocompromised patients with acute onset of focal or diffuse neurologic signs and symptoms. *Aspergillus* species can enter the CNS by hematogenous spread from the lung, extension from the paranasal sinus or nasal cavity, and, least frequently, direct introduction by a neurosurgical procedure. Facial swelling, facial pain, black or brownish nasal secretions, exophthalmos, and cranial nerve abnormalities are suggestive of invasive paranasal sinus infection. While paranasal sinus aspergillosis seems to be less common in children than in adults, primary cutaneous aspergillosis has been preferentially reported in the pediatric setting in association with lacerations by arm boards, tapes, and electrodes and at the insertion site of peripheral or central venous catheters. Primary gastrointestinal aspergillosis is a rare clinical entity; clinical manifestations of this primary luminal infection include pain, ileus, and perforation. Symptoms of disseminated infections are uncharacteristic and determined by the site and extent of infection.

Risk Factors and Populations at Risk

Hypersensitivity Reactions and Saprophytic Aspergillosis

Most hypersensitivity reactions and saprophytic aspergillosis, respectively, occur in patients with underlying chronic destructive pulmonary conditions. These include patients with cystic fibrosis and, much less frequently, asthma or certain congenital immunodeficiency disorders affecting B-cell number or function. However, data on the exact frequency of these entities do not exist.

Invasive Aspergillosis

The most important clinical risk factors for invasive *Aspergillus* infections include prolonged and profound granulocytopenia (granulocyte count <500/mcL for ≥10 days) and functional deficiencies of granulocytes and macrophages, because they commonly occur following myelosuppressive chemotherapy, following treatment with therapeutic doses of glucocorticosteroids, in graft-vs-host disease (GVHD), or, as a primary immunodeficiency, in chronic granulomatous disease, a rare disorder of phagocyte function. Nonimmunologic factors are also important and include damage to protective surfaces of skin and mucosa and comorbidities such as cytomegaloviral diseases.

The risk of developing invasive aspergillosis is highest in patients with acute leukemia, following allogeneic hematopoietic stem cell transplantation (HSCT) until engraftment, during augmented immunosuppression for GVHD and profound T-cell deficiency, following liver transplantation, following lung and

Box 38-1. Pediatric Populations at Risk for Invasive *Aspergillus* Infections

- Low birthweight infants and neonates
- Children
  - o With primary immunodeficiencies
    - – Defects of phagocytic host defenses
  - o With acquired immunodeficiencies
    - – Acute and recurrent leukemia
    - – Bone marrow failure syndromes
    - – Allogeneic HSCT
    - – SOT
  - o With advanced HIV infection
  - o Undergoing immunosuppressive therapy
  - o With acute illnesses or trauma
  - o With chronic airway diseases

Abbreviations: HSCT, hematopoietic stem cell transplant; SOT, solid organ transplant.

heart-lung transplantation, and in patients with AIDS (Box 38-1). Sporadic cases have been reported in patients without one of these conditions receiving treatment in an intensive care unit, patients with chronic destructive lung diseases, and premature neonates. Invasive aspergillosis is rare following high-dose chemotherapy with autologous stem cell rescue and only casuistically reported in patients with solid tumors. This distribution of patients at risk underscores the effect of prolonged granulocytopenia and treatment with glucocorticosteroids on pathogenesis of the disease.

The outcome of invasive aspergillosis is mostly dismal, particularly following allogeneic HSCT, after liver transplantation, and in patients with AIDS. Case fatality rates at 3 months post-diagnosis are between 30% and 50%, with worse prognosis in patients with persisting granulocytopenia or immunosuppression, CNS involvement, and major hemorrhage.

Evaluation

Hypersensitivity Reactions and Saprophytic Aspergillosis

The diagnosis of extrinsic asthma is based on the patient's history, chest radiographic findings, pulmonary function test results, and detection of *Aspergillus*-specific IgE and IgG antibodies and a highly elevated serum IgE concentration (>500 U). Allergic bronchopulmonary aspergillosis needs to be considered in any patient with a chronic pulmonary disorder, recurrent airway obstruction, and pulmonary infiltrates that are not otherwise specified. Further diagnostic criteria include brownish sputum; blood eosinophilia; elevated serum IgE concentration; elevated IgG anti-*Aspergillus* antibody or *Aspergillus* precipitin level; detection of specific IgE antibodies against the recombinant *Aspergillus* Asp f1 and f3 and Asp f4 and f6 antigens, respectively; positive skin test results; and presence of a central bronchiectasis. Detection of *Aspergillus* in sputum is frequent but not essential for diagnosis. In *saprophytic forms,* the diagnosis is mostly based on imaging findings; microbiologic detection and resistance testing is advised when treatment with antifungals is considered.

Invasive Aspergillosis

Early recognition and rapid initiation of effective treatment are paramount for control of invasive aspergillosis. In view of the increasing diversity of fungal pathogens, differences in spectrum of current antifungals, and looming resistance, identification of the causative agent and resistance testing should always be attempted. While microscopic and culture specimens obtained from the clinically affected site remain the standard criteria, technical problems in obtaining an appropriate specimen, the time of culturing, and negative results all limit an efficient and rapid diagnosis. Similarly, the diagnostic yield of histology is also unsatisfactory, having an approximate sensitivity of 50%. Given this background, detection of fungal cell wall antigens and DNA in blood and other tissues may enhance the diagnosis of invasive aspergillosis.

Detection of Cell Wall Antigens

Galactomannan (GM), a heteropolysaccharide of the cell wall of *Aspergillus* species, is released into the extracellular fluid during cell wall turnover and hyphal growth and can be detected by an enzyme immunoassay (EIA). Studies performed in adults show a high sensitivity and specificity of the GM assay in serum in granulocytopenic patients with hematologic malignancies or following allogeneic HSCT, and usefulness for early diagnosis in conjunction with serial computed tomography (CT).

While cross-reactions with other fungal organisms are rare, false-positive results can be caused by contaminating GM in β-lactam antibiotics, dietary GM (in pasta, cereals, and formula), and cross-reactivity with lipoteichoic acids of *Bifidobacteria* of the infantile gut microflora. The GM assay also has high diagnostic utility for analysis of bronchoalveolar lavage fluid of pediatric patients with suspected pulmonary aspergillosis. Similarly, limited data suggest utility of GM assay in the CSF of both children and adults.

In contrast to GM, $(1\rightarrow3)$-β-D-glucan assay is a useful test for preemptive treatment strategies. Cut-off values in pediatric patients are yet undefined, and data in pediatric patients at risk for or diagnosed as having invasive aspergillosis are thus far anecdotal.

Detection of Fungal DNA

Standardized, polymerase chain reaction–based diagnostic methods in blood or serum are currently being evaluated for inclusion as screening methods in the criteria set forth by the Mycoses Study Group and the European Organization for Treatment of Cancer (or MSG/EORTC). The use of polymerase chain reaction on diagnostic aspirates or tissue biopsies has yielded promising performance data in small non-pediatric patient series and may be helpful in individual cases.

Diagnostic Imaging

Modern imaging studies including magnetic resonance imaging and high-resolution CT are essential to investigate clinically suspicious sites and guide diagnostic and surgical interventions. Whereas high-resolution CT is a sensitive screening method of pulmonary mold infections in adult hematologic patients, these characteristic CT findings appear to be of lesser utility in children, particularly in non-hematologic patients. The most frequent radiologic finding of invasive pulmonary aspergillosis is nodules. Computed tomographic findings are variable and mostly nonspecific. As a consequence, any non-diffuse pulmonary CT finding in a high-risk patient needs to be considered to indicate invasive mold infection and should prompt further diagnostic workup. Computed tomographic scans, particularly those for follow-up, should be used judiciously and at the lowest dose rates possible.

Management

Hypersensitivity Reactions and Saprophytic Aspergillosis

Whereas the treatment of extrinsic asthma is symptomatic coupled with avoidance of antigen exposure, options for treatment of allergic bronchopulmonary aspergillosis include the systemic administration of prednisone (starting dose: 2 mg/kg of body weight a day with taper over 2 weeks) and itraconazole (no pediatric label; starting dose: 5 mg/kg of body weight day of the oral suspension in 2 divided doses over several weeks; therapeutic drug monitoring recommended with target trough concentration of ≥0.5 mg/L). Management of aspergilloma depends on the patient's symptoms and severity of the underlying pulmonary condition and may include physical therapy, systemic administration of antifungal triazoles, and surgical resection, if feasible.

Invasive Aspergillosis

Cornerstones for successful management of invasive aspergillosis include the prompt initiation of appropriate antifungal therapy (Table 38-1), reversal of the patient's underlying deficiency in host defenses, and, in select circumstances, surgical interventions. Because of the existing difficulties in obtaining a definite diagnosis rapidly and imminent risk of clinical deterioration, treatment often needs to be started preemptively on the basis of risk profiles, imaging studies, and serologic markers. Nevertheless, all efforts should be made to perform necessary procedures to confirm the diagnosis and obtain information on species and antimicrobial resistance.

On the basis of phase III clinical trials in adults and approved pediatric dosages, options for first-line antifungal treatment of invasive aspergillosis in patients 2 years or older include voriconazole and liposomal amphotericin B; for children younger than 2 years, liposomal amphotericin B is the only first-line option with an existing pediatric dosage. Emerging data suggest a

Table 38-1. Pediatric Doses of Systemic Antifungals Used for Treatment of Invasive Aspergillosis[a]

Antifungal	Daily Dose per Age Group			
	13–18 y	2–12 y	1–24 mo	Neonates
Amphotericin B deoxycholate	0.75– 1.5 mg/kg IV	0.75– 1.5 mg/kg IV	0.75– 1.5 mg/kg IV	0.75– 1.5 mg/kg IV
Liposomal Amphotericin B	3 (–5) mg/kg IV	3 (–5) mg/kg IV	3 (–5) mg/kg IV	3 (–5) mg/kg IV
Amphotericin B lipid complex	5 mg/kg IV	5 mg/kg IV	5 mg/kg IV	5 mg/kg IV
Itraconazole oral suspension[b]	5 mg/kg orally divided in 2 doses	5 mg/kg orally divided in 2 doses	NA	NA
Voriconazole[b]	8 mg/kg (d 1: 12) IV divided in 2 doses for ≥15 y and for 12–14 y weighing ≥50 kg	16 mg/kg (d 1: 18) IV divided in 2 doses for 2–<12 y and for 12–14 y weighing <50 kg	NA	NA
Voriconazole oral suspension/ capsules[b]	400 mg orally divided in 2 doses for ≥15 y and for 12–14 y weighing ≥50 kg	18 mg/kg orally divided in 2 doses for 2–<12 y and for 12–14 y weighing <50 kg	NA	NA
Posaconazole delayed-release tablets	300 mg once/d (d 1: 300 mg twice daily)	NA	NA	NA
Caspofungin	50 mg/m² (d 1: 70) IV (maximum: 70)	50 mg/m² (d 1: 70) IV (maximum: 70)	50 mg/m² (d 1: 70) IV	25 mg/m² IV

Abbreviations: IV, intravenously; NA, not applicable (no or no sufficient data).
[a] For detailed indications, please refer to the text.
[b] Therapeutic drug monitoring recommended.

rationale for therapeutic drug monitoring of voriconazole to optimize outcome with a target trough concentration of greater than 1.0 mcg/mL. It should be noted, however, that little systematic data on the efficacy of both compounds in pediatric patients with invasive aspergillosis exist.

Options for second-line antifungal treatment in patients 2 years or older include amphotericin B lipid complex, caspofungin, and, limited to adolescents

13 years and older, posaconazole delayed-release tablets. These options are based on the existence of approved pediatric dosages and phase II data generated in adults. Efficacy data in children and adolescents are limited with the exception of amphotericin B lipid complex, for which a large published phase II and IV experience exists. Unapproved alternatives may include oral itraconazole, and intravenous (IV) posaconazole for adolescents 13 years and older. Options in children younger than 2 years include amphotericin B lipid complex and caspofungin.

Adjunctive surgical interventions need consideration in skin and soft-tissue infections, sinus infections, impeding erosion of pulmonary arteries, and operable CNS and lung lesions. Granulocyte colony-stimulating factor is indicated in neutropenic patients and reduction, discontinuation, or replacement of steroids in patients receiving these agents.

Duration of treatment is individual and defined by the complete disappearance of all signs and symptoms and resolution of the underlying deficiency in host defenses. Treatment of patients who have responded to initial IV therapy and are clinically stable may be consolidated with oral therapies.

Certain clinical situations bear note. Although not formally investigated, a change in class is advised when a change in antifungal therapy is considered necessary because of refractory disease or a break-through infection on antifungal prophylaxis. While the role of antifungal combination therapies remains to be defined, it may be justified in profoundly compromised patients and those with fulminant or refractory disease. Clinical data collected in adults suggest that voriconazole is the preferred agent for treatment of CNS aspergillosis, with high-dose ($\geq$5 mg/kg/day) liposomal amphotericin B as the next best alternative on the basis of pharmacodynamic animal data. Because of its high solubility in water, voriconazole may also be an option for endophthalmitis, peritonitis, and bone and joint infections.

Multi-azole-resistant *Aspergillus* species, such as *Aspergillus calidoustus* and *A nidulans,* have been reported; *A terreus,* on the other hand, has a reduced susceptibility to amphotericin B and is best treated with voriconazole. Zygomycetes are resistant to voriconazole and caspofungin, and non-*Aspergillus* hyalohyphomycosis and phaeohyphomycosis are considered resistant to caspofungin. Identification to the species level and in vitro susceptibility testing are recommended despite the absence of firm in vitro–in vivo correlations.

Primary chemoprophylaxis of invasive aspergillosis may be indicated in high-risk populations with incidence rates of close to 10% or higher. These may include patients receiving intensive chemotherapy for acute leukemia, patients with bone marrow failure syndromes, and those following allogeneic HSCT, particularly when immunosuppression is augmented for GVHD. On the basis of pivotal clinical trials conducted in adults, patients 13 years or older may receive posaconazole delayed-release tablets at the adult dose of 300 mg once a day (day 1: 300 mg twice daily). Alternatives in patients 2 to 12 years include oral or IV voriconazole or itraconazole oral suspension. Patients younger than

2 years and those unable to take oral medication may receive either amphotericin B liposomal complex at 1 mg/kg every other day (all age groups) or IV voriconazole (≥2 years). This practical algorithm, however, requires careful attention to contraindications, drug interactions, and adverse effects because appropriate clinical trials in pediatric patients are lacking.

Long-term Implications

Beyond a considerable short-term case fatality rate of 30% to 50% and the frequent necessity of treatment for months and sometimes years, the long-term prognostic effect of invasive aspergillosis is difficult to evaluate. Cancer treatment may be delayed in the presence of invasive aspergillosis for fear of progression of infection during neutropenia. Unfortunately, this delay of chemotherapy may also increase the probability of relapsed or progressive leukemia. As a case in point, in one case series, the cure rate in patients who were diagnosed and treated for a minimum of 10 days was 64%. However, overall long-term survival was only 31% after a median of 5.68 years post-diagnosis.

Non-*Aspergillus* Mold Infections

A wide variety of previously uncommon opportunistic filamentous fungi are increasingly encountered as causing life-threatening infections in severely immunocompromised children. The genera of the order Mucorales require initial therapy with amphotericin B. Apart from the agents of mucormycosis, these emerging pathogens include hyaline filamentous fungi (eg, *Fusarium* species, *Paecilomyces* species, *Pseudallescheria boydii*, and *Scedosporium prolificans*) and dematiaceous molds (eg, *Bipolaris*, *Exophiala*, and *Alternaria* species). These filamentous fungi cause infections that are virtually indistinguishable from those of *Aspergillus* species, in clinical presentation and in their appearance in tissue specimens (colorless or lightly pigmented, septate, and branching). However, some of the hyaline molds, most notably *Fusarium* species, *Acremonium* species, and *Paecilomyces* species, disseminate via the bloodstream and can cause fungemia and numerous embolic skin lesions. Infections by the emerging pathogens have extraordinarily high case fatality rates; several of these organisms, including but not limited to *Fusarium* species and *P boydii*, have limited susceptibility to amphotericin B. However, while the echinocandins appear to have no useful activity, limited and uncontrolled data indicate an important role of both voriconazole and posaconazole in the management of these infections. *Scedosporium prolificans* is usually resistant to all licensed antifungals. Treatment of infections by the emerging fungal pathogens is an interdisciplinary challenge and needs to be individualized on the basis of the patient's presentation and response to treatment.

Suggested Reading

Antachopoulos C, Walsh TJ, Roilides E. Fungal infections in primary immunodeficiencies. *Eur J Pediatr.* 2007;166(11):1099–1117

Burgos A, Zaoutis TE, Dvorak CC, et al. Pediatric invasive aspergillosis: a multicenter retrospective analysis of 139 contemporary cases. *Pediatrics.* 2008;121(5): e1286–e1294

Dornbusch HJ, Groll A, Walsh TJ. Diagnosis of invasive fungal infections in immunocompromised children. *Clin Microbiol Infect.* 2010;16(9):1328–1334

Dornbusch HJ, Manzoni P, Roilides E, Walsh TJ, Groll AH. Invasive fungal infections in children. *Pediatr Infect Dis J.* 2009;28(8):734–737

Groll AH, Castagnola E, Cesaro S, et al. Fourth European Conference on Infections in Leukaemia (ECIL-4): guidelines for diagnosis, prevention, and treatment of invasive fungal diseases in paediatric patients with cancer or allogeneic haemopoietic stem-cell transplantation. *Lancet Oncol.* 2014;15(8):e327–e340

Groll AH, Tragiannidis A. Update on antifungal agents for paediatric patients. *Clin Microbiol Infect.* 2010;16(9):1343–1353

Stergiopoulou T, Walsh TJ. Clinical pharmacology of antifungal agents to overcome drug resistance in pediatric patients. *Expert Opin Pharmacother.* 2015;16(2):213–226

Tragiannidis A, Roilides E, Walsh TJ, Groll AH. Invasive aspergillosis in children with acquired immunodeficiencies. *Clin Infect Dis.* 2012;54(2):258–267

Walsh TJ, Anaissie EJ, Denning DW, et al. Treatment of aspergillosis: clinical practice guidelines of the Infectious Diseases Society of America. *Clin Infect Dis.* 2008;46(3):327–360

Walsh TJ, Groll A, Hiemenz J, Fleming R, Roilides E, Anaissie E. Infections due to emerging and uncommon medically important fungal pathogens. *Clin Microbiol Infect.* 2004;10(Suppl 1):48–66

CHAPTER 39

Candidiasis

Emmanuel Roilides, MD, PhD; Charalampos Antachopoulos, MD;
Andreas H. Groll, MD; and Thomas J. Walsh, MD, PhD

Key Points

- Candidiasis causes many patterns of disease in neonates and children. It may present as uncomplicated catheter-related candidemia or disseminated candidiasis in a neutropenic child, potentially leading to septic shock. It can affect neonates, children with hematologic malignancies, patients in critical care, and those having risk factors for candidiasis. It can affect almost all organs and tissues of the body, causing multiple local infections.

- While *Candida albicans* is still the most frequently isolated species in pediatric patients, certain non-*albicans Candida* species, such as *Candida parapsilosis* and *Candida glabrata,* have become more frequent and may cause problems with their differential susceptibilities to antifungals.

- Conventional and lipid formulations of amphotericin B, azoles, echinocandins, and flucytosine are the main antifungals for the treatment of candidiasis.

- Management of candidiasis is sometimes complicated. It starts from 2-week therapy for a catheter-related candidemia and may last several months in a difficult case of candidal endocarditis or spondylodiscitis.

Overview

Candidiasis is the disease caused by the fungus *Candida* species. It mainly affects immunocompromised patients but may also affect other subjects with risk factors.

Those with congenital immunodeficiencies involving T cell immunity and rare genetic syndromes (ie, chronic mucocutaneous candidiasis and autoimmune polyendocrinopathy-candidiasis-ectodermal dystrophy), AIDS, and malignancies treated with cytotoxic chemotherapy are at risk for mucocutaneous candidiasis. Neonates, immunocompromised hosts, and those with vascular catheters are at risk for invasive candidiasis.

Causes and Differential Diagnosis

Candida is the most frequent fungal genus causing disease in humans. Blasto-conidia (yeast cells) are the infecting form of the organism, whereas hyphae/pseudohyphae are the invasive form. Among hundreds of different *Candida* species, *Candida albicans* is the most frequent isolate, accounting for about half of cases. Other *Candida* species are *Candida parapsilosis, Candida tropicalis, Candida glabrata, and Candida krusei. Candida parapsilosis* is especially frequent in neonates, whereas *C glabrata* is more common in patients with hematologic malignancies.

Mucosal or cutaneous candidiasis must be differentiated from other oral lesions and skin exanthemas, such as atopic dermatitis and eczema. Candidal diaper dermatitis is characterized by satellite lesions and appears on regions of skin that are in contact with the diapers of infants around their urogenital area.

Candidemia and other forms of invasive candidiasis are difficult to differentiate from bacterial, other fungal, or even viral infections before microbiologic diagnosis is made. In neonates, candidemia resembles bacterial sepsis, and in older children, it has to be differentiated from other bacterial systemic infections. A typical erythematous papular exanthem of acute disseminated candidiasis may differentiate it from bacterial sepsis.

Clinical Features

Mucocutaneous Candidiasis

In chronic mucocutaneous candidiasis and autoimmune polyendocrinopathy-candidiasis-ectodermal dystrophy (APECED), mucosal candidiasis as well as skin and nail candidiasis are apparent either continuously or intermittently in these patients. In APECED, candidiasis tends to disappear before endocrino-pathies start.

Diaper dermatitis is a common mild exanthema around the urogenital area of infants, which comes in contact with diapers.

Oropharyngeal candidiasis and candidal esophagitis may be seen in HIV-infected children with AIDS who are not under highly active antiretroviral therapy and in children with malignancies and cytotoxic chemotherapy-associated acquired immunodeficiencies, as well as regional radiotherapy. Odynophagia and white plaques on the tongue and buccal surfaces of the mouth can be a problem.

Vulvovaginal candidiasis may be seen in sexually active adolescent girls or those exposed to broad-spectrum antibiotics. It is infection of the vagina's mucous membranes by *C albicans* and presents as vaginal irritation and white discharge.

Invasive and Deep-seated Candidiasis

Candida species are the third to fourth most frequent cause of late-onset sepsis in premature infants. However, they are the second most frequent cause of mortality and most important cause of neurodevelopmental delay as sequelae of neonatal sepsis, especially when candidemia is followed by the characteristic syndrome of hematogenous *Candida* meningoencephalitis. The degree of prematurity (ie, low gestational age, low birthweight) is the most important factor associated with increased incidence of candidiasis. Thus, while neonates with very low birthweight (<1.5 kg) may have as high as 5% probability to contract candidiasis during their stay in the neonatal intensive care unit (NICU), this probability reaches up to 12% to 15% in extremely low birthweight (<1.0 kg) infants. Invasive candidiasis is almost synonymous to candidemia in neonates. Candidemia may be followed in up to 25% by hematogenous meningoencephalitis and in a much higher percentage (up to 60%) by urinary tract infection. Other syndromes that may complicate candidemia in neonates include endocarditis, brain or other organ abscesses, arthritis/osteomyelitis, and renal infection. Neonates are colonized with *C albicans* by their mothers vertically and with *C parapsilosis* by NICU personnel horizontally. Central venous catheters, total parenteral nutrition (TPN), previous bacterial sepsis, and administration of multiple antibacterials are the most important risk factors for candidiasis. Other risk factors are fungal colonization, high glucose concentrations, antibiotic and H_2-receptor antagonist use, endotracheal intubation, congenital conditions, and necrotizing enterocolitis.

The clinical syndromes that *Candida* causes in older children are similar to those in adults. *Candida* species are important causes of health care–associated infections in pediatric cancer patients receiving treatment for hematologic malignancies, pediatric allogeneic hematopoietic stem cell transplant recipients, and children and adolescents with indwelling central venous catheters. Severe sepsis or septic shock occur in approximately 30% of them; mortality ranges within 10% to 25%, and reaches 50% in patients admitted to the pediatric intensive care unit (PICU). Invasive candidiasis is also a clinically important syndrome in solid organ transplant recipients.

Bloodstream infection due to *Candida* occurs in cancer patients with neutropenia; critically ill patients, especially when hospitalization in PICU is prolonged; and those with abdominal surgery, use of immunosuppressants, short gut syndrome, or TPN. It may be central venous catheter associated.

Acute disseminated candidiasis with hemodynamic and inflammatory signs of sepsis, as well as a possible characteristic erythematous papular exanthema, may follow candidemia. *Candida glabrata* and *C tropicalis* are more frequent in children with hematologic malignancies than in other patients, probably because of the increased use of azoles and amphotericin B, respectively, in these patients. The attributable mortality of invasive candidiasis has been estimated to be around 10% in children.

Chronic disseminated candidiasis (hepatosplenic candidiasis) is a well-described syndrome that occurs in children with hematologic malignancies during and after recovery from neutropenia. It is characterized by persistent fever and upper abdominal pain as well as increased inflammatory index, alkaline phosphatase, and γ-glutamyltransferase levels, but not transaminase. Ultrasounds, computed tomography, or magnetic resonance imaging (MRI) (which is more sensitive) can reveal bull's eye–shaped small abscesses throughout the liver and spleen. The disease can last relatively long despite appropriate antifungal therapy and is determined by an ineffective inflammatory response.

Organ- or Tissue-Specific Candidal Infections

Meningoencephalitis frequently occurs in neonates following about as many as 25% of episodes of neonatal candidemia. In contrast, it is rarely diagnosed in older children with malignancies. It can present with nonspecific symptoms, and the cerebrospinal fluid (CSF) may have increased numbers of leukocytes and protein concentrations and possibly decreased glucose concentrations. Cerebrospinal fluid culture may be frequently negative. The abnormal CSF picture and blood culture positivity for *Candida* place the diagnosis. In premature neonates, candidal meningoencephalitis may be followed by calcifications and neurodevelopmental delay.

Chorioretinitis and endophthalmitis occur as a relatively infrequent complication of candidemia, especially when antifungals with suboptimal eye penetration are used, such as echinocandins. Funduscopy can reveal the characteristic picture of chorioretinal infiltrates and purulent vitreous opacity, respectively. Loss of vision may occur.

Endocarditis occurs in 5% of patients with candidemia and presents as persistent fever with refractory candidemia and usually large heart vegetations shown at echocardiography of the heart.

Urinary tract infection can present as cystitis, pyelonephritis, or fungal balls within the kidneys. In addition to urinary culture, imaging including ultrasound and MRI facilitates diagnosis of these syndromes. Fungal balls are usually refractory to antifungal therapy and in some refractory cases may require surgery.

Peritonitis in children with end-stage renal insufficiency who are on continuous ambulatory peritoneal dialysis (CAPD) may also occur. During CAPD *Candida* species or rarely other fungi may be introduced in the peritoneal cavity through the peritoneal dialysis catheter and cause peritonitis that presents with abdominal pain and low-grade fever. Peritoneal fluid neutrophil count is increased, and its culture may be positive for *Candida* species.

Osteoarticular infections are relatively rare infections occurring in neonates and less frequently in children. In neonates, *Candida* can infect the bone and joint simultaneously (osteoarthritis), and the infection is almost always hematogenous. In older children, infection occurs either hematogenously or through contiguous spread of the organism, and it can be either osteomyelitis or arthritis. A recent large series of candidal bone and joint infections also involves a relatively large number of neonates and children. The most frequent bones affected are femur, humerus, and then vertebra/ribs, whereas the joints frequently affected are knee, hip, and shoulder. Spondylodiscitis is a specific form of osteomyelitis that requires particularly careful surgery in conjunction with antifungal therapy.

Evaluation
. . . .

Microscopy and culture of appropriate specimens remain the criterion standards of mycologic diagnosis. Successful management of invasive candidal infections relies on early recognition and rapid initiation of effective treatment.

Blood cultures may not always be positive in cases of invasive candidiasis. However, a positive blood culture should never be considered as contamination, and the patient must receive antifungal therapy. Microscopy of direct smears of blood or other fluids may show yeast-like cells. This is an indication of candidal infection, but culture is the method that yields the definitive diagnosis. It is important to note that not all yeast-like organisms in the bloodstream are *Candida* species. *Trichosporon* and *Cryptococcus* species are yeasts but have different susceptibility profiles and require different treatment strategies. When an organism has grown in culture, it must be identified to the species level, especially when it is derived from a sterile site. As a rapid test for presumptive identification of *C albicans* (and, infrequently, *C dubliniensis*), germ tube test can be performed. *C albicans* is germ-tube positive, whereas other common non-*albicans Candida* species are negative.

Testing of susceptibility to antifungals is necessary, especially for strains isolated from sterile sites that are non-*albicans*. Some of the non-*albicans* isolates, such as *C krusei* and a large proportion of *C glabrata*, are not susceptible to fluconazole. *Candida parapsilosis* may exhibit relatively high minimum inhibitory concentration (MIC) for echinocandins (although this may not be clinically important), and *Candida lusitaniae* may be resistant to amphotericin B.

Non–culture-based methods for diagnosing invasive candidiasis, such as the assay for $(1\rightarrow3)$ β-D-glucan assay and polymerase chain reaction, may be available for use. However, they both have problems of either no definition of normal values of β-D-glucan in pediatrics or no standardization of polymerase chain reaction; thus, they are not currently recommended for routine use in pediatric patients.

It often is a challenge to distinguish surface colonization, such as candiduria and positive endotracheal tube secretions, from invasive disease. In the case of candiduria, consideration of the host immune status, such as neutropenic, deeply immunocompromised, and neonatal; removal of a urinary catheter and repeat urinary culture; ultrasound of kidneys; and blood cultures should be attempted to decide whether candiduria is a sign of invasive disease. Similarly, interpretation of candidal growth in endotracheal tube secretion cultures requires consideration of the immune status of the host, as well as search for lung opacities and other indices of lung inflammation. Almost always it does not correspond to lung infection by *Candida,* and candidal lung infection is rare.

Imaging of organ-specific infections is always important. Ultrasound of heart, liver, spleen, kidneys, or neonatal brain is a very useful and easy diagnostic tool and yields reliable results. In addition, when ultrasound findings are unclear, high resolution computed tomography and MRI are very helpful for diagnosing osteoarticular infections and brain abscesses, as well as other organ infections. Finally, radionuclide scanning, such as technetium scan and leukocyte indium scan, is helpful for diagnosing difficult and multiple organ cases.

Management
· · · · · · · · · · · ·

Therapeutic strategies, apart from targeted treatment of mycologically documented candidal infections, include prophylactic antifungal administration in special patient groups and empiric therapy of critically ill patients, who are at high risk for developing invasive candidiasis.

Important considerations when choosing the antifungal and mode of application include localization of the infection, severity of the disease, impairment of liver and renal functions, previous recent exposure to antifungals, identified *Candida* species, and local or institutional patterns of resistance.

Antifungals

Currently, there are 4 available classes of antifungals: polyenes, triazoles, echinocandins, and flucytosine (Table 39-1). The available polyenes include nystatin, conventional amphotericin B deoxycholate, and lipid formulations, such as liposomal amphotericin B and amphotericin B lipid complex. All amphotericin B preparations are fungicidal and effective against most *Candida* species, with the possible exception of *Candida guilliermondii* and *C lusitaniae*. Nystatin is used only superficially for oral and cutaneous infections.

For decades, amphotericin B deoxycholate has been the cornerstone of antifungal treatment; nevertheless, its use is limited by renal and infusion-related toxicities. The lipid formulations show less nephrotoxicity than amphotericin B deoxycholate, while infusion-related adverse effects such as fever, chills, and rigor are substantially less with liposomal amphotericin B only. The rate of other significant adverse effects does not seem to differ between the various preparations.

The group of triazoles includes fluconazole, itraconazole, and the new-generation triazoles, voriconazole and posaconazole, which are approved for use in children older than 2 and 12 years of age, respectively. All triazoles are fungistatic against *Candida* species, which is a limiting factor in critically ill patients. Although azoles are considered safe and well-tolerated drugs, variable degree of hepatotoxicity is a common adverse effect. They are metabolized through cytochrome P450 isoenzymes, and caution should be implemented with the concomitant use of other drugs sharing the same metabolic pathways, particularly in the case of voriconazole. They are effective against *C albicans*, while non-*albicans* species show increasing resistance to fluconazole, a fact related to the wide use of this agent as antifungal prophylaxis. Fluconazole exhibits no activity against *C krusei* and less activity against *C glabrata*. Voriconazole and posaconazole have a wider therapeutic range, including *C glabrata, C krusei*, and molds such as *Aspergillus* species. Varying degrees of cross-resistance have been recorded among all triazoles. An advantage of azoles is they can also be administered orally with very good bioavailability for fluconazole and voriconazole. Therapeutic drug monitoring is recommended for itraconazole, voriconazole, and posaconazole.

Table 39-1. Antifungals for Neonates and Children: Pharmacokinetic Properties, Treatment Dosages, and Toxicities

Drug	Administration Route	Pediatric Dosage	Cerebrospinal Fluid Penetration, %	Dose Reduction in Renal Failure	Dose Reduction in Liver Failure	Toxicities	Comments
Amphotericin B deoxycholate	IV	1–1.5 mg/kg/d every 24 h	<4	No	No	Infusion-related reactions (eg, fever, chills), nephro-toxicity, potassium loss	None
Liposomal amphotericin B	IV	3 mg/kg/d every 24 h Neonates: up to 7 mg/kg/d	Improved vs amphotericin B deoxycholate	No	No	Less nephrotoxicity vs amphotericin B deoxycholate	Possible low renal tissue distribution
Amphotericin B lipid complex	IV	5 mg/kg/d every 24 h	Poor	No	No	Less nephrotoxicity vs amphotericin B deoxycholate	Possible low renal tissue distribution
Fluconazole	IV; orally	12 mg/kg/d every 24 h Neonates: maybe a loading dose of 25 mg/kg/d	50–90	Yes	No	GI concerns, rash, increased liver enzyme levels	High rates of resistance related to prior use
Itraconazole	(IV); orally	2–5 mg/kg orally every 12 h	Poor	No	No	GI concerns, rash, dizziness, headache	Not licensed for children <18 y TDM needed

Continued

Table 39-1 (cont)

Drug	Administration Route	Pediatric Dosage	Cerebrospinal Fluid Penetration, %	Dose Reduction in Renal Failure	Dose Reduction in Liver Failure	Toxicities	Comments
Voriconazole	IV[a]; orally	9 mg/kg every 12 h on d 1, then 8 mg/kg every 12 h IV	46	No	No	Visual changes, mental status changes, increased liver enzyme levels	Not licensed for use in children <2 y; TDM required
Posaconazole	Orally	400 mg every 12 h	Poor	No	No	Headache, dizziness, abdominal pain, diarrhea	Not licensed for use in children <13 y; TDM needed
Caspofungin	IV	70 mg/m²/d on d 1, then 50 mg/m²/d	2–6	No	Yes	Fever, rash, hypokalemia	US FDA approved in children >3 mo
Micafungin	IV	<40 kg: 2–4 mg/kg/d; >40 kg: 100–200 mg/d; Neonates with HCME: up to 10 mg/kg/d every 24 h; Prophylaxis: 1 mg/kg/d	Poor	No	Yes	GI concerns, headache	EMA warning[b]
Flucytosine	IV; orally	100–150 mg/kg/d in 4 doses	65–90	Yes	No	Headache, rash, GI concerns, bone marrow suppression[c]	Only as part of combination therapy; TDM warranted

Abbreviations: EMA, European Medicines Agency; FDA, US Food and Drug Administration; GI, gastrointestinal; HCME, hematogenous *Candida* meningoencephalitis; IV, intravenous/intravenously; TDM, therapeutic drug monitoring; vs, versus.

[a] Not recommended in patients with creatinine clearance <50% due to carrier (cyclodextrin) accumulation.

[b] Because of tumor development in rats; use only if other antifungals are inappropriate.

[c] Rare in children.

Echinocandins, namely caspofungin, micafungin, and anidulafungin, all available in parenteral preparations only, are fungicidal against most *Candida* species, including azole-resistant strains. They have good penetration into tissues, with the exception of central nervous system (CNS), eyes, and urinary tract. Echinocandins are metabolized in the liver, except anidulafungin, which is metabolized in bile through chemical degradation. Few adverse effects and drug interactions are observed with all echinocandins. Caspofungin is the only echinocandin licensed by the US Food and Drug Administration for pediatric prophylaxis and treatment of invasive disease, while the European Medicines Agency has also approved micafungin for neonatal and pediatric use. Micafungin has shown similar safety and effectiveness to liposomal amphotericin B with fewer adverse effects.

Flucytosine has excellent bioavailability and organ distribution, including CNS, and demonstrates broad antifungal activity. Because of rapid emergence of resistance, it is only used as part of combination therapy with amphotericin B, mainly in disseminated organ involvement.

The combination of antifungals remains restricted for salvage therapy or individual cases. Combination of amphotericin B preparations with flucytosine or fluconazole has been used in disseminated candidiasis.

Prophylaxis in High-risk Patients

Because of the high fatality rates, antifungal prophylaxis has been recommended in high-risk neonates and children.

Prophylaxis in Neonates

In NICUs with high frequency of invasive candidiasis, prophylaxis is recommended for *all* neonates with a birthweight less than 1.0 kg. Fluconazole at 3 or 6 mg/kg twice weekly is administered intravenously or orally (Evidence Level I). This policy leads to reduction in candidal colonization as well as fungal infection, but not to change in overall mortality. There are concerns for emergence of resistant species after continuous use in the NICU.

In NICUs with a lower incidence of invasive candidiasis (ie, <2%) prophylaxis is recommended *for neonates*
- With birthweight less than 1.0 kg
- Who have risk factors (ie, central venous catheters, third-generation cephalosporins and carbapenems) for the development of invasive candidiasis: fluconazole at 3 or 6 mg/kg twice weekly intravenously or orally (Evidence Level II-1). Decision for prophylaxis is on an individual basis.

Prophylaxis in Children

Recommendations for the prevention of invasive candidiasis in children are largely extrapolated from studies performed in adults with concomitant pharmacokinetic data and models in children. Antifungal prophylaxis should be implemented in

- Allogeneic stem cell transplant recipients with neutropenia (<500 cell/mcL)
- Liver and pancreas transplant recipients
- Possibly PICU patients in institutions with a high rate of candidiasis (>10%); who have prior colonization with *Candida* in multiple body sites, TPN, or exposure to broad-spectrum antimicrobials for longer than 3 days, especially those with antianaerobic activity, vancomycin, carbapenems, and others; and those with multiple abdominal surgeries

Prophylactic fluconazole is well-established post-allogeneic hematopoietic stem cell transplantation (Evidence Level I). Alternatives include the use of voriconazole (Evidence Level I) or micafungin (Evidence Level I). In patients with graft-versus-host disease and increased immunosuppression, as well as high-risk hematologic malignancies, posaconazole (Evidence Level II-1) is effective in prevention of invasive fungal infections, but its use is limited for children older than 12 years. In younger children, voriconazole can be an alternative (>2 years), as well as amphotericin B and micafungin. Duration of prophylaxis is not well defined but should probably be extended until resolution of neutropenia (Table 39-2).

Table 39-2. Primary Prophylaxis of Pediatric Patients With Hematologic Malignancies

Clinical Context	Recommendation and Grading	Comments
Allogeneic HSCT, AML, and recurrent leukemia	Fluconazole at 8–12 mg/kg every day IV or orally; studied from d 0 until d +75 posttransplant (Evidence Level I)	Fluconazole should be used only if the institutional incidence of invasive mold infections is low, or if there are active diagnostic and therapeutic algorithms for mold infections.
Allogeneic HSCT	Micafungin at 1 mg/kg every day IV; from start of preparative regimen until d +30 (Evidence Level I)	Spectrum of antifungal activity also extends to *Aspergillus* spp.
Allogeneic HSCT, AML, and recurrent leukemia	Voriconazole at 8 mg/kg twice daily (d 1: 9 mg/kg twice daily) for IV and 9 mg/kg twice daily for oral administration (maximum: 350 mg twice daily) for ages 2–14 y and approved adult dose for patients ≥15 y and 12–14 y weighing >50 kg; studied from d 0 until at least d +100 (Evidence Level I)	Spectrum extends to *Aspergillus* spp and other medically important opportunistic molds. TDM should be performed; dosing target: trough concentration of ≥1 mg/L.

Continued

Table 39-2 (cont)

Clinical Context	Recommendation and Grading	Comments
Allogeneic HSCT, AML, and recurrent leukemia	Itraconazole suspension at 2.5 mg/kg every 12 h for patients ≥2 y; to be started after completion of conditioning regimen; until at least d +100 (Evidence Level II-1)	Spectrum extends to *Aspergillus* spp and other medically important opportunistic molds. Not approved in patients <18 y. TDM is suggested; dosing target: trough concentration of ≥0.5 mg/L.
Allogeneic HSCT, AML, and recurrent leukemia	Posaconazole suspension at 200 mg every 8 h orally for patients with ≥grade II GVHD and ≥13 y (Evidence Level II-1)	Spectrum extends to *Aspergillus* spp and other medically important opportunistic molds. Not approved in patients <18 y. TDM is suggested; dosing target: trough concentration of ≥0.7 mg/L.
AML and recurrent leukemia	Micafungin at 1 mg/kg every day IV; after last dose of chemotherapy until neutrophil recovery (Evidence Level II-2)	Prophylactic efficacy inferred from study in HSCT patients. Alternative for leukemia patients receiving vincristine.
AML and recurrent leukemia	Liposomal amphotericin B at 1 mg/kg every other day IV (Evidence Level II-2)	Spectrum extends to *Aspergillus* spp and other medically important opportunistic molds. Alternative antifungal for leukemia patients receiving vincristine.
Liver and pancreas transplantation	Micafungin at 1 mg/kg every day IV; from transplantation until d +30 (Evidence Level II-2)	Spectrum of antifungal activity also extends to *Aspergillus* spp.
Liver and pancreas transplantation	Liposomal amphotericin B at 1 mg/kg every other day IV (Evidence Level II-2)	Alternative agent.

Abbreviations: AML, acute myeloid leukemia; GVHD, graft-versus-host disease; HSCT, hematopoietic stem cell transplantation; IV, intravenous/intravenously; spp, species; TDM, therapeutic drug monitoring.

Adapted from Hope WW, Castagnola E, Groll AH,et al. ESCMID guideline for the diagnosis and management of Candida diseases 2012: prevention and management of invasive infections in neonates and children caused by *Candida* spp. *Clin Microbiol Infect*. 2012;18(Suppl 7):38–52, with permission from Elsevier.

Empiric Therapy

Empiric therapy is the administration of antifungal treatment in patients with clinical signs or laboratory indications of fungal infection. While colonization with *Candida* does not require therapy, if a patient is colonized at multiple sites (at least 2) and has even nonspecific signs of infection, he may need empiric antifungal therapy.

Clinical scoring systems of prediction of candidemia are used in adults, but they have not been validated in children. A clinical prediction rule for children in the PICU has been recently suggested, based on combinations of various risk factors, most important of which were presence of a central venous catheter or malignancy, use of vancomycin for longer than 3 days in the prior 2 weeks and receipt of agents against anaerobic organisms for longer than 3 days in the prior 2 weeks. As first choice empiric treatment in non-neutropenic children, fluconazole (12 mg/kg/day) or echinocandins can be used. In neutropenic children with fever refractory to administration of broad-spectrum antibiotics for 3 to 4 days, liposomal amphotericin B (3 mg/kg/day) or caspofungin (70 mg/m^2/day on day 1, then 50 mg/m^2/day) is recommended until resolution of neutropenia, because they are also active against *Aspergillus* species. Echino-candins are preferred over azoles in non-neutropenic patients with moderate to severe disease or those with a history of prior azole use as prophylaxis. There are accumulating data for the use of micafungin and anidulafungin in children.

Treatment of Documented Infections

Candidemia

Appropriate therapeutic management depends on

- Assessment of clinical status and comorbidities, prior antifungal use, possible risk factors for non-*albicans* candidemia (eg, *C tropicalis* and *C glabrata* in the context of malignancy and immunosuppression, *C parapsilosis* in central venous catheter–related candidemia)
- Species identification and antifungal susceptibility testing
- Eradication of possible foci of infection, such as infected catheters
- Close observation for evidence of treatment failure or signs of dissemination

Fluconazole is the first treatment option in the case of clinically stable, non-neutropenic patients who have no prior exposure to azoles, while an echinocandin should be chosen for moderate to severe illness or history of prophylaxis with azoles. Amphotericin B preparations (conventional or lipid) are proposed as a second choice, mainly because of either associated nephrotox-icity for conventional amphotericin B or high treatment costs for liposomal amphotericin B in the presence of equivalent less toxic or less costly alterna-tives. Voriconazole is an option when additional coverage for molds is required. Transition (step-down) to fluconazole, in cases of fluconazole-susceptible species, is advised after clinical improvement. In neutropenic patients with candidemia, fungicidal drugs, such as echinocandins or liposomal amphoteri-cin B, are preferred as first-option drugs (Table 39-3).

Azole use is discouraged in cases of infections with *C glabrata* or *C krusei* unless there is confirmation of susceptibility to them. Similarly, echinocandins may not be preferred in cases of documented *C parapsilosis* infection, because *C parapsilosis* has higher echinocandin MICs. However, there should be no treatment modification if echinocandin treatment has been initiated prior to

Table 39-3. Management of Specific *Candida* Infections (For most of the specific indications, the recommendations are Evidence Levels II-2–II-3.)

Candida Infection	First-line Antifungal	Dosage	Duration	Comments	Second-line[a]
Neonatal candidemia ± HCME	Amphotericin B deoxycholate	1 mg/kg/d	14 d (21 d for HCME)	Micafungin at 2–4 (up to 10 for HCME) mg/kg/d is an alternative.	Fluconazole, liposomal amphotericin B
Candidemia in children (non-neutropenic, stable)	Fluconazole	12 mg/kg/d	14 d from 1st negative blood	Echinocandin if critical condition.	Liposomal amphotericin B , voriconazole
Candidemia in children (non-neutropenic, critical)	Caspofungin	70 mg/m²/d on d 1, then 50 mg/m²/d	14 d from 1st negative blood	Micafungin is an alternative.	Liposomal amphotericin B
Candidemia in children (neutropenic)	Caspofungin	70 mg/m²/d on d 1, then 50 mg/m²/d	14 d from 1st negative blood	Micafungin and liposomal amphotericin B are alternatives.	None
Chronic disseminated candidiasis	Fluconazole ± corticosteroid	12 mg/kg/d	Several months		None
CNS candidiasis in children	Liposomal amphotericin B	5 mg/kg/d	At least 21 d	None	Fluconazole or voriconazole
Osteomyelitis/arthritis	Liposomal amphotericin B	5 mg/kg/d	Several weeks to months	Surgery is required.	Fluconazole

Continued

Table 39-3 *(cont)*

Candida Infection	First-line Antifungal	Dosage	Duration	Comments	Second-line[a]
CAPD peritonitis	Fluconazole, liposomal amphotericin B			Removal of the peritoneal catheter.	None
Endocarditis	Liposomal amphotericin B ± flucytosine or echinocandin		Several weeks	Early surgery necessary.	None
Pyelonephritis	Amphotericin B deoxycholate, fluconazole		14 d	Depends on species and susceptibility.	None
Oropharyngeal candidiasis	Local nystatin, oral or IV fluconazole		7 d	Maintenance may be required.	None
Esophagitis	Fluconazole		14 d	Micafungin.	None

Abbreviation: CAPD, continuous ambulatory peritoneal dialysis; CNS, central nervous system; HCME, hematogenous *Candida* meningoencephalitis; IV, intravenous.

[a] For dosages, see Table 39-1.

C parapsilosis isolation, provided the patient is stable with negative follow-up cultures.

Central venous catheters should be removed in candidemic patients, the supporting data being stronger for non-neutropenic patients than neutropenic patients. Prompt removal of other infected catheters (eg, urinary catheter) is also recommended, because candidal biofilm production hampers the efficacy of therapy.

Follow-up blood cultures should be taken to assess treatment efficacy. Treatment should last at least 14 days after documented clearance of infection from the bloodstream and resolution of symptoms, in the absence of dissemination. Funduscopy is recommended for all patients at the first week after initiation of therapy. Abdominal ultrasound imaging as well as cultures from sterile sites other than blood (ie, CSF) can be helpful if dissemination is suspected.

Organ Infections

Distinction between infection and colonization is essential in certain cases, such as candiduria and *Candida* species isolation from respiratory secretions, since it influences the decision to treat. In particular, isolated candiduria of children, in the absence of immunosuppression, usually needs no antifungal therapy, and removal of predisposing factors (ie, urinary catheter) is sufficient. If dissemination is suspected or the patient is a neonate or immunosuppressed, treatment as for candidemia is proposed. Lipid amphotericin B formulations are not preferred for treatment of urinary tract infections because of presumed low concentrations in the urinary tract. In contrast, fluconazole is an appropriate agent for susceptible urinary tract infections. Isolation of *Candida* species in respiratory tract secretions represents colonization in virtually all cases, and no antifungal therapy is required.

Therapy of organ infections usually lasts longer and can extend to months. The degree of immunosuppression and presence of foreign material, such as prosthetic valves, influence the duration and efficacy of treatment, while in many cases surgical intervention might be warranted. In most cases of deep-seated candidal infections, treatment options include fluconazole in stable patients or lipid formulations of amphotericin B alone or in combination with flucytosine. Echinocandins present an option with the exception of CNS and eye infections because of unsatisfactory penetration. Fluconazole consolidation therapy after clinical improvement is recommended in many cases.

For CNS infections such as meningitis or meningoencephalitis or infections related to foreign bodies (eg, shunts), amphotericin B preparations (conventional amphotericin B or liposomal amphotericin B) are the drugs of choice because of their sufficient CNS penetration, possibly combined with flucytosine in refractory cases. Fluconazole can also be used, alone or in combination with flucytosine. In the case of an infected shunt, it is very important that the foreign body is removed. The duration of therapy is at least 21 days.

In hepatosplenic candidiasis, mainly observed in patients with hematologic malignancies after recovery from neutropenia, prolonged therapy is required and the addition of corticosteroids might be beneficial, because an inflammatory reaction is the main driver of its pathogenesis and clinical disease.

Candidal endocarditis requires liposomal amphotericin B or an echinocandin, usually in combination, for several weeks. Early surgery is necessary in most cases. The advent of the new antifungals and use of combination therapy has improved outcome.

Treatment of endophthalmitis often requires combination therapy with fluconazole or liposomal amphotericin B and flucytosine and long-term follow-up. Voriconazole is an alternative agent with good ocular penetration. Amphotericin B intravitreal infusions are occasionally necessary for the treatment of endophthalmitis.

Osteoarticular infections require combinational approach of surgery and antifungal treatment most of the time. Antifungals that can be used are liposomal amphotericin B and fluconazole. Correct identification and susceptibility testing is very important.

Peritonitis caused by *Candida* species in patients on CAPD usually requires both systemic administration of fluconazole or liposomal amphotericin B and removal of the peritoneal catheter. Local infusions of amphotericin B may cause chemical peritonitis and may be painful. An echinocandin (eg, caspofungin), fluconazole, or voriconazole may replace amphotericin B on the basis of species identification and MIC values.

For mucocutaneous infections, such as oropharyngeal, esophageal, and genital infections, oral or local therapy with nystatin oral gel or ointment, respectively, is usually sufficient. In particular for candidal diaper dermatitis, practical measures that reduce exposure to wet diapers, as well as baby powders and zinc oxide paste, are helpful. If local therapy is not sufficient, systemic administration of an azole (fluconazole or itraconazole) is required. For esophagitis, micafungin is an alternative treatment. Because mucocutaneous infections may be refractory on the ground of immunodeficiencies, they may require maintenance therapy for a long time. The treatment of documented candidal infections is summarized in Table 39-3.

Long-term Monitoring

Neonatal candidiasis, especially when it is followed by hematogenous *Candida* meningoencephalitis, has a greater than 50% probability to develop neurodevelopmental delay with all its consequences. Therefore, a long-term neurodevelopmental follow-up is required in patients who survive.

Hepatosplenic candidiasis also needs a long-term antifungal management and follow-up of liver image and function.

Candidal infections of the long bones, especially during early infancy, may also have dismal growth sequelae and necessitate several surgical procedures.

Other organ infections may have implications on specific functions that are difficult to treat. For example, candidal endocarditis may lead to heart function problems, which need long-term follow-up having dismal implications.

Suggested Reading

Blyth CC, Chen SC, Slavin MA, et al. Not just little adults: candidemia epidemiology, molecular characterization, and antifungal susceptibility in neonatal and pediatric patients. *Pediatrics.* 2009;123(5):1360–1368

Gamaletsou MN, Kontoyiannis DP, Sipsas NV, et al. Candida osteomyelitis: analysis of 207 pediatric and adult cases (1970-2011). *Clin Infect Dis.* 2012;55(10):1338–1351

Groll AH, Castagnola E, Cesaro S, et al. Fourth European Conference on Infections in Leukaemia (ECIL-4): guidelines for diagnosis, prevention, and treatment of invasive fungal diseases in paediatric patients with cancer or allogeneic haemopoietic stem-cell transplantation. *Lancet Oncol.* 2014;15(8):e327–e340

Hope WW, Castagnola E, Groll AH, et al. ESCMID guideline for the diagnosis and management of *Candida* diseases 2012: prevention and management of invasive infections in neonates and children caused by *Candida* spp. *Clin Microbiol Infect.* 2012;18(Suppl 7):38–52

Katragkou A, Roilides E. Best practice in treating infants and children with proven, probable or suspected invasive fungal infections. *Curr Opin Infect Dis.* 2011;24(3):225–229

Pappas PG, Kauffman CA, Andes D, et al. Clinical practice guidelines for the management of candidiasis: 2009 update by the Infectious Diseases Society of America. *Clin Infect Dis.* 2009;48(5):503–535

Roilides E. Invasive candidiasis in neonates and children. *Early Hum Dev.* 2011;87(Suppl 1):S75–S76

Steinbach WJ, Roilides E, Berman D, et al. Results from a prospective, international, epidemiologic study of invasive candidiasis in children and neonates. *Pediatr Infect Dis J.* 2012;31(12):1252–1257

Stergiopoulou T, Walsh TJ. Clinical pharmacology of antifungal agents to overcome drug resistance in pediatric patients. *Expert Opin Pharmacother.* 2015;16(2):213–226

Zaoutis TE, Prasad PA, Localio AR, et al. Risk factors and predictors for candidemia in pediatric intensive care unit patients: implications for prevention. *Clin Infect Dis.* 2010;51(5):e38–e45

CHAPTER 40

Endemic Mycoses

Martin Kleiman, MD

Key Points

- Residence within, or visits to, geographic regions native to the endemic mycoses should be considered when patients present with symptoms compatible with infections caused by these agents.

- When exposed to regions in which the endemic fungi are known to exist, immunocompetent children and adolescents may have subclinical or unrecognized infections; disease is more frequent and symptomatic in those exposed to a large fungal inoculum, in infants, and in those whose cellular immunity is impaired.

- Radiographic patterns of infection may be suggestive of disease and prompt diagnostic testing in those who reside within, or travel to, an endemic region.

- Progressive disseminated disease may occur in high-risk groups and may be life-threatening.

- The decision to begin treatment with antifungals is based on confirmation of the diagnosis, disease severity, and underlying host factors that are predictive of severe illness.

- Consultation with an infectious diseases specialist is recommended in settings in which the patient has risk factors predictive of a poor outcome or the infection is accompanied by severe symptoms and a suboptimal response to treatment.

Overview

Both residents and visitors to geographically specific regions of the United States are at risk for acquiring histoplasmosis (Mississippi, Ohio, and Missouri River valleys), blastomycosis (Ohio and Mississippi River valleys, southeastern United States, states bordering the Great Lakes), and coccidioidomycosis (southwestern United States). While self-limited infection is typical in a large proportion of infections in otherwise healthy individuals, each of these pathogens is capable of causing serious illness in infants, individuals with primary or acquired disorders of cellular immunity, or, at any age, following inhalation of a large fungal inoculum. Certain populations (African Americans, those of Filipino ancestry, pregnant women, and those with cardiopulmonary disease or diabetes) have greater risk for developing disseminated infections in the setting of coccidioidomycosis.

Causes and Differential Diagnosis

The etiologic agents of histoplasmosis (*Histoplasma capsulatum*), blastomycosis (*Blastomyces dermatitidis*) and coccidioidomycosis (*Coccidioides immitis* predominant in California and *Coccidioides posadasii* in southwestern states outside of California) are dimorphic fungi.

Differential diagnosis primarily includes tuberculosis as well as noninfectious pulmonary or cardiac diseases, neoplastic disease, and other etiologies of infectious pneumonia. The risk for serious disease is greatest in individuals with immunodeficient states, organ transplant recipients, those with congenital or acquired T-cell deficiency, and those treated with biologic response modifiers (eg, tumor necrosis factor α inhibitors).

Clinical Manifestations

Histoplasmosis

Approximately 90% of histoplasmosis cases are asymptomatic. Clinical manifestations depend on the extent of disease (ie, pulmonary versus disseminated); acute, subacute, and chronic disease may occur. Typical symptoms include cough, chest pain, and fever. Radiographs may show pulmonary nodules, reticulonodular pulmonary infiltrates, and hilar or mediastinal lymphadenopathy. The latter may cause compression of bronchi, the esophagus, or other mediastinal structures. Inflammatory syndromes most commonly associated with primary infections include rheumatologic symptoms; erythema nodosum may be seen in adolescents. Clinical manifestations vary widely and are summarized in Box 40-1.

Blastomycosis

Blastomycosis is asymptomatic in approximately 50% of those infected. Fever, chest pain, fatigue, weight loss, or myalgia are commonly reported in symptomatic children. Radiographic features of infection include pulmonary infiltrates, nodules, cavitation (rare), and, following exposure to a large inoculum or in disseminated infections, diffuse reticulonodular infiltrates.

A subset of patients with pulmonary disease may progress to life-threatening illnesses accompanied by acute respiratory distress syndromes. Disseminated disease occurs in 25% to 40% of patients and most commonly presents as osteoarticular, genitourinary, or central nervous system (CNS) infection. Disseminated infection is seen most commonly in individuals with HIV infections, organ transplant recipients, and those with diabetes.

Box 40-1. Clinical Manifestations of Histoplasmosis in Children

- Asymptomatic infection
- Pulmonary disease
  - o Acute pneumonitis (mild, moderate, or severe)
  - o Mediastinal adenitis
  - o Mediastinal granuloma, fibrosis[a]
  - o Obstruction/dysfunction of mediastinal or (rarely) abdominal structures, resulting from inflammation/impingement of adjacent lymph nodes
  - o Broncholithiasis[b]
  - o Chronic disease with cavitation[b]
  - o Lithoptysis[b]
  - o Diffuse mediastinal fibrosis[b]
- Progressive disseminated infection
  - o Acute: predisposing factors
    - – Infancy (often associated with meningitis)
    - – Acquired (HIV, immunosuppressive therapy) or congenital cellular immune dysfunction
  - o Subacute[c]
  - o Chronic[c]
- Pericarditis
  - o Most commonly induced by pericardial irritation resulting from *Histoplasma*-induced lymphadenitis adjacent to the pericardium
- Presumed ocular histoplasmosis[c]
- Primary cutaneous infection[c]
- Isolated meningitis[c]

[a] Symptoms similar to those resulting from mediastinal adenitis but presentation either unassociated with other signs and symptoms of acute infection or resulting from previously unrecognized infection.
[b] Infrequent manifestation during childhood.
[c] Rare in children.

Verrucous and crusting skin lesions with regional lymphangitis and infections of osseous structures are most commonly described. Cutaneous infection may result from wound contamination or dog bites. Unlike other endemic and opportunistic fungal pathogens, *B dermatitidis* does not appear to have a propensity for causing infections in immunocompromised hosts; however, in instances in which infection occurs, it has been associated with increased mortality.

Coccidioidomycosis

Approximately 60% of primary pulmonary coccidioidomycosis (also called San Joaquin or valley fever) cases in children are subclinical or self-limited. When present, symptoms are usually flu-like and include fever, malaise, myalgia, chest pain, and headache. Erythema nodosum, multiforme, or nonspecific erythematous maculopapular rashes may accompany acute infections. Fatigue and weight loss are common and may persist for up to several months. Disseminated infection occurs in 0.5% of infected individuals and does so most commonly in infants. Additionally, individuals who have diabetes or primary cardiopulmonary disease and pregnant women in the third trimester are at increased risk for dissemination as are other specific populations (African Americans and individuals of Filipino ancestry).

In addition to the lungs, infected sites may include skin, bones, joints, soft tissues, and the CNS. Bones often affected are the spine, hands, feet, cranium, and tibia. Monoarticular joint infections may involve the ankle and knee. Meningitis, frequently accompanied by basilar inflammation and hydrocephalus, is often fatal unless treated. Albeit infrequent, infection may also result from fungal (arthroconidial) contamination of wounds; regional adenitis may accompany cutaneous manifestations.

Evaluation

Histoplasmosis

In patients with compatible symptoms and who have visited or live within endemic regions, the observation of typical yeastlike forms in histopathologic specimens constitutes strong support for the diagnosis. Isolation of *Histoplasma capsulatum* from cultures of tissue or body fluids is confirmatory; growth requires 3 to 4 weeks, thereby making culture less desirable than more rapid diagnostic methodologies. The presence of *Histoplasma* antibody, measured by complement fixation or immunodiffusion techniques performed in experienced laboratories, also offers strong support for the diagnosis. Serologic tests are less useful in patients with primary or acquired immune dysfunction. In the latter instances, quantitation of *Histoplasma* antigen concentration in urine, blood, cerebrospinal fluid, bronchoalveolar lavage fluid, or other body fluids from sites of inflammation provide strong support for the diagnosis, as well as a sensitive parameter, during and following treatment, for assessing the adequacy of response and prompt identification of relapse or reexposure. *Histoplasma* antigen detection is the most sensitive and rapid laboratory parameter for identifying acute or subacute pulmonary or progressive disseminated infections.

Blastomycosis

The diagnosis of blastomycosis is most accurately and promptly confirmed by observation of the distinctive broad-based, thick-walled, budding yeast forms in histopathologic specimens from infected sites. Recovery of *B dermatitidis* in culture is also diagnostic but requires specialized laboratory procedure. Serologic tests (immunodiffusion and complement fixation) used to detect specific antibody are not sufficiently sensitive and also cross-react with those of other endemic mycoses. Their interpretation requires recognition of characteristic disease manifestation as well as exposure to an endemic region.

Coccidioidomycosis

Growth of *Coccidioides* species in culture is definitive evidence of infection; although easily grown in its mycelial form, it poses risk to laboratory personnel. The observation of distinctive spherules within clinical specimens also confirms the diagnosis in patients with compatible illnesses and exposure to an endemic area. Serologic tests are widely used for diagnosis in immunocompetent patients. Immunoglobulin M–specific antibody is measured using tube precipitin or immunodiffusion methodology. Immunoglobulin G–specific antibody can be measured using complement fixation, enzyme immunoassay, or immunodiffusion techniques. A positive result using either method is indicative of acute or recent infection. Radiographic findings are nonspecific and include pulmonary infiltrates, pleural effusions, or micronodular pulmonary lesions. Computed tomography scans are more sensitive than plain radiographs.

Management

If drug treatment is instituted in a patient with an endemic mycosis, the typical agents of choice are amphotericin and azole antifungals (Table 40-1). In general, children tolerate amphotericin B deoxycholate better than adults; therefore, this agent can be used first-line, if an amphotericin product is indicated.

Azole antifungals may be considered for those with moderate disease and in some patients with severe manifestations of disease. Azole antifungals should be avoided in the setting of pregnancy because of teratogenicity concerns. If itraconazole is used for severe manifestations of histoplasmosis or blastomycosis, a loading dose is recommended for 3 days; then a transition should be made to maintenance dosing. If itraconazole is used, levels should be measured in those with severe infection and in patients in whom the clinical response is suboptimal. Random serum levels of greater than 1 mcg/mL are recommended when steady state is reached (approximately 2 weeks). When measured by high-pressure liquid chromatography, the sum of itraconazole and its active

Table 40-1. Drugs and Dosing for Commonly Used Antifungals

Drug	Dose	
	Non-CNS	**CNS**
Amphotericin B deoxycholate	0.7–1 mg/kg/d	1 mg/kg/d
Amphotericin B liposomal complex	3–5 mg/kg/d	5 mg/kg/d
Itraconazole	Loading dose: 10–15 mg/kg/d divided 3 times/d Maintenance dose: 5–10 mg/kg/d divided 2 times/d (maximum: 400 mg/d)	Same as non-CNS
Fluconazole	6–12 mg/kg/d (maximum: 800 mg/d)	12 mg/kg/d (maximum: 800 mg/d)

Abbreviation: CNS, central nervous system.

metabolite, hydroxy-itraconazole, should be considered. If itraconazole is used, many experts prefer the solution formulation because it results in concentrations 30% higher than those associated with use of the capsule; however, wide intersubject variability has been reported.

Histoplasmosis

Most otherwise healthy children with light or moderate fungal exposure and mild illnesses recover without receiving antifungals. Treatment is required for those exposed to large fungal inocula or who have prolonged or moderate to severe symptoms and in all instances in which with there is evidence of acquired or congenital immunodeficiency. Consensus treatment guidelines have been developed and include recommendations for treating children depending on the type of presentation (Table 40-2).

Table 40-2. Summary of Treatment Recommendations for Children/Adolescents With Histoplasmosis

	Treatment	
Manifestation	**Severe Illness**	**Moderate or Mild Illness**
Acute pulmonary	Amphotericin B, 1–2 wk, then itraconazole for 12 wk (Use of concomitant steroids is controversial.)	Persistent symptoms for >4 wk, itraconazole for 6–12 wk
Progressive disseminated (non-HIV)	Amphotericin B for 1–2 wk, then itraconazole for 6–12 mo	Itraconazole for 12 mo or same as for severe
Disseminated (with HIV)	Amphotericin B for 4–6 wk, or amphotericin followed by itraconazole[a]	Same as for severe
CNS	Amphotericin B for 4–6 wk, then itraconazole for 12 mo	Same as for severe because of poor outcome
Pericarditis[b]	NSAID for 2–12 wk	NSAID for 2–12 wk
Rheumatologic	NSAID for 2–12 wk	Same as for severe
Compression of contiguous structures by mediastinal adenitis/granuloma[c]	Prednisone, 2 mg/kg/d, concurrent itraconazole	

Abbreviations: CNS, central nervous system; NSAID, nonsteroidal anti-inflammatory drug (indomethacin, 1–3 mg/kg/d).

[a] Liposomal amphotericin B (3–5 mg/kg/d) may be superior to amphotericin B deoxycholate in patients with HIV. Therapy should continue until *Histoplasma* urinary antigen concentrations are stable and <4 ng/mL; prolonged low-level excretions may persist.

[b] Pericardial drainage for severe tamponade. Prompt administration of NSAID may obviate need for drainage in non–life-threatening manifestation of pericarditis.

[c] If differentiation between mediastinal fibrosis and granuloma is difficult, may consider treatment with itraconazole for 3 mo.

Derived from Wheat LJ, Freifeld AG, Kleiman MB, et al. Clinical practice guidelines for the management of patients with histoplasmosis: 2007 update by the Infectious Disease Society of America. *Clin Infect Dis.* 2007;45(7):807–825, with permission.

Blastomycosis

Amphotericin B deoxycholate, or a lipid preparation of amphotericin B, is recommended for the initial treatment of moderate to severe infections. Following a satisfactory clinical response, oral itraconazole may be substituted and given for a total of 12 months. Infections that are mild to moderate in severity can be treated with itraconazole. Infections that occur during pregnancy are treated with amphotericin B since the azole antifungals may be teratogenic (Table 40-3).

Coccidioidomycosis

Guidelines for treating coccidioidomycosis with antifungals in adults have been developed, but those for use in children are not established. In adults for whom the decision to treat with antifungals was based on the severity of clinical symptoms (Box 40-2), complications were identified only in those for whom treatment was elected and then subsequently discontinued. While it is estimated that 90% or greater of primary infections in otherwise healthy children resolve without antifungal treatment, it has not been determined whether use of antifungals decreases the duration or severity of symptoms. Most experts would treat children with severe infections or those with risk factors that may predispose to severe illnesses. In such settings, expert consultation should be considered (Table 40-4). In all settings, parents and older children should be educated about the activities and sites that may result in reexposure to *Coccidioides.*

Table 40-3. Summary of Treatment Recommendations for Children/Adolescents With Blastomycosis

Manifestation	Treatment	
	Severe Illness	**Moderate or Mild Illness**
Acute pulmonary	Amphotericin B, 1–2 wk, then itraconazole for total of 6–12 mo	Itraconazole for 6–12 wk
Disseminated extrapulmonary	Amphotericin B or amphotericin B for 1–2 wk, then itraconazole for 12 mo	Itraconazole for 6–12 mo[a]
CNS	Amphotericin B, 4–6 wk, then fluconazole, itraconazole, or voriconazole for 12 mo	
Immunosuppressed	Amphotericin B, 1–2 wk, then itraconazole for 12 mo	
Children	Amphotericin B, then itraconazole for 12 mo	Itraconazole for 6–12 mo

Abbreviation: CNS, central nervous system.

[a] If osteoarticular, treat for total of 12 mo.

Box 40-2. Criteria for Classification of Coccidioidomycosis as "Severe Primary Infection" in Adults

1. Complement fixation antibody titer of ≥1:16
2. Infiltrates involving more than half of 1 lung or portions of both lungs
3. Weight loss of >10%
4. Marked chest pain
5. Severe malaise
6. Inability to work or attend school
7. Intense night sweats
8. Symptoms that last more than 2 mo

Table 40-4. Summary of Treatment Recommendations for Children/Adolescents With Coccidioidomycosis

Manifestation	Treatment	
	Severe Illness	Moderate or Mild Illness
Acute pneumonia	Itraconazole or fluconazole for 3–6 mo	None
Diffuse pneumonia	Amphotericin B, then fluconazole or itraconazole for total of 12 mo	Fluconazole or itraconazole for total of 12 mo
Chronic progressive fibrocavitary pneumonia	Itraconazole or fluconazole for 12 mo	NA
Disseminated extrapulmonary[a]	Itraconazole or fluconazole for 12 mo	NA
CNS	Fluconazole indefinitely	

Abbreviation: CNS, central nervous system; NA, not applicable.
[a] Amphotericin B may be used if lesions appear to worsen rapidly or are in critical locations.

For acute coccidioidal pneumonia, fluconazole or itraconazole can be used for 3 to 6 months. In patients with diffuse pneumonia, antifungal initiation with amphotericin B may be warranted. Transition to fluconazole or itraconazole or initial therapy with these azole antifungals should be used for a total of 12 months. Follow-up is as needed every 1 to 3 months for 2 years to assess radiographic improvement or to identify complications of disease.

Oral itraconazole or fluconazole are used for initial treatment of disseminated infections that are not associated with CNS involvement. Amphotericin B deoxycholate may be substituted if improvement is slow or infected sites involve critical areas. Lipid formulations of amphotericin B can be used if the deoxycholate preparation is poorly tolerated. Fluconazole is preferred for treatment of CNS infections, and, in patients who respond to treatment, fluconazole should be continued indefinitely.

Suggested Reading

Ampel NM, Giblin A, Mourani JP, Galgiani JN. Factors and outcomes associated with the decision to treat primary pulmonary coccidioidomycosis. *Clin Infect Dis.* 2009;48(2):172–178

Anstead GM, Graybill JR. Coccidioidomycosis. *Infect Dis Clin North Am.* 2006;20(3):621–643

Bravo R, Pelayo-Katsanis LO, Shehab ZM, Katsanis E. Diagnostic and treatment challenges for the pediatric hematologist oncologist in endemic areas for coccidioidomycosis. *J Pediatr Hematol Oncol.* 2012;34(5):389–394

Chamany S, Mirza SA, Fleming JW, et al. A large histoplasmosis outbreak among high school students in Indiana, 2001. *Pediatr Infect Dis J.* 2004;23(10):909–914

Chapman SW, Dismukes WE, Proia LA, et al. Clinical practice guidelines for the management of blastomycosis: 2008 update by the Infectious Diseases Society of America. *Clin Infect Dis.* 2008;46(12):1801–1812

Chu JH, Feudtner C, Heydon K, Walsh TJ, Zaoutis TE. Hospitalizations for endemic mycoses: a population-based national study. *Clin Infect Dis.* 2006;42(6):822–825

Dotson JL, Crandall W, Mousa H, et al. Presentation and outcome of histoplasmosis in pediatric inflammatory bowel disease patients treated with antitumor necrosis factor alpha therapy: a case series. *Inflamm Bowel Dis.* 2011;17(1):56–61

Fanella S, Skinner S, Trepman E, Embil JM. Blastomycosis in children and adolescents: a 30-year experience from Manitoba. *Med Mycol.* 2011;49(6):627–632

Gaebler JW, Kleiman MB, Cohen M, et al. Differentiation of lymphoma from histoplasmosis in children with mediastinal masses. *J Pediatr.* 1984;104(5):706–709

Galgiani JN. Coccidioidomycosis. *West J Med.* 1993;159(2):153–171

Hage CA, Knox KS, Wheat LJ. Endemic mycoses: overlooked causes of community acquired pneumonia. *Respir Med.* 2012;106(6):769–776

Hage CA, Ribes JA, Wengenack NL, et al. A multicenter evaluation of tests for diagnosis of histoplasmosis. *Clin Infect Dis.* 2011;53(5):448–454

Kaplan JE1, Benson C, Holmes KK, Brooks JT, Pau A, Masur H; Centers for Disease Control and Prevention, National Institutes of Health, HIV Medicine Association of the Infectious Diseases Society of America. Guidelines for prevention and treatment of opportunistic infections in HIV-infected adults and adolescents. *MMWR Recomm Rep.* 2009;58(RR-4):1–207

Kimberlin DW, Brady MT, Jackson MA, Long SS, eds. *Red Book: 2015 Report of the Committee on Infectious Diseases.* 30th ed. Elk Grove Village IL: American Academy of Pediatrics; 2015

Martynowicz MA, Prakash UB. Pulmonary blastomycosis: an appraisal of diagnostic techniques. *Chest.* 2002;121(3):768–773

Powell DA, Schuit KE. Acute pulmonary blastomycosis in children: clinical course and follow-up. *Pediatrics.* 1979;63(5):736–740

Saccente M, Woods GL. Clinical and laboratory update on blastomycosis. *Clin Microbiol Rev.* 2010;23(2):367–381

Schutze GE, Hickerson SL, Fortin EM, et al. Blastomycosis in children. *Clin Infect Dis.* 1996;22(3):496–502

Shehab ZM. Coccidioidomycosis. *Adv Pediatr.* 2010;57(1):269–286

Smith JA, Kauffman CA. Blastomycosis. *Proc Am Thorac Soc.* 2010;7(3):173–180

Smith JA, Kauffman CA. Pulmonary fungal infections. *Respirology.* 2012;17(6):913–926

Wheat LJ. Improvements in diagnosis of histoplasmosis. *Expert Opin Biol Ther.* 2006;6(11):1207–1221

Wheat LJ, Freifeld AG, Kleiman MB, et al. Clinical practice guidelines for the management of patients with histoplasmosis: 2007 update by the Infectious Diseases Society of America. *Clin Infect Dis.* 2007;45(7):807–825

CHAPTER 41

Mucormycosis

Charalampos Antachopoulos, MD; Emmanuel Roilides, MD, PhD;
Andreas H. Groll, MD; and Thomas J. Walsh, MD, PhD

Key Points

- Mucormycosis is a rapidly progressing, life-threatening, invasive mold infection predominantly affecting children with history of uncontrolled diabetes (with or without ketoacidosis), hematologic malignancies, solid organ or hematopoietic stem cell transplantation (particularly in the presence of prolonged neutropenia, corticosteroid use, and graft-versus-host disease), and deferoxamine therapy, as well as premature neonates.

- Mucormycosis may manifest as sinus, pulmonary, cutaneous, and gastrointestinal disease, often extending to adjacent tissues, as well as disseminated infection.

- A high index of suspicion in susceptible hosts together with careful clinical assessment, imaging studies, conventional microbiologic methods, and histopathologic examination of infected tissues helps establish the diagnosis; broad, aseptate hyphae with perpendicular branching are the hallmark of this infection.

- Optimal management includes rapid initiation of treatment as soon as the diagnosis is suspected, reversal of the patient's predisposing underlying condition, appropriate antifungal therapy (lipid formulations of amphotericin B), and extensive surgical debridement.

Overview

The class Zygomycetes includes 2 orders of medically important filamentous fungi, the Mucorales and Entomophthorales. A number of medical conditions have been recognized as risk factors for the development of mucormycosis, such as diabetes (with or without ketoacidosis), hematologic malignancies, solid organ or hematopoietic stem cell transplantation (particularly in the presence of prolonged neutropenia, corticosteroid use, and graft-versus-host disease), deferoxamine therapy, injection drug use, and prematurity.

Causes and Differential Diagnosis

Mucormycosis is an invasive fungal infection with organisms of the genera *Rhizopus* and *Mucor* being most frequently implicated; less commonly, species belonging to *Cunninghamella, Lichtheimia* (formerly *Absidia*), *Apophysomyces,* and other genera are causative agents of human disease. The differential diagnosis includes bacterial and other fungal causes of sinopulmonary and central nervous system (CNS) disease.

Clinical Features

The rapidly growing Mucorales tend to cause rapidly progressive disease in susceptible hosts, which is characterized by angioinvasion, thrombosis, tissue necrosis, and extension to adjacent tissues or dissemination. Common patterns of infection include sinus disease, either localized or extended to the orbit (sino-orbital) or brain (rhinocerebral); pulmonary; cutaneous; gastrointestinal; disseminated; and miscellaneous infection.

Sinus disease is commonly observed in children with diabetes. The paranasal sinuses are initially affected, and the condition may mimic bacterial sinusitis, with nasal discharge, sinus pain, and soft-tissue swelling; fever is not a consistent symptom. Tissue discoloration commonly occurs with changes to red, violaceous, and finally black color, secondary to necrosis. Painful necrotic ulcerations in the hard palate may concomitantly be observed, suggesting extension of the infection to the mouth. Signs of extension to the orbit (sino-orbital disease) include periorbital edema, chemosis, painful eye movements, diplopia, blurring of vision, and exophthalmos. Finally, rhinocerebral disease may be manifested by focal neurologic signs and altered mental status, and complicated by cavernous sinus or internal carotid artery thrombosis.

Pulmonary disease tends to affect patients with hematologic malignancies, solid organ or hematopoietic stem cell transplant recipients, and those on deferoxamine therapy. It may present as pulmonary consolidation, infiltrates, or nodular or cavitary lesions. Rapid evolution of the lesions may be observed, and extension may occur to the chest wall, diaphragm, mediastinum, pericardium, and myocardium. Intraparenchymal bleeding is likely caused by angioinvasion. Associated signs and symptoms are nonspecific; cough, chest pain, fever, dyspnea, hemoptysis, crackles, decreased breath sounds, and wheezing have been reported.

Cutaneous disease is a common manifestation of mucormycosis in children, affecting hosts with or without immunosuppression, diabetes, or other medical conditions. It may follow direct inoculation of sporangiospores through injuries, burns, and postoperative wounds, or, rarely, hematogenous dissemination to the skin from a distant focus. Primary cutaneous mucormycosis may initially present with signs of acute inflammation (eg, erythema, tissue swelling), followed by necrosis and formation of black eschars that may slough and leave large ulcers. Without timely and aggressive therapeutic intervention, the infection extends rapidly to deep tissues, invading muscles, fat, fascial layers, tendons, and bones. Occasionally, it may spread through blood vessels to noncontiguous sites. When cutaneous mucormycosis occurs in the context of disseminated disease from a distant focus, it tends to present as nodular lesions, which may subsequently ulcerate.

Gastrointestinal disease is rare in adults but occurs more frequently in children and, in fact, is the most common clinical presentation of mucormycosis in neonates. In the neonatal population, gastrointestinal mucormycosis most frequently affects premature neonates and mimics necrotizing enterocolitis, a fact that leads to delay in diagnosis and appropriate management. Some clinical features seem to favor the diagnosis of mucormycosis over that of necrotizing enterocolitis, such as an absence of pneumatosis cystoides intestinalis; a more extensive involvement of the gastrointestinal tract, with lesions anywhere from the esophagus to large bowel (as opposed to the distal ileum and proximal colon most frequently affected in necrotizing enterocolitis); and lack of response to antibacterial agents administered for necrotizing enterocolitis. Not infrequently, mucormycosis affects multiple sites of the gastrointestinal tract, with spread of the infection to adjacent tissues and the peritoneal cavity. In a small percentage of cases, dissemination to distal sites may occur.

Disseminated mucormycosis involves at least 2 noncontiguous sites. It is commonly observed in neonates and patients treated with deferoxamine, although it may also occur in the context of severe immunosuppression. Dissemination occurs hematogenously and may originate from any of the above sites of primary infection. It appears to be most frequently associated with pulmonary disease. Common sites of dissemination include the brain and skin.

Miscellaneous manifestations of mucormycosis have also been reported, including endocarditis following cardiac surgery, isolated peritonitis in patients with peritoneal dialysis, renal infection, and malignant otitis externa.

Evaluation

Mucormycosis is a rapidly progressive infection with high death rate; timely diagnosis is essential for prompt initiation of treatment and improved outcome. Therapy should start as soon as the diagnosis is suspected and not await confirmation, which should still be pursued by all available means. The diagnosis of mucormycosis relies on a high index of suspicion in susceptible hosts together with careful clinical assessment and the combination of imaging studies, clinical microbiology, and histopathologic methods.

Clinical assessment requires knowledge of the various clinical manifestations of mucormycosis as well as the underlying conditions that are predisposed to this invasive mycosis. An alarming sign is rapid spread of the infection. Signs and symptoms of mucormycosis are often nonspecific; their prognostic significance, however, is enhanced in susceptible hosts. For example, sinus pain and facial swelling, necrotic eschars in the hard palate, or diplopia in a ketoacidotic patient should raise the suspicion of mucormycosis. Similarly, mucormycosis may be one of the causes of necrotic cutaneous lesions in a child with prolonged neutropenia. A common scenario is the development of mucormycosis in immunocompromised leukemic patients or transplant recipients receiving antifungal therapy, which is not active against the Mucorales (eg, voriconazole or echinocandins).

Imaging findings in children with mucormycosis are generally not specific and should be interpreted in the context of the patient's underlying condition. However, imaging studies help assess burden of the disease, involvement of adjacent tissues, and response to therapy. Computed tomographic scans are helpful in sinus and pulmonary disease, with greater sensitivity compared to conventional radiographs. High-resolution computed tomographic findings in pulmonary mucormycosis may include consolidation, infiltrates, nodules, cavities, and pleural effusion, as well as halo and reverse halo signs (early findings) and air crescent sign (late finding during recovery from neutropenia). Magnetic resonance images are preferred in osseous, cerebral, and cutaneous disease.

Conventional microbiologic methods for diagnosis include direct examination and culture of infected tissues, paranasal sinus secretions, sputum, or bronchoalveolar lavage. Growth of Mucorales in culture is important for identification to the genus or species level and antifungal susceptibility testing. Recovery in culture is enhanced if tissue is sliced into small pieces before inoculation; by comparison, grinding or homogenization of tissue specimens may destroy hyphae, yielding negative culture results.

Histopathologic examination of tissue specimens is often needed to confirm the diagnosis of mucormycosis. Detection of Mucorales in tissue may be difficult, because often only fragments of hyphae are seen and their morphologic characteristics may not be appreciated. It is important that the pathologist is informed regarding the possibility of mucormycosis in a particular patient.

Novel molecular diagnostic approaches, such as in situ hybridization and polymerase chain reaction, may improve the speed and sensitivity of diagnosis of mucormycosis; however, they are still investigational methods.

Management

Optimal management of mucormycosis includes
1. *Prompt initiation of treatment.* Mucorales are rapid-growing organisms in vivo; delay in initiation of appropriate treatment has been associated with increased mortality. Therefore, therapy should be initiated as soon as the diagnosis is suspected.
2. *Reversal of the patient's underlying predisposing condition.* Reversal of the underlying condition predisposing to mucormycosis is important in

improving outcome. Examples include control of diabetes, discontinuation/tapering of steroids, reduction of immunosuppressive therapy, discontinuation of deferoxamine therapy, and administration of hematopoietic growth factors in patients with neutropenia.

3. *Appropriate antifungal therapy.* First-line treatment of mucormycosis includes lipid formulations of amphotericin B, such as liposomal amphotericin B or amphotericin B lipid complex. Limited data suggest greater efficacy of liposomal amphotericin B over amphotericin B lipid complex in the case of CNS infection. Optimal dosages of these 2 agents for treatment of mucormycosis have not been defined. Doses of 5 to 10 mg/kg/day for liposomal amphotericin B and 5 to 7.5 mg/kg/day for amphotericin B lipid complex have been used. Therefore, both agents could be administered at 5 or greater mg/kg/day, with higher doses considered for CNS infections. Data on optimal duration of treatment are lacking; this should be continued until resolution of clinical/imaging findings and immune reconstitution, which may take months or even years. Unapproved options for second-line therapy of mucormycosis, in the case of no response (or intolerance) to amphotericin B, include combination of lipid formulations of amphotericin B with caspofungin (limited clinical data exist only for caspofungin, but promising results have been demonstrated in vivo using micafungin and anidulafungin as well) and posaconazole orally (delayed-release tablets) or intravenously for patients 13 years or older at 300 mg once a day (day 1: 300 mg twice a day). Some experts suggest an overlap of 5 or more days with first-line therapy until steady state concentrations are achieved. Oral posaconazole may also be considered for switch from intravenous amphotericin B therapy in stable or improving patients. Monitoring of posaconazole serum levels is recommended. Isavuconazole, a recently approved triazole for primary treatment of mucormycosis in adults, has not yet been studied in children.

4. *Extensive surgical debridement.* Appropriate surgical debridement has been associated with improved outcome in patients with mucormycosis. It is strongly recommended for sinus (or sino-orbital) and cutaneous disease and should be discussed for localized pulmonary disease. Surgery should be considered early in the course of treatment and aim at "aggressively" removing all infected or possibly infected tissues. It may include excision of infected sinuses, debridement of retro-orbital space, lobectomy/pneumonectomy, or limb amputation. It may be repeated if necessary. If the patient survives, plastic surgery may be needed to correct disfiguring resulting from debridement.

Because of the rarity of this devastating infection, consultation by physicians experienced in the management of invasive mycoses is recommended.

Suggested Reading

Gonzalez CE, Rinaldi MG, Sugar AM. Zygomycosis. *Infect Dis Clin North Am.* 2002;16(4):895–914

Groll AH, Castagnola E, Cesaro S, et al. Fourth European Conference on Infections in Leukaemia (ECIL-4): guidelines for diagnosis, prevention, and treatment of invasive fungal diseases in paediatric patients with cancer or allogeneic haemopoietic stem-cell transplantation. *Lancet Oncol.* 2014;15(8):e327–e340

Roilides E, Zaoutis TE, Walsh TJ. Invasive zygomycosis in neonates and children. *Clin Microbiol Infect.* 2009;15(Suppl 5):50–54

Spellberg B, Edwards J Jr, Ibrahim A. Novel perspectives on mucormycosis: pathophysiology, presentation, and management. *Clin Microbiol Rev.* 2005;18(3):556–569

Spellberg B, Ibrahim A, Roilides E, et al. Combination therapy for mucormycosis: why, what, and how? *Clin Infect Dis.* 2012:54(Suppl 1):S73–S78

Stergiopoulou T, Walsh TJ. Clinical pharmacology of antifungal agents to overcome drug resistance in pediatric patients. *Expert Opin Pharmacother.* 2015;16(2):213–226

Walsh TJ, Gamaletsou MN, McGinnis MR, Hayden RT, Kontoyiannis DP. Early clinical and laboratory diagnosis of invasive pulmonary, extrapulmonary, and disseminated mucormycosis (zygomycosis). *Clin Infect Dis.* 2012;54(Suppl 1):S55–S60

Zaoutis TE, Roilides E, Chiou CC, et al. Zygomycosis in children: a systematic review and analysis of reported cases. *Pediatr Infect Dis J.* 2007;26(8):723–727

PART

1

Infectious Diseases

CHAPTER 42

Intestinal Helminthic Infections

Benjamin R. Hanisch, MD,[a] and Chandy C. John, MD, MS

Key Points

- Inquiry regarding travel, exposures, and country of origin is vital to diagnose helminthic infections.

- Not all helminthic infections present with diarrhea or eosinophilia; some infections may present years after exposure.

- *Enterobius vermicularis* (common pinworm) infection is the most common intestinal helminthic infection in the United States and is diagnosed with the tape test, rather than through examination of stool for ova and parasites.

- Early *Ascaris* infection can cause pulmonary eosinophilia (Löffler syndrome) because of larval migration, with symptoms of cough, fever, and wheezing. Patients with Löffler syndrome may have eosinophilia but typically do not have *Ascaris* eggs on stool examination.

- *Ancylostoma duodenale* and *Necator americanus* (hookworm) infections are a leading cause of anemia in childhood for children of low- and middle-income countries.

- Treatment of a patient with *Strongyloides* infection with steroids or other immunosuppressive medications can lead to hyperinfection, gram-negative sepsis, and death. Any person from an at-risk area should be screened by testing at least 3 stools for *Strongyloides* prior to initiation of steroids or other immunosuppressive therapy.

Overview

Helminths have a disproportionate burden on tropical and subtropical regions where clean water and public sanitation are lacking. In addition to acute illness, chronic infections affect growth and cognitive development. With the dramatic increase in world travel and immigration, awareness of helminthic infections throughout the world is important to provide quality care to children in pediatric practices in the United States and beyond.

[a] Dr Hanisch's work on this paper was supported in part by grant ST32HD068229 (PI: Schleiss, MR) from the Eunice Kennedy Shriver National Institute of Child Health and Development.

Causes and Differential Diagnosis

Helminthic infections that affect humans are generally divided into 3 major groups: nematodes (roundworms), cestodes (tapeworms), and trematodes (flukes). Roundworm agents of importance include *Enterobius vermicularis* (common pinworm), *Ascaris lumbricoides, Ancylostoma duodenale* and *Necator americanus* (hookworm), *Strongyloides stercoralis,* and *Trichuris trichiura* (whipworm). Common tapeworms include *Diphyllobothrium latum* (fish tapeworm), *Hymenolepis nana* (dwarf tapeworm), *Taenia saginata* (beef tapeworm), *Taenia solium* (pork tapeworm), and *Dipylidium caninum.* Intestinal flukes are less frequently encountered.

Pinworm infection, ascariasis, and trichuriasis are most commonly identified in US-born children. Clinicians should be aware that parasitic infections of any type should be considered in foreign immigrants, internationally adopted children, and travelers returning from endemic areas, depending on their clinical exposure history. Clinical disease may be serious if immunosuppressive medications are given in the setting of certain helminths (*Strongyloidiasis*), and disease may be more severe if acquired in the immunocompromised patient.

Given that the primary clinical feature of most helminthic infections is abdominal pain or diarrhea, the differential diagnosis generally includes other gastrointestinal (GI) infectious agents, GI diseases including celiac disease and inflammatory bowel diseases, or other malabsorption syndromes. Many helminthic infections cause eosinophilia, and the differential diagnosis includes hypersensitivity reactions, drug reactions, and certain malignancies (eg, lymphoma, leukemia). For helminths that present with features of central nervous system involvement, epilepsy may be considered if the clinical presentation is an afebrile seizure (ie, neurocysticercosis). If fever and features of meningoencephalitis or eosinophilic meningitis are present, other infectious agents can be considered along with certain neoplasms and drug reactions.

Clinical Features

Intestinal Nematodes (Roundworms)

Common pinworm is the most common gut helminth in US school children aged 5 to 10 years. High worm burden may result in abdominal pain, nausea, and vomiting. Pinworms are occasionally found in the appendix, though it is unclear if it is the cause of appendicitis. It may also cause eosinophilic enterocolitis, which is unassociated with a peripheral eosinophilia. Ectopic migration may give rise to vaginal infections and has been associated with urinary tract infections.

Ascaris lumbricoides is the most common intestinal helminthic parasite worldwide. It is most frequent in tropical countries with areas of poor sanitation. The adult worms live in the ileum and jejunum. Infection is acquired through ingestion of eggs, through contaminated food, or most commonly through dirty hands. The eggs hatch in the intestine and are then are carried hematogenously to the liver or lungs. One to 2 weeks after exposure, the larvae migrate through the lungs up the bronchial tree, which may cause a pneumonitis (Löffler syndrome) or hypersensitivity reaction, particularly in those who have been previously exposed. The larvae are then swallowed and return to the intestine where they mature. The infection is often asymptomatic and noticed when adult worms pass per rectum or are vomited. Early infection (within 4–6 weeks of ingestion) that leads to larval migration may be asymptomatic or manifest as Löffler syndrome, with symptoms of cough, fever, shortness of breath, and wheezing. Late or established infection (6–8 weeks after egg ingestion) may also be asymptomatic or present with abdominal pain (often epigastric), a dry cough, nausea, and vomiting. Chronic infections may lead to malabsorption. Severe disease may result from migration into the biliary tree, causing cholangitis; from migration to the appendix; or from mechanical bowel obstruction (most commonly at the ileocecal valve), sometimes leading to intussusception or volvulus.

Whipworm is primarily found in tropical regions as well as rural areas of the southern United States. Infection occurs after ingestion of ova and larva and then matures in the intestine. Worms may live in the intestine 2 to 3 years, and reinfection is common. Infections are often asymptomatic, but heavy infection may lead to abdominal cramps, nocturnal stooling, diarrhea containing mucus or blood, rectal bleeding, and anemia. Rectal prolapse occurs with heavy worm burden. Growth restriction, pica, and clubbing may be other indications of chronic infection.

Hookworm is a common cause of moderate and severe anemia worldwide. *Ancylostoma duodenale* and *N americanus* are the 2 species responsible for most hookworm infections in humans. Hookworm is most commonly found in tropical and subtropical regions. Areas with poor sanitation and frequent walking barefoot are at highest risk. Both species of hookworm are acquired through larval penetration of the skin in contact with soil contaminated with feces, usually the feet. *Ancylostoma duodenale* may also be acquired by oral ingestion. Penetration of skin may result in a localized erythematous, pruritic rash at the site of entry. This may then develop to a serpiginous rash called cutaneous larva migrans. After skin penetration or ingestion, it travels to the lungs and may result in an eosinophilic pneumonitis similar to that observed with *Ascaris*. The larvae proceed up the bronchial tree and are subsequently swallowed and mature in the intestinal tract. They may live in the gut for a decade and may cause anemia in a matter of months. Infected individuals may develop low protein concentrations in blood, diarrhea, abdominal pain, or midepigastric pain worse with eating, resulting in malnourishment. Growth and cognitive delay in addition to anemia have been associated with chronic illness. Patients may also present in high output heart failure because of progressive anemia.

Strongyloides stercoralis infection is common throughout the world, particularly in warmer climates. Larvae penetrate skin from soil contaminated with feces or through ingestion. After entering the circulation system, the larvae travel to the lungs where they ascend the bronchial tree and are then swallowed. In the intestines, they develop into adults and lay and fertilize eggs. These eggs hatch, and the larvae may be passed in the stool or develop into adults and repeat the life cycle though penetration of the colon or perianal skin. Persistent infection may present years after leaving the endemic area. This infection is most commonly asymptomatic, but it may produce epigastric pain that is similar to a peptic ulcer but aggravated by food consumption. A large parasite burden may cause diarrhea, nausea, and vomiting; protein-losing enteropathy; or edema. In chronic infections, symptoms are often intermittent. Other symptoms include recurring urticaria, particularly on the buttocks and wrists. Larva currens, which is a serpiginous, pruritic, elevated rash, may develop along the tract of larval migration of the skin in the perianal, gluteal, or other body areas. Larval migration in the lungs can cause pulmonary eosinophilia syndrome, with dry cough, fever, and wheezing. A previously asymptomatic host who becomes immunocompromised can develop severe disease with an overwhelming parasite burden and accompanying gram-negative bacteremia and sepsis. A patient's risk of having an unrecognized parasitic infection must be considered prior to prescription of immunosuppressants, including cortico-steroids. This is a particular concern in patients who may have wheezing from tropical pulmonary eosinophilia caused by *Strongyloides* infection.

Capillariasis is attributed in most cases to *Capillaria philippinensis*. It is most common in East Asia and acquired through consumption of raw fresh-water fish or birds that eat freshwater fish. After consumption, the worms dwell in the intestine and lay eggs that pass in the stool; however, autoinfection from eggs hatching that are still in the intestine occurs. Symptoms include watery diarrhea, fever, and abdominal pain. Severe infection may result in edema, muscle wasting, malabsorption, and protein-losing enteropathy. Some cases involve the lung or liver and have been associated with hepatitis, cough, and pneumonia.

Intestinal Trematodes (Flukes)

Fasciolopsis buski infection occurs on ingestion of encysted metacercariae on aquatic plants, which then develop in the intestine. This infection occurs primarily in India and East Asia. Areas where runoff from pigs may contaminate the water supply are at highest risk. Symptoms may develop 3 months after ingestion. Infections are usually asymptomatic unless there is a high parasite burden. This manifests with diarrhea, abdominal pain and fever, ascites, and intestinal obstruction. Intestinal ulcerations and abscesses may develop, compli-cating the course and contributing to malabsorption and anemia.

Intestinal Cestodes (Tapeworms)

Fish tapeworm is acquired through ingestion of cysts in freshwater fish that are consumed raw or undercooked. *Diphyllobothrium latum* is the most common etiology. Symptoms are often minimal and include vague abdominal pain (internal sensation of movement), diarrhea, weakness, and dizziness. Prolonged infection may result in vitamin B_{12} deficiency.

Dwarf tapeworm is acquired though infected humans; it is the only tapeworm transmitted human to human. It is found worldwide, including the southeastern United States. Once established, the tapeworm can complete its life cycle within the host. It presents with mild abdominal discomfort. It may present with diarrhea and vague neurologic symptoms, including headaches, dizziness, and sleep disturbance.

Beef tapeworm is the most common and widespread tapeworm and is acquired through consuming cysts in undercooked beef. On ingestion, larvae penetrate the GI tract, enter circulation, and encyst in muscle. Patients may present with mild abdominal discomfort, though will rarely have severe disease.

Pork tapeworm/cysticercosis. Taenia solium is also known as pork tapeworm and is found in areas where pigs may come in contact with human waste. The infection comes from ingestion of undercooked pork, and the tapeworm sheds eggs in the GI tract. The human host then transmits the infection to others. After ingestion, the larvae proceed to the blood where they may go on to form cysts in muscle, brain, or other organs. Only a small percentage of those infected have symptoms, and incidental diagnosis on imaging for other reasons is common. More severe disease presents with signs of local inflammation and mass effect. Infection of the brain (neurocysticercosis) is the most common clinical presentation of pork tapeworm infection. Patients with neurocysticercosis usually present with seizures, and in more severe cases may develop hydrocephalus and arachnoiditis. Neurocysticercosis may be responsible for approximately 30% of seizures in low- and middle-income countries where pork is eaten.

Dipylidium caninum infection is found worldwide and contracted most commonly by children through close proximity with dogs. Ingestion of an infected flea transmits the infection. The infection is often asymptomatic, though it may result in mild GI symptoms. The worm may pass from the rectum, and motile proglottids may be visualized. The dog may also be symptomatic and show signs of anal pruritus.

Evaluation

Stool examination for ova and parasites is the test of choice to diagnose most helminthic infections with the exception of common pinworm, for which the tape test is preferred (Table 42-1). If a worm is identified in the child's stool by a parent, the relative large size of the worm may be suggestive of a specific agent; the worms of *A lumbricoides* tend to be quite large.

Serologic studies should be considered for diagnosis of strongyloidiasis and neurocysticercosis. Peripheral eosinophilia occurs when the helminths invade tissue. Eosinophilia does not occur if the infection is limited to the intestine.

Table 42-1. Evaluation for Various Helminthic Infections

Pathogen	Stool	Serology	Peripheral Eosinophilia	Anemia	Imaging	Respiratory Secretions	Tape Test
Enterobius vermicularis (common pinworm)							X
Ascariasis	X		X		X GI tract	X Löffler syndrome	
Trichuris trichiura (whipworm)	X		X				
Ancylostoma duodenale (hookworm)	X		X	X			
Strongyloidiasis	X	X	X			X Hyperinfection	
Capillariasis	X						
Diphyllobothrium latum (fish tapeworm)	X						
Hymenolepis nana (dwarf tapeworm)	X						
Taenia saginata (beef tapeworm)	X		X				
Taenia solium (pork tapeworm)	X	X			X Neurologic		
Dipylidium caninum	X						

Abbreviation: GI, gastrointestinal.

Eosinophilia is most common in *Ascaris,* whipworm, and *Strongyloides* infections.

Common pinworm diagnosis. The adult worm is approximately 1 cm long and occasionally visualized near the perianal region while the child is sleeping. The "clear tape test" consists of pressing clear tape against skin around the anus to adhere eggs to the tape that may be visualized under a microscope. The eggs are typically bean shaped. This is most sensitive at night or early in the morning prior to bathing. Repeated 3 times this test is approximately 90% sensitive. Analysis of stool for eggs is unhelpful.

Ascariasis diagnosis. Ascaris lumbricoides infection is usually diagnosed by stool microscopy, looking for *Ascaris* eggs. Adult worms are sometimes seen by patients in excreted stool, and can be quite large. Eggs typically appear in the stool more than 30 days after infection, so testing by stool microscopy is often negative in individuals with Löffler syndrome. Larvae may be found in respiratory secretions during the pulmonary phase. Peripheral eosinophilia may be observed in early infection, when larvae pass through the lungs, but is often absent in individuals with established GI infection. Imaging of the upper GI tract with contrast and small-bowel follow-through, or imaging by ultrasound or computed tomography, may show intestinal worms if there is a high worm burden. Endoscopic retrograde cholangiopancreatography may be needed if biliary involvement is suspected. Serology is not used for clinical diagnosis.

Trichuriasis diagnosis. Examine the stool for eggs. The worm may be visualized on proctoscopy or colonoscopy. Ongoing tissue invasion often leads to a peripheral eosinophilia in patients with heavy infection.

Hookworm diagnosis. Anemia in a person from an area endemic with hookworm should have a stool sample sent to evaluate for hookworm ova. The eggs are detectable in the stool 6 to 8 weeks after initial infection; several specimens are often required. Adult worms are rarely seen in stool samples. There often is a peripheral eosinophilia 1 to 2 months after infection. Reinfection from the environment after treatment is extremely common.

Strongyloidiasis diagnosis. Serial stool samples (up to 7) are needed to identify larvae and are consistently negative in approximately 25% of patients. Serologic evaluation may be helpful in initial diagnosis, and antibodies to *Strongyloides* decline following treatment. Eosinophilia is variable and often minimal or absent in chronic infections and hyperinfections. In cases of suspected hyperinfection, larvae may be found in sputum, cerebrospinal fluid, or other sampled fluid collections.

Capillariasis diagnosis. Examination of stool or histopathology of the intestine for eggs or larvae may establish the diagnosis.

Fasciolopsis diagnosis. The adult worm or eggs may be identified in the stool.

Fish tapeworm diagnosis. Examination of stool showing eggs or proglottids is diagnostic. Contrast studies may be helpful. There are no reliable serologic tests.

Dwarf tapeworm diagnosis. Identification of the eggs or motile proglottids in stool specimens is diagnostic.

Beef tapeworm diagnosis. Eggs and parasite can be identified in the stool. Identification of species is important to assess risk of cystelcosis caused by pork tapeworm and not beef tapeworm. Stool antigen testing is available and may be helpful. Eosinophilia is common.

Pork tapeworm diagnosis. Neuroimaging is required to make a diagnosis of neurocysticercosis. A non-enhancing ring lesion on a computed tomographic scan is the classic finding in neurocysticercosis. Patients may have multiple such lesions. Guidelines have been established for definitive diagnosis and treatment of neurocysticercosis. Characteristic imaging features in individuals from endemic areas are the primary finding used to establish the diagnosis. Antibody assays that detect specific antibody to larval pork tapeworm in serum are important in confirming the diagnosis, and antibodies to pork tapeworm antigens in the cerebrospinal fluid are a helpful additional testing method. Cerebrospinal fluid typically shows a monocytic pleocytosis, elevated protein concentration, and normal glucose concentration. Epidemiology is important: a history of living in endemic areas (eg, Mexico and many countries in Central and South America), travel to these areas, or the presence of a household contact with pork tapeworm infection is key. Surgical pathology is usually not required to make the diagnosis. Examination of stool may be helpful.

Dipylidium caninum diagnosis. Infection is established though observation of the motile proglottid or eggs in the stool.

Management

Common pinworm. Albendazole and mebendazole are available for treatment of pinworms; pyrantel pamoate is an alternative that is significantly less costly and available without a prescription (Table 42-2). There is limited experience with use of pinworm medications in the baby younger than 12 months of age. Most cases resolve after 1 dose, and treatment is nearly 100% effective with 2 doses. Family members are often infected, and treatment of the entire family is indicated. Relapsing infections are common and may require monthly treatment to break the cycle of reinfection due to eggs remaining in the environment. Reinfection risk may be decreased by preventive methods such as washing the anal area in the morning, changing underwear and bed linens regularly, laundering in hot water, avoiding scratching of the infected area, cleaning toilet seats daily, and regular hand washing.

Ascariasis. Albendazole is the recommended therapy (Table 42-2). Antihelminthic treatment is usually not initiated during the pulmonary phase because of concern for exacerbation of hypersensitivity reaction, but inhaled beta-agonists may be helpful at this stage. Surgery or endoscopy may be indicated if symptoms are caused by intestinal, biliary, or pancreatic obstruction. Patients should be reevaluated 2 to 3 months after therapy with stool microscopy to ensure clearance. Testing of other family members may also be beneficial.

Trichuriasis. Albendazole is recommended; ivermectin is an alternative (Table 42-2). Repeat examination of the stool 2 weeks after treatment is recommended.

Hookworm. Albendazole is the treatment of choice along with treatment of the iron deficiency. Repeat examination 2 weeks after treatment is recommended.

Strongyloidiasis. Ivermectin is recommended for treatment (Table 42-2), and has been found to be more effective than albendazole. In immunocompromised patients, prolonged or dual therapy with ivermectin and albendazole may be needed. Serial stool examinations should be continued for weeks to months after therapy to confirm parasite clearance.

Capillariasis. Recommended treatment is albendazole at 400 mg orally for 10 days. Relapse is not uncommon and should be treated with a longer duration of therapy.

Fasciolopsiasis. Praziquantel at 75 mg/kg/day in 3 divided doses for 1 day is the treatment of choice.

Fish tapeworm. Praziquantel is the treatment of choice, and niclosamide is an alternative (Table 42-3). Stool samples should be checked for clearance in 1 month to document clearance.

Dwarf tapeworm. Praziquantel is the recommended therapy, and niclosamide is an alternative (Table 42-3). Praziquantel is not approved by the US Food and Drug Administration for this indication. Stool samples should be checked for clearance in 1 month to document clearance.

Beef tapeworm. Praziquantel is recommended, and niclosamide is an alternative (Table 42-3). Test of cure after 3 months is recommended.

Neurocysticercosis. Patients with only subcutaneous or muscular lesions often do not require treatment. For those with symptomatic lesions, anti-inflammatory medication or excision of the lesion may be required. Treatment of ocular cysticercosis is complex, requiring consultation with an ophthalmologist and treatment with albendazole and corticosteroids. Treatment for neurocysticercosis is likewise complex, and should be done in consultation with an infectious diseases specialist and neurologist familiar with the disease for cysticercosis. Single lesions may be observed or treated with a combination of albendazole and steroids, while multiple lesions (>5) are almost always treated. Concurrent epilepsy should be treated with antiseizure medications. Complex disease with hydrocephalus or increased intracranial pressure requires neurosurgical consultation. An excellent review of treatment guidelines was published in 2002, is available open access through PubMed Central, and is the current standard for recommendations while new guidelines are being promulgated.

Dipylidium caninum. Praziquantel at 5 to 10 mg/kg is the recommended treatment, though it is not approved by the US Food and Drug Administration for this indication. An alternative therapy is niclosamide at 50 mg/kg up to 2 g once.

Table 42-2. Common Intestinal Nematodes (Roundworms)

	Enterobius vermicularis (Common Pinworm)	*Ascaris lumbricoides*	*Trichuris trichiura* (Whipworm)	*Ancylostoma duodenale and Necator americanus* (Hookworm)	*Strongyloides stercoralis*
Route of infection	Ingestion	Ingestion	Ingestion	Percutaneous	Percutaneous or internal with ongoing autoinfection
Adult worm size	0.2–1.3 cm	1.5–4 cm	4 cm	0.5–1.3 cm	2–2.5 mm
Adult worms seen in stool?	Rarely (Use tape test.)	Yes	Yes	Rarely, but eggs seen	Rarely, but larvae seen
Person to person	Yes	No	No	No	Yes
Principal symptoms and signs	Perianal pruritus	Early: cough, wheezing, fever (Löffler syndrome) Late: abdominal pain, GI or biliary tract obstruction, respiratory symptoms	Most infected individuals are asymptomatic; with heavy worm burden, may develop abdominal pain, loose stools, failure to thrive, anemia, growth stunting, or rectal prolapse.	Early: rash at site of entry, abdominal pain, wheezing, fever (Löffler syndrome) Late: anemia	GI symptoms, larva currens, respiratory, disseminated disease, secondary bacteremia
Duration of infection	1 mo	1–2 y	1–3 y	1–10 y	Lifetime of host

Diagnosis	Clear tape test	Eggs in stool or sputum. Upper gastrointestinal tract endoscopy may identify intestinal worms; ultrasound or computed tomography scan may reveal biliary tree involvement.	Eggs in stool, rectal prolapse	Eggs in stool, cutaneous larva migrans	Larvae in stool, aspirate of duodenal, pulmonary fluids, serology
Eosinophilia	–	+ in early infection (Löffler syndrome) – in established GI infection	+ in heavy infection – in light infection	+	±
Recommended treatment	Albendazole: <20 kg, 200 mg orally once; ≥20 kg, 400 mg orally once; repeat in 2 wk	Albendazole: 400 mg orally once OR mebendazole 500 mg orally once	Albendazole: 400 mg orally for 3 days	Albendazole: 400 mg orally once (may repeat if necessary) Treatment of concurrent iron deficiency if present.	Ivermectin: 200 mcg/kg/d orally for 2 d Prolonged or repeated course potentially needed in those with immuno-suppression.
Alternative treatment	Pyrantel pamoate: 11 mg/kg orally once (maximum: 1 g/d); repeated in 2 wk	Ivermectin: 150–200 mcg/kg orally once	Ivermectin: 200 mcg/kg orally for 3 d OR mebendazole 100 mg orally twice daily for 3 d	Pyrantel pamoate: 11 mg/kg (maximum: 1 g/d), orally for 3 d	Albendazole: 400 mg orally twice daily for 7 d

Abbreviation: GI, gastrointestinal.

Drug information adapted from Preferred therapy for specific parasitic pathogens. In: *Nelson's Pediatric Antimicrobial Therapy*. 22nd ed. Bradley JS, Nelson JD, et al, eds. Elk Grove Village, IL: American Academy of Pediatrics; 2016:159–176.

Table 42-3. Common Intestinal Cestodes (Tapeworms)

	Diphyllobothrium latum (Fish Tapeworm)	*Taenia saginata* (Beef Tapeworm)	*Taenia solium* (Pork Tapeworm)	*Hymenolepis nana*	*Dipylidium caninum*
Route of infection	Ingestion	Ingestion	Ingestion	Ingestion	Ingestion
Adult worm size, cm	600	400	200–700	3–4	20
Adult worms seen in stool?	No	Yes	Yes	No	Yes
Person to person	No	No	Yes	Yes	No
Principle symptoms	Abdominal pain, weakness, dizziness	Abdominal pain, nausea, anorexia	Abdominal discomfort, seizures, subcutaneous nodules	Abdominal discomfort, headaches	Abdominal discomfort
Duration of infection	6 mo–10 y	6 mo–20 y	2 mo–lifetime of host	1–3 y	1–3 mo
Diagnosis	Eggs in stool	Eggs or proglottids in stool, stool antigens	Eggs or proglottids in stool, serologic, CT	Eggs in stool, serologic	Proglottids or egg packets in stool
Eosinophilia	No	Yes	No	Yes	No
Recommended treatment	Praziquantel: 5–10 mg/kg orally once	Praziquantel: 5–10 mg/kg orally once	Praziquantel: 5–10 mg/kg orally once Neurocysticercosis: Consult an Infectious disease expert regarding treatment options.	Praziquantel: 25 mg/kg orally once	Praziquantel: 5–10 mg/kg orally once
Alternative treatment				Nitazoxanide[a]: Children aged 12–47 months, 100 mg orally twice daily for 3 d Children 4–11 years, 200 mg orally twice daily for 3 d	

Abbreviation: CT, computed tomography.

[a] Centers for Disease Control and Prevention. Hymenolepiasis: treatment information. *Laboratory Identification of Parasitic Diseases of Public Health Concern* Web site. http://www.cdc.gov/dpdx/hymenolepiasis/tx.html. Updated November 29, 2013. Accessed September 15, 2016.
Drug information adapted from Preferred therapy for specific parasitic pathogens. In: *Nelson's Pediatric Antimicrobial Therapy.* 22nd ed. Bradley JS, Nelson JD, et al, eds. Elk Grove Village, IL: American Academy of Pediatrics; 2016:159–176.

Suggested Reading
• • • • • • • • • • • • • • • • • •

Centers for Disease Control and Prevention. Laboratory Identification of Parasites of Public Health Concern Web site. http://www.dpd.cdc.gov/dpdx. Accessed April 5, 2016

Craig P, Ito A. Intestinal cestodes. *Curr Opin Infect Dis.* 2007;20(5):524–532

Drugs for Parasitic Infections. Vol 11. New Rochelle, NY: The Medical Letter Inc; 2013

García HH, Evans CA, Nash TE, et al. Current consensus guidelines for treatment of neurocysticercosis. *Clin Microbiol Rev.* 2002;15(4):747–756

Jia TW, Melville S, Utzinger J, King CH, Zhou XN. Soil-transmitted helminth reinfection after drug treatment: a systematic review and meta-analysis. *PLoS Negl Tropl Dis.* 2012;6(5):e1621

Keiser J, Utzinger J. Efficacy of current drugs against soil-transmitted helminth infections: systematic review and meta-analysis. *JAMA.* 2008;299(16):1937–1948

Montes M, Sawhney C, Barros N. *Strongyloides stercoralis:* there but not seen. *Curr Opin Infect Dis.* 2010;23(5):500–504

Steinmann P, Utzinger J, Du ZW, et al. Efficacy of single-dose and triple-dose albendazole and mebendazole against soil-transmitted helminths and *Taenia* spp: a randomized controlled trial. *PLoS One.* 2011;6(9):e25003

Suputtamongkol Y, Premasathian N, Bhumimuang K, et al. Efficacy and safety of single and double doses of ivermectin versus 7-day high dose albendazole for chronic strongyloidiasis. *PLoS Negl Trop Dis.* 2011;5(5):e1044

CHAPTER 43

Malaria

Keren Z. Landman, MD, and Paul M. Arguin, MD

Key Points

- Malaria should be considered in all febrile patients returning from malaria-endemic regions.

- Severe disease most commonly occurs with *Plasmodium falciparum* infection, but all malaria species can cause severe infections.

- Microscopy continues to be the diagnostic technique of choice, and rapid antigen testing, if available, can be used in parallel; polymerase chain reaction is the best technique for species confirmation.

- Treatment decisions depend on the infecting species and severity of disease; those with severe disease require intensive care and parenteral treatment.

- Bed nets, mosquito repellents, and chemoprophylaxis are the keys to prevention of mosquito-borne infection.

Overview

In 2015, an estimated 214 million cases of malaria occurred worldwide and 438,000 people died, most of them children. In the United States, malaria is encountered primarily as an imported disease (ie, a disease contracted while the patient is either a resident of or traveler to a malaria-endemic country). In 2013, 1,727 cases of malaria were reported in the United States, 291 (17%) of them in people younger than 18 years. Because these infections are largely preventable, the general pediatrician can play an important role in educating caregivers about malaria prevention and empowering them to provide appropriate chemoprophylaxis to the pediatric traveler.

Causes and Differential Diagnosis

Five species of *Plasmodium* are responsible for human malaria infections: *Plasmodium falciparum, Plasmodium vivax, Plasmodium ovale, Plasmodium malariae,* and *Plasmodium knowlesi. Plasmodium falciparum* is the most common cause of malaria worldwide, and comprises most imported cases in the United States. It is also the most common cause of severe malaria—also known as complicated malaria—and is responsible for the bulk of deaths from malarial infection.

The second most common cause of imported and endemic malaria is *P vivax*. Although malaria caused by *P vivax* is less likely to be fatal than that caused by *P falciparum,* this parasite can cause severe disease. Additionally, it can cause relapses of disease long after initial clearance of the blood-stage parasite if incompletely treated.

Plasmodium ovale, also a cause of relapsing malaria, and *P malariae* have much smaller geographic foci and cause a less severe spectrum of disease, while *P knowlesi* has only recently become recognized as an agent of human disease in parts of Southeast Asia.

Plasmodium infection is overwhelmingly the result of mosquito bites sustained in malaria-endemic areas, although isolated cases of congenital transmission and induced transmission by transfusion and intravenous drug use have been documented. Among travelers returning from endemic areas, malaria is a significant etiology of systemic febrile illness that can have dire consequences if not diagnosed and treated right away.

In the febrile returned traveler with 3 negative malaria smears, other diagnoses should be considered in context of the country visited and presence of other symptoms. Dengue, chikungunya, rickettsial disease, and influenza have considerable clinical overlap with uncomplicated malaria, as do mononucleosis syndromes (Epstein-Barr virus, cytomegalovirus, HIV, and toxoplasmosis), leptospirosis, and many noninfectious syndromes, such as rheumatologic disease and malignancy (Box 43-1).

The findings of severe malaria are similar to those of other critical illnesses: the depressed consciousness characteristic of cerebral malaria can mimic meningoencephalitis; the acute respiratory distress syndrome, which frequently complicates late-presenting severe malaria, can also be mistaken for a primary pneumonia; and acidosis and metabolic derangements of severe malaria are similar to those found in bacterial sepsis.

In patients presenting with signs and symptoms of either uncomplicated or severe malaria, these and other diagnoses should be considered. It is not uncommon for bacterial sepsis or pneumonia to complicate malarial infection. In the patient with severe malaria, evaluation and empiric therapy for secondary infection should be considered.

Clinical Features

The symptoms of uncomplicated malaria are nonspecific and are similar for all species of *Plasmodium.* The diagnosis should therefore be considered in any traveler returning from an endemic area who develops a fever. The presence of splenomegaly and thrombocytopenia increases the likelihood that malaria is the cause of fever; however, the absence of these signs does not decrease its likelihood (Evidence Level II-2).

Severe malaria, which is most commonly caused by *P falciparum,* is defined by hyperparasitemia (parasitemia ≥5%) or the presence of any 1 of the clinical

Box 43-1. Common Non-malarial Diagnoses in the Febrile Returned Traveler (Evidence Level II-2)

Systemic Febrile Illness
- Dengue
- *Salmonella enterica* serovar Typhi or Paratyphi
- Rickettsia

Acute Diarrheal Disease
- Acute traveler's diarrhea
- Bacterial diarrhea due to *Campylobacter* spp and others
- Gastroenteritis due to non-typhoidal *Salmonella* spp or *Shigella* spp

Respiratory Illness
- Acute unspecified respiratory tract infection
- Bronchitis
- Bacterial pneumonia
- Tonsillitis
- Influenza and influenzalike illness
- Acute sinusitis

Genitourinary Diagnosis
Acute urinary tract infection

Dermatologic Diagnoses

Acute Hepatitis

Acute Unspecified Febrile Illness

Vaccine-Preventable Illness
Including hepatitis A and B; influenza A and B; measles; meningococcal, pneumococcal, or *Haemophilus influenzae* meningitis; meningococcal sepsis; mumps; pertussis; rubella; typhoid fever caused by *S enterica* serovar Typhi infection; tick-borne encephalitis; and chickenpox

Abbreviation: spp, species.

Derived from Wilson ME, Weld LH, Boggild A, et al. Fever in returned travelers: results from the GeoSentinel Surveillance Network. *Clin Infect Dis.* 2007;44(12):1560–1568.

or laboratory criteria (Box 43-2). It should be noted that even in a clinically stable patient, hyperparasitemia alone is diagnostic of severe malaria.

Severe malaria caused by *P vivax* can manifest with hematologic symptoms (ie, severe anemia, thrombocytopenia, or pancytopenia), as well as kidney and respiratory failure and splenic rupture.

Older children in endemic countries with frequent exposure to malaria often develop partial immunity to the infection, resulting in lower level parasitemia and less dramatic clinical and laboratory findings with infection. However, this partial immunity wanes rapidly after leaving the endemic area. The cellular and molecular determinants of this phenomenon are as yet unclear.

The incubation period in most cases of malaria ranges from 7 to 30 days. In cases of malaria caused by *P vivax* and *P ovale,* however, the first presentation may be delayed. These species can form hypnozoites, which can become active weeks to months after the initial infection.

Box 43-2. Diagnosis of Severe Malaria

Severe Malaria

Plasmodium hyperparasitemia *or* the presence of 1 or more of the following clinical or laboratory features:

Clinical features
- Impaired consciousness or unarousable coma
- Prostration (ie, generalized weakness causing the patient to be unable to walk or sit up without assistance)
- Multiple seizures—>2 episodes in 24 h
- Acute respiratory distress syndrome
- Circulatory collapse or shock, systolic blood pressure <70 mm Hg in adults and <50 mm Hg in children
- Jaundice
- Hemoglobinuria
- Abnormal spontaneous bleeding

Laboratory findings
- Parasitemia ≥5%
- Hypoglycemia (blood glucose concentration <40 mg/dL)
- Metabolic acidosis (plasma bicarbonate concentration <15 mmol/L or serum lactate level >5 mmol/L)
- Severe normocytic anemia (Hb concentration <7 g/dL, hemoglobinuria)
- Renal impairment (serum creatinine level >3.0 mg/dL)

Abbreviation: Hb, hemoglobin.

Adapted from World Health Organization. *Guidelines for the Treatment of Malaria.* 2nd ed. Geneva, Switzerland: World Health Organization; 2010, with permission.

Evaluation

When malaria is suspected, the diagnosis of *Plasmodium* species parasitemia should be made immediately to aid in choosing therapy and determining the need for further evaluation. Determining the involved species of *Plasmodium* is likewise important, because this affects the choice of therapy and likelihood of clinical deterioration necessitating monitoring during therapy.

Microscopy remains the criterion standard of malaria diagnosis. Initial evaluation of the patient with suspected malaria should include parasite smears both thick (because of higher sensitivity for detecting infection) and thin (for determining the species and calculating the parasitemia). In settings where a skilled microscopist is not immediately available, antigen detection test kits or rapid diagnostic tests (RDTs) may aid in the initial diagnosis of suspected *Plasmodium* infection without delay. One RDT, the Binax NOW, is currently US Food and Drug Administration (FDA)–approved for use in the United States. Although it is sensitive and specific for *P falciparum* infections, it is less so for non-*falciparum* infections, and cannot determine either the species or parasitemia during an acute malaria episode. Additionally, it is less sensitive at levels of parasitemia below 500 parasites/mcL; hence, when there is a high suspicion of malaria, negative results should be interpreted with caution.

All positive and negative RDT results must be followed up with microscopy as soon as it is available, although treatment in the setting of a positive RDT result should not be delayed while awaiting microscopy. The Centers for Disease Control and Prevention (CDC) offers assistance with the microscopic diagnosis of malaria and other parasitic diseases. Further information about this service can be obtained at http://dpd.cdc.gov/dpdx/HTML/Contactus.htm.

Negative parasite smears should be repeated every 12 to 24 hours for a total of 3 sets. If all are negative, malaria can be considered to be ruled out as a cause of infection.

In addition to microscopic diagnosis, a basic metabolic panel and complete blood cell count should be obtained to aid the clinician in detecting renal failure, metabolic acidosis, hypoglycemia, and anemia. If hepatomegaly or jaundice is noted on examination, liver function tests may be obtained to establish a baseline. In patients who present with electrolyte abnormalities, anemia, or abnormal liver function, clinicians should check daily electrolytes, measures of creatinine clearance, and complete blood cell count until they have demonstrated a trend toward normal.

In parallel with these diagnostic efforts, assessment of the severity of clinical disease should be made. Clinical findings suggestive of severe disease should provoke further evaluation, such as arterial blood gas measurement, chest radiograph, and head imaging.

Polymerase chain reaction is a highly sensitive and specific diagnostic technique for malaria, although it is performed only in reference laboratories and hence involves substantial delays in diagnosis. Additionally, it is more costly than microscopy. It should therefore be performed as a confirmatory test or in cases when differentiating species is difficult, such as in mixed infection.

Syndromic and algorithmic methods of malaria diagnosis have been investigated as alternatives to laboratory diagnosis in resource-poor areas (Evidence Level II-2) but have not demonstrated test characteristics that would justify their use. In the developed world, multiple retrospective studies have demonstrated no sign or symptom, singly or in combination, is sufficient to predict the presence of malaria (Evidence Level II-3). Thus, it is essential to have access to and use specific malaria diagnostic tests.

Management

All patients with *P falciparum* parasitemia, regardless of disease severity, should be admitted for monitoring during the first 24 hours of therapy, with rare exceptions made for stable patients who can be carefully and reliably monitored in the outpatient setting. Patients with severe disease caused by any *Plasmodium* species should be admitted to an intensive care unit for cardiorespiratory monitoring and treatment with parenteral therapy.

Choice of therapy (Table 43-1) depends on the infecting species of *Plasmodium,* severity of the disease, and likelihood that the infecting organism is resistant to antimalarial drugs.

Table 43-1. Guidelines for Treatment of Malaria in the United States

Clinical Diagnosis/ Plasmodium Species	Region Infection Acquired	Recommended Drug
Uncomplicated malaria/ Plasmodium falciparum or species unidentified If "species unidentified" is subsequently diagnosed as Plasmodium vivax or Plasmodium ovale, see P vivax and P ovale (below) regarding treatment with primaquine.	**Chloroquine resistant or unknown resistance** All malarial regions except those specified as chloroquine-sensitive are listed in the box below.	A. Atovaquone/proguanil (Malarone) ($\times$ 3 d) B. Artemether/lumefantrine (Coartem) ($\times$ 3 d) C. Quinine sulfate ($\times$ 7 d if malaria acquired in Southeast Asia; $\times$ 3 d if acquired elsewhere) plus 1 of the following drugs: **doxycycline,**[a] **tetracycline,** or **clindamycin**[b] (all $\times$ 7 d) D. Mefloquine (Lariam and generics)[c] ($\times$ 1 d)
Uncomplicated malaria/ P falciparum or species unidentified	**Chloroquine sensitive** Central America west of Panama Canal, Haiti, the Dominican Republic, and most of the Middle East	Chloroquine phosphate (Aralen and generics) ($\times$ 3 d) or Hydroxychloroquine (Plaquenil and generics) ($\times$ 3 d)
Uncomplicated malaria/ Plasmodium malariae or **Plasmodium knowlesi**	All regions	Chloroquine phosphate ($\times$ 3 d) or Hydroxychloroquine ($\times$ 3 d)
Uncomplicated malaria/P vivax or **P ovale**	All regions (For suspected chloroquine-resistant P vivax, see row below.)	Chloroquine phosphate ($\times$ 3 d) plus **primaquine phosphate** ($\times$ 14 d) or Hydroxychloroquine ($\times$ 3 d) plus **primaquine phosphate** ($\times$ 14 d)
Uncomplicated malaria/P vivax	**Chloroquine resistant**[d] Papua New Guinea and Indonesia	A. Quinine sulfate ($\times$ 7 d) plus Either **doxycycline** or **tetracycline** ($\times$ 3 d) plus **Primaquine phosphate** ($\times$ 14 d) B. Atovaquone-proguanil ($\times$ 3 d) plus **primaquine phosphate** ($\times$ 14 d) C. Mefloquine ($\times$ 1 d) plus **primaquine phosphate** ($\times$ 14 d)

Uncomplicated malaria/ alternatives for pregnant women	**Chloroquine sensitive** Central America west of Panama Canal, Haiti, the Dominican Republic, and most of the Middle East	**Chloroquine phosphate** (× 3 d) *or* **Hydroxychloroquine** (× 3 d)
	Chloroquine resistant Papua New Guinea and Indonesia	**Quinine sulfate** *plus* **clindamycin** (× 7 d) *or* **Mefloquine** (× 1 d)
Severe malaria	All regions	**Quinidine gluconate IV** (× 7 d if malaria acquired in Southeast Asia; × 3 d if acquired elsewhere) *plus* 1 of the following drugs: **doxycycline, tetracycline,** or **clindamycin** (× 7 d) *Investigational new drug (Contact the CDC for information.)* **Artesunate** *plus* 1 of the following drugs: **atovaquone/proguanil (Malarone), doxycycline** (**clindamycin** in pregnant women), or **mefloquine**

Abbreviations: CDC, Centers for Disease Control and Prevention; IV, intravenously.

[a] Doxycycline and tetracycline are contraindicated in children <8y.

[b] For option C, because there is more data on the efficacy of quinine in combination with doxycycline or tetracycline, these treatment combinations are generally preferred to quinine in combination with clindamycin.

[c] Treatment with mefloquine is not recommended in persons who have acquired infections from Southeast Asia, because of drug resistance.

[d] For treatment of chloroquine-resistant *P vivax* infections, options A, B, and C are equally recommended.

Adapted from Centers for Disease Control and Prevention. Malaria: malaria diagnosis and treatment in the United States; treatment table. CDC Web site. http://www.cdc.gov/malaria/diagnosis_treatment/index.html. Accessed August 18, 2016.

Uncomplicated malaria may be treated with oral agents. For most *P falciparum* or un-speciated malaria cases, there are 4 equally effective options. Atovaquone/proguanil and artemether/lumefantrine are equally recommended options that are well tolerated and easy to dose. Quinine sulfate plus an additional agent (clindamycin, doxycycline, or tetracycline) has a more complicated dosing schedule and higher rates of adverse effects than the first 2 options. Because of its high rate of severe neuropsychiatric adverse effects at treatment doses, the fourth option, mefloquine, is recommended only if 1 of the first 3 options cannot be used. In cases when *P falciparum* is likely to be chloroquine sensitive and other chloroquine-sensitive *Plasmodium* species are involved, chloroquine can be used.

Standard of care for the treatment of severe malaria in the United States, regardless of species, is parenteral quinidine gluconate combined with either doxycycline, tetracycline, or clindamycin. At least 24 hours of parenteral quinidine therapy are recommended; therapy may be transitioned to an oral regimen at the same dosage as for uncomplicated malaria once the parasitemia is less than 1% and the patient can take oral medication.

Because parenteral quinidine is cardiotoxic, a baseline electrocardiogram should be obtained prior to initiating therapy, and the patient should undergo continuous cardiac and frequent blood pressure monitoring during administration. Additionally, quinidine- (or quinine-) induced hypoglycemia may occur; glucose must therefore be monitored closely. Children with severe malaria should be cared for in a pediatric intensive care unit.

Parenteral artesunate is the preferred first-line therapy for severe malaria in many parts of the world. However, it is not yet FDA approved for use in the United States. Thus, quinidine gluconate remains the only FDA-approved medicine for the treatment of malaria in the United States. Hospitals should maintain supplies of quinidine for this indication or ensure prompt availability of the product within their community. Hospital pharmacists should know their nearest supply points for additional stocks of the medication. If quinidine is contraindicated or unavailable, artesunate can be obtained through the CDC under an investigational new drug protocol. To enroll a patient with severe malaria in this treatment protocol, contact the CDC Malaria Hotline: 770/488-7788 (Mon–Fri, 8:00 am–4:30 pm, Eastern time) or after hours, call 770/488-7100 and request to speak with a CDC Malaria Branch clinician.

In the case of infection with either *P vivax* or *P ovale,* patients should be treated for blood-stage parasites immediately, then receive additional treatment for relapse prevention. The only medicine available that can eliminate hypnozoites from the liver is primaquine. Persons with *P vivax* or *P ovale* infections should therefore receive a 2-week course of primaquine in addition to treatment for blood-stage parasites. Because deficiency of the glucose-6-phosphate dehydrogenase enzyme can result in development of severe hemolytic anemia with administration of primaquine, all patients should have documentation of normal glucose-6-phosphate dehydrogenase activity by laboratory testing prior to first using primaquine.

In uncomplicated malaria, improvement in symptoms is generally seen within the first 24 to 48 hours after initiating therapy. Laboratory abnormalities, which may include elevated C-reactive protein concentration, elevated liver function test results, abnormal electrolyte concentrations, and markers of decreased renal clearance, demonstrate a trend toward normal at 48 to 72 hours. It is common for hemoglobin level and platelet counts to drop in the days following treatment, especially in children with higher levels of parasitemia. The platelet count should begin to recover within 5 days, although anemia may persist for weeks; if the latter occurs, supplemental iron therapy or, if appropriate, a workup for iron deficiency or other causes of anemia should be considered.

Parasitemia may increase over the first 24 to 36 hours after the initiation of appropriate, effective therapy but should trend downward after 48 hours of therapy. Repeat parasite smears may be helpful in the evaluation of patients who are not clinically improving as expected.

In the patient with complicated malaria, clinical status may deteriorate even as the parasitemia clears. This may occur as a complication of the initial immune response to the parasite or, less commonly, as an adverse effect of therapy. Cerebral edema, pulmonary edema, metabolic acidosis, and renal failure may worsen, and improvement in hematologic parameters may be delayed. Management of complications should follow the same parameters as in non-malarial illness. Failure of antimalarial treatment should be considered if the parasitemia is higher at 48 hours than baseline or if at 72 hours parasitemia is greater than 25% of baseline.

No adjunctive measures have demonstrated clinical benefit in the treatment of malaria, and some have demonstrated harm. For example, high-dose cortico-steroids in the treatment of cerebral malaria are harmful (Evidence Level I). Exchange transfusion, which is able to reduce the parasitemia rapidly, has not been shown to improve survival. CDC no longer recommends its use.

Prevention

Caregivers of children planning to visit a malarious area (see www.cdc.gov/malaria/map/index.html) should seek care at least a month prior to travel from a clinician who is knowledgeable about malaria prevention, such as a travel medicine specialist. An individualized risk assessment should be done, taking into consideration the destination, planned duration of stay, past medical history, and other factors. Appropriate recommendations may include avoiding contact with mosquitoes by staying indoors during biting hours (dusk and nighttime for most malaria vectors), wearing long sleeves/pants when outdoors during biting hours, using insect repellants, and taking prophylactic medication appropriate to the area (Table 43-2). Travelers should be aware that mosquito-borne illness related to daytime exposure (dengue and yellow fever) may coexist in malarious regions, so appropriate precautions should be maintained

Table 43-2. Drugs Used in the Prophylaxis of Malaria

Drug	Use	Adult Dose	Pediatric Dose	Comments
Atovaquone/proguanil	Prophylaxis in all areas	1 adult tablet orally, daily (Adult tablets contain 250 mg atovaquone and 100 mg proguanil hydrochloride.)	5–8 kg: ½ pediatric tablet daily >8–10 kg: ¾ pediatric tablet daily >10–20 kg: 1 pediatric tablet daily >20–30 kg: 2 pediatric tablets daily >30–40 kg: 3 pediatric tablets daily >40 kg: 1 adult tablet daily (Pediatric tablets contain 62.5 mg atovaquone and 25 mg proguanil hydrochloride.)	Begin 1–2 d before travel to malarious areas. Take daily at the same time each day while in the malarious area and for 7 d after leaving such areas. Contraindicated in people with severe renal impairment (creatinine clearance <30 mL/min). Atovaquone/proguanil should be taken with food or a milky drink. Not recommended for prophylaxis for children weighing <5 kg, pregnant women, and women breastfeeding infants weighing <5 kg. Partial tablet doses may need to be prepared by a pharmacist and dispensed in individual capsules.
Chloroquine phosphate	Prophylaxis only in areas with chloroquine-sensitive malaria	300-mg base (500 mg salt) orally, once/wk	5 mg/kg base (8.3 mg/kg salt) orally, once/wk, up to maximum adult dose of 300-mg base	Begin 1–2 wk before travel to malarious areas. Take weekly on the same day of the week while in the malarious area and for 4 wk after leaving such areas. May exacerbate psoriasis.
Doxycycline	Prophylaxis in all areas	100 mg orally, daily	≥8 y: 2.2 mg/kg, up to adult dose of 100 mg/d	Begin 1–2 d before travel to malarious areas. Take daily at the same time each day while in the malarious area and for 4 wk after leaving such areas. Contraindicated in children <8 y and pregnant women.
Hydroxychloroquine sulfate	An alternative to chloroquine for prophylaxis only in areas with chloroquine-sensitive malaria	310-mg base (400 mg salt) orally, once/wk	5 mg/kg base (6.5 mg/kg salt) orally, once/wk, up to maximum adult dose of 310-mg base	Begin 1–2 wk before travel to malarious areas. Take weekly on the same day of the week while in the malarious area and for 4 wk after leaving such areas.

Mefloquine	Prophylaxis in areas with mefloquine-sensitive malaria	228-mg base (250 mg salt) orally, once/wk	≤9 kg: 4.6 mg/kg base (5 mg/kg salt) orally, once/wk >9–19 kg: ¼ tablet once/wk >19–30 kg: ½ tablet once/wk >30–45 kg: ¾ tablet once/wk >45 kg: 1 tablet once/wk	Begin ≥2 wk before travel to malarious areas. Take weekly on the same day of the week while in the malarious area and for 4 wk after leaving such areas. Contraindicated in people allergic to mefloquine or related compounds (quinine and quinidine) and in people with active depression, a recent history of depression, generalized anxiety disorder, psychosis, schizophrenia, other major psychiatric disorders, or seizures. Use with caution in persons with psychiatric disturbances or a previous history of depression. Not recommended for persons with cardiac conduction abnormalities.
Primaquine	Prophylaxis for short-duration travel to areas with principally *Plasmodium vivax*	30-mg base (52.6 mg salt) orally, daily	0.5 mg/kg base (0.8 mg/kg salt), up to adult dose orally, daily	Begin 1–2 d before travel to malarious areas. Take daily at the same time each day while in the malarious area and for 7 d after leaving such areas. Contraindicated in people with G6PD deficiency. Also contraindicated during pregnancy and lactation, unless the infant being breastfed has a documented normal G6PD level.
	Presumptive antirelapse therapy (terminal prophylaxis) to decrease the risk for relapses of *P vivax* and *Plasmodium ovale*	30-mg base (52.6 mg salt) orally, daily for 14 d after departure from the malarious area	0.5 mg/kg base (0.8 mg/kg salt), up to adult dose orally, daily for 14 d after departure from the malarious area	Indicated for people who have had prolonged exposure to *P vivax, P ovale*, or both. Contraindicated in people with G6PD deficiency. Also contraindicated during pregnancy and lactation, unless the infant being breastfed has a documented normal G6PD level.

Abbreviation: G6PD, glucose-6-phosphate dehydrogenase.
Adapted from Centers for Disease Control and Prevention. *CDC Health Information for International Travel*. New York, New York: Oxford University Press; 2016.

throughout the day and night. Insect repellants are safe for children of all ages. Further preventive guidance can be found at wwwnc.cdc.gov/travel/yellowbook/ 2012/chapter-2-the-pre-travel-consultation/protection-against-mosquitoes-ticks-and-other-insects-and-arthropods.htm.

Suggested Reading

Cullen KA, Mace KE, Arguin PM; Center for Global Health, Centers for Disease Control and Prevention. Malaria surveillance—United States, 2013. *MMWR Surveill Summ.* 2016;65(2):1–22

Griffith KS, Lewis LS, Mali S, Parise ME. Treatment of malaria in the United States: a systematic review. *JAMA.* 2007;297(20):2264–2277

Taylor SM, Molyneux ME, Simel DL, Meshnick SR, Juliano JJ. Does this patient have malaria? *JAMA.* 2010;304(18):2048–2056

Wilson ME, Weld LH, Boggild A, et al. Fever in returned travelers: results from the GeoSentinel Surveillance Network. *Clin Infect Dis.* 2007;44(12):1560–1568

World Health Organization. *Guidelines for the Treatment of Malaria.* 3rd ed. Geneva, Switzerland: World Health Organization; 2015

World Health Organization. *Management of Severe Malaria: A Practical Handbook.* 3rd ed. Geneva, Switzerland: World Health Organization; 2013

World Health Organization. *World Malaria Report.* Geneva, Switzerland: World Health Organization; 2015

CHAPTER 44

Pneumocystis jiroveci Infection

Navjyot K. Vidwan, MD, MPH

Key Points

- Pneumocystis pneumonia is now known as *Pneumocystis jiroveci* and is classified as an atypical fungus.

- The clinical presentation is generally acute or subacute respiratory illness similar to other pathogens presenting as pneumonia, but generally severe hypoxemia is a feature.

- Consider the diagnosis in immunocompromised patients, including those with HIV or other cell-mediated deficiencies.

- The treatment of choice is trimethoprim/sulfamethoxazole and should be initiated when there is a high level of clinical suspicion prior to final diagnosis.

Overview

Pneumocystis jiroveci, now classified as an atypical fungus, was formally known as *Pneumocystis carinii* when it was previously classified as a protozoan. The organism can exist in 2 forms (cyst and trophozoite), which has made classification challenging. The condition has also been referred to as pneumocystis pneumonia (PCP), which came to great attention during the 1980s, the first decade of the HIV/AIDS epidemic when case reports described "otherwise" healthy patients as having severe opportunistic infections, including fulminant respiratory disease. We now associate PCP with immunocompromised patients, specifically those with cell-mediated deficiencies, including HIV/AIDS; solid organ transplant; bone marrow stem cell transplant; severe combined immunodeficiency; immunodeficiency with hyper-IgM; or cancer; and those on immunosuppressive medications. Pneumocystis epidemics have also been recognized in malnourished children and neonates and infants in resource-poor regions, as well as preterm infants. Per Centers for Disease Control and Prevention statistics, PCP incidence in the United States is around 9% in hospitalized HIV/AIDS patients and 1% in solid organ transplant recipients. The death rate ranges from 5% to 40% in patients who receive treatment to 100% without therapy. The mode of transmission is still unknown in humans, but animal models have indicated airborne spread. The exact incubation period is also unknown.

Differential Diagnosis (Box 44-1)

Box 44-1. Differential Diagnosis for *Pneumocystis jiroveci*

- Bacterial pneumonia
- Viral pneumonia
  - o *Mycoplasma pneumoniae* pneumonia
  - o *Chlamydia pneumoniae* pneumonia
  - o *Chlamydia trachomatis* pneumonia
  - o Legionellosis
  - o Lymphocytic interstitial pneumonia
- Fungal pneumonia
  - o Tuberculosis
  - o MAC disease
- Chemical pneumonitis

Abbreviation: MAC, *Mycobacterium avium* complex.

Clinical Features

The primary clinical syndrome associated with *P jiroveci* is pneumonia or pneumonitis presenting in an acute or subacute fashion with clinical symptoms, including nonproductive cough, fever, decreased oxygen saturation, difficulty breathing/shortness of breath, and tachypnea. Other symptoms can include anorexia, fatigue, diarrhea, night sweats, and weight loss. Sputum production is usually limited. Pneumothorax is a known complication of the disease process, and respiratory failure can also occur.

Evaluation

Noninvasive tests that can help in PCP diagnosis but are not 100% diagnostic include a blood gas analysis (mainly showing respiratory alkalosis), an alveolar-arterial oxygen gradient (used primarily in adults and for treatment regimen), and a pulse oximeter (showing hypoxemia). Radiologically, chest radiographs can reveal bilateral diffuse interstitial or alveolar disease; their findings can also be normal. High-resolution chest computed tomography (CT) shows extensive ground-glass opacities affecting the central lung, interlobular septal thickening with the lung periphery spared. A negative CT finding does not rule out PCP. Of note, a gallium 67 scan can also be used, although it is expensive, may take more time than a CT scan, and is associated with substantial radiation exposure, all of which limit its use.

A recent meta-analysis suggests that measurement of serum 1,3-β-D-glucan may be helpful in establishing diagnosis. The assay has high sensitivity for

P jiroveci pneumonia with high diagnostic accuracy. More important, a negative test result is good evidence that the diagnosis can be excluded. However, if the assay is positive, consider other entities that may be associated with false-positive testing, including intravenous amoxicillin-clavulanic acid, treatment of patients with intravenous immune globulin, use of cellulose membranes, filters made from cellulose in hemodialysis, and use of cotton gauze swabs/packs/pads and sponges.

Definitive diagnosis is made with open lung biopsy or bronchoscopy with bronchoalveolar lavage, with lung samples being sent to a histopathologic specialist. Polymerase chain reaction can also be used to detect *P jiroveci* DNA from these clinical specimens; however, this is not widely available.

Management

Treatment should be initiated before an official diagnosis is made when clinical suspicion is high or in severely immunocompromised patients. Although *P jiroveci* is now classified as a fungus, antifungal treatment is not the drug of choice. Trimethoprim/sulfamethoxazole is the drug of choice and should be given intravenously for moderate to severe infection. However, the oral formulation can be used for patients with mild disease and functional gastrointestinal tract. A typical duration of therapy is 21 days.

An alternative treatment is pentamidine. Oral atovaquone is also approved for mild to moderate PCP in adults, although limited data exist in children. Prednisone/corticosteroid should be included as adjunctive therapy in children with moderate to severe PCP disease.

Chemoprophylaxis
- Patients with AIDS who have CD4 cell counts below 200
- Infants 4 to 6 weeks through 12 months of age who are HIV infected or have indeterminate status (Please refer to Chapter 30, HIV.)
- Bone marrow transplant recipients
- Organ transplant recipients
- People with chronic illness taking high-dose corticosteroids
- Patients with previous episodes of this infection

Long-term Monitoring

Patients with a PCP diagnosis should be considered for HIV or other immunocompromised conditions. Trimethoprim/sulfamethoxazole adverse effects during treatment include pancytopenia, hepatitis, and renal impairment. Pentamidine adverse effects during treatment include pancreatitis, cardiac arrhythmias, neutropenia, and renal impairment with electrolyte abnormalities.

Suggested Reading

American Academy of Pediatrics. Kimberlin DW, Brady MT, Jackson MA, Long SS, eds. *Red Book: 2015 Report of the Committee on Infectious Diseases.* 30th ed. Elk Grove Village, IL: American Academy of Pediatrics; 2015

Centers for Disease Control and Prevention. *Pneumocystis* pneumonia. CDC Web site. www.cdc.gov/fungal/diseases/pneumocystis-pneumonia/index.html. Updated February 13, 2014. Accessed March 18, 2016

CHAPTER 45

Schistosomiasis

Shirley Molitor-Kirsch, RN, MSN, CPNP-AC

Key Points

- Schistosomiasis is prevalent in the tropics and subtropics, affecting several hundred million people per year; generally, school-aged children are the most heavily infected.

- Self-limited cercarial dermatitis, or swimmer's itch, is most common, but severe disease involving the bladder or lower genital tract, intestine, lungs, or central nervous system has significant morbidity.

- Urinary/stool samples have limited sensitivity (approximately 25%), so multiple tests are needed.

- Serologic testing, available through the Centers for Disease Control and Prevention, may be helpful but cannot differentiate between active disease and past infection or reinfection.

- Praziquantel is the only effective anthelmintic against adult worms and must be repeated in 4 to 6 weeks.

Overview

Schistosomiasis, or bilharziasis, is an infection caused by the species *Schistosoma,* a trematode (fluke) helminth that is globally distributed and dependent on freshwater exposure. More than 200 million people are infected across 52 countries in Africa, Asia, the Middle East, and South America, with most infections acquired in sub-Saharan Africa.

Causes and Differential Diagnosis

Infection typically occurs when people come in contact with freshwater contaminated with cercariae (the larval form of the schistosome) while swimming, bathing, washing clothes, fishing, and farming. Over several weeks, the parasites migrate through host tissue and develop into adult worms. Once mature, the worms mate and the females produce eggs; these eggs travel to the bladder or intestine and are passed into the urine (*Schistosoma haematobium*) or stool (*Schistosoma mansoni, Schistosoma japonicum, Schistosoma mekongi,* and *Schistosoma intercalatum*). Freshwater snails act as intermediate hosts in which the parasites develop into sporocysts and produce cercariae. It is when these cercariae are released into freshwater that the cycle continues.

Symptoms of schistosomiasis, and therefore differential diagnosis, vary depending on phase of the disease as well as which species of schistosome is causing the infection (Box 45-1).

Box 45-1. Presenting Symptoms and Potential Differential Diagnoses

Fever and Rash With Eosinophilia	Hematuria	Neurologic Symptoms of Increased Intracranial Pressure	Abdominal Pain With Diarrhea or Hematochezia	Other
• Coccidioido-mycosis • Filariasis • Fascioliasis • *Loa loa* • Leukemia • Strongyloidiasis • Tissue protozoa • Toxocariasis	• Acute nephritis • Renal tuberculosis • Urogenital tract cancer	• Neuroschisto-somiasis • Seizure • Space-occupying lesion • Stroke	• Colorectal cancer • Inflammatory bowel disease • Peptic ulcer • Visceral leishmaniasis	• Acute viral syndrome (including HIV) • Appendicitis • Coinfection with malaria, hepatitis B, hepatitis C, or HIV • Cirrhosis • Drug reaction • Gastroenteritis • Helminthic parasitic diseases • Pancreatitis • *Salmonella* infection • Serum sickness • Urinary tract infection

Derived from Centers for Disease Control and Prevention. *CDC Health Information for International Travel.* New York, New York: Oxford University Press; 2016.

Clinical Features

Schistosomiasis presents in 3 distinct forms: acute, chronic, and advanced disease.

Early

Rash (Cercarial Dermatitis)

Individuals infected may develop cercarial dermatitis, or swimmer's itch, within a few hours after water exposure, although a rash may appear up to a week later. A maculopapular rash consisting of discrete erythematous raised lesions that vary in size from 1 to 3 cm may appear where the schistosome penetrated the skin, but systemic disease does not occur (Figure 45-1).

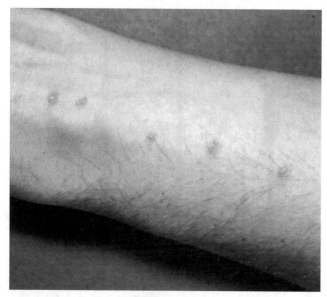

Figure 45-1. Cercarial dermatitis.
From Cercarial dermatitis. Centers for Disease Control and Prevention Web site.
http://www.cdc.gov/dpdx/cercarialDermatitis/dx.html. Updated November 29, 2013. Accessed August 18, 2016.

Acute Schistosomiasis (Katayama Fever)

Symptoms of schistosomiasis are not caused by the worms themselves but mediated by the host's immune response to schistosome eggs and granulomatous reactions evoked by the antigens they secrete. Eggs shed by the adult worms that do not pass out of the body can become lodged in the intestine or bladder, causing inflammation, granuloma formation, and scarring. Patients may present with symptoms resembling serum sickness, including fever, chills, headache, myalgia, malaise, right upper quadrant abdominal pain, diarrhea, dry cough, lymphadenopathy, and hepatosplenomegaly; significant eosinophilia is routinely noted. The combination of contact with freshwater in sub-Saharan Africa followed in a few weeks by fever and eosinophilia is characteristic of the diagnosis of schistosomiasis and specific enough to warrant initiation of appropriate treatment.

Chronic and Advanced Disease

Chronic schistosomiasis is far more common than the acute disease. The symptoms and severity of disease are related to the species, number of eggs trapped in tissues, their distribution, and duration of infection. Rarely, pulmonary hypertension follows embolization of eggs to the lungs, but urogenital, gastrointestinal (GI), liver, and central nervous system disease are more commonly encountered.

Urogenital Disease

Even when parasite burden is relatively low, urinary schistosomiasis is often symptomatic. Urinary tract disease develops after infection with S haematobium and the subsequent local inflammation after eggs are lodged in the tissues. Hematuria appearing 10 to 12 weeks after infection is often the first sign of disease. Dysuria may present in either early or late disease. Progressive involvement, fibrosis, and calcification of the bladder and ureters can result in hydroureter and hydronephrosis. Obstruction can lead to secondary bacterial infections and renal failure. Chronic inflammation may predispose to squamous cell carcinoma of the bladder. Genital disease, or vulval schistosomiasis, is present in about a third of infected women and may also increase the risk of HIV transmission.

Gastrointestinal and Liver Disease

Infection with *S mansoni, S intercalatum, S japonicum,* and *S mekongi* leads to GI disease. Eggs trapped in the gut wall lead to inflammation, ulceration, hyperplasia, microabscess formation, and polyposis. Symptoms of chronic GI schistosomiasis include abdominal pain, blood in the stool, diarrhea (particularly in children), and protein-losing enteropathy.

Eggs of *S mansoni* and *S japonicum* embolize to the liver. Hepatomegaly, secondary to granulomatous inflammation, occurs early in the evolution of chronic disease. Progressive obstruction of blood flow leads to portal hypertension, which ultimately leads to the development of portosystemic collateral vessels. These collateral vessels can lead to varices, variceal bleeding, splenomegaly, and hypersplenism, as well as allow schistosome eggs to embolize to the pulmonary circulation. Eggs lodged in pulmonary arterioles lead to pulmonary hypertension and cor pulmonale; presenting symptoms include dyspnea and pulmonary nodules on chest radiograph.

Neurologic Disease

Neuroschistosomiasis is arguably the most severe disease manifestation of schistosomal infection. Rarely, adult worms can migrate to the brain or spinal cord. The mass effect of thousands of eggs and large granulomas produces symptoms of increased intracranial pressure, neuropathy, and myelopathy. Patients can present with symptoms of encephalopathy, including headache, visual impairment, delirium, seizures, ataxia, and motor deficits. Spinal symptoms include lumbar pain, weakness, paralysis, or spinal cord inflammation. Myelopathy (acute transverse myelitis and subacute myeloradiculopathy) of the lumbosacral region is the most commonly reported neurologic manifestation of both *S mansoni* and *S haematobium.*

Evaluation

Diagnosis of schistosomiasis depends on its infection stage and intensity. A large variety of tests are available for clinical practice, each with its limitations in specificity and sensitivity (Table 45-1). However, microscopic examination of stool or urine for ova remains the criterion standard for diagnosis for suspected schistosomiasis.

Table 45-1. Currently Available Diagnostic Procedures for Schistosomiasis in Travelers and Immigrants

	Schistosoma mansoni	Schistosoma haematobium	Parasite Load	Sensitivity	Specificity	Cost
Schistosome polyclonal antibody tests	+	+	–	Moderate	High[a]	Low
Schistosome antigen detection (CAA)	+	+	+	Low	High[a]	High
Ova detection urine	–	+	+	Moderate	High[b]	Low
Ova detection stool	+	–	+	Low	High[b]	Low
Ova rectal snips	+	–	+	High	High[b]	Low
PCR schistosome DNA in serum, stool, or urine	+	+	Unable to determine parasite load	High	High	Moderate

Abbreviations: CAA, circulating anodic antigen; PCR, polymerase chain reaction.

[a] For *Schistosoma* species.

[b] For *Schistosoma mansoni* and *Schistosoma haematobium* specifically.

Adapted from Clerinx J, Van Gompel A. Schistosomiasis in travelers and migrants. *Travel Med Infect Dis.* 2011;9(1):6–24, with permission from Elsevier.

Microscopy

Careful review of travel and residential history is critical for determining whether infection is likely and which species may be causing infection. Table 45-2 outlines the disease category, associated species, endemic regions, and diagnostic sample recommended for microscopy.

Table 45-2. Parasite Species and Geographic Distribution and Diagnostic Sample Required

	Species	Region	Diagnostic Sample
Intestinal schistosomiasis	*Schistosoma mansoni*[a]	Certain tropical and sub-tropical areas of sub-Saharan Africa, the Middle East, South America, and the Caribbean	Stool[a]
	Schistosoma japonicum	Asia, particularly in China; the Philippines; Thailand; and Indonesia	Stool
	Schistosoma mekongi	Cambodia and the Loa People's Democratic Republic	Stool
	Schistosoma guianensis and related *Schistosoma intercalatum*	Rain forest areas of central Africa	Stool
Urogenital schistosomiasis	*Schistosoma haematobium*[a]	Predominantly in North Africa, sub-Saharan Africa, the Middle East, Turkey, and India	Urine[a]

[a] It is important to remember that both *Schistosoma mansoni* and *Schistosoma haematobium* are endemic in some areas of sub-Saharan Africa; patients with freshwater exposures in those areas should have both stool and urinary samples examined for eggs.

Adapted with permission from Schistosomiasis. World Health Organization Web site. http://www.who.int/mediacentre/factsheets/fs115/en/. Updated February 2016. Accessed August 19, 2016.

Schistosome eggs are easy to detect and identify on microscopy owing to their characteristic size and shape with a lateral or terminal spine as depicted in Figure 45-2. Specificity of microscopy is 100%, but sensitivity varies with burden of illness and therefore number of eggs excreted. To increase the sensitivity of testing, 3 samples should be collected on different days to increase sensitivity. It is important to wait at least 2 months from the last known freshwater contact before looking for eggs, because it takes this long for the worms to produce eggs.

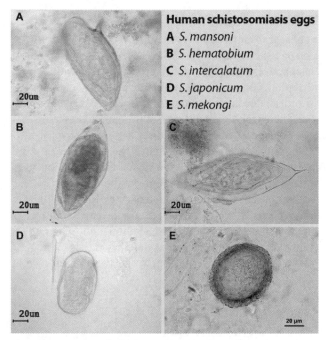

Figure 45-2. Egg morphology of human schistosomiasis.

Urogenital Disease

Schistosoma haematobium adult worms are found in the venous plexus of the lower urinary tract and shed eggs in the urine. Diagnostic urinary samples are ideally collected between 10:00 am and 2:00 pm to coincide with the maximum excretion of eggs. The specimen is concentrated by sedimentation, centrifugation, or filtration and forced over a paper or nitrocellulose filter. Microscopic identification is confirmed with identification of eggs in the urine.

Intestinal Disease

Intestinal schistosomes, *S mansoni*, *S japonicum*, *S mekongi*, and *S intercalatum* reside in the mesenteric venous plexus of infected hosts, and eggs are shed in stool. Diagnosis can be made by observing even a single egg in thick smears of stool specimens (2–10 mcg) with or without suspension in saline. Formalin-based techniques for sedimentation and concentration may increase the diagnostic yield in patients with a light infection, such as seen in returned travelers.

Other Diagnostic Tools

Serologic testing for antischistosomal antibody is available but does not provide reliable information on parasite burden, because it is less sensitive than multiple stool or urinary samples and less specific, owing to cross-reactivity with antigens from other helminths. Most routine techniques detect IgG, IgM, or IgE against soluble worm antigen or soluble egg antigen by enzyme-linked immunosorbent assay, indirect hemagglutination (IHA), or immunofluorescence. A cercarial antigen enzyme-linked immunosorbent assay has been tested recently and proved promising in a non-endemic setting. In new infections, the serum sample tested should be collected at least 6 to 8 weeks after likely infection, to allow for full development of the parasite and antibody to the adult stage. Serologic testing is *not* appropriate for determination of active infection in patients who have been repeatedly infected and treated in the past because specific antibody can persist despite cure. The latest addition in the diagnostic arsenal is the development of polymerase chain reaction–based tests to detect parasite DNA both in excreta and serum, but to date these are not routinely available.

Management

Currently, praziquantel is by far the most cost-effective and widely used antischistosomal compound (Table 45-3). Praziquantel, available in 600-mg tablets, is an acylated quinoline pyrazine that is active against all *Schistosoma* species and (human) cestodes. The timing of treatment is important since praziquantel is most effective against the adult worm and requires the presence of a mature antibody response to the parasite. For travelers, treatment should be at least 6 to 8 weeks after last exposure to potentially contaminated freshwater. Dosing is typically 40 mg/kg/day but species specific (see Table 45-2). The drug acts within an hour after ingestion by inducing a sustained muscular contraction, effectively paralyzing the schistosomes and damaging their tegument. Praziquantel is subject to a first-pass liver clearance, and most (80%) of its inactive metabolites are excreted mainly in the urine within 24 hours after ingestion. Adverse effects may result in part from parasite disintegration, but are usually mild. These include nausea, vomiting, malaise, and abdominal pain. Host immune response differences may affect individual response to treatment

Table 45-3. Treatment of Schistosomiasis

Schistosoma Species Infection	Praziquantel Dosage and Duration
Schistosoma mansoni, Schistosoma haematobium, Schistosoma intercalatum	40 mg/kg/d orally in 2 divided doses for 1 d
Schistosoma japonicum, Schistosoma mekongi	60 mg/kg/d orally in 3 divided doses for 1 d

with praziquantel. In patients with a large disease burden or schistosomal encephalopathy, systemic corticosteroids may be beneficial. Patients that present with seizures will also require conjunctive treatment with anticonvulsants.

Although a single course of treatment is usually curative, the immune response in lightly infected patients may be less robust, and repeat treatment after 6 weeks is recommended to increase effectiveness. If the pretreatment stool or urinary examination was positive for schistosome eggs, follow-up examinations at 1 to 2 months posttreatment is suggested to help confirm successful cure.

Prevention

No vaccine is currently available. Unlike other vector-borne diseases, schistosomiasis is not unavoidable and can thus be prevented by behavioral changes and providing a safe water supply for bathing.

- Avoid swimming or wading in freshwater when you are in countries in which schistosomiasis occurs. Swimming in the ocean and chlorinated swimming pools is safe.
- Vigorous towel drying after an unintentional, very brief water exposure may help prevent the *Schistosoma* parasite from penetrating the skin. However, do not rely on vigorous towel drying alone to prevent schistosomiasis. Applying a 50% DEET solution to the skin immediately after exposure has prevented infection in nonimmune travelers bathing in Lake Malawi.
- Drink safe water. Although schistosomiasis is not transmitted by swallowing contaminated water, one can become infected when the mouth or lips come in contact with water containing the parasites. Because water coming directly from canals, lakes, rivers, streams, or springs may be contaminated with a variety of infectious organisms, it is recommended individuals boil or filter water before drinking it. Bringing water to a rolling boil for at least 1 minute will kill any harmful parasites, bacteria, or viruses present. Iodine treatment alone will not guarantee that water is safe and free of all parasites.
- Water used for bathing should be brought to a rolling boil for 1 minute to kill any cercariae, then cooled before bathing to avoid scalding. Water held in a storage tank for at least 1 to 2 days should be safe for bathing.

Those who have had contact with potentially contaminated water overseas should see their clinician after returning from travel to discuss testing.

Suggested Reading

Carod-Artal FJ. Neurological complications of *Schistosoma* infection. *Trans R Soc Trop Med Hyg.* 2008;102(2):107–116

Clerinx J, Van Gompel A. Schistosomiasis in travelers and migrants. *Travel Med Infect Dis.* 2011;9(1):6–24

Doenhoff MJ, Cioli D, Utzinger J. Praziquantel: mechanisms of action, resistance and new derivatives for schistosomiasis. *Curr Opin Infect Dis.* 2008;21(6):659–667

Gray DJ, McManus DP, Li YS, Williams GM, Bergquist R, Ross AG. Schistosomiasis elimination: lessons from the past guide the future. *Lancet Infect Dis.* 2010;10(10):733–736

Gray DJ, Ross AG, Li YS, McManus DP. Diagnosis and management of schistosomiasis. *BMJ.* 2011;342:d2651

Gryseels B, Polman K, Clerinx J, Kestens L. Human schistosomiasis. *Lancet.* 2006;368(9541):1106–1118

Ross AG, Bartley PB, Sleigh AC, et al. Schistosomiasis. *N Engl J Med.* 2002;346(16): 1212–1220

Ross AG, Vickers D, Olds GR, Shah SM, McManus DP. Katayama syndrome. *Lancet Infect Dis.* 2007;7(3):218–224

World Health Organization. *Preventive Chemotherapy in Human Helminthiasis: Coordinated Use of Anthelminthic Drugs in Control Interventions; A Manual for Health Professionals and Program Managers.* Geneva, Switzerland: World Health Organization; 2006

World Health Organization. *Report of the WHO Informal Consultation on the use of Praziquantel during Pregnancy/Lactation and Albendazole/Mebendazole in Children under 24 months.* Geneva, Switzerland: World Health Organization; 2003. http://apps.who.int/iris/bitstream/10665/68041/1/WHO_CDS_CPE_PVC_2002.4.pdf. Accessed March 30, 2016

CHAPTER 46

Toxoplasmosis

John A. Vanchiere, MD, PhD, and Joseph A. Bocchini Jr, MD

Key Points

- *Toxoplasma* is transmitted by ingestion of the oocyst, which is present in soil, water, and raw food contaminated with cat feces; *Toxoplasma* can also be transmitted in undercooked meats contaminated with viable encysted bradyzoites.

- Following primary infection, encysted bradyzoites remain in multiple tissues.

- Ocular toxoplasmosis in older children is most often the result of congenital infection.

- Immunocompromised patients and congenitally infected neonates and infants are at highest risk for severe toxoplasmosis.

- Prolonged treatment may be necessary in patients with congenital infection or severe disease and in immunocompromised persons.

- *Toxoplasma* should be considered in the differential diagnosis of children with fever of unknown origin and lymphadenopathy.

Overview

Toxoplasmosis is a systemic illness caused by the protozoan parasite *Toxoplasma gondii*, whose definitive host is the cat. Approximately 22% of the US population 12 years and older has been infected with *Toxoplasma*. Infection generally occurs by ingestion of the oocyst of *T gondii*, which can be found in soil, water, and unwashed fruits or vegetables from a garden contaminated with cat feces or inadequately cooked meats (especially pork, lamb, or venison) containing encysted bradyzoites. Congenital infection results from transmission during a maternal primary infection or during reactivation in an immunocompromised pregnant woman. *Toxoplasma* can be transmitted through organ transplantation or blood transfusion.

Causes and Differential Diagnosis

The differential diagnosis of toxoplasmosis is extensive and should take into account the protean manifestations of disease and immune status of the patient with suspected *T gondii* infection, as detailed in Table 46-1.

Clinical Features

Congenital Infection

Like other congenital infections (eg, syphilis, rubella, cytomegalovirus), the manifestations of congenital toxoplasmosis range from asymptomatic to severe multiorgan dysfunction. Small for gestational age, hepatosplenomegaly, chorioretinitis, cerebral calcifications, jaundice, and seizures are common features of congenital toxoplasmosis. Rash, pneumonitis, gastrointestinal symptoms (vomiting and diarrhea), thrombocytopenia, and nephrotic syndrome are observed in more severe cases. The long-term sequelae of congenital toxoplasmosis are primarily related to damage to the central nervous system (CNS), including mental retardation, seizures, spasticity, and severe vision impairment. Neonates born with asymptomatic toxoplasmosis have a high risk of late sequelae occurring months to years after congenital infection, including chorioretinitis, hydrocephalus or microcephaly, developmental delay, deafness, and seizures. As such, close follow-up and regular ophthalmologic examina-

Table 46-1. Differential Diagnosis of Suspected Toxoplasmosis by Patient Group

Patient Group	Clinical Features	Diagnostic Considerations
Congenital infection	IUGR, hepatosplenomegaly, thrombocytopenia, chorioretinitis, leukopenia or leukocytosis, transaminasemia, intracranial calcifications, seizures, hydrocephalus or microcephaly, pneumonitis	Rubella, CMV, syphilis
Late sequelae of congenital infection	Chorioretinitis (typically unilateral), strabismus, nystagmus, blindness, hydrocephalus or microcephaly	Syphilis, toxocariasis, tuberculosis, cat-scratch disease, LCMV
Postnatally acquired in immunocompetent patient	Lymphadenopathy, fatigue, elevated transaminase concentrations, sore throat, myalgia	Infectious mononucleosis, adenovirus, CMV, lymphoma
Postnatally acquired in immunocompromised patient	Encephalitis, chorioretinitis, myocarditis, pneumonitis	CNS tumors, cryptococcal meningitis, CMV disease, aseptic meningitis

Abbreviations: CMV, cytomegalovirus; CNS, central nervous system; IUGR, intrauterine growth retardation; LCMV, lymphocytic choriomeningitis virus.

tions (eg, every 3 months until old enough to report visual changes) are recommended.

Postnatally Acquired Infection

In immunocompetent patients, postnatally acquired *T gondii* infection is usually asymptomatic. Approximately 10% to 15% have a self-limited clinical illness. Lymphadenopathy and fatigue are the most common manifestations, but some patients may have fever, sore throat, and myalgia suggestive of infectious mononucleosis. Elevated serum transaminase concentrations, reflective of mild liver involvement, are observed in some patients. Chorioretinitis is a rare finding in non-congenital toxoplasmosis, but is reported postnatally because of reactivation years after the initial infection in healthy and immunocompromised individuals. Toxoplasmosis should be considered in the differential diagnosis of fever of unknown origin with lymphadenopathy, and life-threatening pneumonia has been reported in patients who acquired primary toxoplasmosis in certain tropical countries in South America.

Infection in Immunocompromised Patients

The primary manifestations of *T gondii* infection in immunocompromised patients are related to CNS disease, which may be due to primary infection or reactivation of latent infection. Patients with acquired immunodeficiency syndrome and other states of T-lymphocyte dysfunction (eg, solid organ transplant recipients and cancer chemotherapy patients) are at highest risk of toxoplasmic disease, including encephalitis, pneumonitis, myocarditis, and disseminated toxoplasmosis. Toxoplasmic meningoencephalitis usually presents as an acute or subacute neuropsychiatric disease with ring-enhancing lesions in the brain parenchyma detected on CNS imaging. Magnetic resonance imaging is generally superior to computed tomography for evaluation of suspected toxoplasmic meningoencephalitis.

Evaluation

The clinical suspicion of toxoplasmic disease relies heavily on an association with exposure to cats or cat feces or consumption of contaminated foods, but these epidemiologic clues are not always present, even in confirmed toxoplasmosis. Therefore, the astute clinician will consider toxoplasmosis in the differential diagnosis of a broad range of symptoms, especially in young children who may be inadvertently exposed to cat feces and in patients who live in areas of high endemicity. The diagnosis of *T gondii* infection is usually made on the basis of serologic testing (Box 46-1), but this may be unreliable in immunocompromised patients. In the absence of specific findings on histopathologic examination of tissues, polymerase chain reaction is commonly used to test blood and body fluids (including amniotic fluid) for the presence of toxoplasmic DNA sequences. The Toxoplasma Serology Laboratory at the Palo Alto Medical Foundation has special expertise in serologic and nucleic acid

Box 46-1. Diagnosis of Acute Toxoplasmosis

- Detection of *Toxoplasma* genomic sequences in blood or body fluids
- Detection of *Toxoplasma*-specific IgM and IgG in serum
- Isolation of *Toxoplasma gondii* from blood or body fluids
- Demonstration of tachyzoites of *T gondii* in tissue or cytologic preparations
- Characteristic lymph node pathology
- Demonstration of *Toxoplasma* cysts in the fetus, neonate, or placenta

amplification assays for diagnosis of toxoplasmosis and provides consultation to physicians on toxoplasmic disease (www.pamf.org/serology; toxolab@pamf.org; 650/853-4828). Congenital toxoplasmosis should be suspected in an infant with a compatible clinical syndrome and any of the following:

- *Toxoplasma gondii* in umbilical cord blood, urine, or peripheral blood or in cerebrospinal fluid (CSF) by mouse inoculation
- *Toxoplasma gondii* DNA polymerase chain reaction in amniotic fluid or in peripheral blood, urine, or CSF of newborn
- IgA and/or IgM antibody to *T gondii* in fetal or newborn blood
- IgG and/or IgM antibody to *T gondii* in the CSF of the newborn
- Fetal or newborn *T gondii*–specific IgG 4 times greater than maternal IgG
- IgG antibody to *T gondii* that increases, or remains positive after 12 months of life

Management

In immunocompetent children, toxoplasmosis is usually self-limited and rarely requires treatment. There have been no controlled clinical trials of treatments for toxoplasmosis. Treatment recommendations are based on data from large case series, particularly from areas of the world with high rates of endemic infection (Evidence Level II-3). Treatment of pregnant women who have acute *T gondii* infection is recommended to reduce the incidence of maternal-to-child transmission in utero. Congenital toxoplasmosis is usually treated for 12 months with sulfadiazine and pyrimethamine. Treatment of neonates and infants with subclinical *T gondii* infection is controversial, because no clinical trial data suggest that such treatment reduces the risk of late sequelae, and the currently available treatments fail to eradicate encysted *T gondii*–containing bradyzoites (Box 46-2). Ocular disease in an older child is treated for 4 to 6 weeks or 2 weeks after symptoms resolve. Prednisone is also given until resolution of sight-threatening active chorioretinitis. Treatment of immuno-compromised patients should continue for at least 4 to 6 weeks after resolution

Box 46-2. Prevention of *Toxoplasma gondii* Infection

- Cook whole cuts of meat to medium done or greater (>62.8°C [>145°F]), ground meat to ≥71.1°C (≥160°F), and poultry to at least 73.9°C (165°F) (smoked or cured meats are also considered unsafe). Freezing meat for several days at subzero temperature greatly reduces infectivity.
- Wash all fruits and vegetables before consumption.
- Disinfect kitchen surfaces, hands, and utensils after contact with raw meat or unwashed fruits and vegetables.
- Avoid contact with materials that may be contaminated by cat feces, or wear gloves while gardening or handling contaminated materials, especially cat litter boxes.
- Change cat litter boxes daily and regularly disinfect with water at approximately 93.3°C (200°F).
- Do not adopt or handle stray cats, especially kittens.
- Keep outdoor sandboxes covered.

of clinical symptoms. Suppressive therapy is commonly given until 6 months after immune restoration or for life if restoration is not possible. Pyrimethamine plus sulfadiazine (or clindamycin for sulfa-allergic patients), trimethoprim/sulfamethoxazole, and atovaquone are effective for secondary prophylaxis in immunocompromised patients. Folinic acid is always given during treatment with pyrimethamine.

Suggested Reading

Centers for Disease Control and Prevention. Parasites: toxoplasmosis (*Toxoplasma* infection); prevention and control. www.cdc.gov/parasites/toxoplasmosis/prevent.html. Accessed March 21, 2016

Jones JL, Dubey JP. Foodborne toxoplasmosis. *Clin Infect Dis.* 2012;55(6):845–851

Robert-Gangeux F, Dardé ML. Epidemiology of and diagnostic strategies for toxoplasmosis. *Clin Microbiol Rev.* 2012;25(2):264–296

PART

2

Dermatology

CHAPTER 47

Acne

Sadaf Hussain, MD, and Albert C. Yan, MD

Key Points

- Mild acne can be successfully managed with topical comedolytic medications, such as benzoyl peroxide, topical retinoids, or both in combination.

- When tolerated, benzoyl peroxide should be incorporated into acne treatment regimens to minimize development of antibiotic resistance among *Propionibacterium acnes*.

- When using topical retinoids for acne treatment, patients may experience irritation during early treatment until their skin becomes conditioned to their use. During the first 1 to 2 weeks of starting retinoid therapy, patients may do better with every-other-day use or short-contact (30- to 60-minute) applications until they become accustomed to their use.

- For those 8 years and older with moderate to severe acne, oral antibiotics should be considered.

- Acne patients with other comorbidities or extracutaneous concerns (especially those with signs of precocious puberty, virilization, menstrual irregularities, alopecia, unwanted hair growth, and joint or bone pain) should be evaluated for associated underlying systemic disease.

Overview

Acne is an inflammatory skin disorder that predominantly affects sebaceous areas of the face, chest, shoulders, and back. The condition is most commonly seen among adolescents and young adults, often heralding the onset of puberty, but variants of acne can be encountered in infants and children as well. The clinical spectrum of disease includes open and closed comedones ("blackheads" and "whiteheads"), papules, pustules, and nodules, as well as secondary changes of pigmentary change and scarring. With appropriate treatments directed at the factors involved in acne pathogenesis, patients can expect to see improvement within the first 6 to 8 weeks, with continued clearance thereafter, with ongoing therapy. Selection of agents is based on several determinants, including the types of acne skin lesions present, their distribution, and their overall severity, as well as the patient's ability to tolerate acne medications.

Causes and Differential Diagnosis

Acne vulgaris has a multifactorial etiology. Androgenic stimulation results in follicular hyperkeratosis and excess sebum production, conditions hospitable to proliferation of resident *Propionibacterium acnes.* A variety of conditions bear a resemblance to acne vulgaris but can be differentiated from acne on clinical grounds (Table 47-1).

Table 47-1. Clinical Differential Diagnosis of Acne Vulgaris

Disease	Characteristics	Differentiating Features
Molluscum contagiosum	Small pearly papules that may resemble closed comedones, while inflamed lesions may resemble acne papules	Older lesions of molluscum contagiosum may display central umbilication. While lesions may occur on the face, chest, and back, these often have a predilection for intertriginous areas (ie, axillae, inguinal, genital) where acne is not typically seen.
Milia	Small, discrete submillimeter papules, usually arising at sites of friction or trauma; often seen around the eyes	Most of those affected usually have 1 or 2, but those with allergic rhinoconjunctivitis may have multiple milia that are often clustered around the eyes. These are often monomorphic in contrast to acne lesions that are often more widespread on the face (as well as chest and back); in acne, comedones are usually seen admixed with papules or pustules.
Periorificial dermatitis	Monomorphic papules and pustules clustered around the eyes, nose, and mouth; may be triggered by antecedent use of topical steroid	Acne is typically a scattered admixture of comedones, papules, and pustules in contrast with the monomorphic and geographically clustered presentations of periorificial dermatitis.
Keratosis pilaris	Keratotic follicular papules, classically located on the cheeks and extensor surfaces of arms and legs	Prickly sandpaper-like quality of keratosis pilaris and geographic distribution at these sites distinguishes this from acne.
Eruptive vellus hair cysts	Often bluish gray cystic lesions concentrated on the mid-chest, axillary, and sometimes inguinal areas	The bluish gray color and geographic distribution differentiates eruptive vellus hair cysts from acne.
Angiofibromas	Reddish brown, rubbery papules concentrated around the nose and on the forehead and cheeks; classically seen in children with tuberous sclerosis complex in whom multiple angiofibromas are present	Angiofibromas are persistent as opposed to the more transient acne lesions; angiofibromas arise in early childhood, an uncommon time for acne vulgaris to appear.

Continued

Table 47-1 *(cont)*

Disease	Characteristics	Differentiating Features
Folliculitis	Gram positive: usually papules and pustules often seen on the torso and buttocks Gram negative: usually seen on the torso or at sites of occlusion beneath swimwear following exposure to contaminated water *Malassezia:* may be seen on the face, chest, and back at sebum-rich sites	The distribution of lesions in folliculitis may provide a clue to the underlying organism. Gram-positive folliculitis is often recurrent and has a characteristic distribution that distinguishes it from acne. Gram-negative folliculitis also arises at stereotypical sites and is often self-limited, needing treatment when patients are especially symptomatic or in immunocompromised patients. *Malassezia* folliculitis is the most difficult to distinguish because it also occurs in typical acne-prone areas. In patients with acne who do not respond to conventional acne treatments, treatment with an antifungal against *Malassezia* may prove useful.

Clinical Features

Acne vulgaris is characterized clinically by the presence of comedones (blackheads and whiteheads), papules, pustules, and nodules in some subset or admixture of these primary lesions. Some patients may also develop secondary pigmentary changes, or evidence of scarring.

Age Variations

Acne is classically a disease of adolescents and young adults and often has its onset around the onset of puberty. However, acne can arise during other developmental periods (Table 47-2).

Neonatal acne, also referred to as neonatal cephalic pustulosis, arises within the first 4 to 6 weeks of life. Some controversy exists regarding its etiology and relationship to true acne vulgaris. Nonetheless, the condition appears to be attributable to some combination of maternal hormones and overgrowth of *Malassezia* species (Evidence Level II-2). The condition is characterized by papules or pustules involving the scalp and face, with some extension onto the upper torso in some. Neonatal acne is self-limited but has, in some cases, responded to topical antifungal therapy such as ketoconazole cream, directed against *Malassezia* (Evidence Level III).

Infantile acne differs from neonatal acne by its later onset, from 1 month to 1 year; its spectrum of clinical findings, including comedones and nodules in addition to papules and nodules; and its potential for permanent scarring. The

Table 47-2. Acne by Age

Acne Category	Clinical Features	Typical Age of Onset	Observations
Neonatal acne	Papules or pustules on the face, scalp, and sometimes upper torso	<6 wk	Self-limited but may respond to topical antifungals.
Infantile acne	Comedones, papules, pustules, or nodules (Underlying systemic disease is rare.)	Usually between 1 mo and 1 y	Conventional acne therapies may be used, except for tetracycline derivatives. Topical agents, either alone or in combination with systemic macrolides, may be considered.
Mid-childhood acne	Comedones, papules, pustules, or nodules (Underlying causes of hormonal excess [eg, adrenal tumor or congenital adrenal hyperplasia] should be considered and screening performed.)	1–7 y	Conventional acne therapies may be used, except for tetracycline derivatives. Topical agents, either alone or in combination with systemic macrolides, may be considered.
Preadolescent acne	Comedones and some mildly inflammatory lesions that may be present, often in a central facial or t-zone distribution	8–12 y	Conventional acne therapies may be used, including tetracycline derivatives. Topical agents, either alone or in combination with systemic agents, may be considered.
Adolescent and young adult acne	Comedones, papules, pustules, or nodules	≥13 y	Conventional acne therapies may be used, including tetracycline derivatives. Topical agents, either alone or in combination with systemic agents, may be considered.

condition is often self-limited but can last for several months or up to 2 to 3 years before remitting (Evidence Level II-2). Most cases are not associated with underlying comorbidities, but a comprehensive history, review of systems, and physical examination should be performed. If an underlying endocrinopathy is suspected, consultation with a pediatric endocrinologist and screening measures (Box 47-1) should be considered. Topical therapies are often effective, but systemic agents may be needed to prevent scarring (Evidence Level II-2). Tetracycline derivatives should be avoided in children younger than 8 years because of their adverse dental effects in this age group.

Box 47-1. Screening Measures for Patients With Infantile or Mid-Childhood Acne Suspected as Having an Underlying Endocrine Disorder

- Bone age radiograph
- Testosterone (free and total)
- DHEA sulphate
- Androstenedione
- Follicle-stimulating hormone
- Luteinizing hormone
- Thyrotropin
- 17-hydroxyprogesterone
- Prolactin
- Consultation with pediatric endocrinologist

Abbreviation: DHEA, dehydroepiandrosterone.

Mid-childhood acne is uncommon and characterized by the onset of acne between 1 and 7 years of age. Patients with mid-childhood acne may present with comedones, papules, pustules, or nodules. Children who demonstrate mid-childhood acne should undergo a comprehensive evaluation that includes a detailed history, review of systems, and physical examination, including assessment of growth velocity and Tanner staging (Evidence Level III). If an underlying endocrinopathy is suspected, screening measures and consultation with a pediatric endocrinologist should be considered (see Box 47-1). Topical therapies may be effective, but systemic agents may also be needed to prevent scarring. Tetracycline derivatives should again be avoided because of their adverse dental effects in this age group.

Preadolescent acne has its onset between 8 and 12 years of age and can represent the first sign of pubertal onset. This form of acne is typified by milder, comedonal presentation with a central facial or t-zone distribution. Most cases are amenable to topical treatment (Evidence Level I).

Severe Phenotypes and Systemic Disease

Acne fulminans represents an acute and severe manifestation of acne characterized by ulcerating acne lesions accompanied by fevers, malaise, and polyarthritis. This type of acne is often recalcitrant to oral antibiotic therapy, and generally requires administration of systemic corticosteroid (Evidence Level III). Acne conglobata is a form of acne represented by numerous comedones admixed with papules, pustules, nodules, and draining sinus tracts that involve the face, chest, back, and buttocks. The condition is often associated with hidradenitis suppurativa, dissecting cellulitis of the scalp, and pilonidal cysts, all of which are distinguished by their shared pathophysiology of follicular occlusion.

Females with severe acne should be evaluated for features of polycystic ovarian syndrome and HAIRAN (hyperandrogenism, insulin resistance, and acanthosis nigricans) syndrome. Other conditions causing an increase or imbalance of androgenic hormones may be associated with acne, including

Box 47-2. Systemic Diseases Associated With Acne

- Polycystic ovarian syndrome
- HAIRAN (hyperandrogenism, insulin resistance, and acanthosis nigricans) syndrome
- Androgen-secreting tumors (gonadal, adrenal, and central)
- Cushing syndrome
- Congenital adrenal hyperplasia
- Gigantism and acromegaly
- SAPHO (synovitis, acne, pustulosis, hyperostosis, and osteitis) syndrome
- PAPA (pyogenic arthritis, pyoderma gangrenosum, and acne) syndrome
- Behçet syndrome
- Apert syndrome

disorders such as Cushing syndrome, congenital adrenal hyperplasia, gigantism, and acromegaly.

Joint symptoms in association with severe acne and other systemic concerns may indicate SAPHO (synovitis, acne, pustulosis, hyperostosis, and osteitis) or PAPA (pyogenic arthritis, pyoderma gangrenosum, and acne) syndrome. Genetic disorders may also have acne as an associated feature. This is true of Apert syndrome and pachydermoperiostosis, in which acne can be particularly severe. Box 47-2 lists systemic diseases associated with acne.

Evaluation

When evaluating a patient with acne vulgaris, a thorough history and physical examination should be performed.

- The onset, distribution, and severity of the acne, as well as prior treatment responses, help direct selection of appropriate therapeutic options.
- Possible exacerbating factors, skin care habits, and medication history should be evaluated to determine if there are avoidable triggers.
- A social history indicating participation in sports that require protective gear may be helpful in identifying reasons for acne arising at unusual locations. Concentration of acne along the forehead often indicates use of a helmet, while localization to the chin suggests frictional influences from a chin strap.
- A family history of scarring acne or acne requiring systemic therapy (eg, antibiotics or isotretinoin) may indicate a greater risk for more severe acne.
- Aggravation of acne during the perimenstrual period in females may be a clue to underlying hormonal imbalances, especially when it is accompanied by other signs, such as menstrual irregularities, unwanted facial hair, unexpected weight gain, or alopecia.

Clinicians caring for patients with acne should be attentive to mood disturbances, which, while common among adolescents and young adults, may also be aggravated by acne and can influence patients' self-esteem as well as school performance and social interactions.

Infants and preadolescent children with acne should be examined for indications of androgen excess. This could include signs of precocious puberty, virilization, or abdominal masses.

Management

Treatment plans should be individualized to each particular patient. A stepwise approach for the treatment of acne has been developed from the recent American Acne and Rosacea Society national pediatric guidelines and endorsed by the American Academy of Pediatrics (Evidence Level III) (Figures 47-1, 47-2, and 47-3). Disease severity is generally based on the number of lesions, their type, their extent, and whether scarring is present. Acne that progresses beyond comedones (namely, moderate to severe acne characterized by papules, pustules, or nodules) generally involves *P acnes* and the patient's host response to the organism, which results in more inflammatory disease. Treatment for moderate to severe acne should include agents directed against *P acnes*, associated inflammation, and hormonal dysregulation.

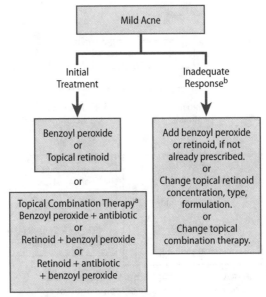

Figure 47-1. Pediatric treatment algorithm for mild acne.
Topical dapsone may be considered as single therapy or in place of topical antibiotic.

[a] Topical fixed-combination prescriptions available.

[b] Assess adherence.

Figures used with permission of the AARS. The AARS makes no representations, endorsements, or warranties related to the information presented by the author(s), AAP, or their affiliates, agents, or representatives.

Figure 47-2. Pediatric treatment algorithm for moderate acne.
Topical dapsone may be considered in place of topical antibiotic.

[a] Topical fixed-combination prescriptions available.

[b] Assess adherence.

[c] Consider dermatologic referral.

Figures used with permission of the AARS. The AARS makes no representations, endorsements, or warranties related to the information presented by the author(s), AAP, or their affiliates, agents, or representatives.

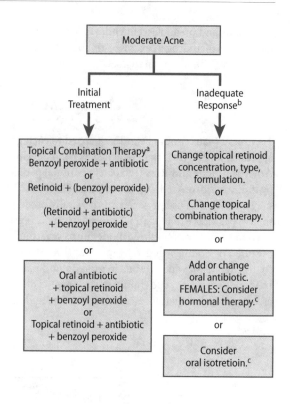

Moderate Acne

Initial Treatment

Inadequate Response[b]

Topical Combination Therapy[a]
Benzoyl peroxide + antibiotic
or
Retinoid + (benzoyl peroxide)
or
(Retinoid + antibiotic)
+ benzoyl peroxide

Change topical retinoid concentration, type, formulation.
or
Change topical combination therapy.

or

Oral antibiotic
+ topical retinoid
+ benzoyl peroxide
or
Topical retinoid + antibiotic
+ benzoyl peroxide

Add or change oral antibiotic.
FEMALES: Consider hormonal therapy.[c]

or

Consider oral isotretioin.[c]

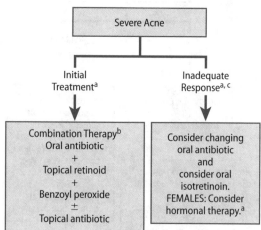

Severe Acne

Initial Treatment[a]

Inadequate Response[a, c]

Combination Therapy[b]
Oral antibiotic
+
Topical retinoid
+
Benzoyl peroxide
±
Topical antibiotic

Consider changing oral antibiotic and consider oral isotretinoin.
FEMALES: Consider hormonal therapy.[a]

Figure 47-3. Pediatric treatment algorithm for severe acne.
Topical dapsone may be considered in place of topical antibiotic.

[a] Consider dermatologic referral.

[b] Topical fixed-combination prescriptions available.

[c] Assess adherence; consider change of topical retinoid.

Figures used with permission of the AARS. The AARS makes no representations, endorsements, or warranties related to the information presented by the author(s), AAP, or their affiliates, agents, or representatives.

Principal Agents (Table 47-3)

Benzoyl Peroxide

Benzoyl peroxide is anti-comedolytic and has activity against *P acnes*. It is available in a wide variety of concentrations ranging from 2.25% to 10%. It can be used as a wash-off cleanser as well as leave-on gel, cream, or lotion, giving it versatility for use on the face, chest, or back. Because of its ability to kill anaerobic *P acnes* by producing oxygen, there has been no documented resistance to benzoyl peroxide, and its use can reduce and prevent the development of antibiotic resistance when used in combination with topical antibiotics (Evidence Level II-2). Its use is limited by irritation and occasionally by contact allergy (hive-like reactions). Patients may also report its tendency to bleach colored fabrics.

Topical Retinoid

Topical retinoids are comedolytic agents that possess mild anti-inflammatory properties. Three commercially available topical retinoids are indicated for acne: adapalene, tretinoin, and tazarotene. Adapalene and tretinoin are often used as first-line treatments for acne because of their relatively good tolerability, while tazarotene is more often reserved for more extensive or recalcitrant comedonal acne. Cream and microsphere-encapsulated gel formulations of retinoids are generally milder than their straight gel counterparts (Evidence Level I). Both adapalene and tretinoin are classified as Pregnancy Category C, while tazarotene is Pregnancy Category X. When first using topical retinoids, they may cause mild chapping or irritation, which usually abates after about a week of use. During the initial week of therapy, it is often helpful to recommend every-other-day use or short-contact therapy (left on for 30–60 minutes and then washed off) until patients are able to tolerate overnight, every night use.

Topical Antibiotic

Topical antibiotics exert their effect in acne by killing *P acnes,* and to some degree by reducing inflammation. They have limited activity against comedonal disease. The agents most commonly used include clindamycin, erythromycin, and sodium sulfacetamide. They are generally well tolerated with a relatively low potential for irritation. Lotion, ointment, and cleanser vehicles are tolerated best by those with dry skin, while those with oilier skin may prefer gels or solutions or foams, which are also easier to spread over large areas. Topical antibiotics are best used in combination with other agents (eg, benzoyl peroxide) to provide synergy and minimize development of antibiotic resistance. For instance, benzoyl peroxide cleanser could be combined with clindamycin gel as a daily regimen for mild to moderate acne. Unopposed use of topical antibiotics as monotherapy should be avoided because of the high likelihood of development of antibiotic resistance (Evidence Level II-2).

Table 47-3. Commonly Prescribed Acne Treatments

Agent	Available Formulations	Vehicles	Comments
Benzoyl Peroxide	2.25%–10% topically applied once or twice daily	Gel, lotion, cream, or cleanser (wash)	Can bleach colored fabrics. Irritation possible. True hypersensitivity is also possible, but uncommon.
Retinoids	Topically applied once daily		
Adapalene	0.1% and 0.3%	Lotion, cream, or gel	Irritation is not uncommon but often self-limited. Use every other day or for 30–60 min and then wash off for 1–2 wk before increasing to daily therapy to improve tolerance.
Tretinoin	0.01%, 0.025%, 0.05%, and 0.1%	Cream, gel, or micro-gel	
Tazarotene	0.05% and 0.1%	Cream or gel	
Topical Antibiotics	Topically applied		
Clindamycin	1%	Lotion, gel, solution, or foam	Usually well-tolerated. Should ideally be used in conjunction with benzoyl peroxide since antibiotic resistance often develops quickly when used as monotherapy.
Erythromycin	2%	Ointment, gel, or solution	
Sodium sulfacetamide (sometimes combined with sulfur)	10%	Cleanser or lotion	
Dapsone	5%	Gel	May be irritating for those with sensitive skin. Dapsone has anti-inflammatory properties and is sometimes used in conjunction with other topical agents.
Fixed Combinations	Topically applied		
Benzoyl peroxide + erythromycin	5%/3%	Gel	These fixed-combination products stabilize both ingredients and may improve ease of use and adherence, but are often more expensive.
Benzoyl peroxide + clindamycin	5%/1%	Gel	
Benzoyl peroxide + adapalene	2.5%/1.2%	Gel	
Tretinoin + clindamycin	2.5%/0.1%	Gel	
	0.025%/1.2%	Gel	

Medication	Dosing	Formulation	Comments
Oral Antibiotics Erythromycin Tetracycline Doxycycline (also, sub-antimicrobial dosing available) Minocycline	Oral 30–50 mg/kg/d divided every 6–8 h 250–500 mg every day–4 times daily 50–100 mg every day–twice daily 20 mg twice daily or 40 mg once daily 50–100 mg every day–twice daily Extended-release formulations available in 45, 55, 65, 80, 90, 105, 115, and 135-mg dosing	Capsule/tablet Capsule/tablet Capsule/tablet Capsule/tablet	Sub-antimicrobial dosing of doxycycline has been used to treat mildly inflammatory acne while reducing the risks of antibiotic resistance and other adverse effects. Extended-release dosing of minocycline is available and may reduce the risk of vestibular effects.
Combination Oral Contraceptives (female patients)	Oral Once daily	Tablet	Use may be associated with increased risk of venous thromboembolism.
Isotretinoin	Oral 10–80 mg once daily or divided twice daily	Tablet	iPledge monitoring program for managing potential adverse effects. Prescribing clinicians, dispensing pharmacies, and patients must be registered to use this medication.

Oral Antibiotic

Oral antibiotics are indicated for moderate to severe acne. They exert their effects through their ability to kill *P acnes* and, in some cases, can demonstrate anti-inflammatory effects (particularly tetracycline and macrolide derivatives).

In children 8 years and older, doxycycline and minocycline are preferred over tetracycline. Rates of antibiotic resistance among *P acnes* to doxycycline and especially minocycline are lower than for tetracycline, and both doxycycline and minocycline can be administered once or twice daily, while optimal effects for tetracycline require taking the medication 2 to 4 times daily. Use of tetracycline derivatives can be associated with adverse effects that include but are not limited to headaches, gastrointestinal issues such as diarrhea or abdominal pain, pill esophagitis, photosensitivity, dizziness or vestibular effects, arthralgias, serum sickness-like syndrome, lupus-like syndrome, and drug hypersensitivity syndrome (Table 47-4).

Erythromycin is a less ideal drug given the high rates of antibiotic resistance among *P acnes*; however, it remains the agent of choice in children younger than 8 years who require systemic therapy because tetracycline derivatives are contraindicated in this age group. While there has been some experience employing other systemic antibiotics for acne, agents such as azithromycin, amoxicillin, cephalexin, trimethoprim, and trimethoprim/sulfamethoxazole are not recommended routinely for acne management (Evidence Level II-3).

Oral Retinoid

Severe nodulocystic acne with scarring or scarring potential requires prompt intervention. If the patient is not responding sufficiently to conventional combination therapy employing topical agents and systemic antibiotics,

Table 47-4. Tetracycline Derivatives for Acne

Effect	Tetracycline	Doxycycline	Minocycline
Propionibacterium acnes antibiotic resistance	+++	++	+
GI effects (eg, diarrhea, abdominal pain)	++	++	+
Pill esophagitis	++	+++	+
Photosensitivity	++	+++	+
Vestibular effects (eg, dizziness)	+	+	+++
Arthralgias	+	+	+++
Serum sickness–like reaction	+	+	+++
Lupus-like syndrome	−	−	+++
Drug hypersensitivity syndrome	+	+	+++

Abbreviation: GI, gastrointestinal.

Number of plus signs (+) indicates likelihood of side effect, and minus sign (−) indicates no association.

isotretinoin should be considered. Isotretinoin (previously available as Accu-
tane until 2009; currently available in other branded generic formulations as
Amnesteem, Claravis, Isotroin, and Sotret) is a systemic retinoid that has
significant effects on the key pathogenic issues contributing to acne, namely,
reducing follicular hyperkeratosis, decreasing inflammation, and decreasing
excess sebum production, which thereby reduces *P acnes* colonization. Patients
with significant acne nearly always show a profound response to isotretinoin
during a half-year course of therapy, which cumulatively equates to approximately 120 to 150 mg/kg total over this time period (Evidence Level I).

Patients taking isotretinoin should be monitored closely for adverse effects
as part of the US Food and Drug Administration (FDA)–mandated iPledge
monitoring program that requires registration of prescribing clinicians,
dispensing pharmacies, and patients to minimize potential adverse effects,
particularly birth defects and mood disorders. Those on the medication
commonly experience xerosis (especially on the forearms and hands) and dry
mucous membranes (dry eyes or nosebleeds). Less commonly, arthralgias or
myalgias, lipid abnormalities (elevated cholesterol or triglycerides), transaminitis, and, rarely, hematologic abnormalities (ie, leukopenia) may be noted. As a
systemic retinoid, isotretinoin is a known potent teratogen, and females of
childbearing age should either maintain abstinence or be offered contraception.
Isotretinoin has also been purported to be a cause of mood disorders (Evidence
Level III) and inflammatory colitis (Evidence Level II-2). Although there are
conflicting data, it is advised that patients receiving isotretinoin be monitored
for changes in mood, as well as for diarrhea and hematochezia.

Mild Acne

Mild acne consists predominantly of comedonal lesions, with a limited extent of
disease. Most cases of mild acne will respond to topical therapy (see Figure
47-1). Over-the-counter agents containing salicylic acid or benzoyl peroxide
may be helpful and are often employed by patients before seeing the pediatric
clinician.

For those who do not respond to over-the-counter options, benzoyl
peroxide or topical retinoid, either one alone or each in combination, should be
considered. Both agents possess comedolytic and anti-comedogenic activity,
which help treat existing and prevent future acne. To optimize results, these
agents should be applied to the entire areas predisposed to acne rather than
individual lesions.

For those with more extensive disease (involving the face, chest, and back),
one tip is to employ a medicated (benzoyl peroxide or sodium sulfacetamide)
cleanser that can be applied easily over large body surface areas; alternatively, a
gel or foam vehicle (for topical retinoids or topical antibiotics, respectively) can
also be considered, since these spread more easily over large areas.

If initial monotherapy is unsuccessful, addition of an adjunct agent is
recommended. For instance, if benzoyl peroxide provides an insufficient
response, a topical retinoid can be added. If benzoyl peroxide and a topical

retinoid are insufficient, a topical antibiotic can be considered. Alternatively, an increase in potency of the benzoyl peroxide or topical retinoid could also be considered.

Moderate Acne

Moderate acne may include comedones, but there is typically an admixture of papules and pustules. Post-inflammatory erythema and pigmentation changes may also be present.

For moderate acne that is predominantly comedonal, topical combination therapy is advised (see Figure 47-2). Topical benzoyl peroxide can be combined with a topical retinoid or antibiotic, or all 3 can be used. Because some compounds are incompatible when used at the same time, a topical benzoyl peroxide can be employed as a cleanser followed by application of a topical antibiotic, and the retinoid can then be used at night. If the response is suboptimal, an oral antibiotic can be added.

For moderate acne that is more inflammatory and consists more of papules and pustules, or when the acne is more extensive and has spread to involve the chest and back, an oral systemic agent is recommended. The oral antibiotic can be combined with a topical regimen consisting of a topical retinoid with a benzoyl peroxide. If there is an insufficient response, the dose of the oral antibiotic or potency of the topical agents may be increased.

For menstruating females, hormonal therapy can be prescribed as an adjunct to therapy. Combination contraceptive pills are indicated for the management of moderate acne (Evidence Level I). Significant effects are generally seen within about 3 to 4 months, and some patients are able to discontinue oral antibiotics and reduce topical therapy while on hormonal therapy. Only certain agents (ie, norgestimate and ethinyl estradiol [Ortho Tri-Cyclen], norethindrone and ethinyl estradiol [Estrostep], and drospirenone and ethinyl estradiol [Yaz]) carry an FDA approval for the treatment of acne. That being said, other generically available hormonal pills, such as desogestrel and ethinyl estradiol (Desogen), have been studied for acne treatment and, while not FDA approved for acne, may also demonstrate benefit for female patients (Evidence Level I).

Spironolactone is an aldosterone antagonist that competes for androgen receptors in target tissues and inhibits androgen biosynthesis. It has the added benefits of treating hirsutism and androgenetic alopecia, and can be considered for adolescent and young adult females for more severe acne. The dose ranges from 50 to 200 mg daily. Menstrual dysfunction may occur and typically resolves over the first 2 to 3 months of treatment. If persistent, alteration of the dosage or addition of an oral contraceptive pill may be beneficial. Because spironolactone may cause feminization of a male fetus, some advocate its use always in combination with an oral contraceptive. While it is used as a potassium-sparing diuretic, recent studies have not indicated a significant risk of hyperkalemia in otherwise healthy patients.

Severe Acne

Severe acne is marked principally by its potential for scarring, or actual scarring, and often consists of a mixture of comedones, papules, pustules, and nodules. Prompt intervention is important to minimize permanent sequelae from scarring (see Figure 47-3).

If the patient is naive to previous therapy, an oral antibiotic such as doxycycline or minocycline could be initiated with combination topical therapy, such as a topical retinoid, benzoyl peroxide, and topical antibiotic. If the patient responds sufficiently promptly within 4 to 8 weeks, this therapy can be continued until the patient clears. If female, hormonal therapy with a combination oral contraceptive can also be considered.

If the patient has already failed maximal conventional therapy, treatment with isotretinoin is advised. Nearly all patients who receive isotretinoin will see their acne remit, although some who relapse may require a second course of therapy (Evidence Level I). Nonetheless, even those who relapse often find that their acne is responsive to treatments that may not have worked previously (Evidence Level III).

Suboptimal Treatment Responses

Patients should be given reasonable expectations about treatment responses. Although some clearing may be noted as soon as a week after starting, patients often do not recognize signs of improvement until about 6 to 8 weeks later, and often some trial and error is involved before arriving at a good response.

For those with more sensitive skin, some patients may become non-adherent if they perceive that the medications prescribed are causing unwanted adverse effects. For instance, topical retinoids often cause some mild irritation or chapping when first initiated. Using a lower concentration, administering the medication every other day for the first 1 to 2 weeks, or applying the medication with short-contact times (30–60 minutes) and washing it off for the first 1 to 2 weeks may reduce the chapping potential and allow patients to become better conditioned to retinoid effects. For those bothered by benzoyl peroxide, limiting concentrations to less than 6% may help reduce irritation. For those allergic to benzoyl peroxide, sodium sulfacetamide cleanser or lotion can be substituted.

Emerging research suggests that diet may be a contributing factor in acne. Diets high in glycemic index (Evidence Level II-3) and increased intake of milk (especially skim milk) have been linked to increased acne (Evidence Level II-2). Further investigations are needed to determine whether specific dietary interventions can effect improvement in acne.

Providing reasonable expectations, anticipating adverse effects, arranging for written treatment plans, and scheduling periodic follow-up can help patients stay on track and remain adherent to prescribed regimens. Table 47-5 shows the recommendations for targeted treatment options based on type of acne.

Table 47-5. Acne Types and Targeted Treatment Options

	Topical Retinoid	Benzoyl Peroxide	Topical Antibiotic	Oral Antibiotic	Hormonal (OCPs and Spironolactone)	Isotretinoin	Other
Comedonal	X	X					Combination products • Topical retinoid + benzoyl peroxide • Topical retinoid + topical antibiotic Salicylic acid cleanser
Mild inflammatory	X	X	X				Combination products • Topical benzoyl peroxide + topical antibiotic • Topical retinoid + benzoyl peroxide • Topical retinoid + topical antibiotic
Moderate inflammatory	X	X	X	X	X		Topical dapsone
Nodulocystic					X	X	

Abbreviation: OCP, oral contraceptive pill.

Long-term Monitoring

While the goal of acne treatment is to prevent scarring, a subset of patients will develop some degree of scarring from their acne. With continued spontaneous remodeling, scars often improve in appearance with time. Topical retinoids may be of modest benefit (Evidence Level III). Chemical peeling, microdermabrasion, laser resurfacing, and surgical procedures (subcisions, excisions, and dermal filler placement) are all effective treatments and may be employed to help reduce the appearance of scars (Evidence Level III). It is important to counsel patients about having realistic expectations from these procedures and to advocate for treatment of active acne lesions to prevent further scarring and its associated psychologic morbidities. In addition, patients with acne should be monitored for signs of underlying comorbidities. Insulin resistance and hormonal disturbances associated with polycystic ovarian syndrome and HAIRAN syndrome, as well as other androgen-driven conditions, may include acne among their manifestations, and clinicians should remain vigilant for other corroborating signs that may develop in the future.

Suggested Reading

Bhate K, Williams HC. Epidemiology of acne vulgaris. *Br J Dermatol.* 2013;168(3): 474–485

Dréno B, Thiboutot D, Gollnick H, et al; Global Alliance to Improve Outcomes in Acne. Large-scale worldwide observational study of adherence with acne therapy. *Int J Dermatol.* 2010;49(4):448–456

Eichenfield LF, Krakowski AC, Piggott C, et al; American Acne and Rosacea Society. Evidence-based recommendations for the diagnosis and treatment of pediatric acne. *Pediatrics.* 2013;131(Suppl 3):S163–S186

Friedlander SF, Baldwin HE, Mancini AJ, Yan AC, Eichenfield LF. The acne continuum: an age-based approach to therapy. *Semin Cutan Med Surg.* 2011;30(3 Suppl):S6–S11

Garner SE, Eady A, Bennett C, Newton JN, Thomas K, Popescu CM. Minocycline for acne vulgaris: efficacy and safety. *Cochrane Database Syst Rev.* 2012;(8):CD002086

Lebrun-Vignes B, Kreft-Jais C, Castot A, Chosidow O; French Network of Regional Centers of Pharmacovigilance. Comparative analysis of adverse drug reactions to tetracyclines: results of a French national survey and review of the literature. *Br J Dermatol.* 2012;166(6):1333–1341

Mancini AJ, Baldwin HE, Eichenfield LF, Friedlander SF, Yan AC. Acne life cycle: the spectrum of pediatric disease. *Semin Cutan Med Surg.* 2011;30(3 Suppl):S2–S5

Patel M, Bowe WP, Heughebaert C, Shalita AR. The development of antimicrobial resistance due to the antibiotic treatment of acne vulgaris. *J Drugs Dermatol.* 2010;9(6):655–664

Thiboutot D, Gollnick H, Bettoli V, et al. New insights into the management of acne: an update from the Global Alliance to Improve Outcomes in Acne group. *J Am Acad Dermatol.* 2009;60(5 Suppl):S1–S50

Yan AC, Baldwin HE, Eichenfield LF, Friedlander SF, Mancini AJ. Approach to pediatric acne treatment: an update. *Semin Cutan Med Surg.* 2011;30(3 Suppl):S16–S21

CHAPTER 48

Alopecia

Kristi Canty, MD

Key Points

- Alopecia areata presents with well-circumscribed, smooth areas of alopecia. Nail pitting and exclamation mark hairs can help confirm the diagnosis. Most isolated, individual patches of hair loss will resolve without treatment.

- The presence of posterior auricular lymphadenopathy, scaling, alopecia, and pruritus are highly suggestive of tinea capitis. High-dose griseofulvin may be used as first-line treatment for *Microsporum* and *Trichophyton* infections. Terbinafine may be used to treat *Trichophyton* infections.

- Trichotillomania is an impulse control disorder that presents as irregular patches of hair loss at varying lengths. Patients with trichotillomania need consultation with a specialist in behavioral medicine that can provide behavior therapy and counseling.

- Traction alopecia is caused by traumatic hairstyles and practices. Discontinuation of these practices can prevent permanent hair loss.

Overview

Hair loss, also known as alopecia, is rare in children but occurs because of many factors. Hair loss can be congenital, acquired, scarring, and non-scarring and can occur in circumscribed or diffuse patterns. Alopecia areata, tinea capitis, trichotillomania, traction alopecia, and telogen effluvium are most commonly encountered in the primary practice setting.

Causes and Differential Diagnosis

There are many causes of alopecia; each is specific to the underlying disorder.

Alopecia areata is classified as an autoimmune disease. It is an acquired, non-scarring type of hair loss in which hair follicles retain the potential for spontaneous recovery. Up to 50% of patients that have alopecia areata will develop it before the age of 21. There may be a family history of this type of hair loss as well as an association with atopic conditions or autoimmune diseases.

Most patients with patchy alopecia enter remission within a year, but a subset of patients have a progressive course.

Tinea capitis, or ringworm of the scalp, is dermatophyte (fungal) infection of the scalp and hair shaft. It is a common form of acquired, non-scarring alopecia. In severe infections, scarring alopecia can result. It is highly contagious and commonly caused by *Trichophyton tonsurans* and *Microsporum canis.*

Trichotillomania is a self-induced, acquired hair loss caused by habitual hair pulling. This type of hair loss is usually non-scarring; however, with repeated trauma, scar formation can occur and hair loss can become permanent. Trichotillomania is classified as an impulse control disorder. Females are more commonly affected than males. Youth typically display automatic pulling, in which the individual is unaware of the behavior. Older individuals often display more focal pulling, in which they are fully cognizant of the action.

Traction alopecia is an acquired, often non-scarring alopecia that results from grooming practices and tight hairstyles. With long-term repetitive trauma, permanent hair loss can result. This is often seen in females and the African American population.

Telogen effluvium is a common acquired, self-limited, diffuse, non-scarring alopecia that results in excessive loss of telogen hairs or hairs that are in a resting stage of the hair cycle. It is usually caused by a prior acute stressful event that abruptly changes anagen hairs (growing phase) into telogen hairs (resting stage) but can occur in response to a variety of disorders (Box 48-1). Telogen hairs are shed 2 to 3 months later, and the process often resolves within 3 to 6 months. The differential diagnosis rests with discrimination from other disorders of hair loss (Box 48-2).

Box 48-1. Causes of Telogen Effluvium

- Acute and severe illness (high fever)
- Surgery/trauma/childbirth
- Thyroid disease
- Iron deficiency anemia
- Malnutrition/malabsorption
- Chronic illness
- Syphilis
- Medications

Box 48-2. Differential Diagnosis of Acquired Childhood Alopecia

- Alopecia areata
- Telogen effluvium
- Tinea capitis
- Trichotillomania
- Traction alopecia

Clinical Features

· · · · · · · · · · · · · · · ·

Clinical features of alopecia are specific to the underlying disorders (Table 48-1).

Table 48-1. Clinical Characteristics of Common Acquired Alopecia of Childhood

Type of Alopecia	Cause	Clinical Presentation	Additional Findings
Alopecia areata	Autoimmune process	Asymptomatic, circumscribed, smooth, hairless patches without scale	• Exclamation mark hairs • Nail pitting • Alopecia at other hair-bearing sites
Tinea capitis	Dermatophyte	Patches of fractured hair, diffuse fine scale, pustules, kerions, history of pruritus	Regional lymphadenopathy
Trichotillomania	Self-induced	Irregular pattern of hair loss with hairs at different lengths	• Scalp excoriations • Follicular petechiae
Traction alopecia	Hairstyling practices	Hair loss at sights of trauma from traction, friction, chemicals	History of styling practices
Telogen effluvium	Acute stressful events (physiologic/ psychologic)	Asymptomatic, diffuse hair loss/ thinning	Microscopic evaluation that shows hairs with club-shaped roots

Alopecia Areata

Alopecia areata presents with well-circumscribed, smooth, hairless patches without scale or erythema. This type of hair loss can occur on any hair-bearing site of the body. There are several patterns of alopecia areata. The most common form is the patch type, which presents with round to oval areas of hair loss that can be an isolated patch or involve multiple areas. The ophiasis pattern presents as a band-like area of hair loss extending from the temporal to occipital area. Loss of hair on the entire scalp is called alopecia totalis, and complete loss of scalp and body hair is coined alopecia universalis. The diffuse type of hair loss presents with widespread thinning of scalp hair.

Examination of hair loss areas will reveal a completely bald, smooth-surfaced patch with a skin color to slightly peachy discoloration. At the periphery, exclamation mark hairs can be found. In active disease, hairs can be pulled easily from the borders of bald areas.

Additional clinical findings can help confirm the diagnosis of alopecia areata. Nail pitting is the primary nail abnormality described, but other nail changes such as trachyonychia (rough longitudinal ridges), onycholysis (detachment of the nail plate from the nail bed), and brittle nails can also be seen. Alopecia areata has been associated with other autoimmune diseases such as thyroiditis, vitiligo, lupus, diabetes mellitus, and celiac disease. A history of asthma, allergies, and atopic dermatitis can be seen in patients as well. Those with a family history of alopecia areata or who have onset in early childhood and an ophiasis pattern of loss, nail changes, and associated atopy or autoimmune diseases are at greatest risk for severe disease.

Tinea Capitis

Tinea capitis can have several clinical presentations, most of which have some form of underlying scaling. The "gray patch" pattern presents with patchy alopecia and scaling. The "diffuse scale" pattern appears as widespread, generalized scaling. The "diffuse pustular" pattern presents with pustules, scaling, and alopecia. A "kerion" pattern appears as a boggy, painful, hairless plaque. "Favus" pattern presents with yellow cup-shaped crusts. The "black dot" pattern presents with a well-demarcated, hairless patch that is studded with fractured hairs giving a speckled appearance. Regional lymphadenopathy is commonly present. The finding of posterior auricular lymphadenopathy, scaling, alopecia, and pruritus is highly suggestive of tinea capitis.

Trichotillomania

Trichotillomania presents with unusual and irregular patterns of hair loss. The hairs are broken and at different lengths with underlying normal scalp. The eyebrows and lashes are additional common sites involved.

Traction Alopecia

Traction alopecia is often obvious on the basis of the patient's hairstyle. Tight braids, weaves, ponytails, barrettes, and other hairstyles produce constant tension, which may lead to fractured hairs, folliculitis, and follicular-based papules.

Telogen Effluvium

Telogen effluvium presents with diffuse thinning of scalp hair. The scalp otherwise appears normal. Hairs from all areas of the scalp can be pulled out with minimal effort. The hairs are all in the telogen stage.

Evaluation

Alopecia Areata

Laboratory investigations are not needed to make the diagnosis of alopecia areata. In some difficult diagnostic cases, such as diffuse hair loss, a scalp biopsy can be helpful to confirm the diagnosis of alopecia areata, but this is rare. Routine screening for autoimmune diseases, such as thyroid disorders, is not recommended at this time because of lack of clinical evidence. However, patients with more severe or persistent forms of alopecia areata are more likely to have thyroid abnormalities.

Tinea Capitis

Evaluation of suspected tinea capitis can be done with a dermatophyte culture. Hair pluck and skin scrapings can also be used to obtain specimen for culture. Dermatophyte cultures often take 7 to 21 days to develop. A microscopic examination of plucked hair and scale with a wet mount of potassium hydroxide can provide a rapid confirmation of infection in clinic. Wood lamp examination is less likely to be helpful since most scalp dermatophyte infections in the United States are caused by *T tonsurans,* an endothrix infection (spores are found within the hair shaft), which does not fluoresce.

Trichotillomania and Traction Alopecia

Trichotillomania and traction alopecia usually do not require extensive workup. In some cases, a scalp biopsy can be useful in differentiating trichotillomania and traction alopecia from other acquired types of hair loss

Telogen Effluvium

Telogen effluvium can often be diagnosed without an excessive workup. Obtaining a history of an inciting event (see Table 48-1), such as high fever that occurred 2 to 3 months prior to the onset of hair loss, can be helpful. A hair pull demonstrating more that 25% of hairs in the telogen phase or daily hair counts of greater than 100 hairs/day can be diagnostic. If etiology of the underlying process is unclear from the history, obtaining blood work to rule out thyroid disease or iron deficiency anemia may be helpful. Additional laboratory workup may be warranted depending on the individual's history and examination.

Management

Alopecia Areata

Not all patients with alopecia areata require treatment, because up to 80% of patients with limited, patchy hair loss will undergo spontaneous remission within a year. It is reasonable to offer most patients a watch-and-wait approach with the anticipation that regrowth of any individual patch can take several months. In patients with extensive, long-standing alopecia, the prognosis is poor. In this group, a wig may be the best option, because treatments are likely to be futile. A subset of patients has progressive hair loss or extensive involvement in which treatment may be desired. Currently, there are no US Food and Drug Administration (FDA)–approved drugs for the treatment of alopecia areata. Several treatments can result in regrowth of hair, but no treatment has been proven to result in long-term remission. A recent Cochrane review summarized that few therapies have been comprehensively evaluated with randomized controlled trials and only topical steroids demonstrated short-term benefit (Evidence Level II).

For the subset of patients with progressive or extensive hair loss that desire treatment, treatment is based on age for implementation by a dermatologist. For children younger than 10 years, suggested first-line treatment is a combination of 5% minoxidil solution twice daily along with a mid-potency topical corticosteroid (Evidence Level II). If patients do not respond to minoxidil and steroids within 6 months, short-contact therapy with anthralin may be helpful. For patients 10 years and older with less than 50% scalp involvement, intralesional injections of triamcinolone acetonide are suggested as first-line therapy. If these patients do not respond to intralesional injections within 6 months, other therapeutic options can be offered, such as 5% minoxidil, potent topical corticosteroids under occlusion at night, and short-contact therapy with anthralin. For patients older than 10 years who also have greater than 50% scalp involvement, suggested therapies include topical immunotherapy with diphenylcyclopropenone alone or in conjunction with intralesional triamcinolone for recalcitrant patches. If these patients remain nonresponders after a 6-month trial, other treatment options include 5% minoxidil solution, topical clobetasol propionate under occlusion, or short-contact anthralin. Modified treatment algorithms for the primary care physician (Figures 48-1 and 48-2)

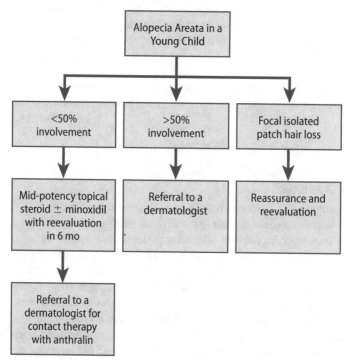

Figure 48-1. Approach to treatment in a young child with alopecia areata.

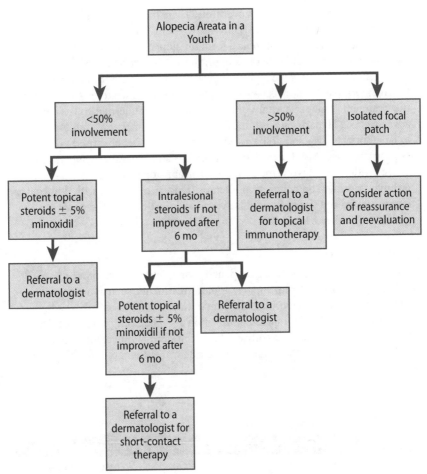

Figure 48-2. Approach to treatment in a youth with alopecia areata.

take into consideration their limited experience with some of the above treatments and offer guidance on when to seek dermatologic consultation (Evidence Level III).

Topical corticosteroids (Evidence Level II) have been used extensively as a first-line treatment for alopecia areata. This treatment is inexpensive, is easy to use, and can cover large surface areas. Folliculitis, atrophy of scalp skin, and rarely systemic adverse effects can be seen.

Intralesional corticosteroids (Evidence Level III) can produce regrowth at the site of scalp injection; however, this requires multiple injections at regular intervals. Clinicians should have previous experience in this technique. Injections are painful, but a topical anesthetic can be helpful. Triamcinolone acetonide (5–10 mg/mL) is commonly used. This type of therapy is limited by the amount of area that can be injected. Scalp skin atrophy is a common adverse effect that often resolves over time. There have been rare case reports of anaphylaxis with triamcinolone acetonide when used to treat alopecia areata.

Minoxidil can be used in topical form for alopecia areata (Evidence Level II). It has been used for years to promote hair regrowth, especially in androgenetic alopecia. Five percent topical minoxidil is used as an adjuvant treatment for patchy alopecia areata. It has not been shown to be effective for the treatment of alopecia totalis or universalis. Contact dermatitis is a common adverse effect. Hypertrichosis (facial hair growth) can occur as well. Application to large surface areas should be avoided because systemic absorption can occur, putting patients at risk for cardiac irregularities and generalized hypertrichosis.

For widespread involvement and recalcitrant alopecia areata, a dermatologist may consider contact immunotherapy (Evidence Level II) with diphenylcyclopropenone and squaric acid dibutylester or short-contact therapy with anthralin (Evidence Level III).

Tinea Capitis

Treatment of tinea capitis requires penetration of medication into the hair follicles (Table 48-2). Unfortunately, topical treatments, such as antifungal shampoos, do not provide adequate penetration and are used only as adjunct therapy in preventing the spread of infection and increasing cure rates. Systemic therapy is required to truly eradicate this dermatophyte infection. Griseofulvin has been the criterion standard for treatment of tinea capitis and

Table 48-2. Tinea Capitis Treatment

Medication	Dosage	Duration	Monitoring
Griseofulvin[a]	20–25 mg/kg/d[b] (maximum: 1 g) (microsized suspension)	Every day–twice daily for 6–8 wk	No baseline studies >8 wk: CBC, LFTs, renal function
Terbinafine[a]	<25 kg: 125 mg 25–35 kg: 187.5 mg >35 kg: 250 mg (granules)	Every day for 4–6 wk	Baseline: LFTs >6 wk: CBC, LFTs
Itraconazole	5mg/kg/d capsule	Every day for 2–4 wk	Baseline: LFTs >4 wk: CBC, LFTs
Fluconazole	6 mg/kg/d	Every day for 3 wk	Baseline: CBC, LFT, renal function Prolonged treatment: CBC, LFTs, renal function

Abbreviations: CBC, complete blood cell count; LFT, liver function test.
[a] US Food and Drug Administration approved for treatment of tinea capitis in the pediatric population.
[b] Current suggested dosage is higher than that of Food and Drug Administration approval.

has a well-known safety profile. However, new antifungals such as terbinafine, itraconazole, and fluconazole may offer shorter treatment durations with similar adverse effects. The newer antifungals are often more expensive, so treatment plans must be tailored to each patient, taking into consideration adherence and affordability. Currently, griseofulvin (≥ 2 years) and terbinafine granules (≥ 4 years) are the only 2 systemic antifungals approved by the FDA for treatment of tinea capitis in the pediatric population.

Griseofulvin is fungistatic against *Trichophyton* and *Microsporum*. It is available in 2 formations, microsized and ultra-microsized. It is best absorbed if taken with a fatty meal. Because of recent concerns about increasing resistance, higher dosage of the microsized formulation (20–25 mg/kg/day) and longer treatment durations have been recommended. Recommendations for dosage and duration are higher than the current FDA-approved label (11–18.3 mg/kg/day for a maximum of 6 weeks). Current recommendation for treatment length ranges between 6 and 12 weeks, but may require longer durations in some cases. The American Academy of Pediatrics endorses the treatment approach of 2 additional weeks of therapy after signs and symptoms of disease have cleared, rather than proving mycological cure (based on culture results), which can be expensive. Routine laboratory work is not required unless treatment duration exceeds several months or dosage is excessively high. The main adverse effects of griseofulvin include headache and gastrointestinal (GI) upset. Hepatic toxicity, leukopenia, hypersensitivity reactions, and severe cutaneous reactions are other rare adverse effects. Griseofulvin is a potent inducer of cytochrome P450 and has the potential for drug interactions. This medication should not be given to individuals with hepatocellular failure and porphyria.

Terbinafine (Evidence Level I compared with griseofulvin for *Trichophyton* infection) is an allylamine that is fungicidal medication and remains in the hair for several weeks even after discontinuation of therapy. Generally 4 to 6 weeks of therapy is required to treat *Trichophyton* infections. It is not currently recommended for *Microsporum* infections because higher doses and longer duration of treatment are required; thus, griseofulvin is still considered first-line treatment for *Microsporum* infections. Adverse effects of terbinafine include headache, GI upset, and rashes. Drug interactions, rare liver enzyme abnormalities, decreased lymphocyte counts, and serious cutaneous reactions can occur. Terbinafine is not recommended for individuals with liver disease.

Itraconazole (Evidence Level I compared with griseofulvin) is a triazole antifungal with fungistatic and fungicidal activities. It can be used to treat both *Trichophyton* and *Microsporum* infections requiring duration of 2 to 6 weeks of therapy. The main adverse effects include headache, GI upset, rash, and liver enzyme abnormalities. Rarely, more serious cutaneous eruptions have been reported. Because itraconazole has a high affinity for cytochrome P450 enzymes, there is significant risk for drug interactions. It is also contraindicated in liver disease and ventricular dysfunction and should not be used in individuals with a history of past sensitivity to other azoles because cross-reactions can occur.

Fluconazole (Evidence Level I compared with griseofulvin) is a triazole medication with fungistatic properties. It has been used for 2- to 4-week regimens to treat *Trichophyton* infections. Common adverse effects include headache, GI upset, and skin rash. Rarely, more serious cutaneous reactions, cardiac abnormalities, hepatic toxicities, and drug interactions can occur. This medication is contraindicated in individuals with liver disease and renal dysfunction and should not be used in individuals with a history of past sensitivity to other azoles because cross-reactions can occur.

Baseline laboratory studies and periodic blood work are recommended with the use of terbinafine, itraconazole, and fluconazole. Prolonged courses of griseofulvin beyond 8 weeks should have blood work assessed as well.

Trichotillomania

Trichotillomania should be further addressed by consultation with a behavioral specialist who can provide counseling and behavior therapy. In recalcitrant cases, a psychiatric consultation may be necessary.

Traction Alopecia

Traction alopecia needs to be addressed early on to prevent permanent hair loss. Avoidance of tight hairstyles, such as braids, cornrows, ponytails, twists, and weaving of artificial hair, and discontinuation of chemicals such as relaxers are the first-line treatment. If there are signs of secondary infection or folliculitis, topical or oral antibiotics may be needed. For significant inflammation, topical corticosteroids can be considered.

Telogen Effluvium

Telogen effluvium is often self-resolving within 3 to 6 months. Gradual improvement should be seen if the underlying cause is corrected. Individuals with hair loss that continues beyond 6 months should be referred to a dermatologist for further evaluation.

Suggested Reading

Alkhalifah A, Alsantali A, Wang E, McElwee KJ, Shapiro J. Alopecia areata update: part I. Clinical picture, histopathology, and pathogenesis. *J Am Acad Dermatol.* 2010;62(2):177–188

Alkhalifah A, Alsantali A, Wang E, McElwee KJ, Shapiro J. Alopecia areata update: part II. Treatment. *J Am Acad Dermatol.* 2010;62(2):191–202

Bedocs LA, Bruckner AL. Adolescent hair loss. *Curr Opin Pediatr.* 2008;20(4):431–435

Chen X, Jiang X, Yang M, et al. Systemic antifungal therapy for tinea capitis in children. *Cochrane Database Syst Rev.* 2016;(5):CD004685.pub3

Hantash BM, Schwartz RA. Traction alopecia in children. *Cutis.* 2003;71(1):18–20

Harrison JP, Franklin ME. Pediatric trichotillomania. *Curr Psychiatry Rep.* 2012;14(3):188–196

Kakourou T, Uksal U; European Society for Pediatric Dermatology. Guidelines for the management of tinea capitis in children. *Pediatr Dermatol.* 2010;27(3):226–228

Kelly BP. Superficial fungal infections. *Pediatr Rev.* 2012;33(4):22–37

Lio PA. What's missing from this picture? An approach to alopecia in children. *Arch Dis Child Educ Pract Ed.* 2007;92(6):193–198

Messenger AG, McKillop J, Farrant P, McDonagh AJ, Sladden M. British Association of Dermatologists' guidelines for management of alopecia areata. *Brit J Dermatol.* 2012;166(5):916–926

Mubki T, Rudnicka L, Olszewska M, Shapiro J. Evaluation and diagnosis of the hair loss patient. *J Am Acad Dermatol.* 2014;71(3):415–431

Nield LS, Keri JE, Kamat D. Alopecia in the general pediatric clinic: who to treat, who to refer. *Clin Pediatr.* 2006;45(7):605–612

CHAPTER 49

Atopic Dermatitis and Eczematous Disorders

Robert Sidbury, MD, MPH

Key Points

- Severe atopic dermatitis and failure to thrive can be a sign of primary immunodeficiency.
- Initial emphasis on good skin care in mild to moderate atopic dermatitis may render allergy questions moot.
- Bleach baths twice weekly can minimize infection risk and improve eczema severity.
- Antihistamines have not been proven to help reduce itch in atopic dermatitis.
- Seborrheic dermatitis and atopic dermatitis have considerable overlap in early infancy.
- Symptomatic seborrheic dermatitis is best treated with topical anti-inflammatories and anti-yeast agents.
- Refractory, severe seborrheic dermatitis should prompt consideration of Langerhans cell histiocytosis.

Atopic Dermatitis

Overview

Essential features of atopic dermatitis include a waxing and waning course and age-related regional areas of involvement. Infants and young children tend toward facial and extensor dermatitis, whereas flexural sites, such as the elbow and knee creases, affect older children. Supportive features include a personal or family history of atopy (eg, atopic dermatitis, asthma, hay fever), related skin findings (eg, keratosis pilaris, ichthyosis, palmar hyper-linearity), and distinctive intraocular skin folds called Dennie Morgan folds. These lines coupled with periorbital darkening, often called "atopic shiners," confer a typical atopic facies. Diagnostic criteria are listed in Box 49-1.

Box 49-1. Features to Be Considered in Diagnosis of Patients With Atopic Dermatitis

- **Essential Features** (must be present)
  - o   Pruritus
  - o   Eczema (acute, subacute, chronic)
    - – Typical morphology and age-specific patterns[a]
    - – Chronic or relapsing history
- **Important Features** (seen in most cases, adding support to the diagnosis)
  - o   Early age of onset
  - o   Atopy
    - – Personal or family history
    - – Immunoglobulin E reactivity
  - o   Xerosis
- **Associated Features**
  The following clinical associations help suggest the diagnosis of atopic dermatitis but are too nonspecific to be used for defining or detecting atopic dermatitis for research and epidemiologic studies:
  - o   Atypical vascular responses (eg, facial pallor, white dermographism, delayed blanch response)
  - o   Keratosis pilaris / hyperlinear palms / ichthyosis
  - o   Ocular / periorbital changes
  - o   Other regional findings (eg, perioral changes / periauricular lesions)
  - o   Perifollicular accentuation / lichenification / prurigo lesions
- **Exclusionary Conditions**
  A diagnosis of atopic dermatitis depends on excluding conditions such as
  - o   Scabies
  - o   Seborrheic dermatitis
  - o   Allergic contact dermatitis
  - o   Ichthyoses
  - o   Cutaneous lymphoma
  - o   Psoriasis
  - o   Immunodeficiencies

[a] Patterns include
 1. Facial, neck, and extensor involvement in infants and children
 2. Current or prior flexural lesions in any age group
 3. Sparing of groin and axillary regions

Adapted from Eichenfield LF, Hanifin JM, Luger TA, Stevens SR, Pride HB. Consensus conference on pediatric atopic dermatitis. *J Am Acad Dermatol.* 2003;49(6):1088–1095, with permission from Elsevier.

Causes and Differential Diagnosis

Atopic dermatitis, commonly called eczema, is an inflammatory dermatosis. Clinicians must exclude other causes of itchy rash, including infections such as tinea and scabies; other inflammatory conditions, such as psoriasis, seborrheic dermatitis, irritant and allergic contact dermatitis, and dermatomyositis; and even malignancies such as cutaneous T-cell lymphoma. Severe infantile eczema in the setting of failure to thrive or unusual or refractory infections should always raise the specter of primary immunodeficiency.

Clinical Features

Atopic dermatitis is typically a clinical diagnosis. Physical examination of acute dermatitis may reveal ill-defined plaques with erythema, papulation, and excoriation at affected areas. Chronic lesions may primarily show thickening of the skin at sites of scratching called lichenification. Nummular eczema presents with more discrete, sharply circumscribed, homogeneous plaques that may be mistaken for psoriasis.

Evaluation

Skin biopsy is supportive but not specific. The histologic hallmark, intraepidermal spongiosis, or edema is also noted in seborrheic dermatitis and contact dermatitis. Allergy tests, including radioallergosorbent tests or skin prick tests, can identify relevant food or environmental triggers that may contribute to eczematous flares, but false-positive rates are high and atopic dermatitis is rarely "cured" by allergen avoidance alone.

As opposed to foods and environmental exposures, such as dust mites, trees, pollen, and grasses, patch testing can identify potential contact allergens such as nickel, fragrance, and neomycin. A high index of suspicion should be maintained in patients who are refractory to standard therapy because contact allergens may be found in emollients and topical steroids otherwise presumed to be beneficial.

Management

A useful approach is to prioritize skin care over allergy care in mild to moderate patients (90%+) because marked improvement without dietary manipulation may render allergic questions moot.

To date, efforts at primary prevention of atopic dermatitis have been unsuccessful. Strategies surrounding maternal and infant diet, breastfeeding, hypoallergenic formulas, and probiotics have not proven fruitful. Clinicians should not recommend restriction diets to prevent atopic dermatitis, nor should solid food introduction beyond 4 to 6 months of age be recommended solely to mitigate atopic dermatitis risk. There is modest evidence that extensively or partially hydrolyzed formulas may be helpful for at-risk neonates and infants not exclusively breastfed, but cost may be prohibitive and benefit uncertain. If a patient has documented IgE-mediated allergy, suspect foods should be avoided to prevent potentially serious health sequelae, but exclusion diets in an unselected atopic dermatitis population are not recommended, and clinicians must remain cognizant of potential iatrogenic malnutrition caused by parental food fears.

Moisturizers are the first and most important treatment recommendation for all patients with atopic dermatitis. Bathing frequency is less critical than the immediate post-bath application of a moisturizing product. In patients who do not bathe daily, emollients should still be used as often as possible and at least twice daily. Thicker petrolatum-based ointments are generally more effective but less cosmetically appealing, particularly in older children or hotter climates. Use of a moisturization product daily is the first of 4 quality performance measures developed by the Physician Consortium for Performance Improvement panel commissioned by the American Medical Association to develop atopic dermatitis measures. Adding Clorox to the bath twice weekly (ie, bleach bath) can help prevent infection and improve eczema severity. For infants, a teaspoon per gallon of bathwater should be used, whereas older children can put a quarter cup of bleach into a full tub. The bleach-containing water should be rinsed off at conclusion.

Topical corticosteroids should be used in patients failing simple emollition. Several factors should be considered including age, distribution, and severity. Steroid vehicle is an important variable; ointments are typically more effective than creams if compatible with patient preference. The least potent effective topical steroid should be used to minimize adverse effects such as skin thinning and hypothalamic-pituitary-adrenal axis suppression. Typically, a class VI or VII (over-the-counter) agent may be used on the face or in the axilla/groin, and a mid-potency class IV to VI product for the trunk or extremities if necessary (Table 49-1). Twice daily use is recommended until flares are controlled, then intermittent use as needed. Patients should treat flares daily for several consecutive weeks if necessary, then attempt to introduce steroid-free breaks as able. Several times' weekly use over the longer term is generally safe given aforementioned parameters. Systemic steroids should be avoided if possible because they seldom lead to sustained benefit and rebound flaring is common. When topical steroids are either ineffective or overused, nonsteroidal alternatives such as topical tacrolimus or pimecrolimus are indicated in patients older than 2 years. These agents are particularly suited to facial and periorbital areas because they do not risk skin atrophy, glaucoma, or cataracts. The US Food and Drug Administration issued a black box warning in 2005 emphasizing appropriate use in older children and as a second-line intermittent therapy. In the wake of this warning, other nonsteroidal products have been promoted for eczema care such as enhanced barrier repair moisturizers or anti-inflammatories; however, these are generally not markedly more effective than standard emollients and considerably more expensive.

Adjunctive therapies such as sedating antihistamines may help with night-time itch in particular, though no evidence supports the use of nonsedating agents in the absence of concurrent allergic rhinitis or conjunctivitis. Topical or

Table 49-1. Treatment for Atopic Dermatitis[a]

First-line	Second-line	Third-line
Babies and Children <2 y		
• Hydrocortisone, 1% (over the counter)	• Class VI topical steroid (eg, hydrocortisone, 2.5%). • Apply twice daily × 2–3 wk as needed for control. • 2–4 times weekly thereafter as needed for maintenance.	• Consider referral.
Children >2 y		
• Class VI topical steroid on face • Class IV–VI topical steroid on trunk or extremities (eg, triamcinolone, 0.1%)	• Tacrolimus, 0.03%, in 2- to 15-year-olds as needed for rash • Tacrolimus, 0.1%, if >15 y as needed for rash • Pimecrolimus, 1%, twice daily as needed for rash • May alternate with topical steroids	• Consider systemic immunomodulators. • Consider phototherapy. • Consider referral.

[a] All patients should engage in proper bathing/emollition as initial treatment and continue throughout treatment course.

systemic antibiotics are indicated when eczema becomes superinfected, as heralded by a flare with accompanying yellow crusting, pustules, or exudative lesions. For refractory atopic dermatitis, wet wrap therapy may be extremely helpful in quieting a flare but its use can be challenging for parents and patients. An online resource produced by University of California, San Diego, provides video tutorials on the use of wet wrap therapy (www.eczemacenter.org).

Atopic dermatitis often improves as children age, though the tendency toward dry skin, irritancy, and superinfection persist. Though bacterial infection is more common, diffuse herpetic infections (ie, eczema herpeticum) can have considerable morbidity and even mortality if untreated. Eczema herpeticum should be considered in a flaring child with signature grouped vesicles or punched-out erosions, particularly if accompanied by fever and anorexia typically not seen in a child with bacterial superinfection. Up to 30% of eczema herpeticum patients have concurrent bacterial superinfection.

General health is typically good, though atopic dermatitis patients are at increased risk for asthma and hay fever. There is emerging evidence that atopic dermatitis may be associated with obesity and attention-deficit/hyperactivity disorder, but these links remain unproven. Severe atopic dermatitis and its intractable itch can take a tremendous psychologic toll on patients and families alike, so ongoing attention to potential effect on quality of life is prudent.

Seborrheic Dermatitis

Overview

Seborrheic dermatitis is a common inflammatory skin condition that can affect all age groups. Often called cradle cap in infants and dandruff in older children, seborrheic dermatitis typically affects sebaceous-rich skin including the scalp, face, upper trunk, axilla, and groin. When involvement is limited to the scalp, there is clinical overlap with psoriasis leading to the catchall term *sebopsoriasis*.

Causes and Differential Diagnosis

The cause of seborrheic dermatitis is unknown, though a role for the commensal yeast *Pityrosporum ovale* (aka *Malassezia furfur*) has long been postulated. The differential diagnosis includes psoriasis, atopic dermatitis, and tinea capitis. Truncal involvement may be mistaken for tinea versicolor. Seborrheic dermatitis affecting the diaper area may mimic many common causes of diaper dermatitis, including "napkin psoriasis" and candidal dermatitis. Both atopic dermatitis and irritant contact dermatitis may confuse, but both classically spare the folds typically affected by seborrheic dermatitis. Langerhans cell histiocytosis must always be considered in refractory seborrheic dermatitis because skin lesions can be identical. Similarly, seborrheic dermatitis, particularly if sudden in onset in a child with risk factors, can be a manifestation of HIV.

Clinical Features

Seborrheic dermatitis presents with a greasy white to yellowish scale diffusely in the scalp. Seborrheic dermatitis is not generally pruritic. Facial involvement manifests as fine whitish scaling at the eyebrows, at the nasal creases, and often behind the ears. The upper trunk may show follicular papules and erythematous plaques.

Evaluation

Diagnosis is clinical. Bacterial and fungal cultures and potassium hydroxide examination can rule out infectious mimics, and when necessary a skin biopsy can rule out Langerhans cell histiocytosis or psoriasis. Histologic features of seborrheic dermatitis are similar to those seen in atopic and contact dermatitis.

Management

When asymptomatic, seborrheic dermatitis may be left untreated. Infants with cradle cap will often improve spontaneously in the first year of life. Vegetable or mineral oils and gentle debridement is often performed by motivated parents, and there is no contraindication to this; however, there is some evidence that olive oil may promote *Pityrosporum* growth, so this is not recommended. When scalp treatment is indicated, 2% ketoconazole and selenium sulfide shampoos among others may be used intermittently for maintenance. Low-potency steroid-containing shampoos and oil preparations can be very effective and should be used once daily to induce remission and then several times weekly or less for ongoing symptoms. Non–hair-bearing areas respond well to 1% to 2.5% hydrocortisone lotion applied twice daily and then as needed. Every effort should be made to limit steroid-containing products to avoid adverse effects such as skin thinning or hypothalamic-pituitary-adrenal axis suppression. No monitoring for long-term implications is necessary, and seborrheic dermatitis often improves spontaneously with time.

Contact Dermatitis

Overview

Contact dermatitis is defined as inflammation in the skin resulting from exogenous exposure to 1 or more substances. There are 2 distinct types: primary irritant and allergic. Irritant contact dermatitis is more common, does not require immunologic sensitization, and is dose dependent. Allergic contact dermatitis requires an initial exposure or sensitizing step, followed by the development of immunologic memory, with any subsequent exposure leading to an adverse effect.

Causes and Differential Diagnosis

Primary irritant contact dermatitis may be caused by numerous exposures ranging from soaps, detergents, and foods to urine and stool in the diaper-wearing infant. Frequent wetting and drying in a susceptible individual can lead to irritant contact dermatitis, as in a lip-licking child. Similarly, the most common cause of diaper dermatitis is irritancy. The differential diagnosis of irritant contact dermatitis includes atopic dermatitis and allergic contact dermatitis. Allergic contact dermatitis is uncommon in children, and nickel, fragrance, and neomycin are the usual suspects, but any refractory pruritic eruption, particularly if patterned or asymmetric in distribution, should prompt consideration of allergic contact dermatitis. The differential diagnosis is similar to irritant contact dermatitis but may also include a distinctive pruritic viral exanthem called unilateral laterothoracic exanthem when rash affects the hip or shoulder girdle areas.

Clinical Features

Both irritant and allergic contact dermatitis look eczematous in appearance with erythema, papulation, and even frank vesiculation. Irritant contact dermatitis will spare protected areas in the diaper where folds, such as the inguinal crease, may be uninvolved, while surrounding skin is acutely inflamed ("affects the peaks, spares the valleys").

Two distinctive presentations of irritant contact dermatitis can easily be mistaken for infection. Jacquet's nodular-erosive diaper dermatitis can present with striking nodules and superficial ulceration that appear volcano-like. Herpes simplex virus infection should be ruled out. A history of recurrent diarrhea, frequent cleaning, and particularly use of cloth diapers is supportive. The same context may produce a different picture characterized by more numerous, smaller, papulopustular lesions without ulceration called pseudoverrucous papules. This is most often mistaken for molluscum or warts. In both cases, minimizing irritancy with barrier protection, topical anti-inflammatories such as hydrocortisone, and elimination of triggers is curative.

Irritant contact dermatitis tends to itch less than allergic contact dermatitis. Allergic contact dermatitis may become impressively edematous and exudative and should present in the distribution and often shape of contact exposure. A potentially misleading feature of allergic contact dermatitis may be the development of an id reaction. An id reaction represents a more diffuse hypersensitivity reaction typically characterized by discrete, monomorphic flesh-colored to erythematous pruritic papules distant from the site of allergic exposure. These papules are most often seen on the extensor arms and hands as well as upper trunk and neck. Because they are present at sites distant from potential allergic trigger, a causal connection may be missed.

Evaluation

Evaluation requires a careful history directed toward any products potentially touching the affected skin, including soaps, emollients, barriers, clothes, wipes, and even prescription medications. A family history with attention to atopy is noteworthy as atopic children are at greater risk for contact dermatitis of all types. A skin biopsy is usually not helpful because it will not distinguish allergic from irritant contact dermatitis, or either from atopic dermatitis, and cannot identify triggers. Allergic contact dermatitis is a delayed-type hypersensitivity (type IV) reaction, and as such IgE-based allergy tests, such as radioallergosor-bent or skin prick tests, are unhelpful. Patch testing is the criterion standard.

Management

Management consists first of identification and avoidance of relevant triggers. It is important to note that any exposure, however brief, may trigger allergic contact dermatitis in a sensitized individual, whereas irritant contact dermatitis tends to be more "dose dependent." This is essential to communicate because children, particularly adolescents forbidden from wearing their favorite earrings or jeans because of nickel allergy, need to understand that absolute avoidance is necessary. Active dermatitis should be treated with topical steroids of appropriate strength, and in rare cases of severe allergic contact dermatitis short courses of prednisone (1 mg/kg/day for 3–7 days) may be necessary. Burows compresses (aluminum acetate) applied several times daily may be soothing when a significant exudative component is present.

Suggested Reading

Aronson PL, Yan AC, Mittal MK, Mohamad Z, Shah SS. Delayed acyclovir and outcomes of children hospitalized for eczema herpeticum. *Pediatrics.* 2011;128(6):1161–1167

Fonacier LS, Aquino MR, Mucci T. Current strategies for treating severe contact derma-titis in pediatric patients. *Curr Allergy Asthma Rep.* 2012;12(6):599–606 (Evidence Level III)

Hanifin JM, Cooper KD, Ho VC, et al. Guidelines of care for atopic dermatitis, devel-oped in accordance with the American Academy of Dermatology (AAD)/American Academy of Dermatology Association "Administrative Regulations for Evidence-Based Clinical Practice Guidelines." *J Am Acad Dermatol.* 2004;50(3):391–404 (Evidence Level III)

Irvine AD, McLean WH, Leung DY. Filaggrin mutations associated with skin and allergic diseases. *N Engl J Med.* 2011;365(14):1315–1327 (Evidence Level III)

Kwan JM, Jacob SE. Contact dermatitis. *Pediatr Ann.* 2012;41(10):422–423, 426–428 (Evidence Level III)

Poindexter GB, Burkhart CN, Morrell DS. Therapies for pediatric seborrheic dermatitis. *Pediatr Ann.* 2009;38(6):333–338 (Evidence Level III)

Schmitt J, Romanos M, Schmitt NM, Meurer M, Kirch W. Atopic eczema and attention-deficit/hyperactivity disorder in a population-based sample of children and adoles-cents. *JAMA.* 2009;301(7):724–726 (Evidence Level II-2)

Siegfried E, Glenn E. Use of olive oil in the treatment of seborrheic dermatitis in chil-dren. *Arch Pediatr Adolesc Med.* 2012;166(10):967 (Evidence Level III)

Williams HC. Clinical practice. Atopic dermatitis. *N Engl J Med.* 2005;352(22):2314–2324 (Evidence Level III)

CHAPTER 50

Diaper Dermatitis

Kristi Williams, MD, and Lori Falcone, DO

Key Points

- Diaper dermatitis is a common pediatric condition of which irritant diaper dermatitis is the most frequent cause.
- History and physical examination findings often lead to the diagnosis, although occasionally further evaluation is needed.
- Treatment includes frequent diaper changes, avoidance of products containing potential allergens, and application of topical barrier ointments.
- Appropriate antimicrobials should be used when an infectious etiology is suspected or confirmed.
- Consultation with a dermatologic specialist may be needed for persistent diaper dermatitis unresponsive to treatment.

Overview

Diaper dermatitis refers to a skin problem in the area covered by a diaper, namely the buttocks, genitalia, upper thighs, and lower abdomen. Diaper dermatitis predominantly affects infants and young toddlers but can affect children of any age who wear diapers.

Causes and Differential Diagnosis

Although diaper dermatitis encompasses any rash in the diaper region, it may not be associated with wearing diapers. The most common cause of diaper dermatitis, and one that is associated with wearing a diaper, is irritant diaper dermatitis (IDD). Exposure of the skin to urine and stool results in wetness, increased pH, and activation of enzymes that causes breakdown of skin. Other causes of IDD include reaction to chemicals in the diapers or diaper wipes, soaps used to wash the skin, and lotions applied to the skin. Friction caused by diapers on the skin, as well as by caregivers during diaper changes, can cause skin breakdown. Exposure to chemicals after ingesting senna-containing laxatives has also been reported to cause contact dermatitis.

While most commonly caused by a chemical irritant, diaper dermatitis can result from infections (*Staphylococcus aureus,* herpes simplex virus, *Candida albicans*), nutritional deficiencies (zinc), metabolic disorders, immunodeficiencies (chronic mucocutaneous candidiasis), malignancies, or structural skin defects. Kawasaki disease in infants may be heralded by a pronounced rash in the diaper region. Occasionally, infants with violent trauma may present with unusually severe diaper dermatitis. Identifying the etiology of diaper dermatitis enables appropriate treatment to be given and prevention strategies to be implemented.

In Jacquet dermatitis, a more severe form of IDD, punched-out erosions and ulcerations with elevated borders are seen. Granuloma gluteale infantum is a rarer form of severe IDD that may be related to inappropriate use of topical fluorinated steroids. It is characterized by asymptomatic, oval, violaceous papules and nodules on the gluteal surfaces sparing the inguinal folds.

Allergic contact dermatitis has a similar appearance to IDD, but the pattern of skin involvement corresponds to areas exposed to potential allergens contained in diapers, such as dyes, rubber, and glue. Tidewater-mark dermatitis involves the skin along the edges of the diaper. Diaper dye dermatitis affects the skin where colored dyes are found in the diapers. Lucky Luke dermatitis (also known as cowboy holster dermatitis) affects the skin of the lateral buttock and upper lateral thighs, resembling a gun holster appearance. This is thought to result from reaction to glue in the diaper.

When skin folds are involved, additional etiologies should be considered. Candidal diaper infections appear as bright red areas with irregular borders that can involve any part of the diaper area and thighs, including the skin folds. Papular satellite lesions are often noted at the periphery of the rash. If the rash does not have the typical appearance of a candidal rash but has lasted more than 3 days, a candidal infection should be suspected. Additional risk factors for candidal diaper infection include gastrointestinal colonization by *Candida,* antibiotic exposure, diabetes mellitus, or an immunodeficiency.

Intertrigo can appear similar to candidal infections except that no papular satellite lesions are noted. Intertrigo is an inflammatory condition induced by heat, moisture, and friction and characterized by moist, sharply demarcated areas of erythema in the skin folds. Although not caused by an infection, intertrigo can become secondarily infected with *Candida* or bacteria.

Seborrheic dermatitis, while often seen on the scalp, face, neck, and axilla, can be seen in the diaper area. Typically, it manifests as salmon-colored plaques with greasy yellow scale in the inguinal folds. Atopic dermatitis, which often spares the diaper region, can resemble seborrheic dermatitis in its presentation with mild erythema and occasional scaling. Patients usually have a history of previous or concurrent rash on the face or extensor limbs; personal and family histories may include allergies, atopic dermatitis, and asthma. Langerhans cell histiocytosis can mimic seborrheic dermatitis in distribution and initial appearance. Erythematous papules can progress to vesicles, pustules, petechiae, erosions, and ulcerations. Systemic manifestations are typically noted, including hepatosplenomegaly and lymphadenopathy. Psoriasis is a less common cause of scaling dermatitis. It appears as sharply demarcated erythematous plaques with silvery scale. In the diaper region, scale may not be noted. Typically, psoriatic lesions are not confined to the diaper region and thus will be noted on other areas of skin.

Bacterial infections, most commonly caused by *Staphylococcus* and *Streptococcus* species, can present in a variety of ways and mimic candidal infections as well as intertrigo. Bright red, well-demarcated patches in the skin folds or perianal region can be seen with streptococcal infections. Additional symptoms that suggest infection with *Streptococcus pyogenes* include perianal pain, pruritus, and rectal bleeding. Bullous lesions and discrete pustular follicular lesions can be seen with staphylococcal and streptococcal infections.

Viral infections can also cause diaper dermatitis. Painful vesicles with or without crust occur with herpes simplex virus infections. Numerous other viral etiologies should be considered when generalized papular or vesicular rashes are noted but not confined solely to the diaper region. Additional symptoms may accompany rashes caused by viruses.

Scabies infections occurring in the diaper area appear as pruritic, raised papules. Additional lesions may be seen in the interdigital spaces of the hands and feet, on the abdomen, and in the axillae.

Additional etiologies of diaper dermatitis can be caused by metabolic disorders, nutritional deficiencies, and genetic disorders. These include biotin deficiency, acquired or congenital zinc deficiency, cystic fibrosis, and Wiskott-Aldrich syndrome. Consideration of these etiologies should occur when a patient presents with diaper dermatitis that is refractory to treatment.

Clinical Manifestations

Regardless of etiology causing IDD, examination reveals sharp, well-demarcated erythema of the convex surfaces. Sometimes vesicles, bullae, and sloughing of the skin are seen. Generally, skin folds do not become affected.

Evaluation

Most cases of diaper dermatitis do not require laboratory evaluation. A complete history, including care of the diaper area and adherence to therapy, should first be assessed. The clinician should also obtain a history for associated symptoms, systemic symptoms, past medical history, and family history, because these are essential for helping to identify an etiology. Physical examination, focusing on morphology and location of the rash, often reveals the diagnosis. Rashes that persist longer than 72 hours are highly suspicious for candidal infections. Microbiologic cultures and scrapings are not routinely performed but may be helpful to confirm the etiology. Rashes that appear atypical or do not improve with conventional therapies warrant further workup.

Management

Topical water-impermeable barrier ointments and creams are the mainstay of treatment for diaper dermatitis and should be applied with each diaper change. A thick layer of petrolatum applied at each diaper change may prevent skin breakdown. Mild diaper dermatitis with erythema and intact skin can often be treated with a cream containing 10% zinc oxide applied as a thick layer; a 40% zinc oxide preparation may be needed for more severe rashes.

If there is evidence of candidal infection or no improvement with standard treatment of presumed IDD, an antifungal topical preparation with a thick barrier cream over it should be applied. Antifungals that are effective against *Candida* include nystatin and any of the -azole drugs. Treatment typically takes 7 to 14 days and should continue for 3 days beyond resolution of the rash. Treatment with oral and topical nystatin is no more effective than topical nystatin alone (Evidence Level II-1).

If there is evidence of a secondary bacterial infection, mupirocin offers both antibacterial and antifungal coverage (Evidence Level I). Low-potency topical corticosteroids should be reserved for moderate to severe cases of diaper dermatitis. No evidence supports or refutes the use of topical vitamin A in diaper dermatitis.

Diaper dermatitis recalcitrant to the interventions mentioned may warrant consideration of metabolic deficiencies, nutritional deficiencies, malignancies, and other cutaneous disorders. Further evaluation and consultation with a pediatric dermatologist may be needed.

The mainstay in preventing diaper dermatitis is keeping the area as clean and dry as possible. Frequent diaper changes, as often as every 2 hours, are crucial, because urine and stool contribute to skin breakdown. Studies with reusable cloth diapers, conventional disposable diapers, and superabsorbent diapers suggest that superabsorbent disposable diapers are superior to conventional disposable diapers and cloth diapers. However, because of the quality of studies and biases within them, not enough evidence supports one type of diaper over another. Emphasis still remains on the frequency of diaper changes. Baby wipes that contain alcohol should be avoided, because they can dry out the skin. Over-the-counter lotions and creams that are applied should be free of fragrances and dyes.

Suggested Reading

Baer EL, Davies MW, Easterbrook KJ. Disposable nappies for preventing napkin dermatitis in infants. *Cochrane Database Syst Rev.* 2006;(3):CD004262

Davies MW, Dore AJ, Perissinotto KL. Topical vitamin A, or its derivatives, for treating and preventing napkin dermatitis in infants. *Cochrane Database Syst Rev.* 2005;(4):CD004300 de Wet PM, Rode H, van Dyk A, Millar AJ. Perianal candidosis—a comparative study with mupirocin and nystatin. *Int J Dermatol.* 1999;38(8):618–622

Friedlander SF, Eichenfield LF, Leyden J, Shu J, Spellman MC. Diaper dermatitis—appropriate evaluation and optimal management strategies. *Contemp Pediatr.* 2009;(Supp):2–14

Munz D, Powell KR, Pai CH. Treatment of candidal diaper dermatitis: a double-blind placebo-controlled comparison of topical nystatin with topical plus oral nystatin. *J Pediatr.* 1982;101(6):1022–1025

Nield LS, Kamat DK. Diaper dermatitis: from "A" to "pee." *Consult Pediatr.* 2006;5(6):373–380

CHAPTER 51

Erythema Nodosum

Cynthia Marie Carver DeKlotz, MD, and Sheila Fallon Friedlander, MD

Key Points

- Erythema nodosum is an uncommon yet most often benign cutaneous hypersensitivity reaction in the skin.

- It is a panniculitis, consisting of inflammation of fat cells and the septal fibrotic structures within fat tissue.

- Clinical presentation is characterized by symmetric, tender, erythematous nodules located most commonly on the anterior and lateral surfaces of the lower legs.

- Evaluation for underlying causes is necessary, with β-hemolytic streptococci representing the most common cause in children.

- Management primarily focuses on treating underlying causes and supportive measures, including bed rest and analgesics as needed.

Overview

Erythema nodosum, also known as erythema contusiformis, is an uncommon self-limited hypersensitivity reaction precipitated by both infectious and noninfectious processes. It classically presents as tender, erythematous nodules primarily located on the bilateral lower anterior legs (pretibial areas); however, more extensive disease can occur.

Erythema nodosum can occur at any age but most commonly develops between the second and fourth decades of life, particularly between 20 and 30 years of age. Boys and girls are reported to be equally affected in the preadolescent period, but later in life the incidence is higher in women.

Causes and Differential Diagnosis

Erythema nodosum is considered a hypersensitivity reaction. Myriad presumed etiologic associations have been identified and include infections, drugs, underlying diseases, and malignancies (Box 51-1). Historically, tuberculosis was the most commonly associated etiologic factor in children. However, streptococcal

Box 51-1. Etiologic Factors Associated With Erythema Nodosum

Idiopathic

Infections

- **Bacterial:** *Streptococcus,* especially β-hemolytic form (primary identified cause in children); less common: *Mycobacterium tuberculosis,* nontuberculous mycobacteria, *Mycoplasma pneumoniae, Yersinia, Salmonella, Campylobacter, Leptospira, Pseudomonas,* cat-scratch disease
- **Viral:** Epstein-Barr virus, mumps
- **Fungal:** coccidioidomycosis, histoplasmosis, blastomycosis, dermatophytes (eg, kerion-associated)
- **Parasitic:** toxoplasmosis

Drugs: sulfonamides, phenytoin, oral contraceptives

Other conditions: sarcoidosis, inflammatory bowel disease (eg, Crohn disease, ulcerative colitis), Behçet syndrome, acne fulminans, celiac disease, hepatitis B vaccine, autoimmune hepatitis

Malignancies: lymphoma (especially Hodgkin disease), leukemia

disease is now the most frequently identified pediatric cause in the United States and Europe. This is in contrast to adults, in whom the most common etiologies are drugs, inflammatory bowel disease, and sarcoidosis. Such underlying causes have been identified but much less frequently in children. Of note, one study in adult patients with sarcoidosis found an association of granulomatous papules on the knees with coexisting erythema nodosum. It is unknown if this association holds true in children.

Differential diagnosis includes other inflammatory diseases of fat, such as Bazin-nodular vasculitis (lobular panniculitis with vasculitis), and cold panniculitis, which may occur in young children following prolonged sucking on cold objects (eg, popsicles, affecting the cheeks). Additionally, patients with Behçet syndrome may develop panniculitis associated with hypersensitivity or lymphocytic vasculitis that clinically mimics erythema nodosum. In other cases, unintentional or violent trauma with resultant contusions may resemble erythema nodosum. Other diagnoses that can be distinguished histopathologically from biopsy tissue include hypersensitivity vasculitis, lupus panniculitis, Henoch-Schönlein purpura, and Wells syndrome.

Clinical Features

Erythema nodosum typically presents with the sudden onset of tender, erythematous, symmetric nodules and plaques on the anterior and lateral surfaces of the bilateral lower legs (Figure 51-1). Clinically, erythematous lesions located on anterior surfaces of the legs are typically larger than those located laterally. Rarely, more extensive disease can present involving upper legs, arms (Figure 51-2), and even the face. Over time, the initially red, raised, tender nodules

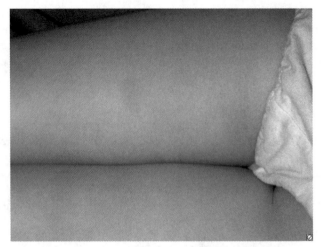

Figure 51-1. Erythema nodosum: erythematous nodule on leg.

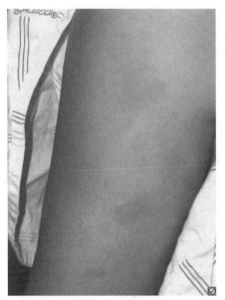

Figure 51-2. Extensive erythema nodosum.

evolve. Within a few days, they flatten and become purplish in color, then subsequently yellowish green, mimicking the appearance of a deep ecchymosis; hence, the name *erythema contusiformis.* Lesions heal without ulceration, scarring, or atrophy. Erythema nodosum may be associated with fever, sore throat, fatigue, arthralgia, malaise, headache, conjunctivitis, cough, abdominal pain, vomiting, or diarrhea. Prodromal symptoms may appear approximately

5 to 15 days prior to the onset of erythema nodosum and often provide clues to the underlying etiologic factor. For example, recent sore throat or concurrent fever are common in patients with underlying β-hemolytic streptococcal infection. Similarly, diarrhea is reported to be a prodromal symptom in some patients with underlying *Yersinia enterocolitica, Leptospira, Campylobacter,* or Crohn disease. Arthralgias may be an accompanying symptom in patients with *Mycoplasma pneumoniae* or *Y enterocolitica* infection.

Typically, the cutaneous eruption persists approximately 1 to 3 weeks in children and 3 to 6 weeks in adults; however, longer duration and recurrence may occur. In one series of erythema nodosum in 35 children, lesions persisted more than 20 days in only 3 patients; underlying causes in the more prolonged cases were Hodgkin disease, Crohn disease, and unknown etiology. This suggests that prolonged cases of erythema nodosum may be caused by an underlying chronic disease with persistent antigenic stimulus.

Evaluation

The diagnosis of erythema nodosum is almost always made clinically. In atypical, persistent, or unclear cases, however, skin biopsy may be necessary to confirm the diagnosis and rule out other possibilities. Workup for underlying processes that might have triggered erythema nodosum is appropriate and should be guided by a detailed history, identifying both prescription and over-the-counter medications, as well as an extensive review of systems and thorough physical examination (Box 51-2). Most experts would recommend tuberculin testing (tuberculin interferon-γ release assays preferred for those older than 5 years) and evaluation of antistreptolysin O titers in any case without a clear cause. Depending on signs and symptoms, as well as duration, any of the following evaluations may be appropriate: complete blood cell count with differential, erythrocyte sedimentation rate, liver function tests, pharyngeal and stool cultures, chest radiograph, urinalysis, antistreptolysin O titer, and serum antibodies for endemic mycoses (depending on geographic exposure). *Mycoplasma pneumoniae* or *Y enterocolitica* infection is uncommon in the United States, but in the right clinical setting, recent infection can be demonstrated using serology (available only in reference or research laboratories).

Box 51-2. Evaluation of Presumed Erythema Nodosum: Diagnostic Considerations

History: medication (prescription and over-the-counter), review of systems

Minimal evaluation in classic cases of typical duration without clear cause: testing for tuberculosis, antistreptolysin O titer

Additional potential studies, particularly in prolonged or atypical disease: complete blood cell count with differential, erythrocyte sedimentation rate, liver function tests, pharyngeal and stool cultures, chest radiograph, urinalysis, and serum antibodies for *Mycoplasma pneumoniae* and *Yersinia enterocolitica*

Management

Management of erythema nodosum should be targeted toward treatment of any underlying diseases or conditions, as well as patient comfort (Box 51-3). Erythema nodosum typically resolves spontaneously within a few weeks. Supportive care, including bed rest for 2 to 3 days, leg elevation, and restriction of physical activity, is the cornerstone of treatment. It has been suggested that restriction of physical activity for a few weeks might prevent exacerbations. Additionally, nonsteroidal anti-inflammatory drugs, or aspirin in older patients, may be helpful. Horio and colleagues demonstrated excellent response in 11/15 adults with erythema nodosum treated with potassium iodide (Evidence Level II-3). Hence, persistently symptomatic lesions in older children, following appropriate evaluation, could be treated with saturated solution of potassium iodide. Potassium iodide is thought to act by either releasing heparin from mast cells, subsequently suppressing delayed hypersensitivity reactions, or inhibiting neutrophil chemotaxis. Rarely, systemic corticosteroids are used in the treatment of erythema nodosum; however, any underlying infection must first be ruled out before initiating administration of corticosteroids.

Box 51-3. Treatment of Erythema Nodosum (Evidence Level III)

- Discontinuation of any possible causative medications
- Treatment of underlying causes
- Supportive care: bed rest for 2–3 d, leg elevation, restriction of physical activity for a few weeks
- NSAIDs/analgesics as needed
- Refractory cases: consideration of potassium iodide or other therapies

Abbreviation: NSAID, nonsteroidal anti-inflammatory drug.

Suggested Reading

Cengiz AB, Kara A, Kanra G, Seçmeer G, Ceyhan M. Erythema nodosum in childhood: evaluation of ten patients. *Turk J Pediatr.* 2006;48(1):38–42

Hoffmann AL, Milman N, Byg KE. Childhood sarcoidosis in Denmark, 1979-1994: incidence, clinical features and laboratory results at presentation in 48 children. *Acta Paediatr.* 2004;93(1):30–36

Kakourou T, Drosatou P, Psychou F, Aroni K, Nicolaidou P. Erythema nodosum in children: a prospective study. *J Am Acad Dermatol.* 2001;44(1):17–21

Kavehmanesh Z, Beiraghdar F, Saburi A, Hajihashemi A, Amirsalari S, Movahed M. Pediatric autoimmune hepatitis in a patient who presented with erythema nodosum: a case report. *Hepat Mon.* 2012;12(1):42–45

Marcoval J, Moreno A, Mañá J. Papular sarcoidosis of the knees: a clue for the diagnosis of erythema nodosum-associated sarcoidosis. *J Am Acad Dermatol.* 2003;49(1):75–78

Requena L, Yus ES. Panniculitis. Part I. Mostly septal panniculitis. *J Am Acad Dermatol.* 2001;45(2):163–183

CHAPTER 52

Pigmented Lesions

Kimberly A. Horii, MD

Key Points

- Worrisome change in a melanocytic nevus warrants evaluation by a dermatologist and possible biopsy for histologic evaluation.

- Pediatric patients with a large number of nevi or many clinically atypical nevi may warrant referral to a dermatologist for evaluation and clinical monitoring.

- Pediatric melanoma may present either with changes in a pigmented lesion or as a new, rapidly growing lesion that can range from pink to dark brown/black.

- It is important to identify patients at risk for the future development of melanoma (light-colored eyes, fair skin that easily burns, family history of melanoma, and many atypical nevi) and monitor them closely over time.

- Pediatricians should counsel all patients and parents, including high-risk patients, regarding UV radiation protection and avoidance of indoor tanning.

Overview

Pigmented lesions are common in children. The most common type of pigmented neoplasm in the pediatric population is the melanocytic nevus, also known as a mole. Melanocytic nevi are composed of nevus cells, which are a type of melanocyte. Melanocytic nevi can be congenital or acquired and may be clinically and histologically banal or atypical. Although melanoma is rare in the pediatric population, it is important for clinicians to be aware of risk factors associated with the development of melanoma and familiar with potentially worrisome features of melanocytic lesions.

Causes and Differential Diagnosis

Cause of pigmented lesions for the individual patient is unknown. The differential diagnosis of pigmented lesions in children is quite broad (Box 52-1). Usually, the clinical history and appearance of a pigmented lesion will allow a

Box 52-1. Differential Diagnoses of Pigmented Lesions in Children

- Acquired melanocytic nevus
- Congenital melanocytic nevus
- Melanoma
- Freckles
- Café au lait spots
- Lentigenes
- Blue nevus
- Mongolian spot
- Postinflammatory hyperpigmentation
- Becker nevus
- Epidermal nevus

clinical diagnosis to be made. Aside from melanocytic nevi, other pigmented lesions may be important to identify because they can be associated with underlying abnormalities. Numerous café au lait spots can be one of the cutaneous markers of neurofibromatosis 1, a relatively common inherited disorder that can have cutaneous, brain, ocular, and bone abnormalities. A large, solitary café au lait spot with a jagged "coast" outline can be associated with McCune-Albright syndrome, a rare disorder with skin, bone, and endocrine anomalies. Finally, multiple lentigines, which are small tan, dark brown, or black flat lesions, may be associated with various syndromes, including Peutz-Jeghers syndrome, a rare inherited disorder with mucocutaneous lentigines and intestinal polyps. Usually, the clinical history and appearance of a pigmented lesion will allow a clinical diagnosis to be made. In certain instances, a skin biopsy may be needed to make a definitive diagnosis through histologic examination.

Clinical Features

Congenital Melanocytic Nevi

Congenital melanocytic nevi (CMN) are usually present at birth or may develop within the first few weeks to months of life. They are relatively common and can occur on any area of the body. The lesions are categorized on the basis of their projected estimated size in adulthood into small, medium, and large size. Most small- and medium-sized CMN do not cause much concern to parents; however, the rarer large nevus can be cosmetically disfiguring and may have significant psychosocial effects on the child and parent. The terms *bathing trunk nevus* or *garment nevus* have been used to describe giant CMN, as they usually encompass a large portion of body surface area.

At birth, CMN may be light brown and flat and can be difficult to distinguish from café au lait spots, or they can be raised with variable texture and pigmentation. Over time, CMN can become more raised and may develop increased hair growth within the lesion.

Large CMN often have clinically atypical areas within the nevus, including pigment irregularity and texture variation, making these nevi difficult to follow. Individuals with large CMN are at a higher risk of developing cutaneous melanoma within the nevus; therefore, these patients should be followed closely by an experienced dermatologist. Patients with large CMN, who also have multiple concomitant smaller CMN scattered on other areas of the body, known as satellite nevi, are also at risk for neurocutaneous melanocytosis. Neurocutaneous melanocytosis is a proliferation of melanocytes within the leptomeninges or brain parenchyma. This proliferation can remain asymptomatic or undergo malignant change leading to symptomatic neurologic deterioration.

Common- or Banal-Acquired Melanocytic Nevi

Acquired melanocytic nevi may appear after the first 6 to 12 months of life and increase in number throughout childhood and adolescence. Both genetic predisposition and environmental factors can play a role in the development of acquired melanocytic nevi. Individuals with a family history of multiple nevi and lighter complexion are at higher risk of developing more acquired melanocytic nevi. Increased sun exposure during childhood may also increase one's number of melanocytic nevi.

Typical "common"- or "banal"-acquired melanocytic nevi may range in color from pink to light brown to dark brown and can be raised or flat. They are generally smaller than 6 mm in diameter, are symmetric, have even pigmentation with a regular outline/border, and can occur on any area of the body. Individuals with many acquired melanocytic nevi often have a predominant nevus type that shares the same general size, shape, and color. A melanocytic nevus that clearly stands out as different from the predominant nevus type, known as the "ugly duckling sign," may warrant evaluation by a dermatologist and excision for histologic examination.

Atypical Melanocytic Nevi and Dysplastic Nevi

Acquired melanocytic nevi that do not have a uniform clinical appearance, as seen in common- or banal-acquired melanocytic nevi, have been labeled as atypical melanocytic nevi. An *atypical nevus* refers to atypical clinical appearance of a nevus, while the term *dysplastic nevus* refers to atypical histologic findings on biopsy. These terms are often used interchangeably even though they refer to different atypical features.

Clinically, atypical nevi often develop during adolescence and frequently occur in "moley" families. The clinical appearance of an atypical melanocytic nevus can include a size larger than 5 mm, irregular border, asymmetric shape, and variable pigmentation. Common locations of atypical nevi in children include the trunk and scalp, but they can occur anywhere on the body. Atypical nevi can range in number from few to many. Studies have shown that individuals with many atypical or dysplastic nevi are at higher risk of developing melanoma. Therefore, recognizing patients with this type of nevus phenotype is important, since these individuals may benefit from being followed by a dermatologist. If an atypical nevus changes or has worrisome features, full excision for histologic evaluation is necessary to rule out melanoma.

Melanoma

Pediatric melanoma is an uncommon but potentially life-threatening malignancy. As the incidence of melanoma in the pediatric population is increasing, specifically in adolescents, clinicians need to be aware of the possible clinical presentation of melanoma in children. Risk factors for the development of melanoma are listed in Box 52-2.

The typical clinical ABCDE features of melanoma are listed in Box 52-3. These ABCDE features, however, may not always apply to melanoma presenting in children. Younger children with melanoma can present with a rapidly enlarging amelanotic (pink or red) raised papule or nodule that may be clinically confused with a pyogenic granuloma or Spitz nevus. Recently, additional ABCD detection criteria for children were proposed that when used with the conventional ABCDE criteria may lead to earlier recognition of melanoma in children (**A**melanotic; **B**leeding and **B**umps; uniform **C**olor; variable **D**iameter and **D**e novo development) Adolescents with melanoma can present with a rapidly growing amelanotic lesion, similar to younger children

---

Box 52-2. Melanoma Risk Factors

- Family history of melanoma
- Light-colored eyes
- Fair skin that burns easily
- Multiple atypical or dysplastic nevi
- Large congenital melanocytic nevus
- History of significant sun exposure and sunburns
- Underlying genetic disorder, such as xeroderma pigmentosum
- History of immunosuppression
- Indoor tanning bed use

Box 52-3. ABCDE of Melanoma (Possible Clinical Features)

A: asymmetry (2 halves of the lesion are not similar.)

B: border irregularity (notched or irregular borders)

C: color variability or change (multiple colors, including black, blue, red, or white)

D: diameter >6 mm

E: evolution (change in appearance of lesion over time)

with melanoma, or they can present with a new or changing pigmented lesion that possesses the ABCDE clinical features of melanoma. Therefore, both the sudden development of an atypical nevus or a change in a melanocytic nevus that follows the ABCDE rules of melanoma is worrisome in an adolescent. Symptoms such as bleeding, itching, ulceration, or pain in a melanocytic nevus are additional worrisome signs. If a lesion appears clinically suspicious for a melanoma, referral to a dermatologist for evaluation and complete excision of the lesion and histologic examination is required.

Evaluation

Most small- and medium-sized CMN are considered to be at low risk of developing malignant change. If melanoma develops within a small- or medium-sized nevus, it usually does not occur until adolescence.

Because large CMN are at higher risk of developing cutaneous and extracutaneous melanoma, these patients should be followed closely by a dermatologist experienced in caring for infants and children with this type of birthmark. Excision of a worrisome lesion within a large nevus is often warranted to rule out melanoma. In some instances, prophylactic removal of part or most of the large nevus by an experienced pediatric plastic surgeon may be considered. Magnetic resonance imaging with contrast of the brain and spine of an infant with a large nevus and multiple satellite nevi will help assess for neurocutaneous melanocytosis.

Individuals with numerous acquired melanocytic nevi need to be followed periodically with full body skin examinations for changes in their nevi. Patients with clinically atypical or dysplastic melanocytic nevi may benefit from evaluation and monitoring by a dermatologist, because these individuals are at higher risk of developing melanoma. Patients or their parents also need to watch and follow their nevi for changes over time, because melanoma is often initially noted by the patients themselves. Patients also need to monitor themselves for the rapid growth of new, clinically atypical lesions, since many cases of melanoma arise de novo.

Management

If a worrisome change is noted in a nevus, referral to a dermatologist for excision of the lesion for histologic evaluation is recommended. Pediatricians should follow head circumference and neurologic examination closely in infants with neurocutaneous melanocytosis. The management of small- and medium-sized CMN is somewhat controversial. Following clinically over time those lesions that are uniform in appearance or in a location that would be difficult to remove is reasonable over routine excision in infancy or childhood. If a change is noted within a nevus, evaluation by a dermatologist and excision of the atypical region or removal of the entire nevus may be needed.

Ultraviolet radiation exposure can increase one's risk of developing acquired melanocytic nevi and melanoma; therefore, pediatricians should counsel patients and parents about UV radiation protection during their health supervision visits as recommended in the 2011 American Academy of Pediatrics policy statement on UV radiation (Box 52-4). Pediatricians also need to recognize which children are at higher risk of developing melanoma and encourage those individuals and their families to routinely perform self-skin examinations (see Box 52-3). Because exposure to artificial UV radiation through indoor tanning is popular among adolescents, discussion about the risks of indoor tanning is also important to begin in the preadolescent years.

Box 52-4. Summary of Recommendations for Pediatricians in the 2011 AAP Policy Statement on UV Radiation

Pediatricians should incorporate advice about UV radiation exposure and education into at least 1 health maintenance visit per year, which includes

- Avoid sunburns and suntanning.
- Wear clothing, hats with brims, and sunglasses when outdoors.
- Limit time outdoors between 10:00 am and 4:00 pm (time of peak UV radiation intensity).
- Promote outdoor physical activity in a sun-safe manner.
- Broad-spectrum sunscreen use of SPF 15 or higher with reapplication every 2 h when outdoors.
- Avoid artificial UV radiation exposure (indoor tanning).
- Babies <6 mo should be kept out of direct sunlight, and limited sunscreen can be applied to exposed areas if sun avoidance is impossible.
- UV radiation protection is needed if taking a photosensitizing medication.
- Vitamin D supplementation should follow AAP recommended guidelines.

Abbreviation: AAP, American Academy of Pediatrics.

Suggested Reading
· · · · · · · · · · · · · · · · · ·

Alikhan A, Ibrahimi OA, Eisen DB. Congenital melanocytic nevi: where are we now? Part I. Clinical presentation, epidemiology, pathogenesis, histology, malignant transformation, and neurocutaneous melanosis. *J Am Acad Dermatol.* 2012;67(4):495. e1–495.e17

Alikhan A, Ibrahimi OA, Eisen DB. Congenital melanocytic nevi: where are we now? Part II. Treatment options and approach to treatment. *J Am Acad Dermatol.* 2012;67(4):515.e1–515.e13

American Academy of Pediatrics Council on Environmental Health, Section on Dermatology. Ultraviolet radiation: a hazard to children and adolescents. *Pediatrics.* 2011;127(3):588–597

Balk SJ; American Academy of Pediatrics Council of Environmental Health, Section on Dermatology. Ultraviolet radiation: a hazard to children and adolescents. *Pediatrics.* 2011;127(3):e791–e817

Cordoro KM, Gupta D, Frieden IJ, et al. Pediatric melanoma: results of a large cohort study and proposal for modified ABCD detection criteria for children. *J Am Acad Dermatol.* 2013;68(6):913–925

Duffy K, Grossman D. The dysplastic nevus: from historical perspective to management in the modern era: part I. Historical, histologic, and clinical aspects. *J Am Acad Dermatol.* 2012;67(1):1.e1–1.e16

Duffy K, Grossman D. The dysplastic nevus: from historical perspective to management in the modern era: part II. Molecular aspects and clinical management. *J Am Acad Dermatol.* 2012;67(1):19.e1–19.e2

Hill SJ, Delman KA. Pediatric melanomas and the atypical spitzoid melanocytic neoplasms. *Am J Surg.* 2012;203(6):761–767

Krengel S, Marghoob AA. Current management approaches for congenital melanocytic nevi. *Dermatol Clin.* 2012;30(3):377–387

Lange JR, Palis BE, Chang DC, Soong SJ, Balch CM. Melanoma in children and teenagers: an analysis of patients from the National Cancer Data Base. *J Clin Oncol.* 2007;25(11):1363–1368

Lazovich D, Isaksson V, Berwick M, Weinstock MA, Anderson KE, Warshaw EM. Indoor tanning and risk of melanoma: a case-control study in a highly exposed population. *Cancer Epidemiol Biomarkers Prev.* 2010;19(6):1557–1568

Lazovich D, Vogel RI, Berwick MI, et al. Melanoma risk in relation to use of sunscreen and other sun protection methods. *Cancer Epidemiol Biomarkers Prev.* 2011;20(12):2583–2593

Rigel DS, Friedman RJ, Kopf AW, et al. ABCDE—an evolving concept in the early detection of melanoma. *Arch Dermatol.* 2005;141(8):1032–1034

Schaffer JV. Update on melanocytic nevi in children. *Clin Dermatol.* 2015;33(3):368-386

CHAPTER 53

Pruritus

Jeana Bush, MD

Key Points

- Pruritus is the most common of all dermatologic concerns and encountered frequently in pediatric practice.
- Pruritus can be classified as dermatologic, systemic, neurologic, or psychogenic.
- Most causes can be identified with a thorough history and physical examination.
- The possibility of a systemic disorder should be considered in patients presenting with generalized pruritus without an obvious source.
- Therapy should be directed toward the underlying cause along with extensive education on appropriate skin care.

Overview

Pruritus can be defined as a sensation that elicits the desire to scratch and is most commonly referred to as *itching*. It is a common symptom but in itself is not a disease. It occurs in the setting of many disease processes and can originate from numerous organ systems. As the most common of all dermatologic concerns, it can interfere with sleep, concentration, and daily function; severity can range from being an annoyance to physically debilitating.

Pruritus is classified as acute (ie, lasting <6 weeks) or chronic (ie, lasting >6 weeks). The International Forum for the Study of Itch divides pruritus into 2 primary tiers, the first tier used when origin of the itch is unknown and the second tier for known etiologies of pruritus (Box 53-1).

Box 53-1. Pruritus Tiers

Tier 1 • Group I: pruritus on diseased skin (ie, inflamed) • Group II: pruritus on non-diseased skin • Group III: pruritus presenting with severe chronic secondary scratch lesions **Tier 2** • Dermatologic: pruritus from a primary skin disorder • Systemic: pruritus with origin from disorders affecting other organ systems • Neurologic: pruritus related to disorders of the peripheral or CNS • Psychogenic: psychiatric disorders in which people report pruritus • Mixed: pruritus attributed to one or more causes

Abbreviation: CNS, central nervous system.

Dermatologic Disorders

Atopic Dermatitis

Atopic dermatitis is a chronic inflammatory disorder of the skin. Pruritus of atopic dermatitis can have a significant effect on quality of life if left untreated. The hallmark of this disease is allokinesis, in which a normally innocuous stimulus induces intense pruritus. Examples of such stimuli can include sweating, temperature change, and skin contact with certain types of clothing or fibers. Another hallmark of this condition is a vicious "itch-scratch" cycle in which excoriations from scratching induce intense pruritus.

Atopic dermatitis is a clinical diagnosis with a broad differential diagnosis. Patients report chronic and relapsing pruritus and dermatitis. Physical findings include sparing of the central face (headlight sign), xerosis (dryness), creases under the lower eyelids (Morgan folds), periorbital darkening, and accentuation of the palmar skin lines. Dermatitis may vary in presentation depending on age of the patient. In infants, it often presents on the cheeks and extensor surfaces of the arms and legs. Older children have the more typical flexural surface involvement of the antecubital and popliteal fossae, back of the neck and hands, wrists, and ankles.

Treatment is directed at decreasing skin dryness using moisturizers, avoiding excessive bathing, and education on appropriate skin products. Avoiding fragrant or dye-containing soaps, detergents, and fabric softeners can be helpful. The inflammation can be treated with topical corticosteroids, preferably ointments over lotions because of the high water concentration and emollience. Starting with low-potency topical steroids and moving up in strength is the standard treatment, being sure to avoid oral or systemic steroids because of rebound flares and long-term adverse effects. Symptomatic treatment with antihistamines (Table 53-1) is important for breaking the itch-scratch cycle of this disease. Children with atopic dermatitis are at high risk for multiple widespread skin infections, including molluscum contagiosum, herpes simplex (specifically, eczema herpeticum), and *Staphylococcus aureus*.

Table 53-1. H₁-Antihistamines With Pediatric Oral Dosing

Trade Name	Generic Name	Typical Usage	Recommended Dosing
First Generation			
Benadryl	Diphenhydramine	Symptomatic relief of allergic symptoms caused by histamine release; anti-motion sickness; antitussive; mild nighttime sedative; adjunct to epinephrine in the treatment of anaphylaxis	2–<6 y: 6.25 mg every 4–6 h, maximum: 37.5 mg/d 6–<12 y: 12.5–25 mg every 4–6 h, maximum: 150 mg/d >12 y and adults: 25–50 mg every 4–6 h, maximum: 300 mg/d
Dramamine	Dimenhydrinate	Treatment and prevention of nausea, vertigo, and vomiting associated with motion sickness	2–5 y: 12.5–25 mg every 6–8 h, maximum: 75 mg/d 6–12 y: 25–50 mg every 6–8 h, maximum: 150 mg/d >12 y and adults: 50–100 mg every 4–6 h, maximum: 400 mg/d
Tavist	Clemastine	Allergic rhinitis and other allergic symptoms including urticaria	Babies and children <6 y: 0.05 mg/kg/d as clemastine base or 0.335 to 0.67 mg/d of clemastine fumarate divided into 2–3 doses 6–12 y: 0.67–1.34 mg clemastine fumarate twice daily, maximum: 4 mg/d >12 y and adults: 1.34 mg clemastine fumarate twice daily, maximum: 8 mg/d
Chlor-Trimeton, Teldrin	Chlorpheniramine maleate	Allergic rhinitis and other allergic symptoms including urticaria	2–5 y: 1 mg every 4–6 h 6–11 y: 2 mg every 4–6 h, not to exceed 12 mg/d or timed-release 8 mg every 12 h >12 y and adults: 4 mg every 4–6 h, not to exceed 24 mg/d or timed-release 8–12 mg every 12 h

Continued

Table 53-1 *(cont)*

Trade Name	Generic Name	Typical Usage	Recommended Dosing
First Generation			
Polaramine	Dexchlorpheniramine	Allergic rhinitis and other allergic symptoms including urticaria	2–5 y: 0.5 mg every 4–6 h, not to exceed 3 mg/d 6–11 y: 1 mg every 4–6 h, not to exceed 6 mg/d >12 y and adults: 2 mg every 4–6 h, not to exceed 12 mg/d
Rynatan	Chlorpheniramine tannate; pyrilamine tannate	Allergic rhinitis and other allergic symptoms including urticaria	2–6 y: 2 mg twice daily, not to exceed 8 mg in a 24-h period 6–12 y: 4–8 mg twice daily, not to exceed 16 mg in a 24-h period >12 y and adults: 8–16 mg twice daily, not to exceed 32 mg in a 24-h period
Atarax, Vistaril	Hydroxyzine	Antipruritic; antiemetic; anxiolytic; preoperative sedation	<6 y: 50 mg/d in divided doses or 2 mg/kg/d divided every 6–8 h >6 y: 50–100 mg/d in divided doses
Phenergan	Promethazine	Symptomatic treatment of various allergic conditions; motion sickness; sedative; antiemetic	(as an antihistamine) Children >2 y: 0.1 mg/kg/dose (not to exceed 12.5 mg) every 6 h during the day and 0.5 mg/kg/dose (not to exceed 25 mg) at bedtime as needed Adults: 6.25–12.5 mg 3 times/d and 25 mg at bedtime

Brand	Generic	Indication	Dosing
Periactin	Cyproheptadine	Allergic rhinitis and other allergic symptoms including urticaria; appetite stimulant; prophylaxis for cluster and migraine headaches; spinal cord damage associated with spasticity	2–6 y: 2 mg every 8–12 h, not to exceed 12 mg/d 7–14 y: 4 mg every 8–12 h, not to exceed 16 mg/d Adults: 4–20 mg/d divided every 8 h, not to exceed 0.5 mg/kg/d
Second Generation			
Zyrtec, All Day Allergy	Cetirizine	Perennial and seasonal allergic rhinitis; uncomplicated skin manifestations of chronic idiopathic urticaria	6–12 mo: 2.5 mg once daily 12–23 mo: initially 2.5 mg once daily; may be increased to 2.5 mg twice daily 2–5 y: 2.5 mg/d; may be increased to maximum of 5 mg/d as single dose or divided doses >6 y–adult: 5–10 mg/d as single dose or divided into 2 doses
Allegra	Fexofenadine	Seasonal allergic rhinitis and chronic idiopathic urticaria	6 mo–<2 y: 15 mg twice daily 2–11 y: 30 mg twice daily >12 y–adult: 60 mg twice daily or 180 mg once daily
Alavert, Claritin, Loradamed, Tavist ND Allergy	Loratadine	Nasal and non-nasal symptoms of allergic rhinitis; chronic idiopathic urticaria	2–5 y: 5 mg daily >6 y–adult: 10 mg daily

Data from Taketomo C, ed. *Pediatric and Neonatal Dosage Handbook.* 21st ed. Hudson, OH: Lexi Comp; 2014.

Xerosis

Xerosis is most commonly referred to as "dry skin." It is a common cause of pruritus in the pediatric population, especially during winter months. Xerosis is characterized by dry, scaly skin and most commonly occurs on the lower extremities. Risk factors for development of xerosis include genetic predisposition, frequent bathing, and ambient high temperatures with low humidity (which is common inside heated homes during cold winter months). Primary treatment of xerosis is limitation of factors that dry the skin and increasing moisture.

Contact Dermatitis

Contact dermatitis arises from direct skin contact with any foreign substance. It may be primary irritant contact dermatitis or allergic contact dermatitis. Primary irritant contact dermatitis is a nonallergic reaction to prolonged or repetitive contact with a variety of irritants, which can include detergents, soaps, saliva, acidic products, or excrement. Common examples of allergic triggers include metals (eg, nickel, chromium), oleoresin from plants (eg, poison ivy, oak, or sumac), and topical medications (eg, neomycin, bacitracin). Treatment depends on the source of dermatitis. Irritant contact dermatitis treatment involves restoring water and lipid to the skin surface using moisturizers at least twice daily (Table 53-2). Allergic contact dermatitis must be treated for at least 14 to 21 days, and the offending allergen must be identified and avoided to prevent recurrence. Dermatitis of less than 10% of skin surface can be treated with topical corticosteroids of moderate potency in ointment preparations for 2 to 3 weeks. If the dermatitis involves greater than 10% of the skin surface, systemic steroids are necessary.

Urticaria

Urticaria is a rash most commonly referred to as *hives*. The typical lesion is well circumscribed, blanchable, raised, and erythematous with central pallor. It is characterized by marked pruritus. The lesions may enlarge and coalesce, transiently appearing and disappearing and resolving most often over a few hours. *Acute urticaria* is defined as lasting less than 6 weeks, while *chronic urticaria* refers to persistent or recurring lesions lasting 6 weeks or more.

Acute urticaria is usually an allergic reaction, while chronic urticaria has various causes including systemic disorders. Common causes of acute urticaria include allergens (eg, foods, medications, pollens, stinging insects), physical factors (eg, cold, heat, pressure as in dermographism, exercise induced), and infections. Papular urticaria is a common cause in children, primarily from stinging insects (eg, fleas, mosquitoes, bedbugs) and characterized by papular or vesicular linear clusters. Chronic urticaria occurs more often in adults than children. Unlike in adults, the association of chronic urticaria with malignancy is not well established in children, so evaluation for malignancy is usually not necessary. However, if malignancy is suspected, the patient should be referred to an oncologist.

Table 53-2. Types of Moisturizers

Type	Mechanism	Indication	Examples	Comments
Occlusive	Blocks trans-epidermal water loss	Xerosis Atopic dermatitis Prevention of irritant contact dermatitis	Petrolatum Zinc oxide Lanolin Mineral oil Silicones	Messy Comedogenic May cause folliculitis (mineral oil) or dermatitis (lanolin)
Humectant	Attracts water to the stratum corneum	Xerosis Ichthyosis	Urea Alpha-hydroxy acids Glycerin Sorbitol Lactic acid	May cause irritation (urea, lactic acid)
Emollient	Smoothes skin	Decreases skin roughness	Cholesterol Squalene Fatty acids	Not always effective
Replacement of deficiencies in "raw materials" of the intact stratum corneum	Claims to replenish essential skin components	Possible skin rejuvenation	Ceramides Natural moisturizing factor	Unproven benefits; may improve skin moisturization and barrier function

Treatment of urticaria focuses on avoiding underlying triggers and histamine blockers (see Table 53-1). If maximal doses of H_1-receptor antagonists do not relieve symptoms, an H_2-receptor antagonist, such as ranitidine or cimetidine, may be added. For severe or refractory cases, oral glucocorticoids may be used in short bursts (0.5–1 mg/kg/day for 5 days). If there are any signs or symptoms of anaphylaxis (eg, angioedema, respiratory distress, or gastrointestinal distress), a self-injectable epinephrine pen should be prescribed. Chronic urticaria or refractory cases should be referred to an allergist for further evaluation and management.

Miliaria Rubra

More commonly referred to as *prickly heat* or *heat rash,* miliaria rubra is caused by blocked eccrine sweat glands at the granular layer of the skin. This leads to leakage of sweat into the surrounding dermis. The rash is characterized by intense erythema with maculopapular vesicles and pruritus. It occurs in hot, humid environments often on intertriginous areas or surfaces of the body covered by clothing.

Infections

Superficial fungal infections caused by dermatophytes (tinea) are common causes of localized pruritus. Tinea cruris (or jock itch) typically presents with bilateral, crescent-shaped lesions extending from the inguinal folds to upper thighs. Tinea pedis (or athlete's foot) typically presents with white macerations; dry, scaly skin; or localized blisters between the toes. Tinea capitis occurs commonly in children and presents with an itchy scalp. Most fungal skin infections are treated with topical antifungal creams (eg, miconazole, clotrimazole, terbinafine). However, tinea capitis requires oral therapy (eg, griseofulvin, fluconazole, terbinafine, or itraconazole).

Viral infections (ie, chickenpox, molluscum) and bacterial infections (ie, folliculitis) are also recognized causes of pruritus.

Insect Bites and Infestations

Insect bites (especially mosquitos, fleas, and scabies) can be markedly pruritic. Some children develop papular urticaria, a delayed hypersensitivity reaction to insect bites that is more common in warmer months. The rash of papular urticaria is characterized by erythematous or umbilicated papules most commonly found in groups on the trunk and extensor surfaces of the extremity.

Scabies is a common infestation in the pediatric population caused by the mite *Sarcoptes scabiei*. The pathognomonic finding is the threadlike burrow (ie, thin gray, red, or brown line 2–15 mm long) produced from the mite traveling through the epidermis. Most often lesions are located on the intertriginous areas of the neck, axillae, groin, and webs of fingers and toes. Patients report intense pruritus worse at night, which is a result of delayed hypersensitivity to the mite protein and may persist for weeks after eradication.

Another common infestation in pediatric patients is pediculoses, more commonly known as lice. Pediculosis capitis (or "head lice"), corporis (or "body lice"), and pubis (or "pubic lice") cause significant pruritus from a delayed hypersensitivity reaction to saliva of the louse. The infecting organism is named on the basis of the body part it infests (*Pediculus humanus capitis, Pediculus humanus corporis,* and *Pediculus humanus pubis*). Diagnosis is clinical. In the case of head or pubic lice, nits are usually visible along the hair shaft. Body lice may present with a pruritic papular rash with excoriations. It is important to search the inner seams of clothing for lice and eggs. Body lice occur most commonly in the setting of poor hygiene, while pubic lice are typically transmitted via sexual contact and occur mainly in adolescents. Pubic lice may be associated with small bluish gray macules around the groin, lower abdomen, and thighs. Treatment options include topical pediculicides such as permethrin, pyrethrin, malathion, lindane, benzyl alcohol, spinosad, and ivermectin. It is important to know resistance patterns of louse in the geographic area of practice.

Lastly, enterobiasis (or pinworms) is a helminthic infection caused by *Enterobius vermicularis* that causes intense perianal pruritus. It is spread by ingestion of eggs, which can be aerosolized or located on surfaces such as contaminated hands and toys. Diagnosis is by visualization of worms in the perianal region or positive "clear tape test" with recovery of worms. Treat the entire family with mebendazole (100 mg) or albendazole (400 mg) in a single dose, and repeat treatment in 2 weeks. All linens and clothes should be laundered in hot water.

Psoriasis

Approximately one-third of initial presentations of psoriasis occur in persons younger than 20 years. Eighty percent of patients with psoriasis report pruritus, most commonly with a cyclic nature worse at night. Interestingly, it tends to be generalized pruritus, rather than localized to the psoriatic plaques, and poorly responsive to antipruritics. The most common form of this condition involves silvery scales over characteristic, erythematous skin lesions. The Koebner phenomenon is common (ie, psoriasis outbreak in the area of an abrasion) and often presents in a linear fashion.

Several forms of psoriasis are seen in the pediatric population. Guttate psoriasis presents with small, scaly papules and plaques on the face, trunk, and proximal extremities. It has been associated with streptococcal infections as a trigger. Erythrodermic psoriasis is an exfoliative-type skin reaction with warmth, erythema, and widespread scaling. It can be associated with difficulty maintaining body temperature (eg, hypothermia/hyperthermia), dehydration, hypoalbuminemia, and anemia of chronic disease. Pustular psoriasis is characterized by numerous small coalescing pustules most often localized to the palms and soles.

The mainstay of treatment for psoriasis is immunomodulators. Plaques are treated with topical glucocorticoids, calcipotriene (vitamin D analog), tazarotene gel (retinoid), tar, or anthralin in combination with UVB therapy. PUVA (oral psoralen and UVA light) is effective but associated with increased risk of skin cancer so generally not recommended in children. Dermatology consultation is recommended for children with a diagnosis of psoriasis.

Systemic Disorders

Renal Disease (Uremic Pruritus)

Pruritus resulting from uremia is more common in the adult population but a markedly disabling symptom in patients with end-stage renal disease. Symptoms tend to be most intense during or at the end of dialysis or in the evening and night.

Gastrointestinal Disease (Cholestatic Pruritus)

The combination of jaundice and generalized pruritus is nearly pathognomonic for biliary obstruction. It can be associated with intrahepatic or extrahepatic biliary obstruction, drug-induced cholestasis (eg, oral contraceptives, anabolic steroids, erythromycin), viral hepatitis, or primary biliary cirrhosis. Choleretic agents (eg, ursodeoxycholic acid), opiate antagonists, antihistamines, and antibiotics (eg, rifampin) have also been found to be effective. The generalized pruritus of liver disease tends to start with an acral distribution over the palms and soles, which is an unusual site in most other forms of pruritus. It is also interesting that the pruritus is unrelated to the degree of hyperbilirubinemia, as patients with intense jaundice are often unaffected.

Endocrine Diseases

Patients with thyrotoxicosis can present with pruritus. Patients with hypothyroidism may also experience pruritus secondary to xerosis. In diabetic patients, infections with *Candida albicans* can predispose to localized pruritus, especially in the genital and perineal areas.

Hematologic and Oncologic Disorders

Iron deficiency, even without anemia, can cause pruritus that improves with iron supplementation. Myeloproliferative disorders such as polycythemia vera may produce pruritus, particularly after a hot bath (known as aquagenic pruritus). Patients may describe a "skin prickling" sensation more so than an itch. The pruritus can last from minutes to hours and tends to be generalized. Aquagenic pruritus has also been associated with myelodysplastic disorders and T-cell lymphomas.

Leukemia and Hodgkin disease can cause pruritus. Itching may be a primary symptom in Hodgkin lymphoma (up to 30% of patients) and may precede presentation of lymphoma by up to 5 years, although this is more common in the adult population.

Rheumatologic Disorders

Patients with dermatomyositis will frequently experience intense pruritus that interferes with sleep and daily activity. Pruritus is also a common concern in systemic sclerosis (ie, scleroderma). Itching is not typically a cutaneous characteristic of lupus erythematosus, so if a patient reports itching with presumed lupus, the diagnosis should be reconsidered.

Neurologic Disorders

Neurologic disorders associated with pruritus are not typically seen in the pediatric population. Brachioradialis pruritus presents with pruritus in the proximal dorsolateral forearm and is typically seen in fair-skinned, middle-aged adults who spend significant amounts of time outdoors. Notalgia paresthetica is characterized by unilateral, localized pruritus. Postherpetic neuralgia is a common phenomenon following infection with herpes zoster and may lead to chronic localized pruritus. Multiple sclerosis can infrequently cause recurrent, severe episodes of generalized pruritus.

Psychiatric Disorders

Psychogenic Pruritus

Pruritus can be a manifestation of stress, anxiety, obsessive-compulsive disorder, personality disorder, depression, or psychosis. Psychogenic/neurotic excoriation is characterized by excessive picking or scratching of normal skin. Patients report significant pruritus, but the source of itch is not apparent. Examination will reveal scattered, linear excoriations anywhere on the body but most often on the extremities. Delusional parasitosis is a manifestation of hypochondriacal psychosis (often presenting with pruritus) that the patient attributes to a nonexistent parasitic infection.

Evaluation and Treatment

The presence of skin lesions usually points towards a dermatologic cause. Itching localized to one anatomic region usually suggests a specific local cause or exogenous exposure. Generalized pruritus often, but not always, points to a systemic etiology. Timing of occurrence and chronicity can be very revealing. Pruritus in general tends to worsen at night, but this is especially true with scabies and pinworms. If pruritus awakens a child from sleep, the cause is most likely organic. Recent, acute onset suggests infection, insect bite, urticaria, contact dermatitis, or sunburn. Chronic dermatitis occurs in the setting of atopic dermatitis and other systemic disorders. Certain associated symptoms such as weight loss, fever, weakness, or polyuria should raise flags for systemic illnesses such as renal failure or malignancy. Social history is important to elicit in recent sick contacts in the case of infestations or foreign travel in the case of certain infections. Family history can be revealing in the case of atopic disease, psoriasis, or thyroid or renal disorders.

The physical examination should be comprehensive, not focusing just on the skin. Weight and height should be plotted on standard growth charts, looking for signs of systemic disease such as growth failure in chronic renal disease. Clues to other disorders include pallor in the case of anemia, hepatomegaly in obstructive biliary disease, nail changes in psoriasis, or goiter in hyperthyroidism. Skin examination should pay close attention to the details of rashes or accompanying findings (eg, excoriations, scars, hypopigmentation or hyperpigmentation). Table 53-3 can be helpful in characterizing skin findings. Last, lack of skin findings can also be very revealing, suggesting other diagnoses such as psychogenic pruritus.

Table 53-3. Pruritic Dermatologic Conditions That Are Usually Apparent on Physical Examination

Physical Findings	Possible Etiology
Erythematous lesion with vesiculation, papulation, oozing, crusting, scaling, and sometimes lichenification	Atopic dermatitis
Erythematous lesion limited to the area of contact with an offending substance	Contact dermatitis
Circumscribed, raised wheals	Urticaria
Minute papulovesicles with intense erythema, usually localized to areas covered by occlusive clothing	Miliaria rubra
Macules, papules, vesicles, pustules appearing in crops with a centrifugal distribution	Chickenpox
Dome-shaped pustules with an erythematous base, lesions centered on hair follicles	Folliculitis
Erythematous, elevated, scaly, annular lesion with central clearing	Tinea corporis (ringworm)
Urticaria wheal with central punctum	Insect bite
Wheals, papules, vesicles, and threadlike burrows	Scabies
Nits on hair shafts	Pediculosis
Dry and cracked skin with fine scales	Xerosis

Reproduced from Leung AKC. Pruritus in children. *JR Soc Promot Health*.1998;118(5):280–286, with permission.

Treatment of pruritus should be tailored to the suspected etiology or diagnosis. Known precipitating or contributing factors should be avoided. In general, H_1-receptor antagonists are the mainstay of treatment (see Table 53-1). Histamine is one of the primary mediators of the itch sensation in the skin. In addition to blocking H_1 receptors in the dermis, many antihistamine medications such as hydroxyzine or diphenhydramine have the added benefit of sedation. This is particularly helpful in most conditions in which pruritus is worse at night. H_2 receptors are not involved with pruritus, so H_2-receptor antagonists are generally not helpful. Behavior therapy such as avoiding long, hot baths is helpful to prevent overdrying of the skin. Soothing lotions or emollients (see Table 53-2) are helpful in most conditions. Fingernails should be kept short to avoid excessive trauma to the skin. Topical steroids such as hydrocortisone can be used in steroid-responsive dermatoses. Consultation with appropriate subspecialists is recommended when the underlying diagnosis warrants expert opinion.

Suggested Reading

Greco PJ, Ende J. Pruritus: a practical approach. *J Gen Intern Med.* 1992;7(3):340–349

Langley EW, Gigante J. Anaphylaxis, urticaria, and angioedema. *Pediatr Rev.* 2013;34(6):247–257

Leung AK, Wong BE, Chan PY, Cho HY. Pruritus in children. *J R Soc Promot Health.* 1998;118(5):280–286

Stander S, Weisshaar E, Mettang T, et al. Clinical classification of itch: a position paper of the International Forum for the Study of Itch. *Acta Derm Venereol.* 2007;87(4): 291–294

CHAPTER 54

Psoriasis and Papulosquamous Disorders

Robert Sidbury, MD, MPH, and Morgan Maier, PA-C

Key Points

- Severe psoriasis is associated with obesity, arthritis, and depression. A targeted review of systems and management of relevant comorbidities should be a part of every psoriasis encounter.

- "Napkin psoriasis" should be considered in cases of refractory diaper dermatitis. It should be recognized that characteristic silvery scale is often absent owing to the uniquely moist regional environment.

- Psoriasis severity assessment should include extent of skin involvement, presence of arthritis, and effect on quality of life. Severe disease may be best managed with either phototherapy or systemic medications.

- Psoriatic arthritis is rare in the pediatric population. Morning back stiffness lasting longer than 30 minutes and nail involvement should heighten index of suspicion.

- Circumscribed pityriasis rubra pilaris is easily mistaken for plaque psoriasis; erythrodermic pityriasis rubra pilaris resembles drug eruption, severe psoriasis, or eczema and may require systemic therapy.

- A large solitary herald patch often precedes the diffuse rash of pityriasis rosea; inverse pityriasis rosea may present only in the axilla or groin.

- Pityriasis lichenoides et varioliformis acuta should be in the differential diagnosis of varicella; pityriasis lichenoides patients have a small risk of lymphoproliferative malignancy.

Psoriasis

Overview

Psoriasis is a multisystem inflammatory disease that typically affects the skin and less commonly joints and occurs in 2% of the population, though it is more prevalent in adults. There is a genetic predisposition, but psoriasis often develops in the absence of known family history. Emerging data link psoriasis with a number of other conditions including metabolic syndrome, adult coronary artery disease, diabetes, inflammatory bowel disease, and depression.

Causes and Differential Diagnosis

The cause of psoriasis is unknown. Psoriasis can be triggered by infections including streptococcal pharyngitis or perianal dermatitis, minor skin trauma, medications, and stress. The differential diagnosis is broad and depends on morphologic subtype. Plaque psoriasis is most often mistaken for atopic dermatitis, particularly nummular eczema, or pityriasis rubra pilaris (PRP). Scalp involvement may closely resemble seborrheic dermatitis; overlap is such that the term *sebopsoriasis* is often employed when only the scalp is affected. Psoriatic nails may have distinctive pits but can present solely with subungual debris; lifting of the distal nail plate, called onycholysis; and yellowish discoloration mimicking onychomycosis. Some patients may have only nail involvement. Pustular psoriasis may be confused with bacterial or candidal infections, a distinctive drug eruption called acute generalized exanthematous pustulosis, and rarely acne. Guttate psoriasis is most often mistaken for pityriasis rosea or a nonspecific viral exanthem. Inverse psoriasis may mimic intertrigo or seborrheic dermatitis. Finally, erythrodermic psoriasis, a rare variant particularly in the pediatric population, has a broad differential including atopic dermatitis, ichthyosis, drug eruption, and cutaneous T-cell lymphoma.

The clinical features of psoriasis are age and subtype dependent. Classic plaque psoriasis presents with thick, hyperkeratotic plaques at the extensor elbows and knees. Itch is variable but not uncommon in pediatric patients. In contrast, guttate psoriasis presents with numerous smaller 0.5- to 2.0-cm scaly red papules and plaques predominantly on the trunk. Streptococcal pharyngitis is a well-recognized trigger. Guttate psoriasis is more common in the pediatric population and may evolve into chronic plaque psoriasis. Psoriasis may koebnerize or spread at sites of trauma. This phenomenon may explain why elbows and knees are so often affected and may be seen at sites of scratching.

The signature psoriatic nail finding is pitting. Unlike alopecia areata, in which pits tend to be ordered and more linear, psoriatic pits are more asymmetric and randomly arrayed. Though evidence is mixed, there has historically been heightened suspicion for psoriatic arthritis in patients with nail changes. Pustular and erythrodermic psoriasis are quite uncommon in children and should be considered in diffuse abrupt erythema if accompanied by fever and leukocytosis.

Clinical Manifestations

Psoriasis is typically a clinical diagnosis. Psoriatic skin lesions are rarely present at birth. Infants may present with well-demarcated erythematous plaques in the diaper area, so-called napkin psoriasis, that are easily mistaken for irritant contact dermatitis. Keys to diagnosis include the well-marginated rash, involvement of the folds often spared by irritant contact dermatitis, and refractoriness to standard therapies. Unlike typical plaque psoriasis, the characteristic silvery scale is absent owing to the moist local environment. Axillary involvement may also be seen and like the diaper does not usually manifest typical psoriatic scale. This pattern is termed *inverse psoriasis.*

When diagnostic uncertainty exists, skin biopsy can be confirmatory. When psoriasis is in the differential, the clinician should perform a full skin examination with attention to extensor elbows and knees, axilla and groin, umbilicus, intergluteal cleft, scalp, palms and soles, and nails (Table 54-1). The pharynx should be visualized and where appropriate cultured for *Streptococcus.* Medication lists should be scrutinized with attention to agents that can induce or exacerbate psoriasis. A careful history should be taken with attention to recent symptoms of sore throat, morning stiffness, or joint pain.

A joint examination should be performed looking for swelling, redness, or pain. Digital dactylitis and enthesitis are characteristic features of psoriatic arthritis, so attention should be paid to fingers, toes, and insertion sites. Other common areas of involvement include the plantar fascia, Achilles tendons, ribs, spine, and pelvis. Plain radiographs of hands and feet may be supportive. Radiographic findings may include joint space narrowing, erosions, periostitis, "pencil in cup" osteolysis, ankylosis, and spondylitis. Laboratories are not routinely drawn but may help distinguish other types of inflammatory arthritis.

Table 54-1. Psoriasis Sites of Involvement

Site	Findings
Extensor elbows/knees	Thickened plaques with overlying silvery scale
Scalp	Adherent scale on an erythematous base with predilection for hairline
Nails	Disorganized pitting, distal onycholysis, oil spot discoloration, nail bed erythema
Palms/soles	Sharply circumscribed scaly plaques
Axilla/groin	Marginated erythema often without scale
Umbilicus/intergluteal cleft	Erythema with variable scale
Concha of ears	Adherent scale with mild erythema
Joints	Erythema, swelling, warmth, dystrophy

Management

Most pediatric patients have mild to moderate disease. In such patients, topical therapy is generally safe and effective (Figure 54-1). Topical corticosteroids are first-line therapy for most types of psoriasis. The exact mechanism of action is unclear but likely acts via anti-inflammatory, antineoplastic, and vasoconstrictive effects. Psoriatic plaques tend to be thicker than those seen in other common inflammatory disorders, such as atopic dermatitis, and as a result, more potent steroids may be required. Mid- to high-potency steroids may be used on affected areas twice a day for several weeks continuously, though no specific safe limit has been established. Topical therapies can be used intermittently and long-term. A general approach is short-term use of more potent products such as corticosteroids to gain control, followed by longer-term use of safer, less potent agents. Therapy can be individualized to optimize safety, efficacy, and adherence. Various "sequential therapy" regimens have been described, typically alternating steroidal and nonsteroidal products to improve both safety and efficacy. This rotation can occur daily, with the topical steroid in the morning and a nonsteroidal agent in the evening, or less often with, for example, "steroid" weekend holidays. Plaques often resolve with postinflammatory dyspigmentation in which the skin looks abnormal but is asymptomatic and there is no palpable scale. In such cases treatment should consist solely of emollition and sun protection. Regular therapy can be resumed at first sign of recurrent skin rash.

Nonsteroidal topical therapies include vitamin D (eg, calcipotriene) and vitamin A (eg, tazarotene) analogues. Combination products are available

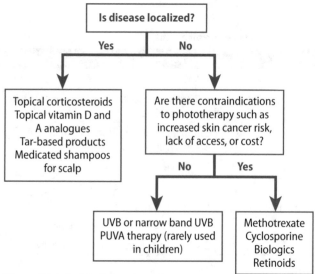

Figure 54-1. Psoriasis treatment.

(eg, calcipotriene/betamethasone) but are more expensive and no more effective than these products used individually, though added convenience likely improves adherence. Topical calcineurin inhibitors, tacrolimus and pimecrolimus, are indicated for atopic dermatitis and less effective treating psoriasis because of thicker scale; however, these products may be quite effective on thinner skin and facial, axillary, or groin skin where there is typically less scale and greater concern for steroid adverse effects.

Systemic therapy should be considered for several reasons: extensive body surface area involvement, concern with efficacy or safety of topical therapy, and significant effect on patient quality of life. Clinicians must also remain cognizant that some patients are terribly debilitated despite objectively having less extensive disease.

Methotrexate is the most commonly used systemic therapy for severe or refractory psoriasis and can be administered as a single weekly dose of 2.5 to 25.0 mg by mouth or subcutaneous injection. Onset of action occurs in 4 to 8 weeks and hepatotoxicity, bone marrow suppression, and gastrointestinal distress are the principal barriers to use. Most clinicians will supplement with folic acid 1 to 5 mg daily to minimize adverse effects. Once disease control has been established, every effort should be made to adjust dosing to maintain control with minimal drug exposure. Liver function tests are checked regularly, but adverse effects are less common in children likely owing to fewer comorbidities.

Cyclosporin is also generally effective and has a more rapid onset of action. Dosing typically starts at 2.5 to 3.0 mg/kg/day in 2 divided doses and is titrated to control. Nephrotoxicity and hypertension are limiting, and guidelines suggest use for up to 1 year. Other systemic treatments such as retinoids and tumor necrosis factor inhibitors are less commonly used in children.

In children intolerant or refractory to topical therapy, phototherapy should be considered second-line when available. Although no long-term pediatric safety studies exist, phototherapy can be employed effectively provided a clinician comfortable treating children is accessible. Broad- or narrow-band UVB (ultraviolet light B) is used almost exclusively in pediatric patients on account of improved safety profiles. Phototherapy units are available at most dermatology offices, but not all clinicians are comfortable treating children. Accessible phototherapy generally begins 2 to 3 times weekly and is tapered once control is achieved. Short-term adverse effects include redness, itch, and burning, while longer-term concerns include skin cancer and photoaging. Caution should be exercised in fairer skin types. Patients with psoriasis should be monitored regularly to guard against adverse effects of medication use. Topical corticosteroid atrophy, or adverse effects from systemic medications, must be monitored by clinical examination and serologies where appropriate. A thorough rheumatologic review of systems should be taken at each visit. Newer data suggest that long-term comorbidities including adult coronary artery disease, dyslipidemia, diabetes, metabolic syndrome, inflammatory bowel disease, and depression should be considered at regular follow-up.

Pityriasis Rubra Pilaris
Overview

Pityriasis rubra pilaris is an uncommon idiopathic inflammatory disorder that primarily affects the skin. It may present in several distinct patterns. The most common pediatric subtype is juvenile circumscribed PRP, which may be easily mistaken for psoriasis given its primary morphology (circumscribed scaly plaques) and distribution (extensor knees, palms, and soles). A less common presentation is generalized exfoliative erythroderma, often with characteristic "island sparing," and these children may have associated edema and arthralgias. Pityriasis rubra pilaris can be triggered by a viral or bacterial illness.

Natural history is one of indolent persistence followed typically by spontaneous remission sometimes in weeks to months. Some cases may persist for years.

Causes and Differential Diagnosis

The cause of sporadic PRP is unknown. Rare families have shown a dominant inheritance pattern that has recently been explained by *CARD14* mutations. The principle differential consideration in circumscribed PRP is psoriasis. Clinical clues suggestive of PRP include a distinctive salmon color, as opposed to the typical pink or red of psoriasis; follicular accentuation that may manifest as goose bump–like papules within an affected plaque; and the absence of the typical silvery scale of psoriasis. Pityriasis rubra pilaris may be mistaken for inherited ichthyosis (erythrokeratodermia), though age of onset, absence of family history, and pattern and distribution of hyperkeratosis are usually quite distinct. Erythrodermic PRP may be more difficult to distinguish from a number of potential mimics, including psoriasis, ichthyosis and atopic dermatitis, drug eruption, and cutaneous T-cell lymphoma. A skin biopsy may be required. Rarely, PRP can be associated with dermatomyositis and inflammatory arthritis.

Clinical Manifestations

Juvenile circumscribed PRP presents with discrete pink to orange plaques often studded with small follicular papules on the extensor knees. These plaques have only a modest degree of overlying scale. Palms and soles are inflamed and hyperkeratotic but generally do not develop thick scales. Other areas of involvement may include the Achilles tendons, ankle, upper trunk, face, and scalp. Erythrodermic PRP is by definition diffuse, involving nearly all skin, but forms strikingly normal-appearing "islands" of sparing. Affected children may have peripheral edema and considerable discomfort because of their taut, inflamed, hyperkeratotic skin. Pityriasis rubra pilaris typically presents in adolescence, though it can occur in much younger children.

Evaluation

A skin biopsy can be helpful. Parakeratosis with alternating zones of orthokeratosis overlying a hyperplastic epidermis with a dermal-mixed lymphohistiocytic infiltrate is specific. Erythrodermic patients may become dehydrated, so attention to fluid and electrolyte balance is important.

Management

Circumscribed PRP is treated similarly to psoriasis. Appropriate-strength topical steroids are first-line; however, more potent agents may be required because affected knee, palm, and sole skin is so naturally thick. This natural thickness provides a margin of safety against cutaneous atrophy caused by steroid overuse. Nonsteroidal agents containing tar or vitamin (A or D) analogues may also be useful.

Erythrodermic PRP may require systemic therapy; retinoids such as acitretin or isotretinoin and immunosuppressive agents have been tried with variable success. Fluid and electrolyte balance and pain control must be maintained. There are no long-term implications, though quality of life can be significantly affected.

Pityriasis Rosea

Overview

Pityriasis rosea is an acute exanthem that typically affects older children and adolescents. Most patients have no associated prodromal symptoms, though headache and malaise occur in some. Pityriasis rosea typically runs a benign self-limited course over several weeks to months. Itch and associated excoriations can potentially become superinfected and even cellulitic, but complications are uncommon and most have a benign course.

Causes and Differential Diagnosis

The cause of pityriasis rosea remains uncertain. A viral etiology is suggested by the occasional occurrence of a prodrome, clustering of cases, and self-limited course. *Human herpesvirus 6* has most often been purported, but definitive proof is lacking. The differential diagnosis typically includes other nonspecific-viral rashes, guttate psoriasis, tinea corporis, pityriasis lichenoides, and drug eruption. Certain medications such as ACE inhibitors and more recently lamotrigine may cause a pityriasis rosea–like drug rash.

Clinical Manifestations

Pityriasis rosea classically presents with a solitary large 1- to 5-cm scaly oval to elliptical red plaque on the trunk called a herald patch. This solitary plaque may easily be mistaken for tinea corporis (ringworm) or nummular eczema, or psoriasis. Days to weeks later, more numerous, smaller elliptical plaques of similar morphology present on the trunk and proximal extremities. These oval lesions typically have their long axes aligned uniformly and parallel to "relaxed skin tension lines" on the trunk, conjuring a "Christmas tree" pattern. Early lesions of pityriasis rosea may show a distinctive "trailing scale," whereby the scaly border lies inside an erythematous rim. When present, this can narrow the differential. Subacute cutaneous lupus and an uncommon hypersensitivity eruption called erythema annulare centrifugum may also manifest trailing scale.

Diagnosis

Serologic and radiographic assessments are generally unnecessary. In cases of persistent or recurrent pityriasis rosea, skin biopsy may help confirm the diagnosis.

Management

Management consists of symptomatic treatment of itching with antipruritics such as Sarna or calamine lotion, antihistamines, and colloidal oatmeal baths when helpful. Topical antibiotics may help prevent superinfection if excoriations are extensive. Topical steroids are generally not helpful. No specific long-term monitoring is required.

Pityriasis Lichenoides

Overview

Pityriasis lichenoides is an inflammatory T-cell–mediated idiopathic dermatosis that spans a clinical spectrum from acute (pityriasis lichenoides et varioliformis acuta, or PLEVA) to chronic (pityriasis lichenoides chronica, or PLC).

Pityriasis lichenoides et varioliformis acuta, also called Mucha-Habermann disease, presents abruptly in otherwise well children with diffuse, often pruritic skin rash that may persist for months to years. Pityriasis lichenoides chronica is more indolent, both in onset and duration, and typically persists for many years. Pityriasis lichenoides is a reactive inflammatory process but can in rare cases develop into lymphoma.

Causes and Differential Diagnosis

The cause is unknown, though pityriasis lichenoides may be triggered by preceding bacterial or viral illness. The differential diagnosis of PLEVA includes bug bites, varicella, viral exanthem, guttate psoriasis, lymphomatoid papulosis, and drug eruption. A rare and dramatic presentation, ulceronecrotic PLEVA, may resemble erythema multiforme and Stevens-Johnson syndrome. Conversely, PLC may be mistaken for tinea versicolor, psoriasis, eczema, pityriasis rosea, vitiligo, drug rash, and even secondary syphilis.

Clinical Manifestations

Pityriasis lichenoides et varioliformis acuta typically presents with discrete 2- to 10-mm erythematous scaly papules that frequently develop central necrosis and eschar. They may vary in number from several lesions to many, predominate on the trunk and proximal extremities, and typically spare the face. Patients feel generally well. Conversely, ulceronecrotic PLEVA often has associated fever and malaise, commonly leading to inpatient admission.

Pityriasis lichenoides chronica presents with small, discrete scaly macules and papules, typically without significant erythema, often healing with striking hypopigmentation. In patients with darker skin types, dyspigmentation may be the most noticeable physical finding with numerous focal areas of hypopigmentation that can coalesce.

Evaluation

Pityriasis lichenoides can be confirmed with a skin biopsy. Histologic features include necrotic keratinocytes, extravasated red blood cells, and a band-like mixed inflammatory infiltrate. Because of potential long-term concern with T-cell malignancy and the likely persistence of skin rash for an extended period, histologic confirmation is advisable. Though the inflammatory infiltrate can be clonal, flow cytometry and further analysis are not routinely recommended because clonality does not have prognostic significance. Persistent enlargement of any skin lesion, regional lymphadenopathy, and unexplained constitutional symptoms should prompt a directed workup to rule out lymphoma. Pityriasis lichenoides chronica patients with extensive dyspigmentation may raise consideration of vitiligo. A Woods light examination will easily distinguish the hypopigmentation of PLC from depigmented patches of vitiligo.

Management

The natural history of pityriasis lichenoides is typically self-limited. The average duration of PLEVA in the pediatric population is 18 months, while PLC may persist much longer. There are no universally effective therapies, and treatment algorithms depend on age of child, extent of involvement, and effect on quality of life. Localized involvement may be treated effectively with mid-potency topical steroids, but care must be taken to prevent overuse given the refractory and persistent nature of pityriasis lichenoides lesions. Clinicians must guide parents to distinguish actively inflamed and scaly lesions from postinflammatory hypopigmentation, which should simply be moisturized. For more extensive involvement, oral erythromycin at 30 to 50 mg/kg/day divided twice daily can be effective. If no response is seen after 4 to 6 weeks, it should be discontinued. Phototherapy, particularly narrow-band UVB, can be very helpful, but access, cost, and inconvenience can be limiting. Phototherapy is usually administered at a dermatologist's office, not all of whom are comfortable treating children, and often requires 2 to 3 times weekly sessions for 1 month or more to obtain response. When these therapies are intolerable or ineffective, methotrexate can be considered. Dosing schedules are largely anecdotal and derived from other inflammatory dermatoses, such as psoriasis, but generally range from 2.5 to 15 mg weekly orally or subcutaneously. Daily folic acid supplementation can improve tolerance. Other therapies that have been tried include prednisone, but lack of efficacy coupled with potential adverse effects limit their use.

Pityriasis lichenoides patients should be seen regularly to manage active symptoms in the short term and monitor for any signs of malignant transformation over time. Particular attention is paid to "B type" symptoms such as fever, night sweats, or weight loss and physical findings such as progressive individual skin lesions, hepatosplenomegaly, or lymphadenopathy.

Suggested Reading

Ersoy-Evans S, Greco MF, Mancini AJ, Subaşi N, Paller AS. Pityriasis lichenoides in childhood: a retrospective review of 124 patients. *J Am Acad Dermatol.* 2007;56(2):205–210 (Evidence Level II-2)

Fuchs-Telem D, Sariq O, van Steensel MA, et al. Familial pityriasis rubra pilaris is caused by mutations in *CARD14*. *Am J Hum Gen.* 2012;91(1):163–170 (Evidence Level II-2)

Luu M, Cordoro KM. The evolving role of biologics in the treatment of pediatric psoriasis. *Skin Therapy Lett.* 2013;18(2):1–4 (Evidence Level III)

Menter A, Gottlieb A, Feldman SR, et al. Guidelines of care for the management of psoriasis and psoriatic arthritis: section 1. overview of psoriasis and guidelines of care for the treatment of psoriasis with biologics. *J Am Acad Dermatol.* 2008;58(5):826–850 (author's note: first of 6-part series) (Evidence Level III)

Mercer JM, Pushpanthan C, Anandakrishnan C, Landells ID. Familial pityriasis rubra pilaris: case report and review of literature. *J Cutan Med Surg.* 2013;17(4):226–232 (Evidence Level III)

Mercy K, Kwasny M, Cordoro KM, et al. Clinical manifestations of pediatric psoriasis: results of a multicenter study in the United States. *Pediatr Dermatol.* 2013;30(4): 424–428 (Evidence Level II-2)

Paller AS, Mercy K, Kwasny MJ, et al. Association of pediatric psoriasis severity with excess and central adiposity: an international cross-sectional study. *JAMA Dermatol.* 2013;149(2):166–176 (Evidence Level II-2)

Rebora A, Drago F, Broccolo F. Pityriasis rosea and herpesviruses: facts and controversies. *Clin Dermatol.* 2010;28(5):497–501 (Evidence Level III)

Shah KN. Diagnosis and treatment of pediatric psoriasis: current and future. *Am J Clin Dermatol.* 2013;14(3):195–213 (Evidence Level III)

CHAPTER 55

Rashes

Charles F. Willson, MD

Key Points

- Examine the entire body, unclothed, to determine distribution.
- Describe the rash to yourself in dermatologic terms (eg, macular, papular, pustular, vesicular).
- Exclude or manage life-threatening conditions. Generalized rashes are likely caused by a systemic infection or reaction.
- Use only mild steroids on areas where the skin is thin (eg, face, eyelids, ears, scrotum).
- Complications caused by prolonged steroid applications may be lessened by applying them only on weekdays and resting the skin on weekends (avoid high-potency steroid preparations).

Overview

Rashes account for about 30% of visits to pediatric offices but are also encountered in nurseries, intensive care units, and pediatric inpatient settings. Developing a systematic approach to a rash will make identification much easier and more accurate. Rashes are often very helpful as a sign at the onset of illness and help direct workup for a sick child.

Causes

The skin is the boundary to our environment, and many rashes are related to external factors such as environmental substances, trauma, heat exposure, infectious agents, and infestations. The skin may also react to internal stimuli brought to it via the blood or lymph. Consider the depth of the skin involvement and what manifestations are the primary rash or secondary to scratching or topical therapy. The condition causing the rash may be localized to the skin, or the rash may be a manifestation of a systemic disease or process. Hair and nails are specialized components of the skin and should be carefully examined.

Age and sex of the child may be important in the differential diagnosis of a rash, especially within the neonatal period.

When considering a child with a rash, a careful history will often focus the differential diagnosis to only a few conditions. Always ask

- When and where did the rash start?
- Has the rash spread?
- Are there any associated symptoms (eg, fever, cough, conjunctivitis, pruritus, pain locally or elsewhere)?
- Is the rash getting better or worse?
- Has the parent given any treatment, topical or systemic?
- Has the rash occurred before in this child or another family member?
- Has the child been exposed to anyone with an illness or rash (always positive for a child in a day care setting)?
- Any recent trauma?
- Have there been environmental exposures?
- Any new foods?
- Any new topical contactants such as soaps, shampoos, bubble baths, lotion, or new clothing?
- Has the child had all recommended vaccines for her age?
- What does the parent or caregiver think is causing the rash?

When examining a child with a rash, it is crucial to examine the entire child, looking for patterns, distribution, and signs of systemic illness or a genetic condition. Also, determine which lesions are the primary lesions or secondary to scratching, medication, or even an infectious disease reaction. A generalized rash is more often caused by internal factors, while a localized rash may reflect a specific trauma or exposure. Figure 55-1 shows typical distribution patterns for common rashes seen in childhood. Once you have come to a preliminary diagnosis, construct a differential diagnosis list and consider why you do not think it is the rash on the differential.

Because many rashes start centrally and spread peripherally, presence of the rash on palms and soles may be helpful in accurately diagnosing the rash. Table 55-1 lists common rashes that are often found in an acral distribution.

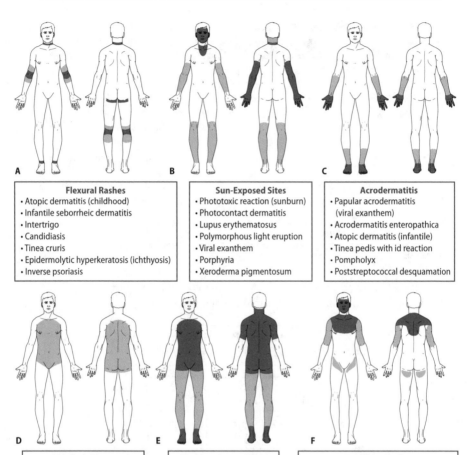

A

Flexural Rashes
- Atopic dermatitis (childhood)
- Infantile seborrheic dermatitis
- Intertrigo
- Candidiasis
- Tinea cruris
- Epidermolytic hyperkeratosis (ichthyosis)
- Inverse psoriasis

B

Sun-Exposed Sites
- Phototoxic reaction (sunburn)
- Photocontact dermatitis
- Lupus erythematosus
- Polymorphous light eruption
- Viral exanthem
- Porphyria
- Xeroderma pigmentosum

C

Acrodermatitis
- Papular acrodermatitis
  (viral exanthem)
- Acrodermatitis enteropathica
- Atopic dermatitis (infantile)
- Tinea pedis with id reaction
- Pompholyx
- Poststreptococcal desquamation

D

Pityriasis Rosea
- Pityriasis rosea
- Secondary syphilis
- Drug reaction (eg, gold salts)
- Guttate psoriasis
- Atopic dermatitis

E

Clothing-Covered Sites
- Contact dermatitis
- Miliaria
- Psoriasis (in summer)

F

Acneiform Rashes
- Acne vulgaris
- Drug-induced acne (eg, prednisone, lithium, INH)
- Cushing syndrome (endogenous steroids)
- Chloracne

Figure 55-1. Pattern diagnosis.

Abbreviation: INH, isoniazid.

Table 55-1. Generalized Rash With Involvement of Palms and Soles

Common	Variable	Rare
Rocky Mountain spotted fever Rubella Scabies Secondary syphilis Staph scalded skin Tinea corporis Toxic epidermal necrolysis Toxic shock syndrome	Lichen planus Meningococcemia Psoriasis (plaques) Urticaria (hives)	Guttate psoriasis Insect bites Keratosis pilaris Lyme disease Miliaria rubra Nummular eczema Pityriasis rosea Scarlet fever Seborrheic dermatitis Varicella Viral exanthems

Abbreviation: staph, staphylococcal.

Reproduced from Ely JW, Seabury Stone M. The generalized rash: part II. Diagnostic approach. *Am Fam Physician.* 2010;81(6):735–736, with permission.

Figures 55-2 and 55-3 outline an approach to the rash of a sick neonate or infant or child older than 2 months in the outpatient setting.

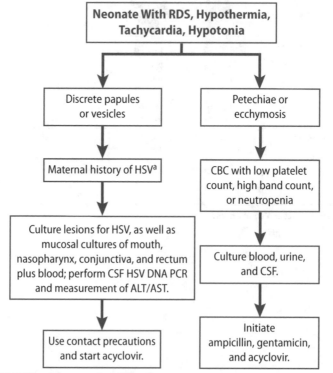

Figure 55-2. The sick neonate with rash.

Abbreviations: ALT, alanine transaminase; AST, aspartate transaminase; CBC, complete blood cell count; CSF, cerebrospinal fluid; HSV, herpes simplex virus; PCR, polymerase chain reaction; RDS, respiratory distress syndrome.

[a] Maternal history is generally negative; HSV disease is more commonly associated with primary HSV infection in the mother, so a negative history is more commonly found.

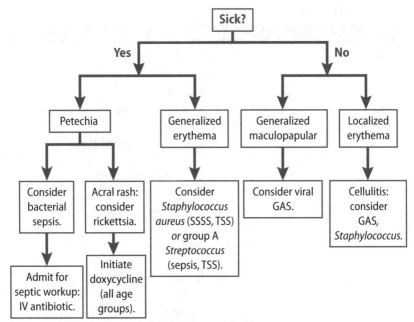

Figure 55-3. The infant or child with fever and rash.

Abbreviations: GAS, group A *Streptococcus*; IV, intravenous; SSSS, staphylococcal scalded skin syndrome; TSS, toxic shock syndrome.

When the cause of the rash is unclear but the patient is stable, fall back on the medical model of a thorough history, comprehensive review of systems, and complete physical examination to further focus the potential diagnoses. Always consider diseases that may cause significant morbidity and even mortality first.

Despite study and experience, some rashes are often confused or misdiagnosed (Table 55-2).

Clinical Features and Management

Neonatal Rashes

In the neonatal nursery, the first consideration of any rash should be for an acute infectious process such as neonatal herpes, group B streptococcal infection, or a congenital infection (eg, toxoplasmosis, syphilis, varicella-zoster virus, parvovirus B19, rubella, cytomegalovirus, herpes simplex, or zika virus). Any vesicle should be cultured for herpes simplex virus. Petechiae on the back after rubbing in the delivery room may signal a group B streptococcal infection or autoimmune thrombocytopenia.

Table 55-2. Often Confused Rashes

Condition	Similar Rashes (Distinguishing Features)
Atopic dermatitis	Contact dermatitis (not associated with dry skin)
	Keratosis pilaris (non-pruritic, involves posterolateral upper arms)
	Psoriasis (well-defined plaques, silvery white scale, flexural areas)
	Scabies (involves genitalia, axillae, finger webs) (Look for burrows.)
	Seborrheic dermatitis (greasy scale, non-pruritic distribution)
Contact dermatitis	Atopic dermatitis (symmetric distribution, family history, allergic triad)
	Dermatitis herpetiformis (vesicles on extensor areas, painful)
	Psoriasis (patches on knees, elbows, scalp, gluteal cleft; silver scale)
	Seborrheic dermatitis (greasy scale on eyebrows, nasolabial folds)
Drug eruption (morbilliform)	Erythema multiforme (target lesions)
	Viral exanthem (more common in children, less intense erythema, less likely to be dusky red, more focal systemic symptoms)
Pityriasis rosea	Drug eruption (no scale, lesions coalesced)
	Erythema multiforme (target lesions)
	Guttate psoriasis (thicker scale, history of GAS)
	Lichen planus (violaceous, involves wrists and ankles)
	Nummular eczema (larger round lesions, not oval)
	Psoriasis (thick white scale, involves extensor surfaces)
	Secondary syphilis (positive serology, involves palms and soles)
	Tinea corporis (+on potassium hydroxide concentration method, scale at periphery rather than within border)
	Viral exanthema (no scale, lesions coalesced)
Psoriasis	Atopic dermatitis (atopic features, flexural areas, lichenification)
	Lichen planus (violaceous, minimal scale, involves wrists and ankles)

Abbreviation: GAS, group A *Streptococcus*.

Adapted from Ely JW, Seabury Stone M. The generalized rash: part I. Differential diagnosis. *Am Fam Physician*. 2010;81(6):726–734, with permission.

A common rash with no significant sequelae, despite its ominous-sounding name, is erythema toxicum neonatorum. Raised, erythematous lesions are often widely distributed and regress after a few hours only to reappear elsewhere. Pustular melanosis may be identified by a superficial bleb that is easily wiped off, leaving a pigmented macule in its place. Maternal systemic lupus erythematosus may cause a rash and arrhythmias in the neonate.

Vascular anomalies are fairly frequent, such as flame nevi, salmon patches, and port-wine stains. Pigmented nevi and mongolian spots are common. Cutaneous angiomas (or strawberry hemangiomas) are often not present at birth, but their development may be predicted by a superficial blood vessel in the neonatal period. Over the ensuing weeks, a classic strawberry hemangioma may develop at that site, enlarging throughout the first year and then regressing. For angiomas that may impair vision or threaten the airway, a course of propranolol may cause early resolution. These lesions may also be ablated by laser treatment. Pigmented nevi and mongolian spots are common. Large "bathing suit" pigmented nevi may be distressing to parents and present a heightened risk of malignancy in adulthood.

Certain inherited or genetic syndromes cause typical rashes that may be the first manifestation of the process of each respective syndrome, such as café au lait spots (as seen in neurofibromatosis), ash leaf macules, shagreen patches, or a port-wine stain in the ophthalmic distribution of cranial nerve V.

Papulosquamous Lesions

Psoriasis is relatively uncommon in childhood but must be considered with a persistent rash that has an acral and extensor surface distribution, often involving the scalp, elbows, knees, and genitalia. It has a pearly scale that bleeds when lifted. Guttate psoriasis is a form of psoriasis often with an onset following a streptococcal infection. Pityriasis rosea is often announced by a herald patch, followed by oval lesions with scales attached at the periphery of lesions that follow the lines of tension of the skin. Gianotti-Crosti syndrome involves polygonal lesions with an acral distribution.

The Dermatitis Group

Atopic Dermatitis

Atopic dermatitis is the most common chronic rash in childhood, found in 10% to 15% of children. There is often an associated familial inheritance pattern of sensitization called atopy: dry skin, asthma, and allergic rhinitis. Presence of atopic dermatitis does not imply that the child will have the other hypersensitivity conditions or that the rash is IgE mediated. There is an infantile presentation and a more typical childhood presentation. Dry skin is the underlying hallmark of atopic dermatitis. Because of the dryness, the skin is pruritic (ie, "the itch that rashes"). As the skin is scratched, the typical pattern of redness, edema, erosions, inflammatory papules, serous drainage, and crusts develops.

Infantile atopic dermatitis often involves the face and exposed areas. The diaper area is typically spared because of the more humid environment and inability of the infant to scratch the area under the diaper.

Childhood atopic dermatitis has characteristic distribution in the flexural creases and behind the neck.

Management of atopic dermatitis. For both infantile and childhood varieties of atopic dermatitis, the critical features of management include

1. A parental understanding that the goal of management is to control symptoms. There is no cure; daily treatment will bring best results.
2. Moisturize the entire skin. Choose an inexpensive product such as Vaseline Intensive Care.
3. Control the itch. Choose a cost-effective antihistamine such as hydroxyzine or cetirizine.
4. Apply an anti-inflammatory medication to the most involved areas. Use low potency on thin skin, such as that of the face, ears, and genitals, and moderate potency on the arms, legs, trunk, and back.
5. Use a mild soap, and make baths a quick dip; many dermatologists advise unscented soap.
6. Consider if excoriated areas are infected. If so, consider a topical antibiotic such as mupirocin or a systemic antibiotic such as erythromycin.

Close follow-up after initiating treatment is essential because many parents become frustrated with a lack of immediate results. To lessen adverse effects of long-term application of topical steroids, parents can apply the steroid on weekdays (after work) and none on the weekends (to allow for rest). Antihistamines and moisturizers are used daily.

Seborrhea

While the cause of seborrhea is still debated and probably multifactorial, it is clearly related to an excess production of oil in the sebaceous glands with a possible fungal component (ie, *Malassezia furfur*). There are infantile and adult presentations. Distribution of the rash overlaps with atopic dermatitis and psoriasis. Unlike atopic dermatitis, bathing with soap and water and mild rubbing to remove scales is the mainstay of treating seborrhea. Also unlike atopic dermatitis, seborrhea is often found in the diaper area. As stimulation of the sebaceous glands by transplacental passage of maternal hormone subsides, infantile seborrhea resolves usually by 3 months of age only to recur during the hormone-rich period of adolescence with dandruff and acne.

Management of seborrhea. Reassurance that excessive oil production will subside over time is a mainstay. Daily care includes gentle brushing during bathing to remove scales. An antiseborrheic shampoo such as Selsun Blue or Head and Shoulders may be used on the scalp. For inflamed areas, a mild-potency steroid may be used on weekdays.

Contact Dermatitis

Contact dermatitis may be divided into irritant dermal effects and allergic dermal reactions. Except for irritant rash caused by diapering and new underclothing, both occur primarily on exposed skin. A detailed history of all possible exposures to agents that may irritate skin (eg, alcohols, hydrocarbons, exposures such as excessive sun or wind that traumatize or dry the skin) should be considered. New clothing is often implicated because of fabric brighteners that will be removed with the first washing. When cloth diapers were used routinely, laundry detergent was a common cause of contact dermatitis and should be considered in some cases. A new disposable diaper brand may contain an irritant that the previous brand did not. Common contacts of an allergic nature in children include plants (which can cause rhus dermatitis), nickel (in items such as jewelry, belts, and metal fasteners on jeans), soaps, shoes, and medications.

Management of contact/irritant contact dermatitis. Once an offending agent is suspected, the management is fairly simple. Remove the offending agent and soothe the irritated skin with emollients and, in more severe cases, topical steroids. For a favorite pair of jeans, a piece of cloth tape may be placed over the metal snap each time the jeans are worn to prevent nickel allergy. For diaper dermatitis, exposure to the air and rapid changing of the wet/soiled diaper is crucial. Because yeast prefer warm, dark, moist areas, an anti-candidal agent is often used and then covered with an ointment to prevent exposure to moisture.

Systemic Allergic Syndromes

Urticaria

Urticaria (or hives) is an IgE-mediated rash that occurs acutely after exposure to an allergen. Intense pruritus and a plaque-like erythematous rash that appears, then disappears within hours, only to reappear in another location, is the hallmark of urticaria. Antihistamines are the treatment of choice acutely. Urticaria should be differentiated from angioedema, which also arises acutely but is not pruritic. Angioedema near the mouth and nose is of immediate concern because of the potential for swelling occluding the airway.

Erythema Multiforme

Like urticaria, erythema multiforme arises acutely with erythema and swelling often in a target pattern. Pruritus is minimal, but vesicles, bullae, and microhemorrhage (ie, ecchymosis) may be present. Unlike urticaria, the erythema multiforme rash stays in one spot and simply enlarges over time. Facial and joint swelling may also occur. A search for the allergen and prompt removal from the environment is critical. Antihistamines and steroids are often used.

Stevens-Johnson Syndrome

Sometimes referred to as erythema multiforme major, Stevens-Johnson syndrome involves not just the skin lesions of erythema multiforme (minor) but also systemic effects with conjunctiva, oral, and recto-genital mucous membranes. Referral to an ophthalmologist is indicated for conjunctival involvement because panophthalmitis may lead to blindness. Reactions to medications and viral infections are the most common triggers for Stevens-Johnson syndrome. Treatment is supportive with nonsteroidal anti-inflammatory drugs and antihistamines. Steroids may be helpful if started early in the course of the hypersensitivity reaction.

Toxic Epidermal Necrolysis

With toxic epidermal necrolysis, the initial rash rapidly progresses to generalized sloughing of the skin. Removal of the offending agent is critical to survival. Prompt admission to an intensive care or burn unit is indicated.

Infectious Rashes and Infestations

Viral

A viral infection is probably the most often implicated diagnosis for a generalized erythematous maculopapular rash accompanied by fever. The astute clinician will always attempt to specify which virus would cause the rash. By specifying which virus, the physician can advise parents how long the rash will last and alert them to other manifestations that may develop. In the case of roseola caused by *Human herpesvirus 6,* the rash develops after resolution of 4 or 5 days of fever, so only clinical suspicion will aid in the initial diagnosis. On the other extreme, Kawasaki disease may be suspected in those with fever, and rash with other clinical criteria (mucositis, extremity changes, isolated cervical lymph node enlargement, bulbar conjunctivitis). If a specific virus cannot be implicated, another causative agent should be suggested (eg, erythroderma caused by staphylococcal infection—staphylococcal scalded skin or toxic shock syndrome). A common mimicker of chickenpox is the vesicles caused by mosquito bites. Other vesicular rashes may be caused by reactivation of chickenpox in a dermatomal distribution (eg, herpes zoster) or in clusters (eg, herpes simplex).

Wart viruses are problematic because of their propensity to spread before finally yielding to host defenses. Local irritants such as liquid nitrogen and the daily application of tape are effective therapies. The vaccine for human papillomavirus should decrease the risk of cervical cancer in sexually active girls and may decrease the incidence of common warts in adolescents.

Bacterial

Staphylococcus aureus and group A *Streptococcus* are common pathogens present on our skin that can invade the dermis because of moisture (around the mouth and nose), friction (caused by excoriation from atopic dermatitis), or burns (thermal or chemical). Once a lesion develops on the skin, the pathogen can quickly spread to surrounding areas and then remotely through scratching. Methicillin-resistant *Staphylococcus aureus* is responsible for an epidemic of deeper cutaneous abscesses that are best treated by incision and drainage.

During warm months in certain locations, ticks may transmit Rocky Mountain spotted fever or ehrlichiosis. A petechial rash that begins on the distal extremities, accompanied muscle aches, and increasingly elevated fever are hallmarks for Rocky Mountain spotted fever. The rash usually appears on the fourth day of fever, with increasing morbidity, and even mortality, if not treated accurately and promptly.

Fungal

Candida albicans is a common colonizer of the mouth (and can lead to thrush) and diaper areas until cellular immunity develops in the second year of life. In older children, the dermatophytes cause tinea in many locations. Most areas can be treated topically, but tinea capitis usually requires oral antifungals such as griseofulvin. Tinea capitis may lead to a localized hypersensitivity reaction called a kerion. Hair loss and pustules along a tight braid line (known as braid dermatitis) may mimic tinea capitis. Tinea pedis, tinea cruris, and tinea versicolor are most commonly found in adolescents.

Infestations

Pediculosis (or lice) and scabies are frequent causes of highly pruritic rashes. Lice prefer the hair-bearing areas, while scabies like the thin skin between the fingers, toes, and axilla. Scabies are suspected with a generalized pruritus, and a careful search for characteristic burrows may confirm the diagnosis. Treatment with an insecticide will eliminate the organism, but the rash is caused by a hypersensitivity reaction to scabies excreta and will persist for a week or more after treatment. Likewise, with pediculosis the nits will persist on the hair shaft long after the organism has been eliminated. Overtreatment with the insecticide is frequent and can cause toxicity.

Cutaneous larva migrans is another infestation but caused by the cat tapeworm. The characteristic linear burrow on the lower extremities is highly pruritic.

Other

In any child with a prolonged fever and rash, Kawasaki disease must be considered. Thought to be a hypersensitivity reaction to an infectious agent, Kawasaki disease may cause dilatation and thrombosis of the coronary arteries, a rare cause of myocardial infarction in a child. The rash is a generalized exanthem that may often be confused with scarlet fever or a common viral exanthema. Fever is present for 5 to 10 days without therapy. Inflammatory markers are extremely elevated, with platelet counts elevated during the second week of illness. Intravenous immune globulin will block the inflammatory response. A pediatric cardiologist should obtain an echocardiogram of the coronary arteries and follow up if they are inflamed. This is one of the rare indications for prolonged aspirin therapy in children.

Vascular Lesions

Superficial hemangiomas often arise within weeks of birth, expanding through-out the first year, then regressing slowly over the next few years. When a hemangioma affects the vision, more aggressive therapy for ablation with lasers may be attempted. Recently, reports indicate that beta-adrenergic blocking agents, such as propranolol, may cause early and complete resolution of large and bothersome angiomas. Deep hemangiomas may persist, and, if closely associated with growth plates of the bone, may cause overgrowth of the bone. Salmon patches on the face in an ophthalmic nerve distribution may indicate intracranial hamartomas (eg, Sturge-Weber syndrome).

Hypopigmented Lesions

Melanocytes are sensitive to disturbances of the skin such as dryness in atopic dermatitis leading to pityriasis alba, blanching from topical steroids applied over a period of time, and immune response to dysplastic nevi with halo nevi. True vitiligo is difficult to miss because of the complete lack of pigment causing a pure white hue. Albinism is rare but must be considered when the hair and eyes also lack pigment.

Disorders of the Hair and Nails

Loss of hair is always troubling to the patient and parent. While alopecia areata is rare in children, other causes such as tineal infections of the scalp, traction, and systemic illness (eg, telogen effluvium) will be routinely encountered. Children may inherit dystrophic nails or hair. Similar to tinea pedis, fungal infection of the nails is rare until adolescence. Psoriasis and albinism have typical patterns of nail involvement.

The Pros and Cons of Topical Steroids

Inflammation of the skin is uncomfortable, and topical steroids help relieve that discomfort. However, proper treatment depends on an accurate diagnosis. Putting a steroid on an undiagnosed rash should be avoided because of the risk of it masking the true diagnosis. It may also cause the rash to acutely worsen if an infection is present. The highest potency steroids should be avoided in most cases and reserved for the dermatologist. Ointments tend to penetrate the skin better and provide a more potent effect. Complications of steroid overuse include thinning of the skin, increased superficial vascularization, acne, and striae formation. Injections of steroids into the superficial dermis can lead to atrophy and subcutaneous tissue loss. One way to avoid complication when a prolonged course of topical steroid is contemplated is to apply the steroid for only 5 days and rest on the weekend to allow for skin recovery. A good strategy may be to choose a product from each potency category and become familiar with it in your practice. Steroid potency is classified on a scale of I to VII, with class I agents as very high potency; class II as high potency; classes III, IV, and V as medium potency; and classes VI and VII as low potency.

Conclusion

Rashes and skin disorders are visible markers of many disorders, some life-threatening that demand immediate and aggressive treatment; some persistent, uncomfortable, or even disfiguring; and some merely inconvenient. When a new rash is encountered or a familiar rash does not respond as expected, the clinician will do well to become familiar with the more common rashes and friendly with an astute dermatologist with a good manner with children and their parents.

Suggested Reading

Chan M, Goldman RD. Erythema multiforme in children: the steroid debate. *Can Fam Physician*. 2013;59(6):635–636

Ely JW, Seabury Stone M. The generalized rash: part II. Diagnostic approach. *Am Fam Physician*. 2010;81(6):735–739

Hurwitz S, ed. *Clinical Pediatric Dermatology.* 2nd ed. WB Saunders: Philadelphia, PA; 1993

Mancini AJ, Krowchuk DP, eds. *Pediatric Dermatology: A Quick Reference Guide.* 3rd ed. Elk Grove Village, IL: American Academy of Pediatrics; 2016

Miller M, Miller AH. Incomplete Kawasaki disease. *Am J Emerg Med*. 2013;31(5):894. e5–894.e7

Zitelli BJ, Davis HW, eds. *Atlas of Pediatric Physical Diagnosis.* 3rd ed. Philadelphia, PA: Mosby-Wolfe; 1997

Zuniga R, Ngyen T. Skin conditions: common skin rashes in infants. *FP Essent.* 2013;407:31–41

CHAPTER 56

Scabies

Michelle Steinhardt, MD, MS, and Rachel Dawkins, MD

Key Points

- Scabies should be suspected when children present with widespread nocturnal pruritus, especially when it spares the head or is out of proportion to visible changes on the skin.

- Atypical presentations may occur in infants. Lesions may appear vesicular or bullous and are more likely to involve the face, head, neck, and scalp.

- Permethrin, 5%, cream (infants >2 months) *or* oral ivermectin (only in those weighing >15.0 kg) is the treatment of choice.

- The topical scabicide must be correctly applied, and all household members must be treated at the same time.

- Expert consultation should be obtained when treating scabies in infants younger than 2 months, in pregnant or breastfeeding women, or when crusted scabies is suspected.

Overview

Scabies is an infestation of the skin caused by the mite *Sarcoptes scabiei*, which is an obligate human parasite. It is transmitted from person to person, usually by direct skin-to-skin contact. Scabies can be contracted by wearing or handling heavily contaminated clothing or if sleeping in an unchanged bed recently occupied by an infested individual. Sexual transmission of scabies is possible. School settings normally do not provide the level of contact necessary to facilitate transmission; however, many schools have exclusion policies for students with scabies.

Causes and Differential Diagnosis

Classic scabies in humans is caused by *S scabiei* subspecies *hominis*. The subspecies *canis*, which may be acquired from direct contact with infected dogs, causes a mild, self-limited infection.

Box 56-1. Differential Diagnosis for Scabies

- Eczema
- Tinea
- Atopic dermatitis
- Systemic lupus erythematosus
- Bullous pemphigoid
- Langerhans cell histiocytosis
- Urticaria pigmentosa
- Seborrheic dermatitis
- Psoriasis
- Infantile acropustulosis

Clinical Features

Signs and symptoms of scabies begin approximately 3 to 6 weeks after primary infestation. In a person previously infested, signs and symptoms will appear as soon as 1 to 3 days. Pruritus is the hallmark of scabies and is usually worse at nighttime. Scabietic lesions can be distributed on the sides and in webs of fingers, on the flexor aspects of wrists, on the extensor aspects of the elbows and knees, and in the axilla. In females, lesions can be found on the skin adjacent to nipples. Additional lesions have been noted to be found in the waist and periumbilical areas, lower half of the buttocks adjacent to the thighs, and lateral and posterior aspects of the feet. The diaper area is a common location of lesions in toddlers. The head is usually spared from lesions except in babies and young children.

The most common presenting lesions of scabies include papules, vesicles, pustules, and nodules with the pathognomic lesion consisting of the burrow. The burrow appears on the skin surface as a short, waxy, and scaly gray line measuring anywhere from 2 to 15 mm. It is far more common to see papules than the more scabies-specific lesions, such as burrows and scabious nodules.

Because of the intensely pruritic nature of scabies, nonspecific secondary lesions are most commonly seen, including excoriation, eczematous eruptions, and even impetigo. If burrows are to be found, they are most easily located on the hands and feet, most notably in finger web spaces, in thenar and hypothenar eminences, and on the wrists. Rarely, the host can have an exaggerated immunologic reaction to scabies. In this case, nodular lesions are common.

It is important to note that eczema can be preexisting or develop from a scabies infection. Eczema can become secondarily infected with *Staphylococcus* species, *Streptococcus* species, or even both. Secondary infections caused by group A streptococci or *Staphylococcus aureus* can confuse the clinical picture by producing impetiginous lesions, ecthyma, paronychia, or lesions classically associated with furunculosis. Extensive eczematization can occur because of constant scratching and irritating medications used to treat the scabies infection. If the skin is excoriated or secondarily infected, the pathognomonic lesion (ie, burrow) can be easily missed.

In young children and infants, scabies rarely involves the palms and soles. Lesions are generally more inflammatory, vesicular, or bullous when compared with lesions found on adults. Very young infants may not actively scratch and may present as being irritable with poor feeding. Another major difference in the presentation of scabies in infants and young children is that the infestation often affects the face, head, neck, and scalp, and has generalized skin involvement. Very young children often have widespread eczematous erythema, particularly on the trunk. Truncal lesions may be more symptomatic in these children than the lesions that occur in typical areas of distribution.

Evaluation

Scabies is usually a clinical diagnosis based on history and distribution of lesions. Scabies should be suspected if widespread itching is present, especially at night; the itching spares the head (except in young children); or the amount of itching seems out of proportion to visible changes existent on the skin. Continue to suspect a diagnosis of scabies if the pruritic eruption has characteristic lesions in the correct distribution and other household members report similar symptoms.

Keep in mind that when making the diagnosis of scabies, the pathognomonic lesion (ie, burrow) may not be present on physical examination. Scabies should be suspected if signs and symptoms persist even if the patient was recently treated, because recurrence can occur as a result of incorrect treatment and reinfection is possible.

Definitive diagnosis is made by microscopic identification of mites, eggs, or mite feces. Definitive diagnosis by microscopy is of the utmost importance in HIV patients with generalized dermatitis and in the homeless population. It is important to establish a diagnosis in HIV or immunocompromised patients because the disease can manifest more severely; additionally, the pruritus may be mild or absent. Ways to definitively diagnosis scabies include epiluminescence microscopy, adhesive tape test, skin scrapings, and, rarely, skin biopsy.

Epiluminescence microscopy involves examining skin surfaces with a handheld dermatoscope to directly visualize mites and eggs for diagnosis or guide placement of skin scrapings. The adhesive tape test is performed by firmly applying tape directly to the suspected lesion and rapidly pulling the tape off. The advantage to this method is that no special equipment is needed. Additionally, it can be utilized in children who are unable to tolerate skin scraping.

Skin scraping has the highest yield in infants and young children when performed from the palms, soles, or torso. A successful skin scraping involves locating a non-excoriated papule with a fine white to gray line across. When this is located, 2 to 3 drops of ink are placed over the papule and left in place for 5 to 10 seconds. Wipe the area clean with an alcohol wipe to allow the ink to seep into the burrows, leaving a fine ink stain present. Next, drop mineral oil on the skin lesion and scrape the area with a blade. Place scrapings on the slide and examine under the microscope at a magnification of $\times$ 10.

Management

According to the Centers for Disease Control and Prevention, 5% permethrin lotion is the primary treatment for scabies. It is safe and effective for children and pregnant women. Permethrin kills not only the mites but also the eggs and is the treatment of choice in the United Kingdom, the United States, and Australia. Additionally, it has been shown in clinical trials to be as effective as lindane and more effective than crotamiton, with less pruritus at 4 weeks than in those treated with lindane.

Five percent permethrin cream is approved by the US Food and Drug Administration (FDA) for treatment in persons older than 2 months. It is applied overnight 1 time/week for 2 applications to the entire body and must be left on for 8 to 12 hours before being washed off. There are few adverse effects. However, a disadvantage of using permethrin is that it is the most expensive of all the topical scabicides.

Ivermectin, an oral antiparasitic, has been shown to be as effective as permethrin for treating scabies; however, it is not FDA approved for this use. Safety has not yet been established in persons weighing less than 15.0 kg and those who are pregnant. Treatment is 0.2 mg/kg in a single dose. It has been found to be extremely useful in patients with a high mite burden.

Sulphur is the oldest anti-scabietic available and preferably used as a 6% ointment. It is extremely inexpensive and can be used in situations when other treatments cannot be tolerated or for pregnant/lactating females and infants and children. Sulphur is applied to the whole body and rubbed into skin over 2 to 3 consecutive nights. Some disadvantages include that it is messy and malodorous, will stain clothing, and can lead to an irritant dermatitis, especially in hot and humid climates.

Crotamiton is used as a 10% cream or lotion and yields best results when applied twice a day for 5 consecutive days after bathing and changing clothes. It is FDA approved for treatment of scabies in adults but not in children. Crotamiton has been historically touted as a great antipruritic, but studies have not supported this claim. Additionally, frequent treatment failures have been described.

Benzyl benzoate works by being neurotoxic to the mites. It is supplied as a 25% emulsion. Application is tedious and involves applying lotion 3 times within a 24-hour period without an intervening bath; these extensive application instructions lead to treatment failure. It is not available in the United States and contraindicated for use in pregnant or breastfeeding females and in children younger than 2 years. It can cause an irritant dermatitis, especially on the face and scrotum, with repeated use, possibly leading to an allergic dermatitis.

Lindane, supplied as a 1% lotion, acts on the central nervous system of insects and leads to convulsions, decreased excitability, and death of the mite. It gets absorbed and distributed to all body compartments, with the highest concentration depositing in lipid-rich tissue and skin. It is metabolized and excreted in the urine and stools. Apply as a single 6-hour application; the application can be repeated 1 week later. This is a cheap and effective alternative to permethrin; however, studies have shown that it can cause central nervous system toxicity, aplastic anemia, and death. A black box warning from the FDA cautions about the risk for neurological toxicity and states that the medication should not be used in premature infants or those with seizure disorder. Lindane is not to be used in patients with psoriasis, eczema, or other severe skin conditions.

In terms of managing adverse effects of scabies, antihistamines can be used to help control pruritus. Coexisting skin infection should be treated after appropriate cultures with targeted antibiotic therapy based on local antibiotic susceptibility data or specific culture results.

Treatment Failures

The goal of management and treatment is to eradicate the mites; however, to maximize treatment success, the topical scabicide must be correctly applied and all household members must be treated at the same time. It is also important to advise your patients that pruritus may continue for 1 to 2 weeks and, in some cases, as long as 6 weeks after correctly applied scabicide therapy.

Scabicide should be applied to clean, dry skin. The therapy should be applied to the whole body with particular attention paid to the groin, fingernails, and toenails and behind the ears. Caution should be used when applying the medicine around the mucocutaneous areas, particularly if using benzyl benzoate. The medicine should also be applied to the face and scalp even if these locations are asymptomatic, because missing these areas could lead to treatment failure. All clothing and bed linens need to be decontaminated by machine washing in water at least to the temperature of 60°C (140°F).

While drug resistance has been reported to lindane, crotamiton, and benzyl benzoate, treatment failure is more commonly associated with failure to use the scabicide properly. Treatment failure can occur if infants remove the treatment from their hands when sucking on fingers or if adults mistakenly wash lotion off the child's hands. To avoid these pitfalls, it is prudent to use mittens and socks when treating children and to reapply the scabicide if washing of hands occurs. Other causes of treatment failure include improper application, with the drug applied only to the affected areas, and inadequate application of scabicide because of dilution of the medicine, which leads to decreased efficacy.

Reinfestation will occur if household members are not treated at the same time. Therefore, close contacts, such as family members, should be treated simultaneously even if they have no signs or symptoms of scabies. Bedding and clothing worn during the 3 days before therapy should be washed in hot water and dried using the hot cycle dryer temperature setting. No environmental disinfection is needed. Dermatology consultation is recommended for patients with crusted scabies and those with complex medical conditions including compromised immune systems.

Suggested Reading

Centers for Disease Control and Prevention. Parasites: scabies; resources for health professionals. CDC Web site. http://www.cdc.gov/parasites/scabies/health_professionals/meds.html. Updated November 2, 2010. Accessed March 23, 2016

Chowsidow O. Clinical practices. Scabies. *N Engl J Med.* 2006;354(16):1718–1727

Currie BJ, McCarthy JS. Permethrin and ivermectin for scabies. *New Engl J Med.* 2010;362(8):717–725

Heukelbach J, Feldmeier H. Scabies. *Lancet.* 2006;367(9524):1767–1774

Johnston G, Sladden M. Scabies: diagnosis and treatment. *BMJ.* 2005;331(7517):619–622

Karthikeyan K. Treatment of scabies: newer perspectives. *Postgrad Med J.* 2005;81(951):7–11

Strong M, Johnstone P. Interventions for treating scabies. *Cochrane Database Syst Rev.* 2007;(3):CD000320

Walter B, Heukelbach J, Fengler G, Worth C, Hengge U, Feldmeier H. Comparison of dermoscopy, skin scraping, and the adhesive tape test for the diagnosis of scabies in a resource-poor setting. *Arch Dermatol.* 2011;147(4):468–473

Stevens-Johnson Syndrome and Toxic Epidermal Necrolysis

Dean S. Morrell, MD; Shelley Cathcart, MD; and Craig N. Burkhart, MD

Key Points

- Removal of the offending medication is the most important part of the management of Stevens-Johnson syndrome/toxic epidermal necrolysis (SJS/TEN).

- Erythema multiforme is a distinct entity and should not be considered part of the SJS/TEN spectrum of disease. It is self-resolving, never fatal, and more likely to be associated with infections than medications.

- Although more research is needed regarding intravenous immune globulin and systemic steroids as treatments for SJS/TEN, both appear to improve the outcome for pediatric patients.

Overview

Stevens-Johnson syndrome (SJS), SJS/toxic epidermal necrolysis (TEN) overlap, and TEN are separate entities within a clinical spectrum of the same severe adverse cutaneous hypersensitivity reaction. The individual distinctions are based on the amount of epidermal detachment that is present. Stevens-Johnson syndrome is defined as less than 10% epidermal detachment, TEN is greater than 30%, and 10% to 30% is classified as SJS/TEN overlap. These entities are now regarded as distinct from erythema multiforme (EM), which is never fatal, always self-resolving, and more likely a result of infectious causes than medications. Further distinguishing features are discussed later in this chapter.

Causes and Differential Diagnosis of the Disease

Over 200 drugs have been reported to cause SJS/TEN, and in 77% to 95% of cases a specific agent can be identified as the cause. The reaction typically occurs 1 to 4 weeks after initiation of the offending medication. While many drugs have been reported to cause SJS and TEN, nonsteroidal anti-inflammatory drugs, antibiotics, and anticonvulsants are by far the most frequently associated groups of medications. Additional causes implicated in a small number of SJS cases include infections such as mycoplasmal pneumonia, vaccines, and several autoimmune and neoplastic diseases.

Other blistering diseases present similarly in the pediatric population. Staphylococcal scalded skin syndrome (SSSS) presents with painful, erythematous skin. The eruption is accentuated in the skin folds but spares mucosa. Following the onset of erythema, superficial bullae and erosions develop within 24 to 48 hours. In contrast to the full-thickness epidermal necrosis in TEN, the blisters in SSSS are more superficial as a result of an intraepidermal cleft seen in SSSS. Differentiation of SJS/TEN from SSSS is easily accomplished on the basis of clinical (morphology and distribution of the eruption; presence or absence of mucosal involvement) or histologic (level of the epidermal separation) grounds.

Erythema multiforme has historically been grouped with SJS/TEN. Erythema multiforme can also have mucosal involvement and bullous lesions, making it difficult to distinguish from SJS/TEN. It can also unfortunately look identical to SJS and TEN on histologic examination; therefore, skin biopsy is not helpful in differentiating the two. However, it is important to note that EM is now thought of as a separate and distinct diagnosis with its own unique causes, clinical presentation, and prognosis.

To assist in the differentiation of bullous EM and SJS/TEN, a consensus classification of 5 categories was proposed by Bastuji-Garin and colleagues in 1993 and is now used by most texts and studies about SJS and TEN (Table 57-1). The original study by Bastuji-Garin included pediatric and adult patients, and further studies have verified its validity in the pediatric population.

Table 57-1. Classification of Erythema Multiforme, Stevens-Johnson Syndrome, and Toxic Epidermal Necrolysis

	Bullous Erythema Multiforme	**Stevens-Johnson Syndrome**	**Stevens-Johnson Syndrome/ Toxic Epidermal Necrosis**	**Toxic Epidermal Necrolysis With Spots**	**Toxic Epidermal Necrosis Without Spots**
Epidermal detachment, %	<10	<10	10–30	>30	>30
Typical targets	Yes	No	No	No	No
Atypical targets	Raised	Flat	Flat	Flat	No
Spots, erythematous or purpuric macules	No	Yes	Yes	Yes	No

The typical target lesions of EM are classified as having a zone of dusky central necrosis surrounded by a middle zone of pale edema and a border of erythema. While SJS may have atypical targetoid lesions, they lack the well-defined zones of EM and often occur in conjunction with purpuric macules and patches. Both entities can present with ulceration of the mucous membranes and hemorrhagic crusting of the lips.

Clinical Features

Patients often present with a prodrome of fever, sore throat, and eye discomfort several days before onset of the rash. The eruption in SJS/TEN starts as erythematous or purpuric macules and atypical target-like lesions that may or may not develop into large sheets of epidermal necrosis. The blisters in SJS and TEN are flaccid and can be spread laterally with central pressure (ie, Asboe-Hansen sign). Normal-appearing but involved epidermis can be sheared away by gentle lateral pressure (ie, Nikolsky sign). Eruption typically starts on the central trunk and then spreads onto the face and extremities. The clinical course can be unpredictable, and mild cases of SJS can evolve rapidly into TEN.

Symptoms of mucosal involvement include eye irritation, painful swallowing, or urination and diarrhea. Stevens-Johnson syndrome/TEN can have internal involvement (eg, gastrointestinal, tracheal, or bronchial erosions; glomerulonephritis; and hepatitis), and initial management should include a systemic evaluation.

Evaluation

Stevens-Johnson syndrome and TEN are often clinical diagnoses, although a skin biopsy can be confirmatory. Pathology will show necrotic keratinocytes at all levels of the epidermis progressing to full-thickness epidermal necrosis and dermoepidermal separation.

On admission, any patient suspected of having SJS/TEN should have a thorough drug history taken with special attention to any medications started within the 4 weeks preceding onset of the condition. Basic chemistries, including serum urea nitrogen, creatinine, liver function studies, and complete blood cell count, should be obtained.

Mortality for SJS is 1% to 5%, and for TEN it is 30% to 50%. The severity of illness score for TEN (SCORTEN) classification system was designed to stratify patients on the basis of their mortality risk and should be performed within 24 hours of a patient's admission. The study that established the validity of the SCORTEN included pediatric patients, and further studies have confirmed its accuracy in the pediatric population.

It is based on the following criteria:
- Age: older than 40 years
- Serum urea nitrogen: greater than 28mg/dl
- Serum bicarbonate: less than 20 mEq/L
- Malignancy
- Heart rate: greater than 120 beats/min
- Blood glucose: greater than 252 mg/dL
- Involved body surface area: greater than 10%

Patients receive 1 point for meeting any of the above criteria, and their score indicates mortality risk as shown below.
- 0–1 factors: 3.2% or greater
- 2 factors: 12.1% or greater
- 3 factors: 35.3% or greater
- 4 factors: 58.3% or greater
- 5 or more factors: 90% or greater

Management

The management of children with SJS and TEN is a subject of substantial controversy and debate but generally focuses on identification and withdrawal of the offending agent, wound care, fluid and electrolyte support, nutrition, analgesia, and anticipation of complications.

The most important first step is a search for and withdrawal of any possible offending medication (typically identified in 77%–95% of cases). Withdrawal of the offending medication can dramatically reduce the risk of mortality, especially in drugs with short half-lives. Once the offending medication has been identified, care should be taken to add it to the patient's allergy list and educate the patient regarding her need to avoid this drug in the future. Subsequent exposures can lead to a more dramatic and deadly recurrence of this drug reaction.

Consultation with a dermatologist or other clinician experienced in the management of SJS/TEN is advised, and patients should be transferred to a burn unit when possible. Management of the fluid/electrolyte balance, environmental temperature regulation, prevention and treatment of infection, respiratory and nutritional support, and adequate analgesia are all important aspects of SJS and TEN patient care. The energy requirements of pediatric SJS and TEN patients are elevated and estimated to be 30% greater than the baseline resting rate.

Intravenous immune globulin (IVIG) (Evidence Level II-3) or systemic steroids (Evidence Level II-3) have both been utilized to try to limit the duration and severity of SJS/TEN. There are few large studies of either treatment and even fewer in the pediatric population. A review of the available data in children was published by Del Pozzo and colleagues. Their review of 128 cases found that both IVIG and systemic steroids shortened the hospital stay and length of fever in children compared with supportive care alone. There was no clinically significant difference in the outcomes of the 2 treatment groups, but both were significantly better than the supportive care groups. Doses of IVIG used ranged from 0.25 to 1.5 g/kg/day for 1 to 5 days. Systemic steroid groups were treated with either prednisone or prednisolone (1 mg/kg/day) or methylprednisolone (4 mg/kg/day) for 5 to 7 days.

Suggested Reading

Bastuji-Garin S, Fouchard N, Bertocchi M, Roujeau JC, Revuz J, Wolkenstein P. SCORTEN: a severity-of-illness score for toxic epidermal necrolysis. *J Invest Dermatol.* 2000;115(2):149–153

Del Pozzo-Magana BR, Lazo-Langner A, Carleton B, Castro-Pastrana LI, Rieder MJ. A systematic review of treatment of drug-induced Stevens-Johnson syndrome and toxic epidermal necrolysis in children. *J Popul Ther Clin Pharmacol.* 2011;18: e121–e133

Forman R, Koren G, Shear NH. Erythema multiforme, Stevens-Johnson syndrome and toxic epidermal necrolysis in children: a review of 10 years' experience. *Drug Saf.* 2002;25(13):965–972

Koh MJ, Tay YK. An update on Stevens-Johnson syndrome and toxic epidermal necrolysis in children. *Curr Opin Pediatr.* 2009;21(4):505–510

Koh MJ, Tay YK. Stevens-Johnson syndrome and toxic epidermal necrolysis in Asian children. *J Am Acad Dermatol.* 2010;62(1):54–60

CHAPTER 58

Warts and Molluscum Contagiosum

Brandon D. Newell, MD

Key Points

- Common warts and molluscum contagiosum are common skin lesions that, in most cases, resolve over time without specific treatment.

- The diagnosis is usually made on clinical examination based on the characteristic features (molluscum contagiosum: umbilicated, 1- to 3-mm pearly pink to tan papules; warts: rough, pink to tan, xerotic skin in 1 mm to >1 cm papules).

- Multiple lesions are notable in immunocompromised hosts, and specific therapies have variable response.

- Genital warts require specific evaluation because they may represent sexual abuse in young children and can predispose to genital cancers.

Common Warts

Overview

Warts, also referred to as *verrucae,* are a common viral infection of the skin and mucous membranes caused by the human papillomavirus (HPV). Warts are ubiquitous in the human population and often seen in children and adolescents, affecting approximately 1 out of 10 individuals. They are spread from person to person or by autoinoculation from other infected areas of one's body. While warts are generally benign, they carry significant comorbidities, including psychosocial trauma from visual stigma, pain, and potential bleeding if the lesions are traumatized or develop in sensitive areas. Treatment of warts is primarily geared toward destruction of the infected skin cells by a variety of potential modalities versus active nonintervention.

There are generally 4 different types of warts, including verruca vulgaris, verruca plantaris, verruca plana, and condyloma acuminatum (Box 58-1). Their names are based on their commonality, location, and sometimes clinical appearance. The following sections will separately cover each group.

Box 58-1. Types of Warts (Verrucae)

Verruca vulgaris	Common or filiform wart
Verruca plantaris	Plantar wart
Verruca plana	Flat wart
Condyloma acuminatum	Genital wart

Causes and Differential Diagnosis

Warts are caused by HPV, a common virus that infects skin and mucous membranes. The virus is well established in the human population, making warts commonplace in any medical care practice. Numerous strains of HPV exist and are responsible for various types of warts.

The differential diagnosis for warts includes but is not limited to melanocytic nevi, corns (clavi), acrochordons (also known as skin tags), lichen planus, seborrheic keratosis, hypertrophic scars, molluscum contagiosum, foreign body, superficial lymphatic malformations (especially in the groin/buttocks area), and even skin cancers (squamous or basal cell carcinomas). Occasionally, traumatized warts can resemble pyogenic granulomas because of their red appearance and tendency to bleed (though not as severe).

Clinical Features

Warts are commonly found in areas of visible trauma or even areas of the body that undergo repetitive microtrauma. Hands, elbows, knees, and feet are some of the most common areas where common warts can be found. Warts display koebnerization, an isomorphic phenomenon in which they are spread along a similarly shaped field that is traumatized or injured. If a solitary wart is scratched through with a fingernail, the wart can spread, forming multiple warts in a linear configuration matching the scratched pattern. Patients with dry skin (ie, xerosis) or an underlying skin disease affecting skin barrier function (ie, atopic dermatitis) are at a higher risk for developing warts. Extensive plantar warts can occur in the setting of active tinea pedis (also known as athlete's foot) and the suspect patient's feet should be cultured and treated with appropriate topical antifungal therapy. Frequent intentional traumatization, such as picking of warts, also contributes to their risk of spreading, often to alternate body sites, and should be discouraged.

If warts are traumatized or injured, bleeding can be quite common. Capillaries in the upper papillary dermis are more prominent within the warts and thus more prone to trauma or bleeding. Pain and discomfort from warts are frequent symptomatic concerns. Periungual or plantar warts can easily form painful fissures and make simple tasks, such as writing or walking, uncomfortable. Exophytic lesions that protrude from the skin can rub on external clothing or objects (eg, jewelry), causing irritation or discomfort. Large and deep plantar warts on the bottom of the foot can be very painful, particularly if they are located in weight-bearing portions of the sole. The visibility and appearance of warts can cause some psychosocial issues, particularly lesions on the face or hands/fingers.

Verruca Vulgaris (Common Wart)

Verrucae vulgaris, or common warts, typically present as raised, xerotic, round, skin-colored to pink papules with a rough or "warty" texture to the surface. They can range in size from 1 to 2 mm to several centimeters in diameter, especially if multiple lesions coalesce together. Common warts can occur as single or multiple lesions. Warts can easily bleed if picked or traumatized, as evidenced by their characteristic thrombosed capillaries that appear as small black macules (resembling "pepper spots"). Lesions are commonly found on the arms, legs, hands, elbows, and knees. Common warts can be found in the perineum, buttocks, and, rarely, genitalia, which usually have a primary source somewhere else on the body. Periungual (around the fingernail) warts often occur in patients who chew their nails or pick the surrounding skin. Filiform warts are an exophytic variant of verrucae vulgaris that commonly occur on the face, nose, neck, and, rarely, trunk. Filiform warts are 1 to 3 mm in diameter and skin colored and have a thin exophytic papular stalk with rough fingerlike verrucous projections that resemble the crown of a pineapple. Filiform warts are commonly mistaken for acrochordons (also known as fibroepithelial polyps or skin tags) and can be distinguished with the help of a magnifying glass.

Verruca Plantaris (Plantar Wart)

Verrucae plantaris occur when HPV infects the epidermis of plantar surfaces of the feet or toes, hence the name *plantar warts*. Plantar warts can be a few millimeters to centimeters in size, solitary or multiple. Multiple lesions can coalesce together forming larger plaques. Lesions are less raised than common warts and often have an endophytic appearance, often flush with the skin. Thrombosed capillaries are commonly present in plantar warts, a useful clinical sign. Plantar warts have a preference for weight-bearing surfaces and can be quite painful as a result, akin to walking on a small stone. Surrounding hyperkeratosis (ie, callus) often occurs around plantar warts. Corn pads, round annular adhesive patches used to relieve pressure off the central portion of the wart, can be useful in minimizing pain associated with plantar warts. Extensive plantar warts should raise suspicion for concomitant tinea pedis.

Verruca Plana (Flat Wart)

Verrucae plana, commonly referred to as *flat warts,* are a commonly overlooked HPV infection that typically occurs on the face and upper extremities. Lesions are typically overall smaller than other warts, ranging 1 to 4 mm in size. Flat warts are small flat-topped papules that can be skin colored, hypopigmented, slightly pink, or light brown. Flat warts tend to cluster in small groups or linear patterns from scratching. Lesions are barely raised from the skin and can be subtle in appearance.

Condyloma Acuminatum (Genital Wart)

Condylomata acuminatum, genital warts, occur when HPV infects skin of the groin or skin and mucous membranes of the genitalia, buttocks, and anal mucosa. Lesions are typically skin colored to tan/brown, soft, verrucous papules ranging in size from 1 to 4 mm to plaques of several centimeters in larger lesions. The anal mucosa is a commonly affected area. Transmission can be horizontal or vertical, and any suspicion of transmission via sexual abuse should be investigated appropriately. Often, lesions in young children are transmitted from an affected mother (non-sexually) who may not have or recall having skin lesions (patients can have and shed the virus without having visible cutaneous lesions). Extensive lesions near the urethra or anus can cause dysuria or dyschezia, respectively. They can bleed if traumatized, particularly perianal lesions. Certain serotypes of HPV can increase an affected patient's risk of cervical cancer, and lesions should be evaluated by a gynecologist when age appropriate.

Evaluation

Warts are identified primarily on clinical examination. Diagnosis is based on appearance, location, and size of the primary lesions. Simple magnification with a handheld magnifying glass can help confirm the diagnosis of a wart clinically, while higher magnification with a dermatoscope can help provide a more detailed visual examination. Rarely, if the diagnosis is in question, a skin biopsy for tissue histopathology may be necessary.

Management

Without treatment, warts can resolve on their own, but can take months to years to do so. Treatment of warts must be practical and tolerable for the individual patient. Primary treatment of warts includes destroying the infected skin cells (Table 58-1). Topical salicylic acid, a common beta-hydroxy acid, is considered first-line for a variety of warts (common and plantar warts). Salicylic acid is available in a variety of strengths (17%–40%) and formulations (solutions, gels, and stick), which represent an affordable and effective

Table 58-1. Treatment Options for Warts

Type of Wart	Treatment Options
Common and plantar warts	Topical salicylic acid (17%–40%) Cryotherapy Intralesional *Candida* antigen Topical imiquimod ± salicylic acid Oral cimetidine
Flat warts	Topical tretinoin Cryotherapy
Filiform warts	Cryotherapy
Genital warts	Topical imiquimod Topical podophyllum resin Cryotherapy

treatment option for non-groin/non-facial areas. Salicylic acid can be applied daily to twice daily to the wart. Tape occlusion of salicylic acid can help enhance penetration and prevent the medication from rubbing off (silver duct tape is often used). For severely thick warts, salicylic acid may be compounded with 10% to 20% urea in white petrolatum to soften the lesion and allow more effective penetration.

Cryotherapy (freezing) is commonly used in treating warts, causing destruction of the virally infected keratinocytes by causing ice crystal formation and subsequent thawing. Liquid nitrogen is the method of choice because of its ability to get down to $-184.5°C$ ($-300°F$). Canned skin refrigerants, while cheaper and readily available, can be used but are generally less effective than liquid nitrogen because they cannot achieve cold enough temperatures to cause adequate skin damage. For thick plantar warts, paring the superficial portion off with a scalpel blade can be done prior to cryotherapy. Pain is the most common adverse effect of cryotherapy and can be lessened using an appropriate amount of topical lidocaine-containing cream with occlusion prior to treatment. Other potential risks of cryotherapy include blistering (including blood-filled blisters), scarring, spreading of the wart (including the formation of a "ring wart"), secondary infection, and nail dystrophy (if performed near a nail). Parents and patients should be properly warned beforehand of the potential risks of cryotherapy.

Intralesional *Candida* antigen therapy can be very effective in recalcitrant cases or cases with a large number of warts. It is performed by injecting 0.3 mL into the base of a solitary wart or divided equally among 2 to 3 warts once monthly for 3 to 6 months. Often, warts distant from the treated ones may resolve as well. A variety of other treatment options have been tried with varying success, including oral cimetidine, oral zinc supplementation, and topical imiquimod cream (often combined with salicylic acid).

The treatment of genital warts requires a different treatment approach, because of the sensitive location of the lesions. Genital warts can be treated with topical imiquimod cream applied 3 times weekly for several months. Irritation at the site of application is a common adverse effect. Topical 25% podophyllum resin can be applied (in an outpatient office by a clinician) with a cotton-tipped applicator and washed off in 4 to 6 hours. Local irritation with podophyllum resin is a common complication of therapy. Cryotherapy can be employed for more recalcitrant cases but can be quite painful and thus is of limited usefulness. Affected adolescent patients should be properly counseled on sexually transmitted infections and preventive measures they can take.

Molluscum Contagiosum
Overview

Molluscum contagiosum is a localized dermatitis more common in toddlers and younger children and less so in adolescents or adults. In adolescents and adults, molluscum contagiosum is often considered a sexually transmitted infection if located in the genital region.

Causes and Differential Diagnosis

Molluscum contagiosum virus (MCV) is a cutaneous infection caused by a DNA-poxvirus that infects keratinocytes of the epidermis. Infection with MCV can last for months to several years and should be discussed with affected families to ensure that proper anticipatory guidance is provided. Molluscum contagiosum virus can often be confused with common warts, flat warts, folliculitis, boils, comedones, milia, and Spitz nevus.

Clinical Features

Lesions are typically characterized by small 1- to 3-mm, dome-shaped, smooth pearly papules, but much larger lesions, called "giant molluscum," have been described. Lesions can be solitary or multiple and are often spread/koebnerized because of scratching. Mature lesions often have a central white cheese-like core that can sometimes be visualized, and once the core has extruded from it, lesions develop the well-known central umbilication. If lesions develop a surrounding red patch of xerotic, pruritic skin, called molluscum dermatitis, this can resemble a patch of eczema. Patients with xerosis or atopic dermatitis are more likely to develop an infection with MCV. Immunocompromised individuals can develop hundreds or thousands of lesions, making therapy challenging.

Evaluation

Diagnosis is typically made by visual appearance of the characteristic pearly papules that have white central cores and sometimes demonstrate central umbilication.

Management

Treatment of molluscum contagiosum is not mandatory because lesions will typically resolve over time (Table 58-2). Despite treatment, smallpox-like/pitted scars can remain after the MCV has resolved. If treatment is desired, several options exist. Cantharidin is a vesicant produced by the meloid beetle (also known as "blister beetle"), available in a 0.7% formulation, and commonly used for treating MCV. Cantharidin is applied (by a clinician in the clinical setting only) atop the molluscum contagiosum lesion (care should be taken to avoid its application to normal skin) with the blunt end of a wooden, cotton-tipped applicator and allowed to dry for 1 to 2 minutes, then washed off 4 to 6 hours later by the parent. This process can be repeated every 4 to 6 weeks until resolution of the molluscum contagiosum is achieved. Occluding cantharidin can worsen the blistering reaction and is unadvised. Cryotherapy can be quite helpful in a few persistent solitary lesions. Topical tretinoin cream has been used for facial lesions, but can cause local irritation and dryness. Other treatment modalities for MCV include topical imiquimod cream (applied 3 times weekly), oral cimetidine (several months), pulsed dye laser, and topical trichloroacetic acid.

Table 58-2. Treatment of Molluscum Contagiosum Virus

Location of Virus	Treatment Options
MCV on trunk or extremities	Nothing (active nonintervention) Topical cantharidin Cryotherapy Topical imiquimod cream Oral cimetidine Curettage Pulsed dye laser
Facial MCV	Nothing (active nonintervention) Cryotherapy Oral cimetidine Topical trichloroacetic acid
Groin/buttocks MCV	Nothing (active nonintervention) Topical imiquimod cream Oral cimetidine Cryotherapy (limited use because of discomfort)

Abbreviation: MCV, molluscum contagiosum virus.

Fomite transmission of the MCV is common and can occur via towels, clothing, and other objects. Bathing with affected individuals can put co-bathers at risk for acquiring MCV. Proper hand-washing hygiene and avoiding digitally manipulating lesions can reduce the risk of autoinoculation of MCV or spreading it to others.

Suggested Reading

Bacelieri R, Johnson SM. Cutaneous warts: an evidence-based approach to therapy. *Am Fam Phys.* 2005;72(4):647–652

Dall'Oglio F, D'Amico V, Nasca MR, Micali G. Treatment of cutaneous warts: an evidence-based review. *Am J Clin Dermatol.* 2012;13(2):73–96

Glass AT, Solomon BA. Cimetidine therapy for recalcitrant warts in adults. *Arch Dermatol.* 1996;132(6):680–682

Jayasinghe Y, Garland SM. Genital warts in children: what do they mean? *Arch Dis Child.* 2006;91(8):696–700

Kim MB, Ko HC, Jang HS, Oh CK, Kwon KS. Treatment of flat warts with 5% imiquimod cream. *J Eur Acad Dermatol Venerol.* 2006;20(10):1349–1350

Kuykendall-Ivy TD, Johnson SM. Evidence-based review of management of nongenital cutaneous warts. *Cutis.* 2003;71(3):213–222

Mammas IN, Sourvinos G, Spandidos DA. Human papilloma virus (HPV) infection in children and adolescents. *Eur J Pediatr.* 2009;168(3):267–273

Mathes FD, Frieden I. Treatment of molluscum contagiosum with cantharidin: a practical approach. *Pediatr Ann.* 2010;39(3):124–130

Silverberg N. Pediatric molluscum contagiosum: optimal treatment strategies. *Paediatr Drugs.* 2003;5(8):505–512

Skinner Jr RB. Treatment of molluscum contagiosum with imiquimod 5% cream. *J Am Acad Dermatol.* 2012;47(4 Suppl):S221–S224

INDEX

Page numbers in *italics* denote a figure, table, or box.

EIA. *See* Enzyme immunoassay (EIA)
Electrolytes, 131
ELISA. *See* Enzyme-linked immunosorbent assay (ELISA)
EM. *See* Erythema multiforme (EM)
Empiric antibiotic therapy, 99
Empiric antimicrobial therapy, 223, 296
Empiric therapy, 41, 155–156, 445–446
Empyema/pneumonia, 148, 190, 306, 404
    antimicrobials, 89–90
    causes and differential diagnosis, *79, 80–82, 82*
        infants, children, and adolescents, 78–82
        neonates, 78
    clinical features, 83
        complications, 84
        parapneumonic effusion and empyema, 84
    clinical manifestations, 224
    common symptoms and signs of, *83*
    community-acquired, *89*
    diagnosis, 224–225
    evaluation, 85–87
    long-term monitoring, 92–93
    management, *89,* 89–92, *90–91, 93*
    microbial causes of, *79, 80–82*
    overview, 77
    with parapneumonic effusion, *93*
    radiographic features of, 88, *88*
Encephalitis, 170, 302–303, 308, 315
    causes and differential diagnosis, 287–290, *288, 289*
    clinical features, 290, *291, 292*
    diagnosis, 290–295, *294*
    initial manifestations of, 290
    management, *295,* 295–298, *297, 298*
    outcome and long-term monitoring, 298–299
    overview, 287
Endemic mycoses
    causes and differential diagnosis, 454
    clinical manifestations, 454–456, *455*
    evaluation, 456–457
    management, *457,* 457–460, *458*
    overview, 453–454
Endocarditis, 438
Endocrine diseases, 588
Endophthalmitis, 438
Enteral therapy, 75
Enteric pathogens, *50*
Enteroviral meningitis, 63
Enteroviruses
    causes and differential diagnosis, 301–302

clinical features, 302–307
evaluation, 309–310
management, 310–311
overview, 301
Enzyme immunoassay (EIA), 373, 402
Enzyme-linked immunosorbent assay (ELISA), 178
Epididymo-orchitis, 371
Epstein-Barr nuclear antigens (EBNA), 319
Epstein-Barr virus (EBV), 48, 138, *138,* 276
    causes and differential diagnosis, 313–315, *314*
    clinical manifestations, 315–318
    evaluation, 318–321, *320*
    overview, 313
    treatment of, 321–322
Erb-Duchenne paralysis, 68, 154
Eruptive vellus hair cysts, *520*
Erysipelas, 97–98, *101, 147*
Erythema contusiformis, 567
Erythema infectiosum, 383, 384
Erythema migrans, 174
    biopsy of, 177
    diagnosis, 177
    single and multiple, 180
Erythema multiforme (EM), 613, 625, 626
    classification of, 626, *626*
Erythema nodosum
    causes and differential diagnosis, 565–566, *566*
    clinical features, 566–568, *567*
    etiologic factors associated with, *566*
    overview, 565
    prolonged cases of, 568
    treatment of, *569*
Erythematous nodule on leg, *567*
Erythematous papules, 560
Erythrocyte sedimentation rate
    erythema nodosum, 568
    osteomyelitis and septic arthritis, 70
    pneumonia and empyema, 84, 87
    Staphylococcus aureus infections, 225
    tick-borne rickettsial diseases, 245
Escherichia coli, 48, *49, 50, 52*
Etiologic agent, 129
Evaluation
    acne, 524–525
    acute bacterial rhinosinusitis (ABRS), 31
    alopecia areata, 540–541
    anaerobic infections, 110
    aspergillosis, 429–430
    atopic dermatitis, 551
    blastomycosis, 456
    bloodstream infections (BSIs), 40–41